2013 EDITION

ICD-10-CM/PCS CODING
THEORY AND PRACTICE

Karla R. Lovaasen, RHIA, CCS, CCS-P
AHIMA Certified ICD-10 Trainer
Coding and Consulting Services
Abingdon, Maryland

Jennifer Schwerdtfeger, BS, RHIT, CCS, CPC, CPC-H
AHIMA Certified ICD-10 Trainer
Partner, Auditing & Coding Experts, LLC
Crofton, Maryland

ELSEVIER

ELSEVIER
SAUNDERS

3251 Riverport Lane
St. Louis, Missouri 63043

ICD-10-CM/PCS CODING: THEORY AND PRACTICE, 2013 EDITION   ISBN: 978-1-4557-4249-3
Copyright © 2013, 2012 by Saunders, an imprint of Elsevier Inc.

Notices

Library of Congress Cataloging-in-Publication Data

Lovaasen, Karla R.
  ICD-10-CM/PCS coding : theory and practice / Karla R. Lovaasen, Jennifer Schwerdtfeger.—2013 ed.
    p. ; cm.
  Includes bibliographical references and index.
  ISBN 978-1-4557-4249-3 (pbk. : alk. paper)
  I. Schwerdtfeger, Jennifer.   II. Title.
  [DNLM: 1. International statistical classification of diseases and related health problems. 10th revision. Clinical modification.   2. International statistical classification of diseases and related health problems. 10th revision. Procedure coding system.   3. Disease—classification.   4. Clinical Coding.
5. International Classification of Diseases.   6. Therapeutics—classification.   WB 15]
  616.001'2—dc23

2012019371

Content Strategy Director: Jeanne R. Olson
Senior Content Development Specialist: Luke Held
Publishing Services Manager: Pat Joiner-Myers
Project Manager: Stephen Bancroft
Designer: Teresa McBryan

Printed in Canada

Last digit is the print number: 9 8 7 6 5 4 3 2 1

Reviewers

Foreword

It is an honor to have an opportunity to share with you my thoughts and feelings about the new edition of *ICD-10-CM/PCS Coding: Theory and Practice.*

Karla and Jennifer have taken the mystery out of ICD-10-CM/PCS coding by preparing a user-friendly book that meets the needs of not only the student but also the busy instructors. The approach taken by the authors is straightforward, clear, concise, and complete. This book contains the latest in coding assignment and covers a wide variety of coding applications by the use of exercises within the text and the accompanying workbook. The use of color illustrations and photographs further enhances the book and will keep the reader interested.

This is the definitive ICD-10-CM/PCS coding text!

Carol J. Buck
Author/Instructor

Preface

Building on the strengths of the first edition, the new edition of *ICD-10-CM/PCS Coding: Theory and Practice* is authoritatively referenced and easy to use for teaching an inpatient coding resource and has been designed with instructors and students in mind. This comprehensive guide presents reliable coverage of ICD-10-CM/PCS in a systematic, straightforward format that guides students through the inpatient coding process. With clear examples, challenging review questions, and outstanding instructor support, this innovative resource is not only a valuable coding tool but also a time-saving teaching tool!

ICD-10-CM/PCS Coding: Theory and Practice is intended for those who are learning to code, as well as experienced professionals who wish to have a reference and/or learn the ICD-10-CM/PCS coding system. Unlike other books in this area, *ICD-10-CM/PCS Coding: Theory and Practice* sets out to help students (1) understand why coding is essential and necessary, (2) understand the basics of the health record, and (3) fully understand the rules, guidelines, and functions of ICD-10-CM/PCS coding. This book can be used in medical insurance, billing, and coding educational programs; in health information management programs; and as a useful reference to practitioners in the field.

As the implementation date of ICD-10-CM and ICD-10-PCS approaches, this textbook will change accordingly. ICD-10-CM and PCS is still in draft form and therefore still evolving. Because it is still a work in progress, there may be omissions, typos, indexing issues, etc. Hopefully, many of these issues will be resolved before implementation. The ICD-10 2012 code sets were used to assign codes in this edition. The 2013 edition will also include the ICD-10-CM guidelines in their respective chapters. The accompanying workbook has been expanded to include more practice exercises. These exercises have been added to help the student with applying the guidelines and selecting the principal diagnosis. Several operative reports have also been added to familiarize the student with different types of operative reports and for more practice in assigning procedure codes.

ORGANIZATION

The organization of *ICD-10-CM/PCS: Theory and Practice* follows the most logical way to learn this material. The early chapters focus on history, the health record as the foundation for coding, and the *Official Guidelines for Coding and Reporting*. A coder must have a basic understanding of this foundational content before moving on to more complicated material. Specifically, Chapter 4 covers the basic steps of ICD-10-CM coding and the correct process for locating codes in the ICD-10-CM manual, whereas Chapter 26 is devoted entirely to reimbursement and the role that ICD-10-CM plays in reimbursement methodologies.

Chapters 8 through 25 cover each chapter of the ICD-10-CM code book. These chapters are sequenced in this book for the following reasons. The assignment of codes for signs, symptoms, infectious diseases, and Z codes may be applied to all chapters in the ICD-10-CM code book; therefore these are the first coding chapters in this book. Each of these chapters follows a very specific template that will help students learn and instructors teach this complex material, beginning with the corresponding coding guidelines from the *ICD-10-CM Official Guidelines for Coding and Reporting*. This reinforces the importance of the guidelines in accurate code assignment. Following this is a section on anatomy and physiology, with full-color illustrations of the body system discussed in the chapter. This allows for more informed decision making when selecting the correct code and also provides an important review of anatomy and physiology. Key disease conditions are covered and illustrated with examples.

Within each coding chapter is a separate list of Z codes. Z codes are used in all sections of the ICD-10-CM code book, and this list gives students, instructors, and practitioners easy reference to the correct Z codes for each section.

Featured in select chapters are common medications and treatment for the related disease conditions. It is important to become familiar with common medications to identify chronic illnesses that may be documented in the health record.

Procedures are another important section of the coding chapters. Common and complex procedures relating to the diagnoses are covered in this section using ICD-10-PCS.

Finally, each coding chapter has a section on documentation and MS-DRG assignment. This feature brings together all of the steps of ICD-10-CM coding for optimal reimbursement, supported by documentation in the health record.

Chapter 27 completes the picture of facility coding by covering ICD-10-CM coding for outpatient facility services. Most healthcare facilities today treat patients on both an inpatient and an outpatient basis. Coders may be required to code both types of services, and it is important for students to understand the differences.

DISTINCTIVE FEATURES

- Full-color design with illustrations. This helps important content such as anatomy and physiology stand out and come alive and provides visual reinforcement of key concepts.
- Numerous and varied examples and exercises within each chapter. These exercises break the chapter into manageable segments and help students gauge learning while reinforcing important concepts.
- Partial answer keys for the textbook and workbook are available on the Evolve website for instant feedback to enhance student learning.

ADDITIONAL RESOURCES

Get the most out of your course with these additional learning and teaching resources.
- Student Workbook. Apply the textbook content and prepare for employment with this study guide! The workbook contains:
  - Application activities that give students hands-on practice applying ICD-10-CM coding to actual health records.
  - Case studies that illustrate common scenarios students will encounter on the job.
- TEACH Instructor Resources. TEACH is the complete curriculum manual, giving instructors everything necessary to enhance an ICD-10-CM course and save time!
  - **Lesson plans** tie together related content in the textbook, workbook, and instructor resources and reduce preparation time.
  - **Lecture slides and notes** presented in PowerPoint guide instructors through class presentations.

- **Complete answer keys** for every exercise, chapter review, and test bank question enable fast, efficient student assessment.
- **Test banks** help prepare exams instantly with chapter-specific test banks presented in ExamView.

◼ Evolve Learning Resources. This companion website contains links to industry updates, reimbursement updates, and important news. The Evolve course management system gives instructors the flexibility of posting course components online.

Acknowledgments

This book was developed to better meet the needs of coding educators, students, and coding professionals.

There are several people who deserve special thanks for their efforts in making this text possible.

Jeanne Olson, Publisher, for stepping in and learning about the world of ICD-9 and ICD-10 coding.

Luke Held, Content Development Specialist, for assisting us with the publishing process and for his incredible attention to detail.

A special thanks to **Kelly Hoefs**, RHIT, for her assistance and support of this textbook and supporting materials. Also, thanks to **Louise Thompson** for her assistance and support of this textbook. Thanks to **Jamie Lovaasen**, PsyD, for her expertise with the mental health case scenarios and to **Randi Wippler**, RN, BSN, for her expertise in home health.

Thanks to all our colleagues who participated in coding discussions and debates about coding issues.

Thanks to **Carol Buck** for her advice and encouragement during this project.

The authors and publisher would like to acknowledge and thank the contributors to the TEACH Instructor Resources and all the textbook reviewers for their constructive comments.

Contents

1

The Rationale for and History of Coding

CHAPTER OUTLINE

LEARNING OBJECTIVES

1. Describe the application of coding
2. Define nomenclature and classification
3. Identify the historical timeline of coding
4. Explain the difference between ICD-9-CM and ICD-10-CM
5. Delineate coder training needs for transitioning to ICD-10-CM
6. Describe different coding organizations and credentials
7. Recognize the importance of the Standards of Ethical Coding
8. Define compliance as it relates to coding
9. Explain confidentiality as it applies to coding

ABBREVIATIONS/ ACRONYMS

AAPC American Academy of Professional Coders

A&P anatomy and physiology

AHA American Hospital Association

AHIMA American Health Information Management Association

CCA Certified Coding Associate

CCS Certified Coding Specialist

CCS-P Certified Coding Specialist—Physician Based

CEUs continuing education units

CMS Centers for Medicare and Medicaid Services

CPC Certified Professional Coder

CPC-H Certified Professional Coder—Hospital Based

CPT *Current Procedural Terminology*

DRGs diagnosis-related groups

HIPAA Health Insurance Portability and Accountability Act

ICD-9-CM *International Classification of Diseases, 9th Revision, Clinical Modification*

ICD-10-CM *International Classification of Diseases, 10th Revision, Clinical Modification*

ICD-10-PCS *International Classification of Diseases, 10th*

Revision, Procedure Coding System

IS information systems

MS-DRG Medicare Severity diagnosis-related group

NCHS National Center for Health Statistics

OIG Office of the Inspector General

RHIA Registered Health Information Administrator

RHIT Registered Health Information Technician

SNOMED Systematized Nomenclature of Medicine

UR utilization review

WHO World Health Organization

BACKGROUND OF CODING

What Is Coding and What Are Its Applications?

As a student in this field, you will often be asked these questions. Why does one study this subject? What type of work does a "coder" do? Basically, medical coding consists of translating **diagnoses** and **procedures** into numbers for the purpose of statistically capturing data. This process is done for us every day in all aspects of daily life. If you buy a banana at the grocery store, the cash register captures that banana as a number, which, in turn, provides data on the number of bananas sold in that store or by that grocery chain; it also yields data of importance to the store on replenishing their inventory, details regarding what time of year the greatest number of bananas are sold, and so forth.

Translation of a disease and/or a procedure into an ICD-10 code is not as simple as it may seem. This process requires a thorough knowledge of anatomy and physiology, disease processes, medical **terminology**, laboratory values, pharmacology, surgical procedures, and last but not least, a myriad of coding rules and guidelines. Diseases and procedures are translated into a coding system known as the *International Classification of Diseases, 10th Revision, Clinical Modification* ICD-10-CM and ICD-10-PCS. This **classification** system has been used worldwide and has been clinically modified for the United States.

Coded data are used for many purposes. Prior to the advent of diagnosis-related groups (DRGs), which are used by Medicare and other payers as the basis for hospital **reimbursement** (payment), coding was used for research and planning. A healthcare provider or facility could use this data to find out how many cases of appendicitis were treated in a year. This information could be used by a healthcare facility in decisions about the possible purchase of more equipment, the addition of an operating room, the hiring of additional staff, or by the provider to gain additional skills. Since the implementation of DRGs—now known as MS-DRGs—coded data are also used for reimbursement purposes, and they are increasingly used for risk management and quality improvement, as well as in nursing clinical pathways. Coded data were important from the start, but use of this data for reimbursement has elevated the importance of accurate coding to new heights.

Capture of health data through ICD-10 codes that are used worldwide has proved useful for the study of patterns of disease, disease epidemics, causes of mortality, and treatment modalities. Without the use of a classification system, comparison of data would be impossible.

Nomenclature and Classification

A nomenclature and a classification of diseases are required for development of a coding system. A **nomenclature** is a system of names that are used as preferred terminology, in this case, for diseases and procedures. Often, diseases in different areas of the country or in different countries are identified by dissimilar terminology, which makes the capture of comparative statistical data next to impossible. For example, another name for "amyotrophic lateral sclerosis" is "Lou Gehrig's disease," which is also known as a "motor neuron disease." Nomenclatures of disease were first developed in the United States around 1928. The Systematized Nomenclature of Medicine (SNOMED), published by the College of American Pathologists, is the most up-to-date system in current use.

Classification systems group together similar items for easy storage and retrieval. Within a classification system, items are arranged into groups according to specific criteria. The history of classification systems goes back as far as Hippocrates. During the 17th century, London Bills of Mortality represented the first attempts of scientists to gather statistical data on disease. The ICD-10-CM classification system is a closed system that comprises diseases, injuries, surgeries, and procedures. In a closed classification system a disease, condition, or procedure can be classified in only one place.

HISTORY OF CODING

ICD-9-CM is the coding classification system that is currently in use in the United States. This classification system dates back to Bertillon's Classification of Causes of Death, which was developed in 1893. This system was adopted by the United States in 1898 under the recommendation of the American Public Health Association. System revisions were scheduled to take place every 10 years, and the classification was maintained by the World Health Organization (WHO). Revisions became known as the International Classification of Causes of Death. Over the years, this system has been changed to allow its use not only in mortality (death) reporting but in morbidity (disease condition) reporting as well. Since its inception, this classification has been revised 10 times. The Clinical Modification (CM) was developed in 1977 by the United States to more accurately capture morbidity data for study within the United States, as well as information on operative and diagnostic procedures that were not included in the original publication of ICD.

Currently, many countries are using ICD-10, which was published in 1993 by the WHO. ICD-10-CM has been clinically modified for use in the United States with proposed implementation set for October 1, 2014. ICD-10-CM will replace the 30-year-old ICD-9-CM. The final rule for adoption of ICD-10-CM and ICD-10-PCS was released in January of 2009.

Work on ICD-10 was begun in 1983. The tabular volume was published in 1992, and the instructional volume followed in 1993; the Alphabetic Index was published in 1994. In 1994, the United States began the process of determining whether a clinical modification (CM) would be necessary. A draft version was made available in 2002, updated in July 2007, and updated again in 2009 and will continue to be updated yearly until it is final. The latest version can be found at the National Center for Health Statistics website.

Clinical modifications made to ICD-10 allow a higher level of specificity. Since 1999, ICD-10 has been used in the United States for the reporting of mortality data. A total of 90 countries, including Canada and Australia, are currently using ICD-10.

ICD-9-CM may be updated biannually in April and October. Updates contain additional codes, revised codes, and codes that are deleted. These updates are published in the *Federal Register* (the official daily publication for rules, proposed rules, and notices of U.S. federal agencies and organizations) as a proposed rule and then as a final rule. They are available at the Centers for Medicare and Medicaid Services (CMS) website (www.cms.gov). It is of the utmost importance that code books and coding software (**encoder**) be updated to ensure that coding is accurate and to facilitate accurate reimbursement. The ICD-9-CM Coordination and Maintenance Committee meets twice a year and is used as a forum for proposals to update ICD-9-CM. Upon full implementation of ICD-10-CM/PCS this will become the ICD-10 Coordination and Maintenance Committee. This Committee serves in an advisory capacity. Two Federal agencies are responsible for maintenance of ICD-9-CM. The classification of diagnoses is the responsibility of the NCHS (National Center for Health Statistics) and the classification of procedures is the responsibility of CMS (Centers for Medicare and Medicaid Services). The Coordination and Maintenance Committee meetings are open to the public and comments are encouraged. All comments and recommendations are evaluated before a final decision on new codes is issued.

The development and maintenance of the guidelines of ICD-9-CM is the responsibility of the National Center for Health Statistics (NCHS), CMS, the American Hospital Association (AHA), and the American Health Information Management Association (AHIMA), which are also known as the Cooperating Parties. Many publications provide coding advice and information, but only one publication is official. This publication, *AHA Coding Clinic for ICD-9-CM* (referred to as *Coding Clinic*), which is published quarterly by the AHA, provides coding advice and guidelines that have been approved by the Cooperating Parties and must be followed by coders.

COMPARISON OF ICD-10-CM AND ICD-9-CM

As noted in Table 1-1, considerable differences can be seen between ICD-10-CM and ICD-9-CM. Most notable is the increase in the number of codes and code categories, the change

TABLE 1-1 COMPARISON OF ICD-10-CM AND ICD-9-CM*

ICD-9-CM	ICD-10-CM
14,000 codes	69,000 codes
Codes begin with number except for V&E supplementary classification	Codes begin with a letter
Maximum 5 number code	3 to 7 characters
All codes end in a number	Codes may end in a number or a letter
Morphology codes begin with M	Both morphology and musculoskeletal codes begin with M
Three tables: Neoplasms, Drugs and Chemicals, Hypertension	Two tables: Neoplasms, Drugs and Chemicals
17 chapters with 2 supplements	21 chapters
1 chapter for Diseases of the Nervous System, Eyes, Ears	3 chapters for Nervous System, Eyes, Ears
No laterality included in codes	Laterality included in codes
Sometimes combine NEC (not elsewhere classified) and NOS (not otherwise specified)	Never combine NEC and NOS
No 7th character extensions	7th character extensions
No placeholder letter X	Placeholder letter X
Excludes notes	Excludes notes 1 and 2

*The index and the tabular of ICD-10-CM are very similar in style to ICD-9-CM.

from numeric to alphanumeric codes with an increase in digits from 5 to 7, and the increase from 17 chapters to 21 chapters.

The best way to appreciate these differences is to view code assignments for the same disease process from both classification systems.

EXAMPLE

Newborn baby delivered via c-section	V30.01 (ICD-9-CM)
Newborn baby delivered via c-section	Z38.01 (ICD-10-CM)

EXAMPLE

Displaced spiral closed fracture shaft of left femur, initial encounter	821.01 (ICD-9-CM)
Displaced spiral closed fracture shaft of left femur, initial encounter	S72.342A (ICD-10-CM)

PREPARATION FOR TRANSITION TO ICD-10-CM

The steps necessary for transition to ICD-10-CM and ICD-10-PCS involve many different areas within the healthcare system, including Information Systems (IS), Billing, healthcare providers, Utilization Review (UR), Researchers, Compliance, and Accounting, to name a few. Most articles written on the subject recommend a team approach across the facility. Existing coding staff will need to be trained on both ICD-10-CM and ICD-10-PCS.

Reports suggest (Practice Brief Destination 10: Healthcare Organization Preparation for ICD-10-CM and ICD-10-PCS)[1] that the knowledge base of coders must be broadened so they have detailed knowledge of anatomy and medical terminology, enhanced comprehension of operative reports, and a greater understanding of ICD-10-PCS definitions. It may be necessary to assess the skills of coders before selecting the type of training needed. It has been suggested that training should not take place too early, and probably around 3 months before implementation would be preferable. Aside from more intensive training in anatomy and physiology (A&P) and terminology, the following education on ICD-10-CM is recommended by AHIMA:

- Structure change
- Disease classification
- Definitions
- Guidelines
- ICD-10-PCS

AHIMA is currently offering ICD-10 courses via the Web. *ICD-TEN* is a monthly newsletter to assist in the transition to ICD-10-CM and ICD-10-PCS. The need is great for qualified instructors to teach both of these classification systems to the many users who will need to know them.

AHIMA's Commission on Certification for Health Information and Informatics (CCHIIM) has implemented a new recertification policy specific to ICD-10-CM/PCS. This policy requires that CEU education hours based on ICD-10-CM/PCS content will be required and will be part of the existing CEU requirement. The CEUs required are based on the credential held and are as follows:

RHIT	6 CEUs
RHIA	6 CEUs
CCS-P	12 CEUs
CCS	18 CEUs
CCA	18 CEUs

If a person holds more than one credential, the CEUs necessary are based on the credential requiring the highest number of ICD-10-CM/PCS CEUs. These CEUs should be earned from January 1, 2011 to December 31, 2013. All AHIMA Certified Professionals who completed AHIMA's Academy for ICD-10 prior to January 1, 2011 will be allowed to use those CEU hours to fulfill the ICD-10-CM/PCS CEU requirement.

CODING ORGANIZATIONS AND CREDENTIALS

Coders come from a variety of educational backgrounds. Many coders have attended 4-year college programs in Health Information Administration; others have completed 2-year college programs in Health Information Technology. Some community colleges offer programs geared only to medical coding. Whatever their background, most coders take certification examinations to earn **credentials** (which are certificates that recognize a course of study taken in a specific field and acknowledge that competency is required) and become members of a professional organization. Many employers include a requirement for certification as part of their coding job description.

Coders can work in a variety of settings; most often, they are employed by hospitals, physician offices, outpatient surgical centers, long-term care facilities, and insurance companies. It is predicted that the demand for coding professionals will far exceed the number of coders in the workforce.

The two most well-known professional associations for coders are AHIMA (www.ahima .org) and the American Academy of Professional Coders (AAPC) (www.aapc.com). Both of these organizations offer a variety of coding credentials. AHIMA, which has been in existence for over 75 years, has undergone several name changes along the way to keep up with the ever-changing technological skills, educational requirements, and roles of its members. It boasts a membership of over 60,000. Traditionally, this organization has provided support for facility coders, but in recent years, it has expanded to include coders who provide services in physician's offices and outpatient settings. AHIMA offers the following credentials:

CCA	Certified Coding Associate
CCS	Certified Coding Specialist
CCS-P	Certified Coding Specialist—Physician Based
RHIT	Registered Health Information Technician
RHIA	Registered Health Information Administrator

TABLE 1-2 CREDENTIALS AND CONTINUING EDUCATION UNIT REQUIREMENTS

Credential	Organization Offering Credential	Education Required	CEUs Required per 2-Year Cycle
CCA	AHIMA	High school diploma or equivalent	20
CCS	AHIMA	High school diploma or equivalent	20
CCS-P	AHIMA	High school diploma or equivalent	20
RHIT	AHIMA	2-Year degree in accredited HIM program	20
RHIA	AHIMA	4-Year degree in accredited HIM program	30
CPC	AAPC	High school diploma or equivalent and 2 years coding experience	36
CPC-H	AAPC	High school diploma or equivalent and 2 years coding experience	36
CPC-P	AAPC	High school diploma or equivalent and 2 years coding experience	36
CPC-A	AAPC	High school diploma or equivalent	36
CPC-H-A	AAPC	High school diploma or equivalent	36
CPC-P-A	AAPC	High school diploma or equivalent	36

AAPC has over 100,000 credentialed members and was started in 1981. It was founded to assist coders in providing services to physicians and offers the following credentials:

CPC	Certified Professional Coder
CPC-H	Certified Professional Coder—Hospital
CPC-P	Certified Professional Coder—Payer
CPC-A	Certified Professional Coder—Apprentice
CPC-H-A	Certified Professional Coder—Hospital Apprentice
CPC-P-A	Certified Professional Coder—Payer Apprentice

To obtain credentials from either organization, a coder must sit for a certification examination and complete college coursework in several areas such as medical terminology and anatomy and physiology. To maintain their credentials, coders must earn continuing education units (CEUs). The number of CEUs required is dependent on the credential(s) of the coder (Table 1-2).

CODING ETHICS

Along with providing credentials, both AHIMA and AAPC have set standards for Coding **Ethics,** which are reprinted in Figures 1-1 and 1-2. (Please see the Evolve companion website for "How to Interpret the Standards of Ethical Coding.") Members of these organizations are expected to abide by these coding standards. A coder who is asked to disregard a guideline to facilitate payment should decline on the basis of these standards, by which coders are bound.

COMPLIANCE

Compliance is defined as "acting according to certain accepted standards or, in simple terms, abiding by the rules." In health care, this requires following the rules and guidelines as set forth by the government through Medicare and Medicaid and all professional organizations which a facility or provider may belong to or is participating with, and following the policies and procedures of that organization.

Standards of Ethical Coding

Coding professionals should:

1. Apply accurate, complete, and consistent coding practices for the production of high-quality healthcare data.
2. Report all healthcare data elements (e.g., diagnosis and procedure codes, present on admission indicator, discharge status) required for external reporting purposes (e.g., reimbursement and other administrative uses, population health, quality and patient safety measurement, and research) completely and accurately, in accordance with regulatory and documentation standards and requirements and applicable coding conventions, rules, and guidelines.
3. Assign and report only the codes and data that are clearly and consistently supported by health record documentation in accordance with applicable code set and abstraction conventions, rules, and guidelines.
4. Query provider (physician or other qualified healthcare practitioner) for clarification and additional documentation prior to code assignment when there is conflicting, incomplete, or ambiguous information in the health record regarding a significant reportable condition or procedure or other reportable data element dependent on health record documentation (e.g., present on admission indicator).
5. Refuse to change reported codes or the narratives of codes so that meanings are misrepresented.
6. Refuse to participate in or support coding or documentation practices intended to inappropriately increase payment, qualify for insurance policy coverage, or skew data by means that do not comply with federal and state statutes, regulations, and official rules and guidelines.
7. Facilitate interdisciplinary collaboration in situations supporting proper coding practices.
8. Advance coding knowledge and practice through continuing education.
9. Refuse to participate in or conceal unethical coding or abstraction practices or procedures.
10. Protect the confidentiality of the health record at all times and refuse to access protected health information not required for coding-related activities (examples of coding-related activities include completion of code assignment, other health record data abstraction, coding audits, and educational purposes).
11. Demonstrate behavior that reflects integrity, shows a commitment to ethical and legal coding practices, and fosters trust in professional activities.

Revised and approved by the House of Delegates 09/08

FIGURE 1-1. AHIMA's Standards of Ethical Coding.

AAPC Code of Ethics

Commitment to ethical professional conduct is expected of every AAPC member. The specification of a Code of Ethics enables AAPC to clarify to current and future members, and to those served by members, the nature of the ethical responsibilities held in common by its members. This document establishes principles that define the ethical behavior of AAPC members. All AAPC members are required to adhere to the Code of Ethics and the Code of Ethics will serve as the basis for processing ethical complaints initiated against AAPC members.

AAPC members shall:

- Maintain and enhance the dignity, status, integrity, competence, and standards of our profession.
- Respect the privacy of others and honor confidentiality.
- Strive to achieve the highest quality, effectiveness and dignity in both the process and products of professional work.
- Advance the profession through continued professional development and education by acquiring and maintaining professional competence.
- Know and respect existing federal, state and local laws, regulations, certifications and licensing requirements applicable to professional work.
- Use only legal and ethical principles that reflect the profession's core values and report activity that is perceived to violate this Code of Ethics to the AAPC Ethics Committee.
- Accurately represent the credential(s) earned and the status of AAPC membership.
- Avoid actions and circumstances that may appear to compromise good business judgment or create a conflict between personal and professional interests.

Adherence to these standards assures public confidence in the integrity and service of medical coding, auditing, compliance and practice management professionals who are AAPC members.

Failure to adhere to these standards, as determined by AAPC's Ethics Committee, may result in the loss of credentials and membership with AAPC.

FIGURE 1-2. AAPC's Code of Ethical Standards.

Compliance officers and programs are found in many industries. It wasn't until after the passage of the Health Insurance Portability and Accountability Act of 1996 (HIPAA) that compliance officers became a standard presence in healthcare facilities. HIPAA gave additional funding to the U.S. Department of Health and Human Services, the Office of the Inspector General (OIG), and the U.S. Department of Justice to increase penalties for healthcare fraud and abuse. Ongoing investigations in healthcare institutions across the United States are exploring violations of the False Claim Act and other laws.

As explained in an article by Joette Hanna that appeared in the *Journal of AHIMA*, entitled "Constructing a Coding Compliance Plan,"[2] several steps must be taken if a coding department wishes to ensure that it is in compliance. Coding departments must do the following:

■ Abide by AHIMA's Standards of Ethical Coding
■ Develop coding policies and procedures
■ Develop a working relationship with the billing department
■ Develop a coding compliance work plan
■ Conduct coding audits
■ Develop an action plan based on audit results

Likewise, a practice brief published by AHIMA in 2001, entitled "Developing a Coding Compliance Policy Document,"[3] states that the following bulleted items should be included in a coding compliance plan:

■ Policy statement regarding the commitment of the organization to correct assignment and reporting of codes
■ The Official Coding Guidelines used by the facility
■ The people responsible for code assignment
■ What needs to be done when clinical information is not clear enough to assign codes
■ If there are payer-specific guidelines, where these may be found
■ A procedure for correcting codes that have been assigned incorrectly
■ Plan for education on areas of risk as identified by audits
■ Identification of essential coding resources that are available and to be used by coding professionals
■ Procedure for coding new and/or unusual diagnoses or procedures
■ A policy for which procedures will be reported
■ Procedure for resolving coding/documentation disputes with physicians
■ Procedure for processing claim rejections
■ Procedure for handling requests for coding amendments
■ Policy that requires coders to have available coding manuals and not just encoder
■ Process for review of coding on those records coded with incomplete documentation

CONFIDENTIALITY

Employees in a healthcare setting must be aware of the confidentiality of the information surrounding them. When they take the Hippocratic Oath, physicians swear to maintain patient confidentiality. Likewise, in the Patient Bill of Rights as prepared by the AHA, the patient's right to privacy is stated. The Code of Ethics of the AHIMA also addresses confidentiality when it says, "Members will promote and protect the confidentiality and security of health records and information."

Coders must read a patient's personal medical information before they can code the encounter and/or patient admission. It is important that this information not be shared with anyone, including other employees, unless they have a legitimate need to know to perform their job; patient information should never be discussed in a place where any visitor could overhear.

CHAPTER REVIEW EXERCISE

Write the correct answer(s) in the space(s) provided.

1. What does a coder do?

   _____

2. What coding system is currently used in the United States for diagnosis coding?

   _____

3. What does the CM of ICD-10-CM stand for?

   _____

4. List three uses for coded data.

   1. _____

   2. _____

   3. _____

5. What payment system does Medicare use for inpatient reimbursement?

   _____

6. Describe the difference between a nomenclature and a classification system.

   _____

7. What nomenclature of disease is used in the United States?

   _____

8. Define a closed classification system.

   _____

9. When was the International Classification of Diseases first adopted by the United States?

   _____

10. When and how often is this system (ICD-10-CM) updated?

    _____

11. What four groups constitute the Cooperating Parties?

    1. _____

    2. _____

    3. _____

    4. _____

12. Who publishes official coding advice and guidance?

    _____

13. What organizations award coding credentials?

    _____

14. What is another word that is used in the industry for "following the rules"?

    _____

15. If you were coding a neighbor's record, would it be okay for you to tell your other neighbors the reason the patient was hospitalized?

    _____

16. What does HIPAA stand for?

    _____

17. Most industrialized countries do not use ICD-10.
   A. True
   B. False

18. Coders will require greater technical skill if they are to master ICD-10-CM and ICD-10-PCS.
   A. True
   B. False

CHAPTER GLOSSARY

Classification: grouping together of items as for storage and retrieval.

Compliance: adherence to accepted standards.

Credential: degree, certificate, or award that recognizes a course of study taken in a specific field and that acknowledges the competency required.

Diagnosis: identification of a disease through signs, symptoms, and tests.

Encoder: coding software that is used to assign diagnosis and procedure codes.

Ethics: moral standard.

Federal Register: the official daily publication for rules, proposed rules, and notices of U.S. federal agencies and organizations.

Nomenclature: system of names that are used as the preferred terminology.

Procedure: a diagnostic or therapeutic process performed on a patient.

Reimbursement: payment for healthcare services.

Terminology: words and phrases that apply to a particular field.

REFERENCES

1. American Health Information Management Association. Destination 10: healthcare organization preparation for ICD-10-CM and ICD-10-PCS, *J AHIMA* 75:56A-556D, 2004.
2. Hanna J. Constructing a coding compliance plan, *J AHIMA* 73:48-56, 2002.
3. AHIMA Coding Practice Team. Developing a coding compliance policy document (AHIMA practice brief), *J AHIMA* 72:88A-888C, 2001.

2

The Health Record as the Foundation of Coding

LEARNING OBJECTIVES

1. Explain the purpose of the various forms or reports found in a health record
2. Define "principal diagnosis"
3. Define "principal procedure"
4. Identify reasons for assigning codes for other diagnoses
5. List the basic guidelines for reporting diagnoses/procedures
6. Identify types of documentation acceptable for assigning codes
7. Explain the query process

ABBREVIATIONS/ ACRONYMS

AHQA American Health Quality Association

BPH benign prostatic hypertrophy

CBC complete blood count

CC chief complaint

CMS Centers for Medicare and Medicaid Services

CPT *Current Procedural Terminology*

COPD chronic obstructive pulmonary disease

DOB date of birth

ED Emergency Department

EEG electroencephalogram

EGD esophagogastroduodenoscopy

EKG electrocardiogram

ER Emergency Room

GERD gastroesophageal reflux disease

H&P history and physical

ABBREVIATIONS/
ACRONYMS—*cont'd*

HPI history of present illness

ICD-9-CM *International Classification of Diseases, 9th Revision, Clinical Modification*

ICD-10-CM *International Classification of Diseases, 10th Revision, Clinical Modification*

ICU intensive care unit

MAR medication administration record

MRA magnetic resonance angiography

MRI magnetic resonance imaging

MS-DRGs Medicare Severity diagnosis-related groups

MVP mitral valve prolapse

NPI National Provider Identifier

OP note operative note

POA present on admission

SOAP Subjective/Objective/ Assessment/Plan

TJC The Joint Commission

TPR temperature, pulse, and respiration

UHDDS Uniform Hospital Discharge Data Set

UPIN Unique Physician Identification Number

UTI urinary tract infection

THE HEALTH RECORD

A health record must be maintained for every individual who is assessed or treated. Although Edna Huffman's classic *Health Information Management*[1] book is no longer in print, her definition of the purpose and use of a health record still holds true today. She states, "The main purpose of the medical record is to accurately and adequately document a patient's life and health history, including past and present illnesses and treatments, with emphasis on the events affecting the patient during the current episode of care." Huffman goes on to say, "The medical record must be compiled in a timely manner and contain sufficient data to identify the patient, support the diagnosis or reason for health care encounter, justify the treatment and accurately document the results." According to Abdelhak's *Health Information: Management of a Strategic Resource,*[2] the health record serves five purposes:

1. Describes the patient's health history
2. Serves as a method for clinicians to communicate regarding the plan of care for the patients
3. Serves as a legal document of care and services provided
4. Serves as a source of data
5. Serves as a resource for healthcare practitioner education

The patient's health record in today's environment may be maintained in several formats or **hybrids**. The traditional health record consists of documentation on paper prepared by **healthcare providers** that describes the condition of the patient and the plan and course of treatment. As the world advances through electronic forms of documentation, paper notes become more and more obsolete. Most health records are currently in a state of transition. Some paper documentation and some transcribed or electronically stored documentation may be available. Some facilities have actually achieved a predominantly electronic health record. One of the advantages of storing the record electronically is that many users are able to access the record at the same time. Whether in electronic, paper, or hybrid form, documentation serves as the basis of a health record.

The Centers for Medicare and Medicaid Services (CMS) has provided physicians with *General Principles of Medical Record Documentation.*[3]

■ Medical records should be complete and legible
■ The documentation of each patient encounter should include:
  • Reason for encounter and relevant history
  • Physical examination findings and prior diagnostic test results
  • Assessment, clinical impression, and diagnosis
  • Plan for care
■ Date and legible identity of the observer
■ The rationale for ordering diagnostic and ancillary services (if not documented, should be easily inferred)
■ Past and present diagnoses should be accessible for treating and/or consulting physician
■ Appropriate health risk factors should be identified

■ Patient's progress, response to changes in treatment, and revision of diagnosis should be documented

■ *Current Procedural Terminology* (CPT) and *International Classification of Diseases, 9th Revision, Clinical Modification* (ICD-9-CM) codes reported on health insurance claim forms should be supported by documentation in the medical record

SECTIONS OF THE HEALTH RECORD

Every facility has its own policies and procedures regarding the organization of the health record. Records will differ slightly depending upon the course of the patient's condition and treatment. If a record were to be organized similarly to a novel that tells a story, the elements discussed in the next sections would be included.

Administrative Data

■ Demographic
■ Personal data
■ Consents

Information contained in this section will facilitate identification of the patient. Some of the UHDDS data elements included are personal identification, date of birth, sex, race, residence, admit date, and discharge date. See Figure 2-1.

Clinical Data

Inpatient records may be organized in a reverse chronological order. The discharge summary may be found at the beginning of the record.

■ Emergency room record (when applicable) (see Figure 2-2)
■ Admission history and physical (see Figure 2-3)
■ Physician orders (see Figures 2-4 and 2-5)
■ Progress notes recorded by healthcare providers (see Figure 2-6, *A* and *B*)
■ Anesthesia forms (when applicable) (see Figure 2-9)
■ Operative report (when applicable) (see Figure 2-10)
■ Recovery room notes (when applicable)
■ Consultations (when applicable)
■ Laboratory test results (when applicable) (see Figure 2-8)
■ Radiology report (when applicable) (see Figure 2-11)
■ Miscellaneous ancillary reports (when applicable)
■ Discharge summary (see Figure 2-12)

Data are collected from the health record as mandated by governmental and nongovernmental agencies. The Joint Commission (TJC) places data requirements and time frames for documentation within the health record. The federal government and state licensing agencies may have similar requirements. Medical staff bylaws often include these documentation requirements. In 1974, the Uniform Hospital Discharge Data Set (UHDDS) mandated that hospitals must report a common core of data. Since that time, the requirements have been revised and will continue to change as necessary. The UHDDS required data elements are listed in Figure 2-1.

Emergency Room Record

The emergency room record is a mini health record. It contains a **chief complaint (CC)**, which is the reason, in the patient's own words, for presentation to the hospital. It contains a history, physical examination, laboratory results, radiology reports (if applicable), plan of care, physician orders, and documentation of any procedures performed. Last but not least, it contains a list of working diagnoses and information on the disposition of the patient. See Figure 2-2 for a sample of an ED (Emergency Department, or also called ER for Emergency Room) record.

Uniform Hospital Discharge Data Set

01. **Personal identification**
02. **Date of birth (month, day, and year)**
03. **Sex**
04. **Race and ethnicity**
05. **Residence (usual residence, full address, and zip code [nine-digit zip code, if available])**
06. **Hospital identification number**
    Three options are given for this institutional number, with the Medicare provider number as the recommended choice. The federal tax identification number of the American Hospital Association number is preferred to creating a new number.
07. **Admission date (month, day, and year)**
08. **Type of admission (scheduled or unscheduled)**
09. **Discharge date (month, day, and year)**
10. **Attending physician identification (NPI)**
11. **Operating physician identification (NPI)**
12. **Principal diagnosis**
    The condition established after study to be chiefly responsible for occasioning the admission of the patient to the hospital for care.
13. **Other diagnoses**
    All conditions that coexist at the time of admission or that develop subsequently that affect the treatment received and/or the length of stay. Diagnoses that relate to an earlier episode and have no bearing on the current hospital stay are excluded.
14. **Qualifier for other diagnoses**
    A qualifier is given for each diagnosis coded under "other diagnoses" to indicate whether the onset of the diagnosis preceded or followed admission to the hospital. The option "uncertain" is permitted.
15. **External cause-of-injury code**
    Hospitals should complete this item whenever there is a diagnosis of an injury, poisoning, or adverse effect.
16. **Birth weight of neonate**
17. **Procedures and dates**
    a. All significant procedures are to be reported. A significant procedure is one that (1) is surgical in nature, (2) carries a procedural risk, (3) carries an anesthetic risk, or (4) requires specialized training.
    b. The date of each significant procedure must be reported.
    c. When multiple procedures are reported, the principal procedure is designated. The principal procedure is one that was performed for definitive treatment rather than one performed for diagnostic or explanatory purposes or was necessary to take care of a complication. If two procedures appear to be principal, then the one most related to the principal diagnosis is selected as the principal procedure.
    d. The UPIN of the person performing the principal procedure must be reported.
18. **Disposition of the patient**
    a. Discharged home (not to home health service)
    b. Discharged to acute care hospital
    c. Discharged to nursing facility
    d. Discharged to home to be under the care of a home health service
    e. Discharged to other health care facility
    f. Left against medical advice
    g. Alive, other; or alive, not stated
    h. Died
19. **Patient's expected source of payment**
    a. Primary source
    b. Other source
20. **Total charges**
    List all charges billed by the hospital for this hospitalization. Professional charges for individual patient care by physicians are excluded.

FIGURE 2-1. Uniform Hospital Discharge Data Set elements.

Date: _____ Room: _____ Time in room: _____ AM/PM

Hx source: (Patient) / spouse / family / friend / EMS / other   ☐ History & ROS limited by medical or other condition

Time seen: // ___ (AM/PM)   PMH: None   PSH: None

CC: Renal (Tx) – now advanced nephropathy

HPI: S/p (o) ₹ Clupus & failing renal tx (prept.   Lupus nephritis   DM   prept
last Cr 8), needle on 7/14/06 for rejection of tx,   h fa   last Cr 8
now presents ₹ 1 d h/o trouble speaking. Pt has   cluster HA
had trouble getting words out x 2 weeks. Now ₹   8 LE
acute stuttering since this am. 9AM ⊕ HA – same pain   fibromyalgia
frontal, band like ⊕ eye pain. on Gabapentin x 2 weeks   s/p cholecystectomy
⊕ cough, ⊕ chills ⊕ twitching x 1 month. ⊕ diplopia   Meds: None   See triage/nursing sheet
⊖ fever x 2 weeks   calcitriol   FeSO4   Prograf
                                                           aranesp   Nexium   Toprol
                                                           gabapentin 800 folic acid Furosemide
                                                           phoslo   Prednisone
                                                           nifedical   Azathioprine
                                                           MVI

FH: (None) / CAD / CVA / Cancer / DM / HTN / Other: Allergies: NKDA (other): Zantac Bactrim
SH: Tobacco: (None) / Current / Past / _____ Pack-year   anti-seizure med?
    Alcohol: (None) / Occ / Mod / Heavy:
Drugs: None / Current / Past / Type: _____ chronic   Lives In: Home (family) / Home (alone) / NH / Homeless / Other

ROS: CIRCLE ALL THAT APPLY, CROSS OUT NEGATIVE COMPLAINTS OR SYSTEMS, LIST OTHERS

Gen	Eyes	ENT	Resp	CV	GI	GU	Skin	MS	Psych	Neuro	All/IM
Fever	Blur vision	Hearing prob	Cough	Chest pain	Abd pain	Dysuria	Rash	Neck pain	Depression	HA	Allergies
Chills	Less vision	Rhinitis	Wheezing	DOE	N/V/D	Flank pain	Itching	Back pain	Hallucination	Weakness	Hives
Weight loss	Diplopia	Nose bleed	Dyspnea	Edema	Melena	Vag bleed	Bruising	Arm pain	Suicidal	Gait prob	Poor healing
Weakness	Pain	Throat pain	Hemoptysis	Palpitations	Rectal blood	Discharge	Wounds:	Leg pain	Homicidal	Speech prob	
	Photophobia	Voice change	Pleuritis	Lightheaded	Vomit blood	Testicle pain					

Heme	Endo	Other ROS: dry mouth	LMP:	☐ All other systems reviewed are negative	Pain Score (1-10): ___
Anemia	Weight loss	⊕ eye pain x 2 weeks			
Bruising	Polyuria	⊕ diplopia – occasional			
Bleeding	Polydipsia				
Lymph nodes					

PE: (X) VS reviewed   BP: 147 / 88   HR: 82   RR: 16   T: 98.5   O2 sat: 97 % on RA   Normal/Hypoxia

Gen	Appearance	NAD	Pt stuttering. Not in respiratory distress. Cushingoid
Eyes	Conjunctiva	Normal	
	Pupils	Normal	EOM Normal Fundi Normal
ENT	Head/Face	Atrauma	
	Ear	Normal	
	Nose	Normal	
	Oropharynx	Normal	
Resp	Effort	Normal	
	Auscultation	Normal	
CV	Auscultation	Normal	
	Jugular	Normal	
	Edema	None	2+ edema to mid calf
GI	Bowel sound	Normal	obese – n
	Palpation	NT / ND	(L) LQ scar where transplant
	Rectal exam	Normal	
GU	CVA Tender	None	
	External	Normal	
	Pelvic	Normal	
Skin		Normal	
MS	Extremity	Normal	
	Neck	Normal	
	Back	Normal	
Lymph	Neck: Normal	Groin: Normal	Axilla: Normal
Psych	Judgment	Normal	Orientation: 0 x 3
	Mood/Affect	Normal	Speech: Normal
Neuro	CN: II - XII	Normal	Gait: Normal
	Motor	Normal	Cerebellar: Normal
	DTRs	Normal	Sensation: Normal

AG 18   5.0 10.6
              34.2   182

143 101 66   (137)
3.7 24   7.8

9.1 6.5 0.2 25
     3.5   14   81

Baseline INR 0.9
          aPTT 0.8

Pt stuttering spontaneously resolves & then recurs
⊕ tremulous occasional having full body
twitching – stops when pt hold extremities
Strength 4/5 (B) LE
⊕ Rhomberg. pt very unsteady when closes
her eyes
Reflexes 1+ throughout

Resident/PA/NP _____   ID #

Resident/PA/NP _____

MEDICAL RECORD

FIGURE 2-2. Emergency Room record.

Continued

MEDICAL DECISION MAKING

PLAN

Head CT
labs

Differential Dx:

1. Stroke
2. uremia
3. infection
4. drug side effect

1745
Renal (XU) 39842 cooled. will come to eval.

Radiology Results: ☐ ED interpretation ☐ Discussed with Radiologist

CT -. NoCT evidence of acute ischemia

EKG/Rhythm: NSR / Arrythmia: _____

☒ Discussed history, plan or diagnosis with other provider.
☐ Prior medical records reviewed.
☐ Nursing / EMS notes reviewed.
☐ The patient was given: *IM / IV* medications or *IV fluids.*
☐ Patient referred for further care.

ATTENDING PHYSICIAN NOTE: Time seen: 11⊃○ AM / PM

☐ I was present with the resident/midlevel during the patient's history and physical and discussed their management with the resident. I have reviewed the resident's note above and agree with the documented findings and plan of care.
☒ I saw and evaluated the patient. I reviewed the resident/midlevel's note above and agree, in addition to/except that:
Additional findings:

s/p Mul 2+

ī unit duly clipping
⊖ dlf
⟶ √ ct

Procedure / Progress Note: Time:_____ AM / PM   **Consult:** _____ **Called:** _____ AM / PM

No acute neurosissues perkeepo
Pt accepted to Medicine For uremic

Provider: _____ ___ ___ ___ ___ ___

Procedures: Central Venous / Intubation / LP / Suture / Chest tube / Nasal Pack / Sedation / Splint / I&D / Other: _____

Diagnosis:
1. Uremia
2. _____
3. _____
4. _____
5. _____
6. _____

☐ **See procedure documentation**
☐ **See additional documentation**

Critical Care Time: _____ minutes

Dispo: Discharge / Admit / Transfer / AMA
Condition: Stable / Good / Fair / Serious / Expired

Admission/Transfer Location: _____
Discharge time: _____ AM / PM   Date:

Attendings: _____ _____

MEDICAL RECORD

FIGURE 2-2, cont'd. Emergency Room record.

Admission History and Physical Examination

Admission history and physical documentation normally contains the following elements:

- Chief complaint (CC)
- History of the present illness (HPI)
- Past medical history
- Family medical history
- Social history
- Review of systems
- Physical examination
- Impression/Assessment
- Plan

  See Figure 2-3 for an example of a history and physical form (H&P).

Physician Orders

This is the area of the record in which the attending **physician**, as well as physician **consultants**, gives directives to the house staff and to nursing and ancillary services. Physician orders are dated, timed, and signed and become part of the record. Verbal orders by physicians are guided by medical staff regulations. See Figure 2-4 for an example of handwritten physician orders and Figure 2-5 for an electronic physician order.

Progress Notes

Progress notes are a record of the course of a patient's hospital care. They are usually written by the attending physician (Figure 2-6, *A*). Academic medical centers may have notes written by medical students, interns, and residents, as well as attending physicians and consultants. Some facilities have integrated progress notes, which allow individuals from several disciplines to write in the same area of the record. An integrated progress note may include notes written by dietitians, physical therapists, respiratory therapists, and nurses.

Progress notes written by the attending physician are recorded on a daily basis; the frequency of such note taking is governed by medical staff regulations. These notes describe how the patient is progressing and put forth the plan of care for the patient. In an electronic patient record, these notes may be dictated and transcribed or typed by physicians themselves. Physicians are usually taught to document progress notes according to the SOAP format. SOAP stands for the following:

Subjective—The problem in the patient's own words (chief complaint)
Objective—The physician identifies the history, physical examination, and diagnostic test results
Assessment—Where the subjective and objective combine for a conclusion
Plan—Approach the physician is taking to solve the patient's problem
See Figure 2-6, *B,* for an example of a progress note written in SOAP format.

Nursing Notes

If nursing notes are not integrated, they are often found in their own section of the record on forms that lend themselves to the type of information nurses are required to document. Nursing notes usually consist of an admission note, graphic charts, medication/treatment records, and temperature, pulse, and respiration (TPR) sheets. See Figure 2-7 for an example of an electronic medication administration record (MAR) and Figure 2-8 for an example of laboratory results.

Anesthesia Forms

The anesthesiologist is required to write preanesthesia and postanesthesia notes. The anesthetic agent, amount given, administration technique used, duration of the procedure, amount of blood loss, fluids given, and any complications or additional procedures performed by the anesthesiologist must be documented. See Figure 2-9 for an example of anesthesia documentation.

Text continued on p. 23

ADMISSION NOTE

M.D.:   Pager:

Date: Time:

Chief Complaint:
twitching

History of Present Illness:
This is a 51 year old woman with a history of lupus, lupus nephritis, and cadaveric renal transplant in 2000 who now presents with 2 weeks of worsening twitching. The patient describes starting neurontin for headaches approximately 3 weeks ago. She subsequently noted first subtle twitching of an extremity or her face. The movements have progressed to include difficulty speaking, dysarthria ("I couldn't say what I was thinking") and difficulty walking.

The patient has also noticed worsening fatigue, a change in her skin ("It's ashy") and worsening edema (including LE and peri-orbital).

On Friday the patient called the transplant nurse who recommended she come to the Emergency room. There, she was seen by neuro, who felt most of her symptoms were most likely related to worsening renal failure with gabapentin. They also noted b/l ptosis and findings suggestive of a peripheral neuropathy.

The patient reports no improvement in symptoms since arrival.

ED Course:
As above.

Primary MD:

Emergency Contact:

Code Status:

Review of Systems: ⬭ positive
Constitutional: A̶B̶C̶ negative
F̶e̶v̶e̶r̶s̶, C̶h̶i̶l̶l̶s̶, N̶i̶g̶h̶t̶ S̶w̶e̶a̶t̶s̶, (Fatigue)
Weight Loss, Weight Gain, Heat Intolerance, Cold Intolerance

Neuro:
(Headache,) S̶e̶i̶z̶u̶r̶e̶s̶, S̶y̶n̶c̶o̶p̶e̶, L̶i̶g̶h̶t̶h̶e̶a̶d̶e̶d̶, V̶e̶r̶t̶i̶g̶o̶, D̶i̶z̶z̶i̶n̶e̶s̶s̶, T̶r̶e̶m̶o̶r̶, W̶e̶a̶k̶n̶e̶s̶s̶, N̶u̶m̶b̶n̶e̶s̶s̶, T̶i̶n̶g̶l̶i̶n̶g̶

HEENT:
V̶i̶s̶i̶o̶n̶ c̶h̶a̶n̶g̶e̶, (Diplopia,) Cataracts, Glaucoma, Hearing Loss, Tinnitus, Sinusitis, S̶o̶r̶e̶ T̶h̶r̶o̶a̶t̶, Polydipsia, Lymphadenopathy

CV:
C̶h̶e̶s̶t̶ P̶a̶i̶n̶, P̶a̶l̶p̶i̶t̶a̶t̶i̶o̶n̶s̶, O̶r̶t̶h̶o̶p̶n̶e̶a̶, PND Claudication, Exercise Intolerance

Respiratory:
S̶O̶B̶, Pleuritic Pain, Wheezing, C̶o̶u̶g̶h̶ S̶p̶u̶t̶u̶m̶, Hemoptysis

GI:
A̶b̶d̶o̶m̶i̶n̶a̶l̶ P̶a̶i̶n̶, N̶a̶u̶s̶e̶a̶, V̶o̶m̶i̶t̶i̶n̶g̶, D̶i̶a̶r̶r̶h̶e̶a̶, C̶o̶n̶s̶t̶i̶p̶a̶t̶i̶o̶n̶, Jaundice, M̶e̶l̶e̶n̶a̶, BRBPR, Dysphagia, Odynophagia, Reflux, Hematemesis

GU:
D̶y̶s̶u̶r̶i̶a̶, Frequency, Urgency, Hesitancy, Incontinence, Hematuria, polyuria
LMP _____

Skin/Skeletal:
(Rashes) (Bruising,) Joint Stiffness/Pain, Myalgias

Psych:
D̶e̶p̶r̶e̶s̶s̶i̶o̶n̶, Mood Changes, SI, HI, Plan

X All other systems negative

FIGURE 2-3. History and physical.

M.D.:   Pager:

Date: Time:

Past Medical History:
Lupus diagnosed 1991, h/o lupus arthritis and muscle pain
- No prior lupus involvement in brain
- No recent flairs

Social History:

Tobacco: none

Alcohol: none

Illicits: none

Residence: lives with daughter

Occupation: owned her own hair salon, now not working

Family: son and daughter in area

Other:

Allergies:
Zantac –> decreased muscle tone

Medications:
Imuran 150mg po qd
Prednisone 10mg po qd
Prograf 4mg po bid
nexium 40mg po qd
stresstab + zinc
folate 1mg po qd
Fe 300mg po tid
Toprol XL 100mg po qd
Calcitriol 0.5mg po q.o.d.
PhosLo 2 tab po TID
Aranesp 100 q.o.week
Lasix 40mg po bid
Clonidine 0.1mg po bid

Family History:
Mo - Kidney stones
No lupus, no renal failure

T_c afeb		HR 72		BP $\frac{140}{80}$	
T_m					
RR 20		SaO$_2$ 98%		FiO$_2$ None	
Pain 0					
Wt		I/O ———		Dexi	
				Stool	

FIGURE 2-3, cont'd. History and physical.

Continued

ADMISSION NOTE

M.D.: Pager:

Date: Time:

General:	Pleasant, NAD. Periodic jerking movements of large muscles, small muscles, and facial muscles	**Affect:**	full

HEENT: B/L ptosis, no scleral icterus. MM sl dry. OP clear.

Neck: Neck supple. No LAD.

Chest:	CTA B/L	**Skin:**	dry

Heart:	RR, soft SM at LUSB	**Vasc:**	

Abd: Soft, full. BSNA. No ascites

Ext:	Warm, + edema	**Joints:**	no effusion or erythema

GU/Rectal: deferred

Neuro: Sensation:

Mental Status: attentive, oriented   Motor: grossly intact. sustained clonus b/l

Cranial Nerves: intact   Coordination:

Reflexes

RDW: 15.4%   MCV: 87.7 FL

	Hgb 10.6 G/DL		Na 143 MEQ/L	Cl 101 MEQ/L	BUN 66 MG/DL		Ca 9.1 MG/DL	TP 6.5 G/DL	TB 0.2 MG/DL	AST 25 U/L	
5030 #/cu mm		182 K/CU MM				137¯ MG/DL					51 U/L
	34.2%		3.7 MEQ/L	24 mEq/L	7.8 MG/DL			3.5 G/DL		14 U/L	
WBC		Plat	K	CO_2	Cr	Glu	Mg	Alb	DB	ALT	AlkP
11:25 2006/08/18	HCT		11:25 2006/08/18				11:25 2006/08/18				

L 28.6%	M 5.8%	N 62.6%	E 2.4%	B 0.6%	PT 9.4 SECONDS	INR: 0.9*	APTT:SECONDS 23.9	APTTr: 0.8 PAT/NORM
11:25 2006/08/18						11:25 2006/08/18		

EKG:
NSR

Chest XR:
obesity, otherwise clear

FIGURE 2-3, cont'd. History and physical.

ADMISSION NOTE

M.D.: Pager:

Date: Time:

Radiographic Data:

Impression

51 year old woman with worsening renal failure and muscle twitching.

Plan:

1. Neuro-Muscle twitching is likely due to uremia in the setting of worsened renal function. Suspect contribution of gabapentin, which can cause twitching and is correlated in time. Plan is to start dialysis Monday. Continue prograf (can stop monday per renal).
2. Renal-Continue prograf, nephrovite, phoslo. Renal diet. Renal has seen patient.
3. Rheum-Continue Imuran. No evidence of acute flair, but check ESR & CRP. Continue prednisone.
4. HTN-Continue clonidine, toprol, nifedipine qd.
5. Dispo-See PMD.

DVT Prophylaxis? heparin 5000 units sq bid, stop Sun for dialysis Monday

1. 332.0: Trembling paralysis
2. 586: Renal failure, unspecified
3. 401.9: HTN [Hypertension]
4. 710.0: Lupus nephritis

Date:

FIGURE 2-3, cont'd. History and physical.

ORDER SHEET

Page____4____

Ordered		Order	Read-Back & Verified	Noted by	Order Completed		Initials
Date	Time	**SIGN EACH ENTRY - INCLUDE ID NUMBER** use a ball point pen, press firmly			Date	Time	
10/19/00		⁰⁰ Kaletra ꝯ tablets po bid					
	6pm	⁰¹ lamivudine 150mg po bid					
		⁰² Abacavir 300mg po bid					
		⁰³ Ranitidine 150mg po bid					
		⁰⁴ Vitamin C 500mg po qday					
		⁰⁵ ~~NRI~~					
		⁰⁶ Zinc sulfate 220mg po q8h					
		⁰⁷ ~~finasteride 5mg po qday~~					
		⁰⁸					
		⁰⁹					
		¹⁰					
		¹¹					
10/19/00		¹² U/A, urine culture, c diff,			done 10/19/00 12:15pm		✓
	11PM	¹³ fecal leuks, lactoferrin					
		¹⁴					
		¹⁵					
		¹⁶ ~~oxycodone~~					
10/19/00		¹⁷ morphine 2mg IV q4h prn pain	✓				
	11PM	¹⁸					
		¹⁹					
		²⁰					
10/19/00		²¹ Lovenox ✓					
		²²					
		²³					

FIGURE 2-4. Handwritten physician orders.

Cumulative Order Summary				

Orders: _____

Med Rec No: _____

Location: _____   Birth date: _____   Age: _____

Atn: _____   Sex: _____

ALLERGIES: Swelling-dexamethasone

Ord #	Order name/description	Start date	Ord status	Stop date
001BXMXJH	**Immunofixation-Electro, Serum LAB**		1 or more final results received	
	Entered DT/TM: _____ _____			
	Auth prescriber: _____ Auth prescriber number: _____			
001BXMXJJ	**Immunoglobulins, Serum LAB**		1 or more final results received	
	Entered DT/TM: _____ _____			
	Auth prescriber: _____ Auth prescriber number: _____			
001BXNBHF	**Transfuse Red Blood Cells**	_____	Completed _____	
	Start date: _____ , urgency: when available, transfuse 2 consent obtained units. Transfuse each unit over 2 hours, in dialysis. When the patient is ready and the product is available, call or fax blood bank for delivery. with dialysis _____			
	Entered DT/TM: _____			
	Auth prescriber: _____ Auth prescriber number: _____			

FIGURE 2-5. Electronic physician order.

Operative Report

An operative report must be included in the health record for patients who undergo surgical procedures. The operative report should include a preoperative diagnosis, a postoperative diagnosis, dates, names of surgeons, descriptions of findings, procedures performed, and the condition of the patient at completion of the procedure. The operative report should be dictated and in the record within 24 hours of completion of surgery. See Figure 2-10 for a sample of a dictated operative report.

Consultations

Consultations are requested by the attending physician who wishes to gain an expert opinion on treatment of a particular aspect of the patient's condition that is outside the expertise of the attending. A preoperative consultation may be requested as part of the determination of the surgical risk of the patient. Information acquired during consults may be integrated within progress notes or recorded on a separate consult form.

Laboratory, Radiology, and Pathology Reports

Laboratory data are often captured electronically and may or may not appear in the paper health record. Laboratory data would include such items as complete blood count (CBC), urinalysis, and metabolic levels. Radiology reports are increasingly captured electronically, and the physician may often find the actual image available electronically. Pathology reports, which are also increasingly found in electronic transcribed reports, consist of a gross description of the tissue removed and microscopic evaluation that includes the diagnosis. See Figures 2-8 and 2-11 for examples of these types of reports.

Text continued on p. 33

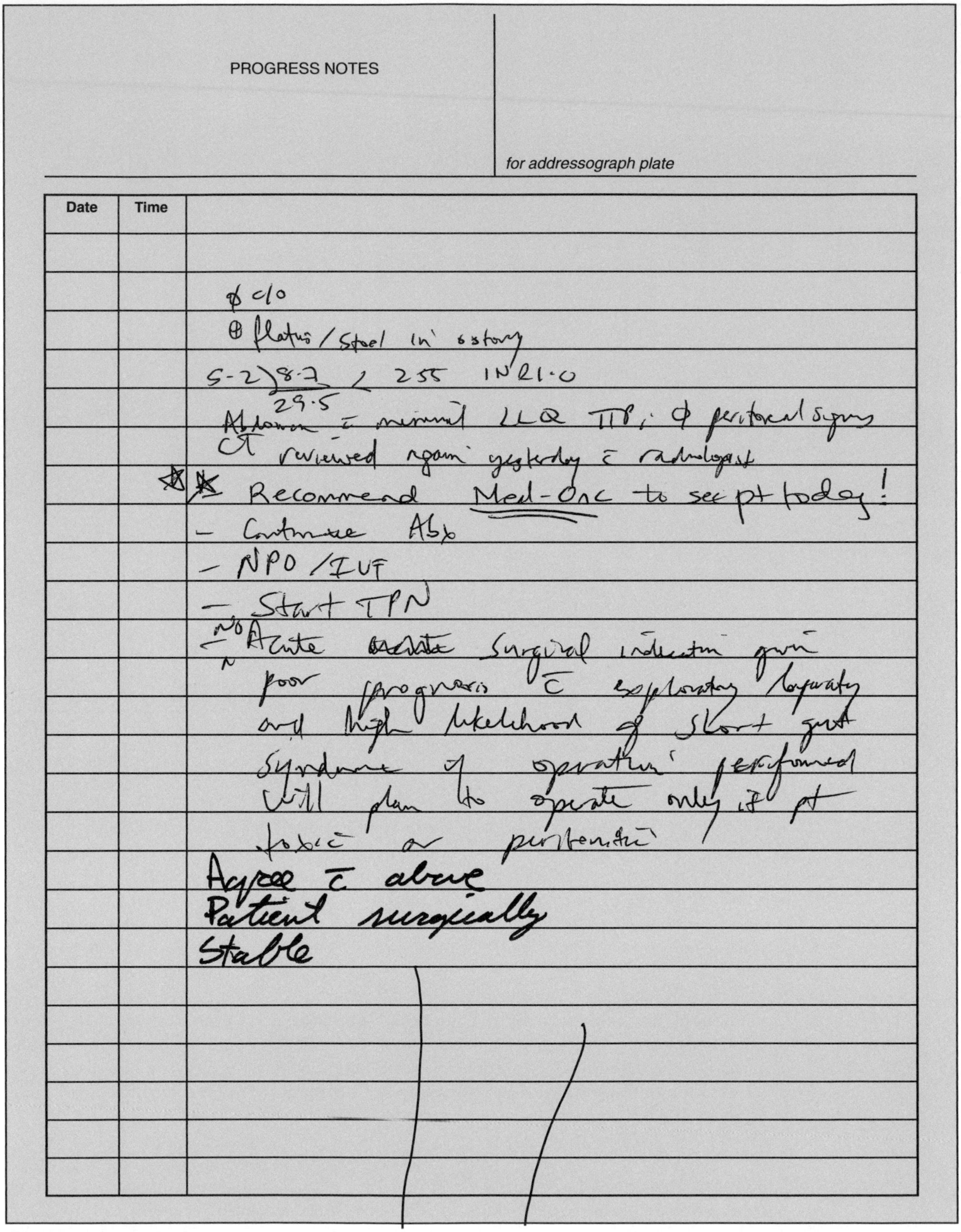

PROGRESS NOTES

for addressograph plate

Date	Time	
		∅ c/o
		⊕ flatus / stool in' ostomy
		5-2)8·7 ⟨ 255 INR 1·0
		29·5
		Abdomen c̄ minimal LLQ TTP; ∅ peritoneal signs
		CT reviewed again yesterday c̄ radiologist
		✳ Recommend <u>Med-Onc</u> to see pt today!
		— Continue Abx
		— NPO / IVF
		— Start TPN
		— No Acute surgical indication given
		poor prognosis c̄ exploratory laparotomy
		and high likelihood of short gut
		syndrome if operation performed
		will plan to operate only if pt
		toxic or peritonitic /
		Agree c̄ above
		Patient surgically
		stable

A

FIGURE 2-6. A, Progress notes.

Page 1

Inpatient Progress Note

┌─────────────────────────────────┐
│ Patient information   │
│   │
│   │
│   [can use hospital plate]│
└─────────────────────────────────┘

Evaluation type: ☒ Followup care   ☐ Discharge note

Meds
Lepirudin
Protonix
Odansetron
Dilaudid PCA
Aspart Insulin sliding scale

Clinical information

S| Tearful ; c/o pain in abd.

O| VS: 37.1   18 95   108/71   97%

Icterus

Abd: distended (mod).
     Well appearing Incision
     c/ o/i c̄ steristrips

Ext: Edema

Assessment & plan:

HD # 10 c̄ Budd chiari 2° PCV s/p surgical shunt (mesocaval) c̄ bx.
  - cont. current management bridging anticoag c̄ Lepirudin
    given h/o HIT. until ok to start umd̄ c̄ therapeutic INR

Assistant: _____ (Signature) _____ (Print) MD #: _____ Date: _____
(If involved)   ☐ Fellow   ☐ Resident   ☐ NP   ☐ PA

Attending: _____ (Signature) _____ (Print) MD #: _____ Date/time _____

(7/03)

B

FIGURE 2-6, cont'd. B, SOAP progress note.

Medication Administration Record

Med Rec No: _____
Visit ID No: _____

Location: _____   Age: _____   Sex: _____

Atn DR: _____   Birthday: _____

ALLERGIES: Swelling-dexamethasone

Scheduled

Medications	Doses	Comments
Routine Hydroxychloroquine enteral 200 mg PO bid routine. Administer with food or milk. **Start:** _____ **Stop:** _____	Ord #: 001BXCBQV (Continued...) Performed _____ 13:00 _____ (RN) Performed _____ 22:00 _____ (RN)	
Routine Labetalol enteral 400 mg PO bid, routine **Start:** _____ **Stop:** _____	Ord #: 001BXTZQD Not performed– _____ 13:00 _____ (RN) Physician request... Canceled	
Routine Levothyroxine enteral 100 mcg PO daily routine **Start:** _____ **Stop:** _____	Ord #: 001BXBJST Performed _____ 13:00 _____ (RN)	
Routine Lisinopril enteral 40 mg PO daily routine **Start:** _____ **Stop:** _____	Ord #: 001BXTKKD Performed _____ 13:00 _____ (RN)	

FIGURE 2-7. Medication administration record.

Laboratory Results

Component	Low range	High range	Range units	16:00:00
Sodium	135	148	mEq/L	140
Potassium, serum	3.5	5.0	mEq/L	4.3
Chloride	99	111	mEq/L	104
Urea-nitrogen	7	22	mg/dL	11
Glucose	60	99	mg/dL	91*
Creatinine, serum	0.5	1.2	mg/dL	0.5
Calcium	8.4	10.5	mg/dL	9.6
Total protein	6.0	8.2	g/dL	7.4
Albumin	3.5	5.3	g/dL	4.6
Total bilirubin	0.1	1.2	mg/dL	0.3
Alanine amino trans	0	31	U/L	5
Aspartate amino tran	0	31	U/L	16
Alkaline phosphatase	100	320	U/L	92
CO_2	21	31	mEq/L	27
Anion gap	11	20	mEq/L	13
Sun/creat ratio				22
Ast/alt ratio				3.2
Est Gfr (Afr Amer)			mL/min/A	Text*
Est Gfr (non-Afr-Am)			mL/min/A	Text*

FIGURE 2-8. Laboratory results.

Anesthesia Preoperative Assessment

PLEASE WRITE LEGIBLY

PROCEDURE _FEMORAL INTRAMEDULLAR ROD_

DIAGNOSIS _(L) leg shortening_

MEDICATIONS _none_

for addressograph plate

ALLERGIES (drug/environmental/food) _NKDA_

PAIN HISTORY ☒ **Negative**
Intensity (0-10) _____
Location _____
Affect quality of life? ☐ Y ☐ N
Pain meds effective? ☐ Y ☐ N
Alleviating / Aggravating factors _____

Quality: Sharp / dull / other ____

Onset / duration _____

Anesthesia Issues ☐ **Negative**
☐ Difficult Airway
☐ ☐ By exam ☐ By history
☐ TMJ problems
☐ Snoring ☐ OSA _d_
☐ Hoarseness _mild_
☐ Nasal obstruction
☐ Stridor/croup
☐ Fam Hx Anesth Problems
☐ Malignant Hyperthermia
☐ Obesity
☐ Post-op nausea/vomiting
☐ Organ transplant _____

Cardiovascular ☒ **Negative**
☐ Myocard infarct: Date _____
☐ Hypertension
☐ Arrhythmia: type _____
☐ Pacemaker ☐ AICD
☐ Angina: ☐ stable ☐ unstable
☐ CHF: Date ____ EF ___ %
☐ Valve disease: _____
☐ ☐Mod ☐Severe
☐ Peripheral vascular disease,
☐ Past cardiac surgery _Denies_
☐ Angioplasty _Cyanosis_
☐ Deep vein thrombus _Diaphoresis_
☐ Pulmonary embolus
☐ Heart murmur _c Activity_
☐ Stress test/cardiac cath
☐ Detail results below

Pulmonary ☒ **Negative**
☐ Smoking hx ☐ current ___ ppd
☐ Asthma
☐ ☐ Hospitalized ☐ Steroid use
☐ Recent wheezing
☐ COPD/BPD
☐ Cough: active / chronic
☐ Other

Renal ☒ **Negative**
☐ Renal insufficiency
☐ Dialysis
☐ Other

Hepatic ☒ **Negative**
☐ Hepatitis
☐ Cirrhosis
☐ Other

Endocrine ☒ **Negative**
☐ Diabetes
☐ Thyroid
☐ Steroid usage
☐ Other

Infections ☐ **Negative**
☐ SBE prophylaxis _Immunized to date_
☐ HIV ☐ Sepsis ☐ URI
☐ VRE
☐ MRSA: contact / resp.

Neurologic ☒ **Negative**
☐ Seizure
☐ Elevated ICP ☐ Shunt
☐ Spinal cord injury
☐ CVA/TIA
☐ Cerebral palsy
☐ Mental retardation
☐ Chronic pain
☐ Neuropathy/paresthesia
☐ Myopathy/muscular dystrophy
☐ Syncope
☐ Hearing loss
☐ Blind: right / left
☐ Other

Gastrointestinal ☒ **Negative**
☐ GE reflux / hiatal hernia
☐ Bowel obstruction ☐ Ascites
☐ Ulcers
☐ GI bleed
☐ Dysphagia
☐ Other

Hematol/Onc ☒ **Negative**
☐ Sickle cell disease ☐ Trait
☐ Coagulopathy
☐ Anemia
☐ Past transfusion
☐ Refuses transfusion
☐ Tumor _____
☐ Chemo/Rad therapy

Obstetrics ☐ **Negative**
☐ Preeclampsia/eclampsia
☐ Placenta previa/abruptio
☐ LMP _7/9_ ☐ HCG _____
☐ Other

Drug Use ☒ **Negative**
☐ ETOH ☐ Daily
☐ Never ☐ Occasional
☐ IVDA ☐ Cocaine
☐ Other

Activity Level
☐ Bedridden
☐ Assistance with self-care
☐ <1 flight of stairs
☐ 1–3 flights of stairs
☒ >3 flights of stairs
☐ Able to lie flat one hour

Pediatrics ☐ **Negative**
☐ Prematurity _FTVD_
☐ Congenital abnl. _in clinic_
☐ Apnea
☐ Passive smoking
☐ Other

Day of Surgery:
NPO since _10 p.m._

DETAILS OF PRESENT ILLNESS AND PAST MEDICAL HISTORY _16 y.o. ♀ for leg length shortening, Ø PMH._

PREVIOUS SURGERY AND ANESTHESIA ☒ NONE _____

140 | 104 | 11 | < 91   4.7 ⟩ 124 ⟨ 232
4.3 | 27 | 0.5   ⟩ 37.4   hcg ⊖

LABS / ECG _____

BP Range (R) 104/60 103/51 (L) P 86 R ___ T 36.9 WT 46.4 (lbs/kg) HT 5'0" (in/cm) Room Air Sat 100% Age 16 M (F)

HISTORY PERFORMED BY: _____ ID Number _____ DATE _____ TIME _____

CHART COPY   page 1 of 2

FIGURE 2-9. Anesthesia record.

Continued

PRE-ANESTHESIA / PRE-OPERATIVE ASSESSMENT
PAGE 2

PLEASE WRITE LEGIBLY

Physical Examination

HEENT _Normocephaly_ , _NO oral lesions MP=I_   for addressograph plate

Neck: _supple c̄ FRom midline trachea_

Cardiovascular _RRR S₁ S₂ NO murmurs or clicks._

Lungs _Bib CTA_

Pain sites / Pertinent other _A OX3 accompanied by Father NAD._
NPO p̄ 13mn Instructions and directions to CrOO were given to
pt's Father instructions to avoid NSAIDS preop were given as
well to Father

Physical exam performed by: _____ ID Number _____ Date _____ Time _____

ANESTHESIA ATTENDING PRE-ANESTHESIA ASSESSMENT AND CONSENT

Medical record and laboratory data reviewed ☑   Patient examined ☑

Patient is appropriate for the planned anesthesia:
    General ☑
    Regional / block ☐   Spinal ☐
    Monitored anesthesia care ☐   Epidural/caudal ☑
    Special monitoring ☐   Other ☐ _____

Planned post-operative care: PACU ☑   ICU ☐   Other ☐

ASA STATUS   1 2 3 4 5 6 E

Airway Assessment:
  Oral excursion: FB   1☐   2☐   3☐   4☐
  T-M distance: FB   1☐
  Dentition: Upper nl☐   dentures☐   caps☐   decayed☐   loose☐
           Lower nl☐   dentures☐   caps☐   decayed☐   loose☐
  Mallampati: I☐   II☐   III☐   IV☐
  Neck   Extension: nl☐   7☐   77☐
        Flexion: nl☐   7☐   77☐

16 y.o. for R leg shortening   _NO Au_
R leg length discrepancy   _NO MODS_
otherwise healthy ⊖ heart/lung hx
ASA I for GOTA / epidural for postop analgesia

☐ Informed consent not obtained due to the emergent condition of the patient.

The plan for anesthesia and postoperative pain management, their alternatives, and the risks and benefits of these plans and alternatives have been explained to me and my questions have been answered to my satisfaction. I give my consent.

_____   _____
Signature of Patient / Parent / Guardian, Health Care Agent   Telephone consent witness   Signature of health care provider securing consent

Anesthesiologist Signature _____ ID Number _____ Date _____ Time _____

SURGICAL ATTENDING PRE-OPERATIVE ASSESSMENT–to be completed by surgeon if used as a surgical history and physical

CHIEF COMPLAINT _____

FAMILY HISTORY _____ SOCIAL HISTORY _____

Pre-operative history, physical exam, and pertinent laboratory data reviewed by me with amendments as follows: ☐ NONE

_____

_____

Preoperative diagnosis: _____

Planned procedure: _____

Surgeon Signature _____ ID Number _____ Date _____ Time _____

CHART COPY   page 2 of 2

FIGURE 2-9, cont'd. Anesthesia record.

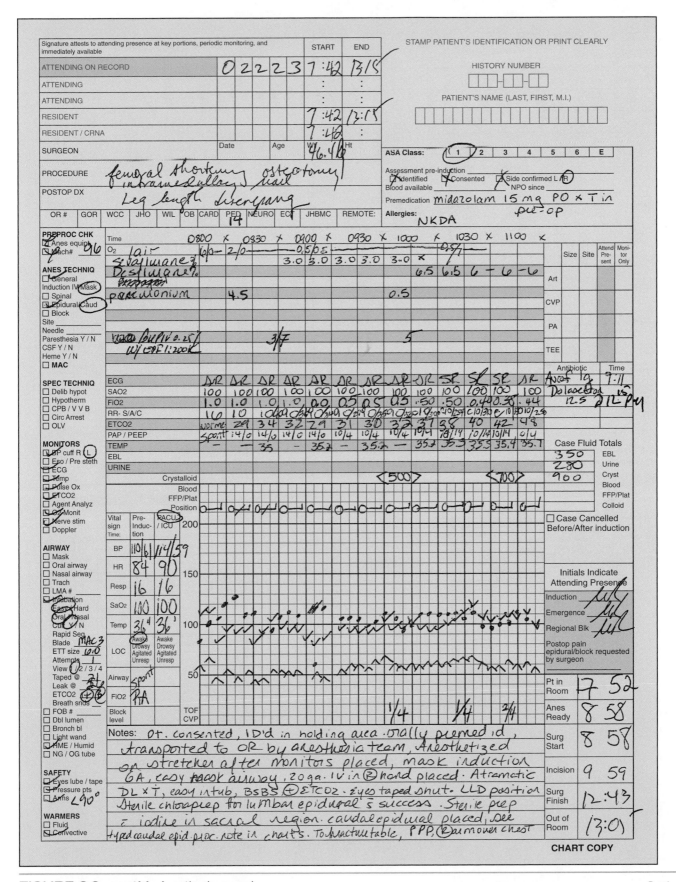

FIGURE 2-9, cont'd. Anesthesia record.

Continued

Signature attests to attending presence at key portions and immediately available				START	END	STAMP PATIENT'S IDENTIFICATION OR PRINT CLEARLY
ATTENDING ON RECORD				:	:	
ATTENDING				:	:	
ATTENDING				:	:	
RESIDENT				:	:	
RESIDENT / CRNA				:	:	PATIENT'S NAME (LAST, FIRST, M.I.)

PROCEDURE DATE

PAGE *2* OF ___

TIME		1115	1130	X	1200	X	1230	X						
O2 / air		0.5	0.5	.5	.5	.5	.5	.5	.5	.5	6/6			
Desflurane %		6	6	4	4	X/6								
pancuronium				1										
Glycopyrolate						0.4								
Neostigmine						2 mg								
Bupivacaine 0.25% 2 epi 1:200 K		3				10								
Fentanyl (mcg)						50								
ECG		JR	JR	JR	JR	JR	SR							
SAO2		100	100	100	100	100	100							
FiO2		.43	.43	.43	.43	.46	1.0							
RR- S/A/C		10/260	10/270	10/260	10/280	10/274	SV							
ETCO2		48	46	45	.45	.45	40							
PAP / PEEP		10/4	10/4	10/4	10/4	10/4								
TEMP		35.7	—	35.7	—	35.7								
EBL														
URINE		‹205›				‹75›								
Crystalloid		‹900›												

Blood
FFP/Plat
Position

200

150

100

50

TOF
CVP

REMARKS

CONTINUATION SHEET

FIGURE 2-9, cont'd. Anesthesia record.

Patient name ____________________ History # ____________________

TIME	pH	pCO2	pO2	HCO3	Na	K	Ca	Glu	HGB				

AS A Physical Status Classification

1: A normal, healthy patient
2: A patient with mild systemic disease
3. A patient with severe systemic disease
4: A patient with severe systemic disease that is a threat to life
5. A moribund patient, not expected to survive without the operation
6: A declared dead patient for organ donation
E: An emergency operation

SYMBOLS		POSITION	TABLE FLAT	OTHER POS.
NIBP	X	Supine		Sitting
PULSE		Prone		Lithotomy
ART BP		Lateral L down		Jackknife
MAP		Lateral R down		

CRITERIA FOR DISCHARGE DIRECTLY TO NURSING UNIT	CRITERIA MET	RETURN TO BASELINE
Level of consciousness–awake, alert appropriately conversant or baseline		
Return to usual pattern of mobility or as appropriate per procedure		
BP within normal range. There is no evidence of severe hyper- or hypotension		
Pulse rate (60–100 adults / 80–150 pediatrics) and rhythm regular or baseline		
Respiratory rate: 12–20 (>3 years); 20–40 (<3 years) and pattern normal		
Oxygen saturation >93% or comparable to baseline		
Ability to swallow secretions or baseline		
Dressings, tubes and drains intact with amount of drainage appropriate for procedure		

DISCHARGE TO: Signature Dr. # Date Time

Intraop and Post Anesthesia Notes:

Stable during procedure
Extubated/extubated in OR
after reversal of paralysis —
Given 2/4 twitches on TOF
(R) sust. tetanus, follows commands, strong hand grip.
Alert/awake to PACU O2 FM. Spont vent
Mild pain (R) leg. Epidural had just been reloaded + is now connected to infusion.
Report given. No complications

☐ Responsibility for patient management and monitoring after transport and report transferred to: PACU / ICU / Other ______

Signature ______ Provider No. ______ Date ______ Time ______

☐ Transfer of care accepted in ICU:

Signature ______ Provider No. ______ Date ______ Time ______

FIGURE 2-9, cont'd. Anesthesia record.

Operative Report

PATIENT NAME: Sonia Sample
ROOM NUMBER: 222 West
MR NUMBER: 12-34-56

DATE OF PROCEDURE: 04/22/00
PREOPERATIVE DIAGNOSIS: Acute cholecystitis
POSTOPERATIVE DIAGNOSIS: Acute cholecystitis
NAME OF PROCEDURE: 1. Laparoscopic cholecystectomy
                         2. Intraoperative cystic duct cholangiogram
SURGEON: Claude St. John, M.D.
ASSISTANT: Mark Weiss, D.O.
ANESTHESIOLOGIST: Angela Adams, M.D.
ANESTHESIA: General

DESCRIPTION OF THE OPERATION:

The patient was placed in the supine position under general anesthesia. The oral gastric tube was placed. The Foley catheter was placed. The patient received appropriate antibiotics. The abdomen was prepped with iodine and draped in the usual fashion. Using a midline subumbilical incision, we entered the subcutaneous fat to find the aponeurosis of the rectus abdominis. Two stay sutures were placed 0.5 cm from the midline bilaterally and we left on these sutures, creating an opening in the linea alba.

Under direct vision, the catheter was placed. The Hasson cannula was placed in the abdominal cavity and all was normal except an acute necrotizing and probably gangrenous gallbladder. There were multiple omental adhesions. Three other trocars were placed in the right subcostal plane in the midline, midclavicular line, and midaxillary line using a #10, #5, and #5 mm trocar, respectively. The gallbladder was punctured and emptied of clear white bile indicating a hydrops of the gallbladder. It was grasped at its fundus and at Hartmann's pouch retracted cephalad and to the right, respectively. We found the cystic duct and the cystic artery after circumferential dissection and isolated the cystic duct completely.

When we were sure that this structure was a deep cystic duct, the clip was placed at this most distal aspect to make an opening immediately proximally and we placed a Reddick cholangiocatheter into it via #14 gauge percutaneous catheter. The cholangiogram showed normal arborization of the liver radicals. Normal bifurcation of the common hepatic duct. Normal common hepatic duct. Long large cystic duct. The common bile duct had numerous stones within it. They could not be emptied from the common bile duct. There was good flow into the duodenum.

The impression was choledocholithiasis. This was corroborated by the radiologist. The decision was made to prepare the patient most probably for endoscopic retrograde cholangiopancreatography postoperatively, and no further intervention of the common bile duct was done in this setting.

The cholangiocatheter was removed. An attempt was made to milk the bile out but no stones came out. Three clips were placed on the proximal aspect of the cystic duct and the duct was then cut distally. The artery was isolated and double clipped proximally and single clipped distally and cut in the intervening section. We then peeled the gallbladder off the gallbladder bed with some difficulty because of the intense edema and inflammation. It was then removed from the liver bed completely. Cautery, suctioning and irrigation were used copiously to create a bloodless field. A last check was made and there was no bleeding and no bile leaking. A #15 Jackson-Pratt type drain was placed into Morrison's pouch and brought out through the lateral most port. We then removed, with great difficulty, the gallbladder from the umbilicus. Because of its enormous size and a 3 cm stone within it that was very difficult to macerate, the opening of the umbilicus had to be enlarged.

As this was done, we removed the gallbladder completely and sent it for pathologic section. Two separate figure-of-eight 0 PDS were used to close the abdominal fascia. The Jackson-Pratt drain was then sutured in place with 2.0 nylon. The skin was closed throughout with subcuticular 3-0 PDS after copious irrigation of the subcutaneous plane. Mastisol and Steri-Strips were placed on the wound. The patient remained stable although she did have bigeminy during surgery and was on a Lidocaine drip. She will be going to the intensive care unit but as she left, she was extubated in the recovery room and was fully alert. She is moving all limbs.

I will discuss with the gastroenterologist postoperative endoscopic retrograde cholangiopancreatography.

SPECIMEN: Gallbladder.

Claude St. John, M.D.
CSJ/ld:
D: 04/22/00
T: 04/25/00 9:21 am
CC: Maria Acosta, M.D.

FIGURE 2-10. Operative report.

Radiology Report

EXAM DATE:
HISTORY NUMBER:
AGE: SEX: RACE:
REQUESTER:

EXAM: MHM 1006-MRI, brain w/wo cont w/diff
RESULT:
SYMPTOMS: Acuto change in mental status.
MEDICAL/SURGICAL HISTORY: Pancreatic cancer, bacteremia.
SUSPECTED DIAGNOSIS: Mets.

TECHNIQUE: Sagittal T1, axial T2, axial FLAIR, and post-contrast axial and coronal T1 through brain. Magnevist (0.1 mmol/kg) injected intravenously without complication. Diffusion images obtained.

FINDINGS:
Minimal cerebral atrophy with expected ventricular dilatation appropriate for age.

Minimal scattered foci of increased T2 signal are noted in the periventricular and subcortical white matter and brainstem, cerebellar peduncles which are nonspecific but likely reflective of small vessel ischemia. Old lacunar infarcts noted in the posterior limb of the right internal capsule/right thalamus.

No evidence of mass, hemorrhage, midline shift, or abnormal enhancement. Ventricles and sulci are normal in size, shape, and position. No abnormal intra or extra axial fluid collection. Normal flow voids in carotid and basilar arteries. Normal scalp, calvarium, orbits. Trace ethmoid and maxillary sinus disease. Minimal left mastoiditis.

IMPRESSION:
Minimal cerebral atrophy with expected ventricular dilatation appropriate for age.

Chronic ischemic disease.
Old lacunar infarcts.

Minimal left mastoiditis.

FIGURE 2-11. Radiology report.

Discharge Summary

The discharge summary (Figure 2-12) is a summary of the patient's stay in the hospital. It should include the following:

- History of the present illness
- Past medical history
- Significant findings
- Pertinent laboratory data
- Procedures performed or treatment rendered
- Final diagnosis
- Discharge instructions; medications and the condition of the patient on discharge

Discharge Summary

PATIENT NAME: Sonia Sample
MR NUMBER: 12-34-56

ADMISSION DATE: 04/19/00
DISCHARGE DATE: 04/27/00
ADMITTING IMPRESSION: Acute abdominal pain, rule out diverticulitis.
HISTORY OF PRESENT ILLNESS:

The patient is a 57-year-old white female who has history of hypertension, valvular heart disease, and cardiomyopathy, who was seen in the emergency room with complaints of acute abdominal pain. On evaluation, she was found to be very tender in the abdomen. She had white blood cell count of 19,000 and was admitted with a diagnosis of rule out diverticulitis.

HOSPITAL COURSE:

CT scan of the abdomen was consistent with cholecystitis and ultrasound of the gallbladder was consistent with cholelithiasis. She was cleared for surgery by cardiologist Dr. Chen and was treated preoperatively with intravenous antibiotics, intravenous fluids, and pain medication. On 4/22/00, the patient underwent laparoscopic cholecystectomy. On 4/26/00, she underwent an endoscopic retrograde cholangiopancreatography. The postoperative course was remarkable for some shortness of breath, otherwise the patient was doing well. She remained very stable, afebrile, and was discharged home.

DISCHARGE DIAGNOSES

1. Cholelithiasis with acute cholecystitis; status post laparoscopic cholecystectomy
2. Mitral valve disorder
3. Hypertensive heart disease with history of angiopathic cardiomyopathy

MEDICATIONS

1. Cozaar
2. Hytrin
3. Lasix
4. Potassium
5. Lanoxin

DIET: The patient is to be on a low-fat diet.

ACTIVITIES: The patient is to be ambulating at home p.r.n.

FOLLOW-UP: Follow-up in two weeks with Dr. St. John and Dr. Glasser.

Medications, diet, activities, and follow-up have all been discussed with the patient and she showed a good understanding

---

Maria Acosta, M.D.
MA/jw: 11931
D: 05/05/00
T: 05/13/00 1:36 pm

FIGURE 2-12. Discharge summary.

EXERCISE 2-1

Choose the correct answer option or write the correct answer(s) in the space(s) provided.

1. Does every patient encounter have a health record?
   A. Yes
   B. No

2. Is the discharge summary always found in the same place in a health record?
   A. Yes
   B. No

3. List five purposes of a health record.

   1. _____

   2. _____

   3. _____

   4. _____

   5. _____

4. Name an advantage of an electronic patient record.

   _____

5. Name the nonfederal organization that requires reporting of data collected from the health record.

   _____

6. List five elements required by the UHDDS.

   1. _____

   2. _____

   3. _____

   4. _____

   5. _____

7. Where in the record would you find the chief complaint?

   _____

8. If a physician was treating a patient with an antibiotic, where in the record would you look to see that treatment had been discontinued?

   _____

9. Where in the record would you expect to see how the patient was progressing on a daily basis?

   _____

10. Where in the record might you look to find how much blood was lost during surgery?

   _____

UHDDS REPORTING STANDARDS FOR DIAGNOSES AND PROCEDURES

It is the responsibility of a coder to extract from the health record the diagnoses for which a patient is being treated and the procedures that have been performed. The extracting of data from the health record may also be referred to as **abstracting**. To complete this task, a coder must rely on definitions as developed by UHDDS for principal diagnosis, secondary diagnoses, principal procedure, and secondary procedures.

Principal Diagnosis

The **principal diagnosis** is defined as the condition established after study to be chiefly responsible for occasioning the admission of the patient to the hospital for care. This definition is one, if not the most important, concept that a coder must understand and apply. The principal diagnosis, along with the principal procedure, determines the assignment of the Medicare Severity diagnosis-related groups (MS-DRGs), which, in turn, affects reimbursement. Physicians are often not aware of this definition or how it is applied; therefore, the coder must take care to select the correct principal diagnosis after record review.

EXAMPLE
> A patient presents to the emergency room with a cough and fever. After the chest x-ray is reviewed, it is determined that the patient has pneumonia.
> The principal diagnosis is pneumonia.

EXAMPLE
> A patient presents to the emergency room with acute abdominal pain. After the patient is evaluated, he is taken to the OR for an appendectomy. The pathology report reveals an acute appendicitis, which is confirmed by the physician in the discharge summary.
> The principal diagnosis is acute appendicitis.

Sometimes, the principal diagnosis is not as easily identifiable as it is in the above two examples. There may be a secondary diagnosis that utilizes more resources during a patient stay but is not the principal diagnosis.

EXAMPLE
> A patient is admitted for coronary artery bypass surgery with a diagnosis of coronary artery disease. The surgery is successful, and on the fourth postoperative day, pneumonia develops. The pneumonia is severe, and the patient goes into respiratory failure and must be intubated and treated in the intensive care unit (ICU). The patient remains in the ICU for 10 days because he cannot be weaned from the ventilator. The patient undergoes a tracheostomy procedure and is discharged to a rehab facility.
> The principal diagnosis is coronary artery disease, even though most of the treatment was focused on postoperative pneumonia.

Principal Procedure

A **principal procedure** is defined as one that is performed for definitive treatment rather than for diagnostic or exploratory purposes, or a procedure that is necessary to take care of a complication. The principal procedure is sequenced first. If two procedures meet the definition of principal procedure, then the one that is most closely related to the principal diagnosis is the one designated as the principal procedure.

Other Diagnoses

UHDDS requires reporting of other diagnoses that have significance for the specific hospital encounter. Reportable diagnoses are "conditions that coexist at the time of admission, or develop subsequently or affect the treatment received and/or the length of stay. Diagnoses which relate to an earlier episode which have no bearing on the current hospital stay are to be excluded."

Other diagnoses are defined as additional conditions that affect patient care because they require one or more of the following:

- Clinical evaluation, or
- Therapeutic treatment, or
- Diagnostic procedures, or

- Extended length of hospital stay, or
- Increased nursing care and/or monitoring

Second only to an understanding and application of the definition of "principal diagnosis" is the definition of when to code "other diagnoses." Once again, the importance of these secondary diagnoses comes into play in the MS-DRG reimbursement system. Other diagnoses may be identified as complications and/or **comorbidities** under the MS-DRG system, which may affect payment.

Clinical Evaluation

If the condition of a patient is being clinically evaluated, the coder would expect to see some testing and clinical observations, or perhaps a consultation.

EXAMPLE

During the course of a hospital stay, a patient develops low sodium levels. The physician makes note of this condition and documents that continued laboratory values will be watched. This would constitute clinical evaluation.

Therapeutic Treatment

Medications, physical therapy, and surgery are forms of therapeutic treatment.

EXAMPLE

The physician documents in the patient's past medical history that the patient has a history of a seizure disorder. The medication list contains the drug Dilantin. The fact that the patient is currently being treated for a seizure disorder with this medication constitutes a reportable secondary diagnosis. Physicians often list conditions in the patient's past medical history for which he or she is currently being treated. The coder should be familiar with medications and the conditions they treat.

Diagnostic Procedures

Often in the course of an inpatient hospital stay, physicians are trying to determine the cause of a sign, symptom, or patient complaint; in these cases, tests are often done to determine the underlying cause. A few examples of types of diagnostic procedures are provided here:

- EKG or ECG (electrocardiogram)
- EEG (electroencephalogram)
- EGD (esophagogastroduodenoscopy)
- Colonoscopy
- Echocardiogram
- MRI (magnetic resonance imaging)
- MRA (magnetic resonance angiography)
- X-rays

EXAMPLE

A patient presents to the emergency room with pain in the leg after a fall down the stairs. An x-ray is performed that reveals a fracture of the tibia.

Extended Length of Hospital Stay

In some cases, a patient is ready to be discharged from the hospital, but develops a condition that requires more intensive investigation, monitoring, or watchful waiting; this may require an additional night's stay.

Increased Nursing Care and/or Other Monitoring

An example of a situation in which increased nursing care or monitoring might be needed is an electrolyte imbalance that is not significant enough to require treatment, although a physician may order additional laboratory draws for monitoring of this condition. In other cases, a patient may have a decubitus ulcer that requires no physician treatment but does require more intensive nursing care. It is important to remember that if the physician does not document the diagnosis for which care is being rendered, the coder must query the physician before adding the code.

Previous Conditions

Often, in a discharge summary or a history and physical, a physician will list diagnoses and/or procedures from previous admissions that are not applicable to the current hospital stay. These conditions are generally not reported. V codes may be used if this historical condition has an impact on current care or influences treatment.

EXAMPLE

A patient is admitted with acute bronchitis. The patient was admitted 2 years ago for an appendectomy and has a history of shingles. In the discharge summary, the physician documents acute bronchitis, status post appendectomy, and a history of shingles. In this case, the only diagnosis to be coded is acute bronchitis. V codes may be assigned for any history of or status post conditions.

Reporting of Coexisting Chronic Conditions

Often, patients may have multiple chronic conditions when they are admitted to a hospital. These chronic conditions may not be specifically treated with medications or procedures; however, they are reported because they may be evaluated and/or monitored, or affect the way a patient is treated.

EXAMPLE

A patient is admitted with benign prostatic hypertrophy (BPH) for a transurethral prostatectomy. The anesthesiologist in the preoperative note documents that the patient has mitral valve prolapse and requires antibiotics prior to undergoing dental procedures. The fact that the patient has mitral valve prolapse and requires antibiotics is a significant factor for the anesthesiologist. This condition is under clinical evaluation by the anesthesiologist and is being treated simultaneously. Therefore, both BPH and mitral valve prolapse (MVP) are reported.

EXAMPLE

A patient is admitted with acute appendicitis. The anesthesiologist and the preoperative consultation indicate that the patient has a history of chronic obstructive pulmonary disease (COPD). The acute appendicitis and the COPD are coded. COPD is a chronic condition that affects patients for the rest of their lives. This, in turn, affects the monitoring and evaluation of this patient.

Integral versus Nonintegral Conditions

Conditions that are an **integral** part of the disease process are not coded.

EXAMPLE

A patient is admitted to the hospital with a cough. After performing a diagnostic evaluation, the physician determines that the patient has pneumonia. Coughing is a symptom of pneumonia and is not coded.

EXAMPLE

A patient is admitted to the hospital with hypotension, fever, and an elevated white blood count. A blood culture comes back positive, and the physician determines that the patient has sepsis. In this case, only the sepsis is coded; hypotension, fever, and an elevated white blood count are all symptoms of sepsis and are therefore not coded.

Likewise, conditions that are NOT an integral part of the disease process may be coded. Additional conditions that may **not** be associated routinely with a disease process should be coded when present.

EXAMPLE

> A patient is admitted to the hospital with a metastatic brain cancer for surgical removal. The patient's history reveals that he has had lung cancer that was surgically removed and now is presenting with seizures, metastatic brain cancer, and headache. Brain cancer is the principal diagnosis, and seizures and history of lung cancer are coded as secondary diagnoses; headache is not reported because it is a symptom of metastatic brain cancer.

Abnormal Findings

Abnormal findings (laboratory, x-ray, pathologic, and other diagnostic results) should not be assigned codes and reported unless the provider indicates their clinical significance. If the findings are outside the normal range and the provider has ordered other tests to evaluate the condition or prescribed treatment, it is appropriate to query the provider as to whether the abnormal finding should be assigned codes.

EXERCISE 2-2

Write the correct answer(s) in the space(s) provided.

1. What is the most important definition a coder should know?

   _____

2. What determines an MS-DRG?

   _____

3. What is the principal diagnosis in the following scenario?
   A patient is admitted to the hospital with extreme indigestion. A workup ensues, and the patient is found to have GERD (gastroesophageal reflux disease). Three days later, on the day of discharge, the patient is unable to speak. After undergoing MRI, the patient is found to have had a stroke.

   _____

4. A patient is admitted to the hospital with an asthma attack. On his last admission 3 years ago, the diagnosis was community-acquired pneumonia. Is the pneumonia coded, and why or why not?

   _____

5. List five reasons why a secondary diagnosis might be reported.

   1. _____

   2. _____

   3. _____

   4. _____

   5. _____

6. The physician documents seizure disorder in the patient's past medical history. The patient is receiving Tegretol, according to the list of medications. Should the seizure disorder be coded, and why or why not?

   _____

7. A patient has low urine output after undergoing surgery. The attending writes an order for the nursing staff to record urine output. Should the low urine output be coded, and if so, why or why not?

   _____

8. If a patient is not on any drugs for Parkinson's, should this diagnosis be coded and why or why not?

    _____

9. If a patient has nausea and vomiting that the attending physician determines to be gastroenteritis, what diagnosis/diagnoses should be coded?

    _____

CODING FROM DOCUMENTATION FOUND IN THE HEALTH RECORD

The usual advice given to a new coder is to begin to code a record by reading the discharge summary. This, in theory, is the summation of what took place during this patient's hospital admission. The discharge summary is similar to a synopsis of a book. By reading this document, the coder should be able to determine the principal diagnosis. However, the caveat is that the documenting physician may not be aware of the definition of a principal diagnosis and may list a diagnosis that does not meet the requirements of this definition.

Following a review of the discharge summary, the coder should move to the ER record (if applicable), which is the beginning of the patient's story. This will reveal the patient's chief complaint. The chief complaint is expressed in the words of the patient and gives the reason why he or she is presenting to the ER. The ER record generally provides to the coder the **admission diagnosis**. The admitting diagnosis may be a symptom, and after examination, a working diagnosis may become apparent. By the time the patient leaves the ER to go to the floor, the emergency room physician will have a working diagnosis or will be aware of a symptom that needs additional workup. If this diagnosis is not clear from the ER record, the admission orders should be reviewed for a diagnosis that is listed as the reason for admission.

If no ER record is available, or after the coder has read the ER record, he or she should move on to the admission history and physical (H&P). Generally, the progress notes are reviewed, followed by the OR reports, laboratory results, radiology reports, consults, and orders. Some documents such as the discharge summary, operative report, or pathology report may not be available at the time of coding. Hospitals may have a policy on whether an inpatient record should be coded without these reports or put on hold until the reports are completed. The following examples show documentation inconsistencies. When documentation inconsistencies are present the attending should be queried for clarification.

EXAMPLE
The ER form has a listing of common medical conditions. The ER physician will circle any pertinent diagnoses. The physician has circled ESRD (end-stage renal disease) on the ER form. Throughout the body of the health record, no documentation of ESRD is found, nor does any documentation state that the patient is on dialysis or that the patient is awaiting a transplant. The only documentation in the chart is for chronic renal insufficiency (CRI).
- Differences in coding: N18.6 versus N18.9

EXAMPLE
Throughout a patient's inpatient chart, it is documented that the patient has a history of pneumonia. This is also documented in the past medical history.
No chest x-ray was performed. Physical exam showed that the lungs were clear. On the discharge summary, pneumonia is documented instead of history of pneumonia.
- Differences in coding: J18.9 versus Z87.01

EXAMPLE
Throughout a patient's chart, documentation of ESLD (end-stage liver disease) is found, along with the fact that the patient is awaiting a liver transplant. The patient has a history of cirrhosis and hepatitis C.
One progress note reads:
Cirrhosis/hep C/ESKD (end-stage kidney disease)
No documentation in the chart describes any abnormal kidney function. It appears that the physician may have meant to write ESLD instead of ESKD.

It is acceptable to code from any documentation provided by a physician. Physicians (individuals qualified by education and legally authorized to practice medicine) may be referred to as attendings, consulting physicians, interns, and residents. Physicians may include surgeons, anesthesiologists, oncologists, internists, hospitalists, intensivists, family practitioners, and interventionalists. Medical students have not completed their education and are not included in the category of physician. Some medical staff bylaws may accept documentation by other healthcare providers such as nurse practitioners or physician assistants.

Some confusion has arisen as to what exactly may be coded from radiology and pathology reports. The coder cannot assign codes from these reports without obtaining documentation by the attending. For example if the attending physician documents lung mass and the pathologist documents carcinoma of the lung, this would be conflicting documentation and the attending must clarify. Additional details (e.g., area of fracture, location of mass) related to confirmed diagnoses may be taken from the x-ray report. For example if the physician has already documented an ulnar fracture, the coder may pick up additional details on the site of the fracture from the radiology report.

THE USE OF QUERIES IN THE CODING PROCESS

In 2001, AHIMA published a Practice Brief entitled *Developing a Physician Query Process*,[4] which describes the goal of the query process as "to improve physician documentation and coding professionals' understanding of the unique clinical situation, not to improve reimbursement." A well-established and managed query process ensures data integrity. This Practice Brief was updated in October 2008 with a new Practice Brief entitled *Managing an Effective Query Process*.[5]

Each facility should prepare its own policies and procedures regarding the query process. Some of the best practices for query forms have been recommended by the American Health Quality Association (AHQA). In the October Practice Brief, AHIMA details many items that may be included in a facility policy.

When to Query

A healthcare provider should be queried when documentation is conflicting, incomplete, or ambiguous. The Practice Brief lists six reasons a provider may need to be queried.

1. Clinical indicators of a diagnosis but no documentation of the condition

EXAMPLE | In the provider's daily documentation, there is a lab value circled K2.8, and orders are given for potassium supplementation to be added to the IV fluids. It may be necessary in this case to query for a condition.

2. Clinical evidence for a higher degree of specificity or severity

EXAMPLE | Physician documents obesity and lists the patient's weight as 345 and height as 5′2″. It may be necessary to query for a patient's BMI or degree of obesity.

3. A cause and effect relationship between two conditions or organisms

EXAMPLE | Patient has documented cirrhosis of the liver. There is also documentation of history of alcoholism. The physician may be queried as to whether there is a relationship between the cirrhosis and alcoholism.

4. An underlying cause when admitted with symptoms

> **EXAMPLE** A patient is admitted with chest pain for workup of the underlying cause. The discharge summary lists atypical chest pain as the principal diagnosis. There is evidence in the chart that the patient has and is being treated for GERD. The provider may be queried as to the underlying cause of the chest pain.

5. Only the treatment is documented (without a diagnosis)

> **EXAMPLE** The MAR shows administration of levothyroxine (Synthroid), but no documentation is provided by the provider of a diagnosis. It is noted that a medication is given, but no diagnosis is documented to correspond with the treatment.

6. Present on admission (POA) indicator status is unknown or unclear

> **EXAMPLE** On the third hospital day, the provider documents that the patient's diabetes is uncontrolled. A query is initiated to determine whether the patient's diabetes was uncontrolled at the time of admission.

When Not to Initiate a Query

Do not query a provider's clinical judgment. It is not the coder's responsibility to question a provider's clinical judgment because the documentation in the record does not support the condition.

> **EXAMPLE** Patient presents to the hospital with a cough and fever. The physician documents pneumonia on the discharge summary. The chest x-ray is negative.

Who to Query

The query should be directed to the provider who supplied the documentation in question. This may mean that the query is directed to a consultant, anesthesiologist, or surgeon, among others. Abnormal lab finding queries should be addressed to the attending physician. If there is conflicting documentation between a consultant and an attending physician, the attending physician should be queried for clarification.

Elements of a Query Form

A query should contain the following elements:
- Date of query
- Patient name
- Medical record number
- Account number
- Admission date/date of service
- Specific question needing clarification along with clinical indicators
- Identification of the coder asking the question
- Contact information for the coder initiating the query
- Area for response from provider
- Place for provider signature and date of response
- Instruction for documentation or any correction or addendum in the body of the record

PHYSICIAN QUERY FORM

Patient Name: _____

Patient Number: _____

Admission Date: _____ Discharge Date: _____

Query Date: _____

Dear Dr. _____ :

In order to assign the most appropriate codes that reflect the conditions of your patient, more clarification is required.

From a coding perspective "urosepsis" is a nonspecific term. It may mean that the patient has sepsis localized in the urinary tract, or it may signify that the urinary tract infection has now become generalized sepsis. Please document in the space below or write an addendum to the patient's record the diagnosis that best represents your use of the term "urosepsis."

Physician Response:

_____

_____

_____

_____

_____

_____   _____

Physician signature   Date

Thank you.

Coder Name: _____ Contact #: _____

FIGURE 2-13. Physician query form.

Queries can be forms (Figure 2-13) placed in charts, faxes, and/or electronic communications transmitted via secure e-mail or IT messaging. Facility policy will control where queries are maintained. It is preferable that they become part of the official health record, whether paper or electronic.

It is not advised to use sticky notes, scratch paper, or any note that can be removed and discarded. It is acceptable to use a single query form for multiple queries.

Unacceptable Types of Queries

It is unacceptable to lead a provider to document a particular response. The query should not be directing, prodding, probing, or presumptive. The provider should not be led to make an assumption.

AHIMA in the Practice Brief *Managing an Effective Query Process*[5] has given the following examples of leading queries.

Leading/Unacceptable

EXAMPLE

> Dr. Smith:
>
> Based on your documentation, this patient has anemia and was transfused 2 units of blood. Also, there was a 10 point dip in hematocrit following surgery. Please document "Acute Blood Loss Anemia," as this patient clearly meets the clinical criteria for this diagnosis.

Acceptable

EXAMPLE

> Dr. Smith:
>
> In your progress note on 6/20, you documented anemia and ordered transfusion of 2 units of blood. Also, according to the lab work done on xx/xx, the patient had a 10 point drop in hematocrit following surgery. Based on these indications, please document, in the discharge summary, the type of anemia you were treating.

Leading/Unacceptable

EXAMPLE

> Dr. Jones:
>
> This patient has COPD and is on oxygen every night at home and has been on continuous oxygen since admission. Please document "Chronic Respiratory Failure."

Acceptable

EXAMPLE

> Dr. Jones:
>
> This patient has COPD and is on oxygen every night at home and has been on continuous oxygen since admission. Based on these indications, please indicate if you were treating one of the following diagnoses:
> - Chronic Respiratory Failure
> - Acute Respiratory Failure
> - Acute on Chronic Respiratory Failure
> - Hypoxia
> - Unable to determine
> - Other _____

In both of the unacceptable examples, the coder was asking for a provider to document a particular diagnosis. No other documentation options were provided other than the one listed. These queries were already assuming a diagnosis, rather than giving the clinical facts and allowing the provider to make a clinical determination. The nonleading way to ask is with open-ended queries or multiple-choice answers with clinically reasonable choices, as well as an "other" option that allows the provider to input something entirely different from the multiple-choice answers given.

It is inappropriate to introduce new information not previously documented in this record. For example, if on a previous admission the provider documents that the patient is HIV positive, but during this stay that diagnosis is not documented, it would be inappropriate to query for "new information" that is not documented during the encounter.

Query forms should steer away from "yes" and "no" answer questions. For POA purposes, when a diagnosis has already been documented, a "yes" or "no" query is acceptable. Impact on reimbursement should never be indicated on a query form.

Qualifications for Individuals Submitting Queries

In the Practice Brief *Managing an Effective Query Process*,[5] AHIMA suggests that individuals performing queries should be very familiar with the AHIMA Standards of Ethical Coding, as well as have competencies in the following areas:

- Knowledge of healthcare regulations, including reimbursement and documentation requirements
- Clinical knowledge with training in pathophysiology
- Ability to read and analyze all information in a patient's health record
- Established channels of communication with providers and other clinicians
- Demonstrated skills in clinical terminology, coding, and classification systems
- Ability to apply coding conventions, official guidelines, and *Coding Clinic* advice to health record documentation

CHAPTER REVIEW EXERCISE

Write the correct answer(s) in the space(s) provided or choose the correct answer option.

1. When coding a record, where is the best place to begin?

_____

2. If the discharge summary includes a list of diagnoses, should the coder choose the first in the list as the principal diagnosis?
   A. Yes
   B. No

3. What does TJC stand for?

_____

4. What does UHDDS stand for?

_____

5. Which report in the record must be on the record within 24 hours?

_____

6. What does the term "integral" mean?

_____

7. Where in the record would a coder find the admitting diagnosis?

_____

8. Name one reason why a coder would query a physician.

_____

9. The best place in the record to find the patient's history is in the _____

_____.

10. The beginning of the patient's story is usually the discharge summary.
    A. True
    B. False

11. It is permissible for a coder to use documentation provided by an interventionalist.
    A. True
    B. False

12. Once a physician answers a coding question, it should be thrown in the trash.
    A. True
    B. False

13. Physician queries should have only enough room for a physician to sign and date.
    A. True
    B. False

14. When a coding question is asked, it is very important that the financial impact of the response is included.
    A. True
    B. False

15. It is important that the date and the identity of the physician be included for every note.
    A. True
    B. False

16. Is it important for the record to include documentation that supports a code used in billing?
    A. Yes
    B. No

17. Documentation from a physician consultant cannot be used to assign codes.
    A. True
    B. False

18. A principal diagnosis is one of the elements that determine an MS-DRG.
    A. True
    B. False

19. An example of a diagnostic procedure is an MRI.
    A. True
    B. False

20. Surgery is a form of therapeutic treatment.
    A. True
    B. False

CHAPTER GLOSSARY

Abstracting: extracting data from the health record.

Admission diagnosis: diagnosis that brings the patient to the hospital. This will often be a symptom.

Chief complaint: the reason, in the patient's own words, for presenting to the hospital.

Comorbidities: preexisting diagnoses or conditions that are present on admission.

Consultant: healthcare provider who is asked to see the patient to provide expert opinion outside the expertise of the requester.

Healthcare provider: person who provides care to a patient.

Hybrid: a combination of formats producing similar results (i.e., paper and electronic records).

Integral: essential part of a disease process.

Physician: licensed medical doctor.

Principal diagnosis: the condition established after study to be chiefly responsible for occasioning the admission of the patient to the hospital for care.

Principal procedure: procedure performed for definitive treatment, rather than for diagnostic or exploratory purposes, or one that was necessary to take care of a complication.

Progress notes: daily recordings by healthcare providers of patient progress.

REFERENCES

1. Huffman E. Health Information Management, 10th ed. Berwyn, IL, Physicians' Record Company, 1994, p 30.
2. Abdelhak M, Grostick S, Hanken MA, Jacobs E (eds). Health Information: Management of a Strategic Resource, 2nd ed. St. Louis, WB Saunders, 2001.
3. Medicare 1995 Documentation Guidelines. General Principles of Medical Record Documentation. Centers for Medicare and Medicaid Services, U.S. Department of Health and Human Services, 1995.
4. Prophet S. Developing a physician query process (AHIMA practice brief). *J AHIMA* 2001;72:88I-88M.
5. AHIMA. Managing an effective query process. *J AHIMA* 2008;79:83-88.

3

ICD-10-CM Format and Conventions

CHAPTER OUTLINE

ICD-10-CM Official Guidelines for Coding and Reporting
    Format of Tabular List of Diseases and Injuries
    Format of Alphabetic Index to Diseases and Injuries
Coding Conventions
    Abbreviations
    Punctuation
    Instructional Notes
Chapter Review Exercise
Chapter Glossary

LEARNING OBJECTIVES

1. Identify the format of the ICD-10-CM code book
2. Explain and apply the conventions and guidelines

ABBREVIATIONS/ ACRONYMS

AHFS American Hospital Formulary Service

CPT Current Procedural Terminology

DSM-IV Diagnostic and Statistical Manual of Mental Disorders, Fourth Edition

ICD-9-CM International Classification of Diseases,

9th Revision, Clinical Modification

ICD-10-CM International Classification of Diseases, 10th Revision, Clinical Modification

ICD-10-PCS International Classification of Diseases, 10th Revision, Procedure Coding System

ICD-O International Classification of Diseases for Oncology

MS-DRG Medicare Severity diagnosis-related groups

NEC not elsewhere classifiable

NOS not otherwise specified

WHO World Health Organization

ICD-10-CM

Official Guidelines for Coding and Reporting (2012)

2012
Narrative changes appear in bold text
Items <u>underlined</u> have been moved within the guidelines since the 2011 version
Italics are used to indicate revisions to heading changes

The Centers for Medicare and Medicaid Services (CMS) and the National Center for Health Statistics (NCHS), two departments within the U.S. Federal Government's Department of Health and Human Services (DHHS) provide the following guidelines for coding and reporting using the International Classification of Diseases, 10th Revision, Clinical Modification (ICD-10-CM). These guidelines should be used as a companion document to the official version of the ICD-10-CM as published on the NCHS website. The ICD-10-CM is a morbidity classification published by the United States for classifying diagnoses and reason for visits in all health care settings. The ICD-10-CM is based on the ICD-10, the statistical classification of disease published by the World Health Organization (WHO).

These guidelines have been approved by the four organizations that make up the Cooperating Parties for the ICD-10-CM: the American Hospital Association (AHA), the American Health Information Management Association (AHIMA), CMS, and NCHS.

These guidelines are a set of rules that have been developed to accompany and complement the official conventions and instructions provided within the ICD-10-CM itself. The instructions and conventions of the classification take precedence over guidelines. These guidelines are based on the coding and sequencing instructions in the Tabular List and Alphabetic Index of ICD-10-CM, but provide additional instruction. Adherence to these guidelines when assigning ICD-10-CM diagnosis codes is required under the Health Insurance Portability and Accountability Act (HIPAA). The diagnosis codes (Tabular List and Alphabetic Index) have been adopted under HIPAA for all healthcare settings. A joint effort between the healthcare provider and the coder is essential to achieve complete and accurate documentation, code assignment, and reporting of diagnoses and procedures. These guidelines have been developed to assist both the healthcare provider and the coder in identifying those diagnoses and procedures that are to be reported. The importance of consistent, complete documentation in the medical record cannot be overemphasized. Without such documentation accurate coding cannot be achieved. The entire record should be reviewed to determine the specific reason for the encounter and the conditions treated.

The term encounter is used for all settings, including hospital admissions. In the context of these guidelines, the term provider is used throughout the guidelines to mean physician or any qualified health care practitioner who is legally accountable for establishing the patient's diagnosis. Only this set of guidelines, approved by the Cooperating Parties, is official.

The guidelines are organized into sections. Section I includes the structure and conventions of the classification and general guidelines that apply to the entire classification, and chapter-specific guidelines that correspond to the chapters as they are arranged in the classification. Section II includes guidelines for selection of principal diagnosis for non-outpatient settings. Section III includes guidelines for reporting additional diagnoses in non-outpatient settings. Section IV is for outpatient coding and reporting. It is necessary to review all sections of the guidelines to fully understand all of the rules and instructions needed to code properly.

Section I. Conventions, general coding guidelines and chapter specific guidelines

The conventions, general guidelines and chapter-specific guidelines are applicable to all health care settings unless otherwise indicated. The conventions and instructions of the classification take precedence over guidelines.

A. Conventions for the ICD-10-CM

The conventions for the ICD-10-CM are the general rules for use of the classification independent of the guidelines. These conventions are incorporated within the Alphabetic Index and Tabular List of the ICD-10-CM as instructional notes.

1. The Alphabetic Index and Tabular List

The ICD-10-CM is divided into the Alphabetic Index, an alphabetical list of terms and their corresponding code, and the Tabular List, a chronological list of codes divided into chapters based on body system or condition (Figures 3-1 and 3-2). The Alphabetic Index consists of the following parts: the Index of Diseases and Injury, the Index of External Causes of Injury, the Table of Neoplasms and the Table of Drugs and Chemicals.

See Section I.C2. General guidelines
See Section I.C.19. Adverse effects, poisoning, underdosing and toxic effects

2. Format and Structure:

The ICD-10-CM Tabular List contains categories, subcategories and codes. Characters for categories, subcategories and codes may be either a letter or a number. All

---

Disease, diseased *(Continued)*
  breast *(see also* Disorder, breast) N64.9
    cystic (chronic) – *see* Mastopathy,
      cystic
    fibrocystic – *see* Mastopathy, cystic
    Paget's (M8540/3)
      female, unspecified side C50.91- ←———
      male, unspecified side C50.92-
    specified NEC N64.8
  Breda's – *see* Yaws
  Bretonneau's (diphtheritic malignant
    angina) A36.0

FIGURE 3-1. Alphabetic Index entry for Paget's disease, female breast.

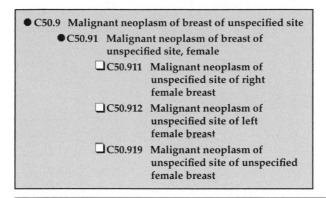

FIGURE 3-2. Tabular List entry for Paget's disease, female breast.

categories are 3 characters. A three-character category that has no further subdivision is equivalent to a code. Subcategories are either 4 or 5 characters. Codes may be **3**, 4, 5, 6 or 7 characters. That is, each level of subdivision after a category is a subcategory. The final level of subdivision is a code. Codes that have applicable 7th characters are still referred to as codes, not subcategories. A code that has an applicable 7th character is considered invalid without the 7th character.

The ICD-10-CM uses an indented format for ease in reference.

3. Use of codes for reporting purposes

For reporting purposes only codes are permissible, not categories or subcategories, and any applicable 7th character is required.

In the Alphabetic Index of ICD-10-CM a dash (-) is used to indicate that there are further digits that need to be assigned for a valid code. In Figures 3-1 and 3-2, note that C50.91 would be an invalid code. A sixth digit is necessary to identify left, right, or unspecified breast. All codes must be assigned to the final level of subdivision. A valid code is at least three characters, but could be four, five, six, or seven characters.

4. Placeholder character

The ICD-10-CM utilizes a placeholder character "X". The "X" is used as a placeholder at certain codes to allow for future expansion. An example of this is at the poisoning, adverse effect and underdosing codes, categories T36-T50.

Where a placeholder exists, the X must be used in order for the code to be considered a valid code (Figure 3-3).

5. 7th Characters

Certain ICD-10-CM categories have applicable 7th characters. The applicable 7th character is required for all codes within the category, or as the notes in the Tabular List instruct. The 7th character must always be the 7th character in the data field. If a code that requires a 7th character is not 6 characters, a placeholder X must be used to fill in the empty characters (see Figure 3-3).

6. Abbreviations

a. Alphabetic Index abbreviations

NEC "Not elsewhere classifiable"

This abbreviation in the Alphabetic Index represents "other specified". When a specific code is not available for a condition, the Alphabetic Index directs the coder to the "other specified" code in the Tabular List.

NOS "Not otherwise specified"

This abbreviation is the equivalent of unspecified.

b. Tabular List abbreviations

NEC "Not elsewhere classifiable"

This abbreviation in the Tabular List represents "other specified". When a specific code is not available for a condition the Tabular List includes an NEC entry under a code to identify the code as the "other specified" code.

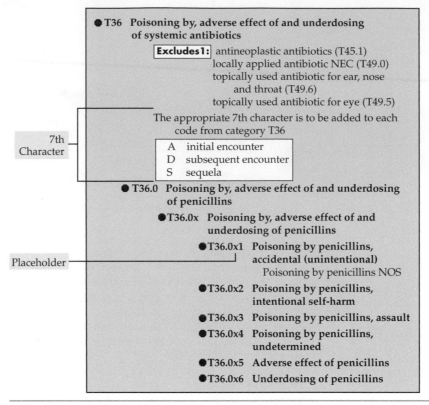

FIGURE 3-3. Placeholder in ICD-10-CM, 7th character.

NOS   "Not otherwise specified"
This abbreviation is the equivalent of unspecified.

7. Punctuation
[ ]   Brackets are used in the Tabular List to enclose synonyms, alternative wording or explanatory phrases. Brackets are used in the Alphabetic Index to identify manifestation codes.

( )   Parentheses are used in both the Alphabetic Index and Tabular List to enclose supplementary words that may be present or absent in the statement of a disease or procedure without affecting the code number to which it is assigned. The terms within the parentheses are referred to as nonessential modifiers.

:   Colons are used in the Tabular List after an incomplete term which needs one or more of the modifiers following the colon to make it assignable to a given category.

8. Use of "and"
When the term "and" is used in a narrative statement it represents and/or.

9. Other and Unspecified codes
   a. "Other" codes
   Codes titled "other" or "other specified" are for use when the information in the medical record provides detail for which a specific code does not exist. Alphabetic Index entries with NEC in the line designate "other" codes in the Tabular List. These Alphabetic Index entries represent specific disease entities for which no specific code exists so the term is included within an "other" code.

   b. "Unspecified" codes
   Codes titled "unspecified" are for use when the information in the medical record is insufficient to assign a more specific code. For those categories for which an unspecified code is not provided, the "other specified" code may represent both other and unspecified.

10. Includes Notes
This note appears immediately under a three character code title to further define, or give examples of, the content of the category.

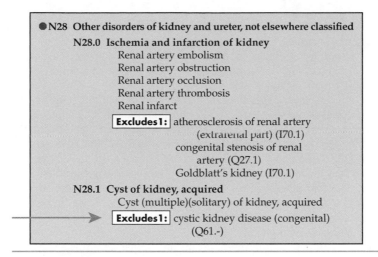

FIGURE 3-4. Example of Excludes1 note.

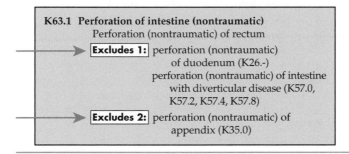

FIGURE 3-5. Example of Excludes1 and Excludes2 notes.

11. Inclusion terms

List of terms is included under some codes. These terms are the conditions for which that code is to be used. The terms may be synonyms of the code title, or, in the case of "other specified" codes, the terms are a list of the various conditions assigned to that code. The inclusion terms are not necessarily exhaustive. Additional terms found only in the Alphabetic Index may also be assigned to a code.

12. Excludes Notes

The ICD-10-CM has two types of excludes notes. Each type of note has a different definition for use but they are all similar in that they indicate that codes excluded from each other are independent of each other.

a. Excludes1

A type 1 Excludes note is a pure excludes note. It means "NOT CODED HERE!" An Excludes1 note indicates that the code excluded should never be used at the same time as the code above the Excludes1 note. An Excludes1 is used when two conditions cannot occur together, such as a congenital form versus an acquired form of the same condition (Figures 3-4 and 3-5).

b. Excludes2

A type 2 excludes note represents "Not included here". An excludes2 note indicates that the condition excluded is not part of the condition represented by the code, but a patient may have both conditions at the same time. When an Excludes2 note appears under a code, it is acceptable to use both the code and the excluded code together, when appropriate (see Figure 3-5).

13. Etiology/manifestation convention ("code first", "use additional code" and "in diseases classified elsewhere" notes)

Certain conditions have both an underlying etiology and multiple body system manifestations due to the underlying etiology. For such conditions, the ICD-10-CM has a coding convention that requires the underlying condition be sequenced first followed by the manifestation. Wherever such a combination exists, there is a "use additional code" note at the etiology code, and a "code first" note at the manifestation code. These instructional notes indicate the proper sequencing order of the codes, etiology followed by manifestation.

In most cases the manifestation codes will have in the code title, "in diseases classified elsewhere." Codes with this title are a component of the etiology/manifestation convention. The code title indicates that it is a manifestation code. "In diseases classified elsewhere" codes are never permitted to be used as first-listed or principal diagnosis codes. They must be used in conjunction with an underlying condition code and they must be listed following the underlying condition. See category F02, Dementia in other diseases classified elsewhere, for an example of this convention.

There are manifestation codes that do not have "in diseases classified elsewhere" in the title. For such codes a "use additional code" note will still be present and the rules for sequencing apply.

In addition to the notes in the Tabular List, these conditions also have a specific Alphabetic Index entry structure. In the Alphabetic Index both conditions are listed together with the etiology code first followed by the manifestation codes in brackets. The code in brackets is always to be sequenced second.

An example of the etiology/manifestation convention is dementia in Parkinson's disease. In the Alphabetic Index, code G20 is listed first, followed by code F02.80 or F02.81 in brackets. Code G20 represents the underlying etiology, Parkinson's disease, and must be sequenced first, whereas codes F02.80 and F02.81 represent the manifestation of dementia in diseases classified elsewhere, with or without behavioral disturbance.

"Code first" and "Use additional code" notes are also used as sequencing rules in the classification for certain codes that are not part of an etiology/manifestation combination.

See Section I.B.7. Multiple coding for a single condition.

14. **"And"**

The word "and" should be interpreted to mean either "and" or "or" when it appears in a title.

15. **"With"**

The word "with" should be interpreted to mean "associated with" or "due to" when it appears in a code title, the Alphabetic Index, or an instructional note in the Tabular List.

The word "with" in the Alphabetic Index is sequenced immediately following the main term, not in alphabetical order.

16. **"See" and "See Also"**

The "see" instruction following a main term in the Alphabetic Index indicates that another term should be referenced. It is necessary to go to the main term referenced with the "see" note to locate the correct code.

A "see also" instruction following a main term in the Alphabetic Index instructs that there is another main term that may also be referenced that may provide additional Alphabetic Index entries that may be useful. It is not necessary to follow the "see also" note when the original main term provides the necessary code.

17. **"Code also note"**

A "code also" note instructs that two codes may be required to fully describe a condition, but this note does not provide sequencing direction.

18. **Default codes**

A code listed next to a main term in the ICD-10-CM Alphabetic Index is referred to as a default code. The default code represents that condition that is most commonly associated with the main term, or is the unspecified code for the condition. If a condition is documented in a medical record (for example, appendicitis) without any additional information, such as acute or chronic, the default code should be assigned (Figure 3-6).

Several publishers have a variety of ICD-10-CM and ICD-10-PCS code books available. Physicians use CPT codes to bill for services and procedures—and therefore will not use ICD-10-PCS. Expert versions may contain reimbursement edits, color-coded information, Medicare code edits, and age and sex edits. Some books are updated with replacement pages quarterly and may include references to *Coding Clinic* articles. At the beginning of a code book, information is usually provided that explains the conventions used in that version.

The **ICD-10-CM** code book is also divided into two parts: an Alphabetic Index and a Tabular List. The Alphabetic Index lists terms and corresponding codes in alphabetic order. The main index is the Index to Diseases and Injuries, and there is an additional index to External Causes of Injury. There are two tables located in the main index: the Neoplasm table and the Table of Drugs and Chemicals. The Tabular List is an alphanumeric listing of codes that are divided into chapters based on body system or conditions.

There is an additional book for procedures, which is entitled **ICD-10-PCS**.

Format of Tabular List of Diseases and Injuries

In ICD-10-CM, the Tabular List of Diseases and Injuries consists of 21 chapters (Table 3-1). Most of the chapters are based on body systems; however, some are based on conditions. Within each chapter, codes are divided as follows:

Failure, failed (*Continued*)
  respiration, respiratory J96.9 ←
    acute J96.0
      with chronic J96.2
    center G93.8
    chronic J96.1
      with acute J96.2
    newborn P28.5
    postprocedural J95.82

FIGURE 3-6. Alphabetic Index default code for respiratory failure.

TABLE 3-1 ICD-10-CM TABLE OF CONTENTS FOR TABULAR LIST

ICD-10-CM Tabular List of Diseases and Injuries
Certain Infectious and Parasitic Diseases (A00-B99)
Neoplasms (C00-D49)
Diseases of the Blood and Blood-Forming Organs and Certain Disorders Involving the Immune
    Mechanism (D50-D89)
Endocrine, Nutritional, and Metabolic Diseases (E00-E90)
Mental and Behavioral Disorders (F01-F99)
Diseases of the Nervous System (G00-G99)
Diseases of the Eye and Adnexa (H00-H59)
Diseases of the Ear and Mastoid Process (H60-H95)
Diseases of the Circulatory System (I00-I99)
Diseases of the Respiratory System (J00-J99)
Diseases of the Digestive System (K00-K94)
Diseases of the Skin and Subcutaneous Tissue (L00-L99)
Diseases of the Musculoskeletal System and Connective Tissue (M00-M99)
Diseases of the Genitourinary System (N00-N99)
Pregnancy, Childbirth, and the Puerperium (O00-O99)
Certain Conditions Originating in the Perinatal Period (P00-P96)
Congenital Malformations, Deformations, and Chromosomal Abnormalities (Q00-Q99)
Symptoms, Signs, and Abnormal Clinical and Laboratory Findings (R00-R99)
Injury, Poisoning, and Certain Other Consequences of External Causes (S00-T88)
External Causes of Morbidity (V01-Y99)
Factors Influencing Health Status and Contact with Health Services (Z00-Z99)

TABLE 3-2	**BLOCKS FOR THE NERVOUS SYSTEM CHAPTER OF ICD-10-CM**
G00-G09	Inflammatory diseases of the central nervous system
G10-G13	Systemic atrophies primarily affecting the central nervous system
G20-G26	Extrapyramidal and movement disorders
G30-G32	Other degenerative diseases of the nervous system
G35-G37	Demyelinating diseases of the central nervous system
G40-G47	Episodic and paroxysmal disorders
G50-G59	Nerve, nerve root, and plexus disorders
G60-G64	Polyneuropathies and other disorders of the peripheral nervous system
G70-G73	Diseases of myoneural junction and muscle
G80-G83	Cerebral palsy and other paralytic syndromes
G89-G99	Other disorders of the nervous system

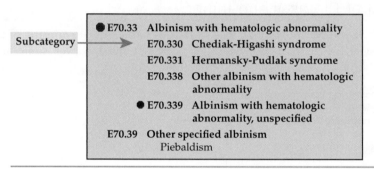

FIGURE 3-7. Example of subcategory in ICD-10-CM.

- Blocks/Sections
- Categories
- Subcategories
- Valid codes

Blocks/Sections

Each chapter in ICD-10-CM is divided into blocks. A block is a group of three-digit categories that represent diseases or conditions that are similar (Table 3-2). A *block* is also known as a *subchapter*.

Categories

In ICD-10-CM, the first character of a three-digit category is a letter, and each letter is associated with a particular chapter except for D and H. The letter D can be found in ICD-10-CM Chapters 2 and 3, the letter H can be found in both ICD-10-CM Chapters 7 and 8, and ICD-10-CM Chapter 19 uses two letters, S and T. The second and third characters are numbers. Most three-character categories are divided into four- or five-character subcategories. If a three-character category is not subdivided, it is a valid three-digit code.

Subcategories

In ICD-10-CM, subcategories can be either four or five characters; every subdivision after a category is a subcategory (Figure 3-7). Subcategory characters can be either letters or numbers. Codes in ICD-10-CM can be three to seven characters in length. The last level of subdivision becomes the final code. The final character may be a number or a letter.

EXERCISE 3-1

Identify the following as a chapter, block, category, or subcategory.

1. Diseases of Veins, Lymphatics Vessels, and Lymph Nodes of NEC (I80-I89) _____
2. Diseases of the Circulatory System (I00-I99) _____
3. I81 Portal vein thrombosis _____
4. I82 Other venous embolism and thrombosis _____
5. I82.0 Budd-Chiari syndrome _____

Placeholder Character

The letter *x* (lowercase) in ICD-10-CM is a dummy placeholder. It is used in the fifth character position and in certain six-character code positions. These dummy placeholders are to be used for future code expansion. When a placeholder exists, the X must be used for the code to be considered valid.

EXAMPLE   T36.0x1A, Poisoning by penicillins, accidental, initial encounter

Some categories have seventh-characters, and this seventh character is required for all codes in that category. These seventh-characters are widely used in Chapter 19, Injury, poisoning, and certain other consequences of external causes. If a code in these categories is not six characters in length, a dummy placeholder of "x" must be added before the seventh character.

EXAMPLE   Sprain of ribs, subsequent encounter, S23.41xD.

EXERCISE 3-2

Using Figure 3-8, select the appropriate seventh-character.

1. Displaced transverse fracture of the shaft of the right ulna, subsequent encounter for closed fracture with nonunion, S52.221 _____
2. Displaced transverse fracture of the shaft of the right ulna, initial encounter for closed fracture, S52.221 _____
3. Displaced transverse fracture of the shaft of the right ulna, initial encounter for open fracture type IIIB, S52.221 _____
4. Displaced transverse fracture of the shaft of the right ulna, subsequent encounter for open fracture type IIIB with a nonunion, S52.221 _____
5. Displaced transverse fracture of the shaft of the right ulna, subsequent encounter for open fracture type IIIB with a malunion, S52.221 _____

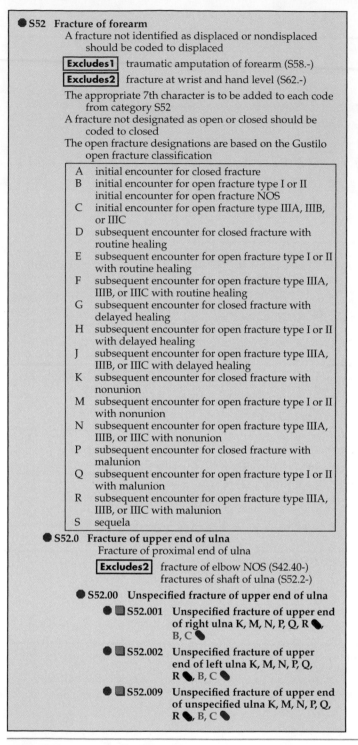

FIGURE 3-8. Example of 7th character.

Format of Alphabetic Index to Diseases and Injuries

The Alphabetic Index in ICD-10-CM contains the following:

- The Index to Diseases and Injuries
  - Neoplasm Table
  - Table of Drugs and Chemicals
- Index to External Causes

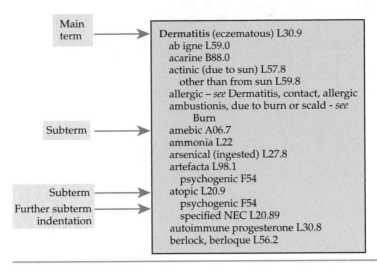

Main term → **Dermatitis** (eczematous) L30.9
ab igne L59.0
acarine B88.0
actinic (due to sun) L57.8
other than from sun L59.8
allergic – *see* Dermatitis, contact, allergic
ambustionis, due to burn or scald - *see*
Burn
Subterm → amebic A06.7
ammonia L22
arsenical (ingested) L27.8
artefacta L98.1
psychogenic F54
Subterm → atopic L20.9
Further subterm indentation → psychogenic F54
specified NEC L20.89
autoimmune progesterone L30.8
berlock, berloque L56.2

FIGURE 3-9. Various levels of indentation in the index. The bold term is the main term.

Deficiency, deficient
3B hydroxysteroid dehydrogenase
E25.0
5-alpha reductase (with male pseudo-
hermaphroditism) E29.1
11 hydroxylase E25.0
21 hydroxylase E25.0
abdominal muscle syndrome Q79.4
accelerator globulin (Ac G) (blood)
D68.2

FIGURE 3-10. Numerical entries in the Alphabetic Index.

Index to Diseases and Injuries

Three levels of indentation are used in the Alphabetic Index. These include the following:

■ Main terms
■ Subterms
■ Carryover lines

The **main terms** are identified by bold print and are set flush with the left margin of each column (Figure 3-9). Alphabetization rules apply in locating main terms and subterms in the Alphabetic Index. Numerical entries appear first under the main term or subterm (Figure 3-10). Main terms usually are identified by disease conditions and nouns. The main term is not a body part or site.

EXAMPLE   The patient has been admitted with deep vein thrombosis. The main term is "thrombosis." "Deep" is a location and "vein" refers to a body part.

EXAMPLE   The patient is being treated for adhesive bursitis of the shoulder.
The main term is "bursitis." "Adhesive" describes the type of bursitis and "shoulder" is a body part.

EXERCISE 3-3

Underline the main terms to be located in the Alphabetic Index in the following diagnosis statements.

1. Decubitus ulcer of the heel   _____
2. Acute anterior wall myocardial infarction   _____
3. Respiratory anthrax   _____
4. Endometriosis of the ovary   _____
5. Gouty arthritis   _____

The subterms are indented to the right under the main term. They are not bolded and begin with a lowercase letter. Subterms modify the main term and sometimes are called essential modifiers. These terms provide greater specificity to the disease or injury. It is possible for a subterm to be followed by additional subterm(s). These additional subterms are indented even farther to the right than are subterms (refer to Figure 3-9).

Some subterms are called connecting words. This means that there is a relationship between a main term or a subterm and an associated condition or etiology. Connecting words "with" and "without" are located before any other subterms (Figure 3-11). Additional connecting words include the following:

- Associated with
- Due to
- In
- With
- With mention of

EXERCISE 3-4

Using the Alphabetic Index only, assign codes to the following conditions.

1. Asthma due to detergent   _____
2. Cholelithiasis with acute cholecystitis   _____
3. Parkinsonism associated with neurogenic orthostatic hypotension _____
4. Cystocele in pregnancy   _____
5. List the subterms for coryza.   _____

```
Abscess (connective tissue) (embolic) (fistu-
    lous) (infective) (metastatic) (multiple)
    (pernicious) (pyogenic) (septic) L02.91
  with
      diverticular disease (intestine) K57.80
          with bleeding K57.81
          large intestine K57.20
              with
                  bleeding K57.21
                  small intestine K57.40
                      with bleeding K57.41
          small intestine K57.00
              with
                  bleeding K57.01
                  large intestine K57.40
                      with bleeding K57.41
      lymphangitis - code by site under
          Abscess
```

FIGURE 3-11. Connecting term "with" follows the main term.

Fenestration, fenestrated - *see also* Imperfect, closure
    aortico-pulmonary Q21.4
    cusps, heart valve NEC Q24.8
       pulmonary Q22.2
    pulmonic cusps Q22.2

FIGURE 3-12. Carryover line.

Mycosis, mycotic B49
    cutaneous NEC B36.9
    ear B36.8
    fungoides (extranodal) (solid organ)
       C84.0-
    mouth B37.0
    nails B35.1
    opportunistic B48.8
    skin NEC B36.9
    specified NEC B48.8
    stomatitis B37.0
    vagina, vaginitis (candidal) B37.3
Mydriasis (pupil) H57.04
Myelatelia Q06.1
Myelinolysis, pontine, central G37.2
Myelitis (acute) (ascending) (childhood)
    (chronic) (descending) (diffuse)
    (disseminated) (idiopathic) (pressure) (progressive) (spinal cord)
    (subacute) (*see also* Encephalitis)
    G04.91

FIGURE 3-13. The Index entry for mycosis, skin "not elsewhere classifiable" (NEC) is assigned code B36.9.

Carryover lines are used when an entry will not fit on a single line. These are indented to the right even farther than a subterm to avoid confusion (Figure 3-12).

CODING CONVENTIONS

Coding **conventions** are addressed by the Official Guidelines for Coding and Reporting in ICD-10-CM. It is important for coders to understand these conventions so that accurate assignment of codes can be ensured. It is important to remember that the instructions and conventions of the classification take precedence over guidelines.

Conventions include some of the following:

- Abbreviations
- Punctuation/symbols
- Instructional notes
- Linking terms
- Cross-references

Abbreviations

In ICD-10-CM, the two main abbreviations are

- NEC—not elsewhere classifiable
- NOS—not otherwise specified

The abbreviation NEC stands for not elsewhere classifiable, which represents "other specified." If a code for a specific condition is not available in the Index, the Index will direct the coder to the "other specified" code in the Tabular. Likewise, in the Tabular the NEC represents "other specified" (Figure 3-13).

NOS is a Tabular List abbreviation that means "unspecified" (Figure 3-14). These codes are to be used only when the documentation in the health record does not provide adequate

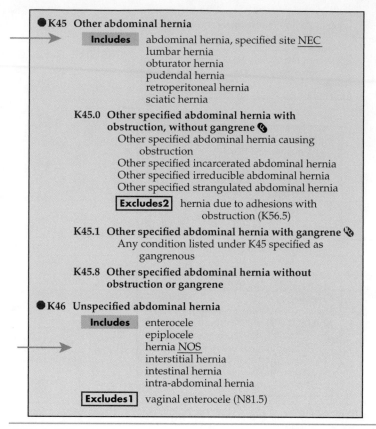

FIGURE 3-14. Examples of NEC and NOS from the Tabular.

information. The unspecified code often appears as the code following the main term in the Alphabetic Index. The subterms should be reviewed to determine whether a more specific code is available.

Punctuation

Brackets

Brackets are used in the Tabular List to enclose synonyms, alternative wording, or explanatory phrases (Figure 3-15). Brackets are used in the Alphabetic Index to identify manifestation codes (Figure 3-16). The code in brackets is always sequenced second.

Parentheses

Parentheses are used in both the Alphabetic Index and the Tabular List to enclose supplementary words. The presence or absence of these terms does not affect code assignment, so they are called nonessential modifiers. A **nonessential modifier** is a term that is enclosed in parentheses following a main term or a subterm, whose presence or absence has no effect on code assignment. These are "take it or leave it" terms. Sometimes, the subterm can be found among the nonessential modifiers (Figures 3-17 and 3-18).

If the diagnostic statement is "double pneumonia," (see Figure 3-17), since "double" is a nonessential modifier, it is assigned the same code as "pneumonia" J18.9. The word "double" makes absolutely no difference in assignment of the code for "double pneumonia."

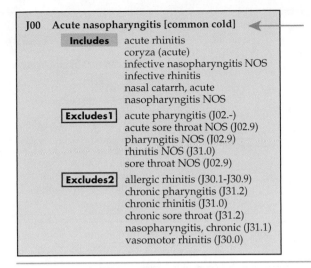

J00   Acute nasopharyngitis [common cold]

Includes	acute rhinitis
	coryza (acute)
	infective nasopharyngitis NOS
	infective rhinitis
	nasal catarrh, acute
	nasopharyngitis NOS

Excludes1	acute pharyngitis (J02.-)
	acute sore throat NOS (J02.9)
	pharyngitis NOS (J02.9)
	rhinitis NOS (J31.0)
	sore throat NOS (J02.9)

Excludes2	allergic rhinitis (J30.1-J30.9)
	chronic pharyngitis (J31.2)
	chronic rhinitis (J31.0)
	chronic sore throat (J31.2)
	nasopharyngitis, chronic (J31.1)
	vasomotor rhinitis (J30.0)

FIGURE 3-15. Brackets for synonyms or alternative wording.

Lichen L28.0
  albus L90.0
    penis N48.0
    vulva N90.4
  amyloidosis E85.4 *[L99]*
  atrophicus L90.0
    penis N48.0
    vulva N90.4
  congenital Q82.8

FIGURE 3-16. Brackets for manifestation codes.

Pneumonia (acute) (Alpenstich) (benign)
    (bilateral) (brain) (cerebral) (circum-
    scribed) (congestive) (creeping) (de-
    layed resolution) (double) (epidemic)
    (fever) (flash) (fulminant) (fungoid)
    (granulomatous) (hemorrhagic)
    (incipient) (infantile) (infectious)
    (infiltration) (insular) (intermittent)
    (latent) (migratory) (organized)
    (overwhelming) (primary (atypical))
    (progressive) (pseudolobar) (puru-
    lent) (resolved) (secondary) (senile)
    (septic) (suppurative) (terminal)
    (true) (unresolved) (vesicular)
    J18.9
  with
    lung abscess J85.1
      due to specified organism - *see*
          Pneumonia, in (due to)
  adenoviral J12.0
  adynamic J18.2
  alba A50.04
  allergic (eosinophilic) J82

FIGURE 3-17. The use of parentheses in the Index for the diagnosis of pneumonia. Multiple nonessential modifiers are used.

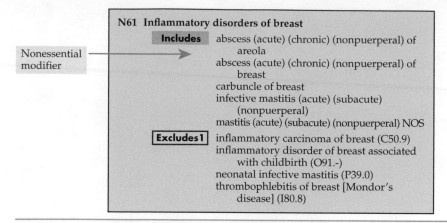

FIGURE 3-18. The nonessential modifier in the Tabular.

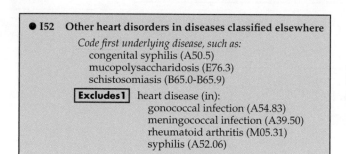

FIGURE 3-19. Colon used within an "Excludes" note.

Using the Alphabetic Index, locate the following main terms, and identify whether the bolded subterm is an essential or a nonessential modifier.

1. **Immature** cataract _____

2. **Nuclear** cataract _____

3. **Essential** hypertension _____

4. **Filarial** infestation _____

5. **Thyrotoxic** exophthalmos _____

Colons

Colons are used in the Tabular List. They are used after a term that requires one or more modifiers that follow the colon to make it assignable to a particular category (Figure 3-19).

Instructional Notes

General notes may be found in the Alphabetic Index and the Tabular List. These notes provide additional information (Figure 3-20). Other types of instructional notes are Inclusion; Exclusion; code first; use additional code; and code, if applicable, any causal condition first.

Inclusion Notes

An Includes note is an instructional note that appears immediately under a three-digit code title or category. The purpose of the Includes note is to give examples or further define the content of the category (Figure 3-21).

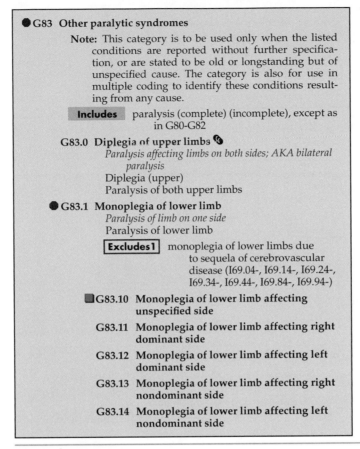

FIGURE 3-20. General notes found in the Tabular.

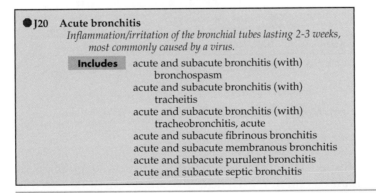

FIGURE 3-21. This "Includes" note is found under category J20.

Inclusion Terms

According to the guidelines, Inclusion terms are a list of terms that are found under some fourth- and fifth-digit codes (Figure 3-22). These terms may be synonyms or various other conditions that are assigned to the code. Inclusion terms do not necessarily constitute a comprehensive list. Additional terms found only in the Alphabetic Index and not in the Tabular List may be assigned a code without mention in the Inclusion terms. In these instances, the Index should be trusted.

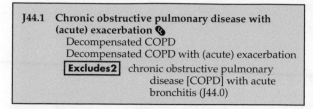

> **J44.1** **Chronic obstructive pulmonary disease with (acute) exacerbation** 🔵
> Decompensated COPD
> Decompensated COPD with (acute) exacerbation
> | Excludes2 | chronic obstructive pulmonary disease [COPD] with acute bronchitis (J44.0)

FIGURE 3-22. Inclusion terms.

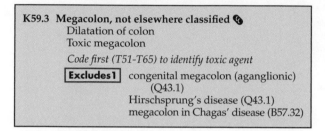

> **K59.3** **Megacolon, not elsewhere classified** 🔵
> Dilatation of colon
> Toxic megacolon
> *Code first (T51-T65) to identify toxic agent*
> | Excludes1 | congenital megacolon (aganglionic) (Q43.1)
> Hirschsprung's disease (Q43.1)
> megacolon in Chagas' disease (B57.32)

FIGURE 3-23. Example of Excludes1 Note.

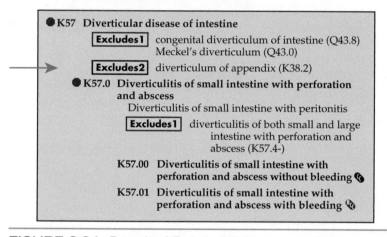

> ⚫ **K57** **Diverticular disease of intestine**
> | Excludes1 | congenital diverticulum of intestine (Q43.8)
> Meckel's diverticulum (Q43.0)
> → | Excludes2 | diverticulum of appendix (K38.2)
> ⚫ **K57.0** **Diverticulitis of small intestine with perforation and abscess**
> Diverticulitis of small intestine with peritonitis
> | Excludes1 | diverticulitis of both small and large intestine with perforation and abscess (K57.4-)
> **K57.00** **Diverticulitis of small intestine with perforation and abscess without bleeding** 🔵
> **K57.01** **Diverticulitis of small intestine with perforation and abscess with bleeding** 🔵

FIGURE 3-24. Example of Excludes2 Note.

Exclusion Notes

ICD-10-CM has two types of "Excludes" notes:

- Excludes1

  An Excludes1 note is used to indicate that two conditions cannot occur together. If a certain condition is excluded, it means it cannot be coded here (Figure 3-23).

EXAMPLE Patient presents to the hospital with severe constipation. The doctor diagnoses the patient with congenital megacolon. Code K59.3 excludes congenital megacolon, directing the coder to Q43.1

- Excludes2

  An Excludes2 note is used to indicate that the condition is not represented by the code, "not included here." In the case of the Excludes2 note, it would be acceptable to use two codes as appropriate (Figure 3-24).

EXAMPLE Patient presents to the hospital with stomach pain. The doctor diagnoses the patient with diverticulitis of the colon and the appendix. This would require two codes, one for the colon and one for the appendix. See the Excludes2 note under K57.

EXERCISE 3-6

Using the Tabular List, answer the following questions.

1. Is bronchitis due to fumes and vapors assigned code J40?   _____
   If not, what code is assigned?   _____

2. Is chronic sinusitis assigned code category J01?   _____
   If not, what code is assigned?   _____

3. Is gangrenous tonsillitis assigned to code category J03?   _____
   If not, what code is assigned?   _____

4. Is hypertensive cardiomegaly included in code category I11?   _____
   If not, what code is assigned?   _____

5. Is aseptic peritonitis included in code category K65?   _____
   If not, what code is assigned?   _____

Etiology and Manifestation Convention

Some disease conditions may have both an underlying etiology as well as many body system manifestations that are the direct cause of the underlying etiology. In ICD-10-CM the underlying condition is sequenced first, followed by the manifestation. There will be two sets of instructions for these conditions. The etiology code will have an instruction to use an additional code while the manifestation code will have a note to code first the etiology code (Figure 3-25). In Figure 3-25 under the code category F02 for Dementia, the instructions advise to code first the underlying condition. If the patient had Alzheimer's, code category G30 (Figure 3-26) would become the first sequenced code, and the instructional note under G30 likewise advises the coder to assign an additional code for dementia. In most cases the manifestation codes will have in the title "in diseases classified elsewhere" (Figure 3-27). When this terminology is used these codes are NEVER to be used first. These codes must

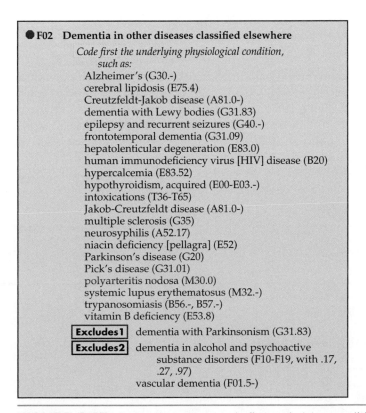

FIGURE 3-25. Instruction note to code first underlying condition.

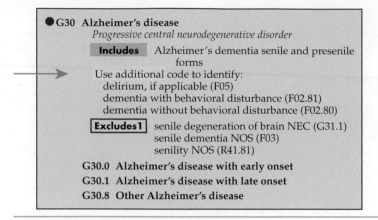

FIGURE 3-26. Use additional code note.

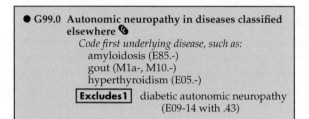

FIGURE 3-27. Example of manifestation code "in diseases classified elsewhere."

Parkinsonism (primary) G20
  with neurogenic orthostatic hypoten-
    sion (idiopathic) (symptomatic)
    G90.3
  arteriosclerotic G21.4
  dementia G31.83 *[F02.80]*
    with behavioral disturbance G31.83
      [F02.81]

FIGURE 3-28. Manifestation code in brackets.

be sequenced after the underlying condition code. If the manifestation code does not have "in diseases classified elsewhere" in the title but does have a "use additional code" note, the same sequencing rules apply as for "in diseases classified elsewhere."

In the Alphabetic Index, manifestation codes will be listed together with the etiology code first followed by the manifestation code in brackets. The code in brackets is always sequenced second (Figure 3-28).

When there is not an etiology/manifestation combination but the terms "code first underlying cause" and "use additional code" are used, the same sequencing rules apply (Figure 3-30).

EXAMPLE | A patient with idiopathic gout of the right foot has a calculus of the urinary tract, M10.071, N22 (Figure 3-29).

EXAMPLE | Patient has ulcer of right ankle with diabetes, type 2, E11.622, L97.319, codes must be sequenced in this order.

Code category L97 includes an instructional note to code first any associated underlying condition.

EXAMPLE | Patient has a urinary tract infection due to *Escherichia coli*, must be sequenced in this order, N39.0, B96.20.

●**M10 Gout**
  Accumulation of uric acid that results in swollen, red, hot,
    painful, stiff joints.
  Acute gout
  Gout attack
  Gout flare
  Gout NOS
  Podagra

  Use additional code to identify:
    Autonomic neuropathy in diseases classified elsewhere
      (G99.0)
    Calculus of urinary tract in diseases classified
      elsewhere (N22)
    Cardiomyopathy in diseases classified elsewhere (I43)
    Disorders of external ear in diseases classified
      elsewhere (H61.1-, H62.8-)
    Disorders of iris and ciliary body in diseases classified
      elsewhere (H22)
    Glomerular disorders in diseases classified elsewhere
      (N08)
    | **Excludes1** | chronic gout (M1a-)

FIGURE 3-29. Instructional note to use additional code.

●**D89.81 Graft-versus-host disease**
  Code first underlying cause, such as:

    complications of transplanted organs
      and tissue (T86.-)
    complications of blood transfusion
      (T80.89)

  Use additional code to identify associated
    manifestations, such as:
    desquamative dermatitis (L30.8)
    diarrhea (R19.7)
    elevated bilirubin (R17)
    hair loss (L65.9)

FIGURE 3-30. Instructional note to code first underlying cause.

The "use additional code" note instructs the coder to assign an additional code for the organism (Figure 3-31).

EXERCISE 3-7

Using the Tabular List and instructional notes, assign and sequence the following code(s).

1. See category G30 and assign code(s) for a patient who has Alzheimer's disease and dementia with behavioral disturbances.   _____

2. See code E84.0 and assign code(s) for a patient with cystic fibrosis and pseudomonas.   _____

3. See category J13 and assign code(s) for a patient with a lung abscess who also has pneumonia due to streptococcus pneumoniae.   _____

4. See code N40.1 and assign code(s) for a patient with hyperplasia of the prostate with urinary retention.   _____

5. See code I85.11 and assign code(s) for a patient with bleeding esophageal varices and cirrhosis of the liver.   _____

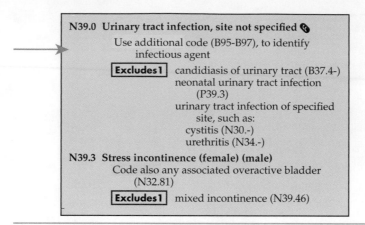

N39.0 **Urinary tract infection, site not specified** 🐾

Use additional code (B95-B97), to identify infectious agent

| Excludes1 | candidiasis of urinary tract (B37.4-)
neonatal urinary tract infection (P39.3)
urinary tract infection of specified site, such as:
cystitis (N30.-)
urethritis (N34.-)

N39.3 **Stress incontinence (female) (male)**

Code also any associated overactive bladder (N32.81)

| Excludes1 | mixed incontinence (N39.46)

FIGURE 3-31. Instructional note to use an additional code.

Diabetes, diabetic (mellitus) (sugar) E11.9
with
    amyotrophy E11.44
    arthropathy NEC E11.618
    autonomic (poly)neuropathy E11.43
    cataract E11.36
    Charcot's joints E11.610
    chronic kidney disease E11.22
    circulatory complication NEC
        E11.59
    complication E11.8
        specified NEC E11.69
    dermatitis E11.620
    foot ulcer E11.621
    gangrene E11.52
    gastroparesis E11.43
    glomerulonephrosis, intracapillary
        E11.21
    glomerulosclerosis, intercapillary
        E11.21
    hyperglycemia E11.65
    hyperosmolarity E11.00
        with coma E11.01
    hypoglycemia E11.649
        with coma E11.641

FIGURE 3-32. Diabetes with hypoglycemia.

Linking Terms

As in the Index, terms such as "and," "with," "due to," and "in" are used to link terms. These terms have special definitions within ICD-10-CM.

The term "and" means "and" or "or" when it appears in a title. The code category J35, chronic disease of tonsils and adenoids, could mean any of the following:

- Chronic disease of tonsils
- Chronic disease of adenoids
- Chronic disease of tonsils and adenoids

The term "with" indicates that both elements in the title must be present and documented for this code to be assigned. The word "with" in the Alphabetic Index is sequenced right after the main term, not in alphabetical order.

EXAMPLE | Diabetes with hypoglycemia and coma is assigned E11.641.

Hereditary - *see* condition
Heredodegeneration, macular - *see* Dystrophy, retina
Heredopathia atactica polyneuritiformis G60.1
Heredosyphilis - *see* Syphilis, congenital
Herlitz' syndrome Q81.1
Hermansky-Pudlak syndrome E70.331

FIGURE 3-33. Under the main term "Hereditary," mandatory instructions are given to *"see"* condition.

Angioblastoma - *see* Neoplasm, connective tissue, uncertain behavior

FIGURE 3-34. Cross-reference to *"see"* another main term.

Hydrarthrosis - *see also* Effusion, joint
  gonococcal A54.42
  intermittent M12.40
    ankle M12.47-
    elbow M12.42-
    foot joint M12.47-
    hand joint M12.44-
    hip M12.45-
    knee M12.46-
    multiple site M12.49
    shoulder M12.41-
    specified joint NEC M12.48
    wrist M12.43-
  of yaws (early) (late) (*see also* subcategory M14.8-) A66.6
  syphilitic (late) A52.77
    congenital A50.55 *[M12.80]*

FIGURE 3-35. *"See also"* instruction to go to the main term "Effusion."

Cross-References

Cross-reference terms are used in the Alphabetic Index to instruct a coder to look elsewhere prior to code assignment. These terms include *"see," "see also," "see* category," and *"see* condition" (Figure 3-33).

The term "see" is a mandatory instruction that advises the coder to go to another main term (Figure 3-34).

The term "see also" instructs the coder about the possibility that a better main term may appear elsewhere in the Alphabetic Index. If the specific diagnosis cannot be completely identified by the subterms, it may be necessary to follow the "see also" instruction (Figure 3-35).

A "code also" note instructs the coder that two codes may be required to fully describe a condition. "Code also" notes do not give sequencing instruction.

Default Codes

In the ICD-10-CM Alphabetic Index, if a code is listed next to the main term, it is the default code. A default code may represent a condition that is most commonly associated with the main term or is the unspecified term for that condition. For example, if pneumonia is documented in a medical record, and no additional information or specificity is supplied, such as aspiration or viral, the default code is J18.9.

Syndromes

To code syndromes, the guidance supplied by the Alphabetic Index must be followed. Should there be no guidance in the Index, codes should be assigned for all the manifestations of the syndrome that have been documented.

EXERCISE 3-8

Using the Alphabetic Index, answer the following questions.

1. Locate the main term "arthropathy" in the Index. Is there another term for "arthropathy" that may be located in the Index, and if so, what is the term?   _____

2. Locate the main term "climacteric" in the Index. Is there another term for "climacteric" that may be located in the Index, and if so, what is the term?   _____

3. Locate the main term "lathyrism" in the Index. Is there another term for lathyrism, and if so, what is the term?   _____

4. Locate the main term "enteric" in the Index. Is there another term for "enteric" that may be located in the Index, and if so, what is the term?   _____

5. Locate the main term "late effect "in the Index. Is there another term for late effect that may be located in the Index, and if so, what is the term?   _____

CHAPTER REVIEW EXERCISE

Match the term, symbol, or punctuation with the appropriate description.

_____ 1. Stands for "not otherwise specified"

_____ 2. Used in both the Index and the Tabular to enclose supplementary words that may be present or absent in the statement of a disease or procedure, without affecting the code number to which it is assigned

_____ 3. This note appears immediately under a three-digit code title to further define, or give examples of, the content of the category

_____ 4. A note under a code indicates that the terms excluded from the code are to be coded elsewhere

_____ 5. A word that should be interpreted to mean either "and" or "or" when it appears in a title

_____ 6. Stands for "not elsewhere classifiable"

_____ 7. Term that is used to indicate that no code should be assigned

A. Omit code	**E.** NEC	**I.** Excludes
B. ( )	**F.** See category	**J.** And
C. NOS	**G.** See also	**K.** Use additional code
D. Includes	**H.** Etiology	

Using ICD-10-CM, Volume 1, Tabular List, locate the first pages of Chapter 10, and answer the following questions about the chapter.

8. The name of the chapter: _____

9. The name of the first section block: _____

10. The description of the first category: _____

11. The description of the first subcategory: _____

12. The description of the first subclassification: _____

13. What instructional note applies to category J01?   _____

14. What Excludes note applies to the first section block?   _____

Underline the main terms to be located in the Alphabetic Index in the following diagnostic statements.

15. Profound anemia   _____

16. Chronic prostatitis   _____

17. Mild protein-calorie malnutrition   _____

18. Granuloma lung   _____

19. Pain in shoulder   _____

Using the Alphabetic Index, locate the following main terms and identify whether the bolded subterm is an essential or a nonessential modifier.

20. Immature cataract   _____

21. Senile cataract   _____

22. Contact dermatitis   _____

23. Classical migraine   _____

24. Congential strabismus   _____

Using the Alphabetic Index, answer the following questions.

25. Locate the main term "acquired immune deficiency syndrome" in   _____
the Index. Is there another term for "acquired immune deficiency
syndrome" that may be located in the Index, and if so, what is the
term?

26. Locate the main term "malarial" in the Index. Is there another   _____
term for "malarial" that may be located in the Index, and if so,
what is the term?

Using the Tabular List, answer the following questions.

27. Is decompensated chronic obstructive pulmonary disease with   _____
acute exacerbation assigned J44.9?
If not, what code is assigned?   _____

28. Is rupture of the esophagus assigned code K22.3?   _____
If not, what code is assigned?   _____

Using the Tabular List and instructional notes, assign and sequence the following code(s).

29. See category G31 and assign code(s) for a patient who has Pick's   _____
disease with behavioral disturbances.

30. See code L62 and assign code(s) for a patient with   _____
pachydermoperiostosis with nail dystrophy of the right hand.

31. Assign code(s) for a patient with atherosclerosis of the lower   _____
extremities with a left ankle ulcer with fat layer exposed.

CHAPTER GLOSSARY

Carryover line: used when an entry will not fit on a single line.

Category: a single three-digit code that describes a disease or a similarly related group of conditions.

Connecting words: subterms that denote a relationship between a main term or a subterm and an associated condition or etiology.

Conventions: general rules for use in classification that must be followed for accurate coding.

Etiology: cause or origin of a disease or condition.

ICD-10-CM: *International Classification of Diseases, 10th Revision, Clinical Modification.*

ICD-10-PCS: *International Classification of Diseases, 10th Revision, Procedure Coding System.*

Main terms: term that identifies disease conditions or injuries, it is identified in bold print and set flush with the left margin of each column in the Alphabetic Index.

Manifestation: symptom of a condition that is the result of a disease.

Morphology: the study of neoplasms.

NEC: abbreviation for "not elsewhere classifiable" that means "other specified."

Nonessential modifier: term that is enclosed in parentheses; its presence or absence does not affect code assignment.

NOS: abbreviation for "not otherwise specified" that means "unspecified."

Section: consists of a group of three-digit categories that represent diseases or conditions that are similar.

See: a mandatory cross-reference that advises the coder to go to another main term.

See also: cross-reference that instructs the coder about the possibility that there may be a better main term elsewhere in the Alphabetic Index.

Subcategory: a fourth-digit code that provides additional information or specificity.

Subclassification: a fifth-digit code that provides even greater specificity.

Subterms: give more specific information about a main term. Subterms identify site, type, or etiology of a disease condition or injury. Also, modifiers that are indented to the right of the main term.

4

Basic Steps of Coding

LEARNING OBJECTIVES

1. Assign a diagnosis or procedure from the Alphabetic Index using main terms, subterms, and essential modifiers
2. Explain the necessity of referencing the Alphabetic Index and the Tabular List
3. Describe basic steps of coding
4. Explain how to use both the Alphabetic Index and the Tabular List

ABBREVIATIONS/ ACRONYMS

CC chief complaint   ER Emergency Room
DS discharge summary   OR Operating Room

BASIC STEPS OF CODING

1. Review the health record.
2. Identify the diagnoses and procedures to be coded.
3. Identify the principal diagnosis and the principal procedure.
4. Identify main term(s) in the Alphabetic Index.
5. Review any subterms under the main term in the Alphabetic Index.
6. Follow any cross-reference instructions, such as *"see also."*
7. Verify in the Tabular List the code(s) selected from the Alphabetic Index.
8. Refer to any instructional notation in the Tabular List.
9. Assign codes to the highest level of specificity.
10. Assign codes to the diagnoses and procedures, reporting all applicable codes, and sequence in accordance with the guidelines.

REVIEW OF THE HEALTH RECORD

As described in Chapter 2 of this textbook, the first step in coding the **principal diagnosis** (condition established after study to be chiefly responsible for occasioning admission of the patient to the hospital for care), other reportable diagnoses, and procedures is review of the health record.

The discharge summary (DS), if available, may be the first document to be reviewed for code selection. The coder reads the summary to understand the highlights of this encounter. The **discharge summary** is a synopsis of the events included in a patient's hospital stay. Most pertinent information is contained in the discharge summary. A physician should list the diagnoses and the procedures that were performed during this encounter. The coder should not solely rely on the discharge summary to capture all diagnoses and procedures that occurred during this encounter.

For many reasons, the discharge summary is not the only document from which codes are captured.

- Coders may not have a discharge summary at the time of coding.
- If the patient is in the hospital for a long stay, often the attending physician will focus only on those diagnoses that were treated during the latter part of the stay.
- Physicians list conditions that are not currently under treatment and that appear only in the patient's history.
- Likewise, physicians describe diagnoses as "history of" when, in fact, they represent conditions that are being currently treated.

Most coders start the coding process as they begin their document review. A coder is continually trying to determine the principal diagnosis during the record review. Clues to determination of the principal diagnosis can be found in the ER record or in the admitting orders. Physicians, in their admitting orders, give a reason for admitting the patient. When evaluating an ER record, a coder first looks for the **chief complaint** (CC), which is the reason in the patient's own words for presenting to the hospital.

EXAMPLE

> CC: I have a bad cough, fever, and headache, and my throat is so sore I can't even swallow liquids.

As the coder continues the review of the ER document, the ER physician provides a diagnosis for admission to the hospital. The **admitting diagnosis** is the condition that requires the patient to be hospitalized. This condition may be a sign or a symptom that requires testing and evaluation to determine a diagnosis. This may be a known diagnosis or a probable diagnosis, or it may include a differential diagnosis. In the previous example, the ER physician might document, "Admit patient to the hospital for possible pneumonia and dehydration." In this case, the pneumonia has not yet been confirmed, but the dehydration is known.

A **differential diagnosis** occurs when a patient presents with a symptom that could represent a variety of diagnoses. During the patient's stay a variety of studies may be conducted to rule out or confirm the differential diagnoses.

EXAMPLE

> A patient presents with abdominal pain, and the physician suspects that this might represent appendicitis, gastroenteritis, or cholecystitis. Appendicitis, gastroenteritis, and cholecystitis are differential diagnoses.

A coder continues on through the health record, reviewing all progress notes, operative reports, anesthesiology notes, and consults to arrive at all diagnoses and procedures that need to be captured or reported.

The second most important concept that a coder must remember (after the definition of principal diagnosis and principal procedure) is that once a term has been located in the Alphabetic Index, the code must then be verified in the Tabular Index. This is not the case in ICD-10-PCS, in which you do not need to refer to the Index before referring to the tables.

ALPHABETIC INDEX

The **Alphabetic Index** consists of an Alphabetic Index to Diseases and an Alphabetic Index to Procedures. In ICD-10-PCS, the purpose of the Alphabetic Index is to locate the appropriate table.

Locate the Main Term in the Index to Diseases

Once the coder begins to establish diagnoses and procedures, the first task in selecting a code is to locate the **main term**, which is always identified by bold type, in the Alphabetic Index.

EXAMPLE   Using pneumonia as the principal diagnosis, locate this term in the Alphabetic Index. The code for pneumonia is J18.9 (Figure 4-1).

EXERCISE 4-1

Using Figure 4-1, assign codes to the following diagnoses:

1. Aspiration pneumonia   _____
2. Pneumonia due to *Klebsiella pneumoniae*   _____
3. Mycoplasma pneumonia   _____
4. Varicella pneumonia   _____
5. Viral pneumonia   _____

After the main term, "pneumonia," in the Alphabetic Index, is a long list of nonessential modifiers (words in parentheses). Remember that nonessential modifiers have no effect on the main term. They are "take it or leave it" terms. Sometimes, the subterm that a coder is searching for can be found among the nonessential modifiers.

EXAMPLE   Granulomatous pneumonia is coded to J18.9.
Acute pneumonia, J18.9.
Fulminant pneumonia, J18.9. (See Figure 4-1.)

In locating the main term, the coder must remember that main terms are usually identified by disease conditions and nouns. They are not body parts or sites. If a physician documents *Klebsiella pneumoniae* pneumonia, the noun is the main term and the one to be located in the Alphabetic Index. To find *Klebsiella pneumoniae* in the Alphabetic Index, the coder goes to "pneumonia" and looks for the subterm, *"Klebsiella"* (Figure 4-2).

Subterms are modifiers of main terms, and in contrast to nonessential modifiers, they do have an effect on the appropriate code assignment. To determine the main term, the coder must decide what condition the patient has (in this case, pneumonia), which is the main term; subterms are modifiers of the main term, which in this case is *Klebsiella pneumoniae.*

EXAMPLE   If a patient has a diagnosis of hiatal hernia, the main term is "hernia," and the subterm is "hiatal."
The main terms usually are nouns and/or disease conditions. The main terms below are underlined.
Gastric <u>upset</u>
Chronic <u>mastoiditis</u>
<u>Herpes</u> simplex

EXAMPLE   The patient has a diagnosis of appendicitis, and the operative report (OR) describes the procedure as a laparoscopic appendectomy.
In ICD-10-PCS, look up "appendectomy," and the Index directs the user to either "excision or resection." Under "resection, appendix," the user is referred to table 0DTJ.

Main Term ———→ **Pneumonia** (acute) (Alpenstich) (benign)
       (bilateral) (brain) (cerebral) (circum-
       scribed) (congestive) (creeping) (de-
       layed resolution) (double) (epidemic)
       (fever) (flash) (fulminant) (fungoid)
Nonessential   (granulomatous) (hemorrhagic)
modifiers   (incipient) (infantile) (infectious)
       (infiltration) (insular) (intermittent)
       (latent) (migratory) (organized)
       (overwhelming) (primary (atypical))
       (progressive) (pseudolobar) (puru-
       lent) (resolved) (secondary) (senile)
       (septic) (suppurative) (terminal)
Code for   (true) (unresolved) (vesicular)
pneumonia   J18.9
   with
      lung abscess J85.1
         due to specified organism - *see*
            Pneumonia, in (due to)
   adenoviral J12.0
   adynamic J18.2
   alba A50.04
   allergic (eosinophilic) J82
   alveolar - *see* Pneumonia, lobar
   anaerobes J15.8
   anthrax A22.1
   apex, apical - *see* Pneumonia, lobar
   Ascaris B77.81
Subterm ———→ aspiration J69.0
      due to
         aspiration of microorganisms
           bacterial J15.9
           viral J12.9
         food (regurgitated) J69.0
         gastric secretions J69.0
         milk (regurgitated) J69.0
         oils, essences J69.1
         solids, liquids NEC J69.8
         vomitus J69.0
      newborn P24.81
         amniotic fluid (clear) P24.11
         blood P24.21
         liquor (amnii) P24.11
         meconium P24.01
         milk P24.31
         mucus P24.11
         food (regurgitated) P24.31
         specified NEC P24.81
         stomach contents P24.31
   atypical NEC J18.9
   bacillus J15.9
    specified NEC J15.8
   bacterial J15.9
    specified NEC J15.8
   Bacteroides (fragilis) (oralis) (melanino-
      genicus) J15.8
   basal, basic, basilar - *see* Pneumonia,
      lobar
   bronchiolitis obliterans organized
      (BOOP) J84.8
   broncho-, bronchial (confluent) (croup-
      ous) (diffuse) (disseminated)
      (hemorrhagic) (involving lobes)
      (lobar) (terminal) J18.0
    allergic (eosinophilic) J82
    aspiration - *see* Pneumonia,
      aspiration
    bacterial J15.9
      specified NEC J15.8
    chronic - *see* Fibrosis, lung
    diplococcal J13
    Eaton's agent J15.7
    Escherichia coli (E. coli) J15.5
    Friedländer's bacillus J15.0

Pneumonia (*Continued*)
   broncho-, bronchial (*Continued*)
    Hemophilus influenzae J14
    hypostatic J18.2
    inhalation (*see also* Pneumonia,
      aspiration
      due to fumes or vapors (chemical)
        J68.0
      of oils or essences J69.1
    Klebsiella (pneumoniae) J15.0
    lipid, lipoid J69.1
      endogenous J84.8
    Mycoplasma (pneumoniae) J15.7
    pleuro-pneumonia-like-organisms
      (PPLO) J15.7
    pneumococcal J13
    Proteus J15.6
    Pseudomonas J15.1
    Serratia marcescens J15.6
    specified organism NEC J16.8
    staphylococcal - *see* Pneumonia,
      staphylococcal
    streptococcal NEC J15.4
      group B J15.3
      pneumoniae J13
    viral, virus - *see* Pneumonia, viral
   Butyrivibrio (fibriosolvens) J15.8
   Candida B37.1
   caseous - *see* Tuberculosis, pulmonary
   catarrhal - *see* Pneumonia, broncho
   chlamydial J16.0
    congenital P23.1
   cholesterol J84.8
   cirrhotic (chronic) - *see* Fibrosis, lung
   Clostridium (haemolyticum) (novyi)
     J15.8
   confluent - *see* Pneumonia, broncho
   congenital (infective) P23.9
    due to
      bacterium NEC P23.6
      Chlamydia P23.1
      Escherichia coli P23.4
      Haemophilus influenzae P23.6
      infective organism NEC P23.8
      Klebsiella pneumoniae P23.6
      Mycoplasma P23.6
      Pseudomonas P23.5
      Staphylococcus P23.2
      Streptococcus (except group B)
        P23.6
       group B P23.3
      viral agent P23.0
      specified NEC P23.8
   croupous - *see* Pneumonia, lobar
   cytomegalic inclusion B25.0
   cytomegaloviral B25.0
   deglutition - *see* Pneumonia, aspiration
   desquamative interstitial J84.8
   diffuse - *see* Pneumonia, broncho
   diplococcal, diplococcus (broncho-)
    (lobar) J13
   disseminated (focal) - *see* Pneumonia,
    broncho
   Eaton's agent J15.7
   embolic, embolism - *see* Embolism,
    pulmonary
   Enterobacter J15.6
   eosinophilic J82
   Escherichia coli (E. coli) J15.5
   Eubacterium J15.8
   fibrinous - *see* Pneumonia, lobar
   fibroid, fibrous (chronic) - *see* Fibrosis,
    lung
   Friedländer's bacillus J15.0

FIGURE 4-1. Alphabetic Index entry for "pneumonia."

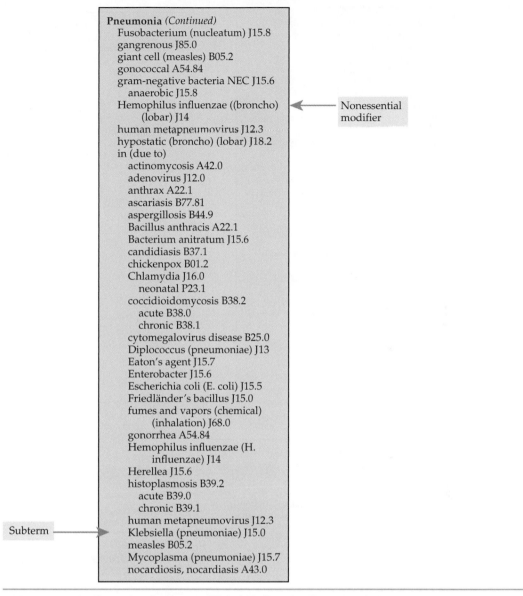

Pneumonia *(Continued)*
 Fusobacterium (nucleatum) J15.8
 gangrenous J85.0
 giant cell (measles) B05.2
 gonococcal A54.84
 gram-negative bacteria NEC J15.6
  anaerobic J15.8
 Hemophilus influenzae ((broncho) ← Nonessential
  (lobar) J14   modifier
 human metapneumovirus J12.3
 hypostatic (broncho) (lobar) J18.2
 in (due to)
  actinomycosis A42.0
  adenovirus J12.0
  anthrax A22.1
  ascariasis B77.81
  aspergillosis B44.9
  Bacillus anthracis A22.1
  Bacterium anitratum J15.6
  candidiasis B37.1
  chickenpox B01.2
  Chlamydia J16.0
   neonatal P23.1
  coccidioidomycosis B38.2
   acute B38.0
   chronic B38.1
  cytomegalovirus disease B25.0
  Diplococcus (pneumoniae) J13
  Eaton's agent J15.7
  Enterobacter J15.6
  Escherichia coli (E. coli) J15.5
  Friedländer's bacillus J15.0
  fumes and vapors (chemical)
   (inhalation) J68.0
  gonorrhea A54.84
  Hemophilus influenzae (H.
   influenzae) J14
  Herellea J15.6
  histoplasmosis B39.2
   acute B39.0
   chronic B39.1
  human metapneumovirus J12.3
Subterm → Klebsiella (pneumoniae) J15.0
  measles B05.2
  Mycoplasma (pneumoniae) J15.7
  nocardiosis, nocardiasis A43.0

FIGURE 4-2. Example of subterm "Klebsiella," under "pneumonia."

   Sometimes, a main term may be found under more than one Index entry (Figure 4-3). This is most often true of eponyms (a disease, syndrome, or a procedure, named for a person). Adjectives and anatomic sites do appear as main terms, but they instruct the coder to see the condition (Figure 4-4).

EXAMPLE   Diagnosis of ischial fracture: The Index for "ischial" would direct the coder to go to the condition or, in this case, fracture.
   Ischium, ischial—*see* condition

EXAMPLE   Chronic otitis media—look up "chronic" in the Alphabetic Index.
   Chronic—*see* condition

   The term *"see"* is a mandatory direction to look elsewhere in the Alphabetic Index.

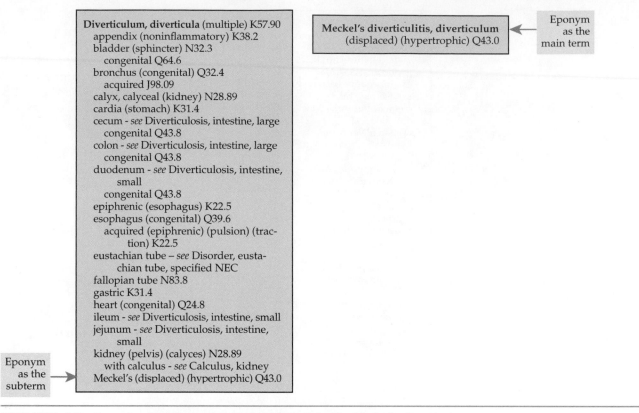

FIGURE 4-3. Example of multiple Alphabetic Index entries for Meckel's diverticulum.

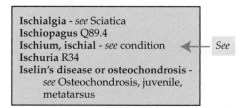

FIGURE 4-4. Example of an anatomic site instructing coder to *see* condition.

Sometimes the Index will direct the coder to *see also*. This instruction means that if the term cannot be located under the Index entry, the user should go to the suggested Index entry.

The general rule that main terms identify disease conditions has some exceptions. One of these exceptions is Z codes, which can be found under main terms such as "admission," "examination," and "status." These will be fully covered in Chapter 8 on Z codes. Likewise, obstetric conditions can be found under main terms such as "pregnancy" and "puerperal" and will be covered in Chapter 21 in the section on obstetrics and gynecology. There is also a main term for Sequelae that can be used to identify residuals of various disease conditions and complications.

Locating a main term may be difficult because of the terminology used by the physician or because an eponym is used. For example, physicians often describe arterial lines used for monitoring as Swan Ganz (pulmonary artery wedge pressure monitoring). If the user were to look under "Swan Ganz" in the procedural Alphabetic Index, no listing would be found. In these cases, the user should try alternative terminology.

EXAMPLE | Swan Ganz is a type of catheter. In ICD-10-PCS, monitoring, arterial, pressure, pulmonary directs the user to see "measurement" in cardiac table 4A0Z.

Locate the Main Term in the Index to Procedures

The purpose of the Alphabetic Index in ICD-10-PCS is to locate the appropriate table. Once the table is located the user will find that it contains the information necessary to develop a procedure code. The PCS tables must always be consulted to find the appropriate valid code. To locate a procedure code in ICD-10-PCS it is not necessary to consult the Index first. This information will be explained in detail in Chapters 6 and 7 in this text.

EXAMPLE   Removal of a skin lesion on the back, (OHB6XZZ) (Figure 4-5). To locate removal of a skin lesion in ICD-10-CM, locate "excision, skin" in the Alphabetic Index. This entry refers the user to table OHB.

   Needle biopsy of the right lobe of the liver, 50.11 (OFB13ZX) (Figure 4-6). In ICD-10-PCS locate biopsy in the Index, which directs the user to either drainage or excision, diagnostic.

EXERCISE 4-2

Underline all main terms to be located in the Alphabetic Index.

1. Esophageal reflux
2. Tourette's disease
3. Iatrogenic thyroiditis
4. Infantile eczema
5. Coronary artery disease
6. Congestive heart failure
7. Rheumatoid arthritis
8. Atrial fibrillation
9. Sickle cell anemia

Excision *(Continued)*
  Sinus
    Accessory 09BP
    Ethmoid
      Left 09BV
      Right 09BU
    Frontal
      Left 09BT
      Right 09BS
    Mastoid
      Left 09BC
      Right 09BB
    Maxillary
      Left 09BR
      Right 09BQ
    Sphenoid
      Left 09BX
      Right 09BW
  Skin
    Abdomen 0HB7XZ
    Back 0HB6XZ
    Buttock 0HB8XZ
    Chest 0HB5XZ
    Ear

FIGURE 4-5. Example from entry for "excision skin lesion" in the Index to Procedures.

SECTION: 0 MEDICAL AND SURGICAL
BODY SYSTEM: F HEPATOBILIARY SYSTEM AND PANCREAS
OPERATION: B EXCISION: Cutting out or off, without replacement, a portion of a body part

Body Part	Approach	Device	Qualifier
0 Liver 1 Liver, Right Lobe 2 Liver, Left Lobe 4 Gallbladder G Pancreas	0 Open 3 Percutaneous 4 Percutaneous Endoscopic	Z No Device	X Diagnostic Z No Qualifier
5 Hepatic Duct, Right 6 Hepatic Duct, Left 8 Cystic Duct 9 Common Bile Duct C Ampulla of Vater D Pancreatic Duct F Pancreatic Duct, Accessory	0 Open 3 Percutaneous 4 Percutaneous Endoscopic 7 Via Natural or Artificial Opening 8 Via Natural or Artificial Opening Endoscopic	Z No Device	X Diagnostic Z No Qualifier

FIGURE 4-6. Table for "needle, biopsy liver" in ICD-10-PCS.

TABULAR LIST

Once the code has been selected from the Alphabetic Index, it must then be verified in the **Tabular List.** Sometimes a code that is selected from the Alphabetic Index does not seem to match what is described in the Tabular List. If this is the case, the user should review the Alphabetic Index and the Tabular List for all exclusion notes and other instructional notes. It may require that the user browse the category in the Tabular List for a more representative code. It also may require that the user access *Coding Clinic* for any advice on how to code a specific diagnosis.

EXAMPLE

Documentation in the chart describes the patient as having anorexia. She has been admitted to the psychiatric unit of the hospital.
Look up "Anorexia" in the Alphabetic Index, R63.0.
Go to the Tabular List and review the Excludes notes.
  Because this is a psychiatric admission, reviewing the codes excluded may assist in assigning the correct code.

The rule of never coding directly from the Alphabetic Index without reviewing the Tabular also applies to never coding from instructional notes within the Tabular without first reviewing the actual Tabular Listing of the code.

CHAPTER REVIEW EXERCISE

Using the Alphabetic Index and the Tabular List, code all the following diagnoses and underline the main term.

1. Acute subendocardial infarction, initial episode of care   _____

2. *Clostridium difficile* enteritis   _____

3. Refractory megaloblastic anemia   _____

4. Acute suppurative appendicitis   _____

5. Stage 3 pressure ulcer of the sacrum   _____

6. Abdominal aortic aneurysm   _____

7. Colon obstruction _____

8. Intractable epilepsy with status epilepticus _____

9. Paroxysmal supraventricular tachycardia _____

10. Streptococcal group A pneumonia _____

11. Deep vein thrombosis of the right femoral vein _____

12. Congenital syphilitic laryngotracheitis _____

13. Dysphagia as a late effect of a stroke _____

14. Adhesive bursitis of the right shoulder _____

15. History of cardiovascular disease in the family _____

CHAPTER GLOSSARY

Admitting diagnosis: the condition that requires the patient to be hospitalized.

Alphabetic Index: the index found in the ICD-10-CM book for both disease conditions and procedures.

Chief complaint: the reason, in the patient's own words, for presenting to the hospital.

Differential diagnosis: when a symptom may represent a variety of diagnoses.

Discharge summary: a review of the patient's hospital course. This summary details the reason for admission or tests or procedures performed and how the patient responded.

Eponym: term for a disease, structure, procedure, or syndrome that has been named for a person.

Main term: term that identifies disease conditions or injuries; it is identified in bold print and set flush with the left margin of each column in the Alphabetic Index.

Nonessential modifier: term that is enclosed in parentheses; its presence or absence does not affect code assignment.

Principal diagnosis: condition established after study to be chiefly responsible for occasioning admission of the patient to the hospital for care.

Subterm: gives more specific information about a main term. Subterms identify site, type, or etiology of a disease condition or injury. Also, modifiers that are indented to the right of the main term.

Tabular List: section of the ICD-10-CM book that contains the code listing, along with exclusion or inclusion notes.

5

General Coding Guidelines for Diagnosis

CHAPTER OUTLINE

ICD-10-CM Official Guidelines for Coding and Reporting
General Coding Guidelines
Selection of Principal Diagnosis
Reporting Additional Diagnoses
Chapter Review Exercise
Chapter Glossary

LEARNING OBJECTIVES

1. Apply ICD-10-CM Official Guidelines for Coding and Reporting
2. Sequence ICD-10-CM diagnosis codes as directed by coding guidelines or ICD-10-CM conventions
3. Determine whether signs, symptoms, or manifestations require separate code assignments
4. Assign ICD-10-CM diagnosis codes for sequela

ABBREVIATIONS/ ACRONYMS

AHA American Hospital Association

AHIMA American Health Information Management Association

CABG coronary artery bypass graft

CMS Centers for Medicare and Medicaid Services

DHHS U.S. Department of Health and Human Services

GPO Government Printing Office

HIPAA Health Insurance Portability and Accountability Act

ICD-9-CM *International Classification of Diseases, 9th Revision, Clinical Modification*

ICD-10-CM *International Classification of Diseases, 10th Revision, Clinical Modification*

ICD-10-PCS *International Classification of Diseases, 10th Revision, Procedure Coding System*

NCHS National Center for Health Statistics

ICD-10-CM OFFICIAL GUIDELINES FOR CODING AND REPORTING

The ICD-10-CM Official Guidelines for Coding and Reporting were developed by the Cooperating Parties to provide further guidance regarding coding and sequencing that is not provided in the ICD-10-CM manual. These guidelines do not cover every situation and have been formatted in a manner that will allow for expansion as new guidelines are developed. The guidelines may be changed each year, and changes may have greater impact in some years than in others.

In this chapter, the coder will review the general guidelines and coding examples as applicable. The convention guidelines with examples were presented in Chapter 3, "ICD-10-CM, Format and Conventions." Chapter-specific guidelines are provided and explained in the respective disease or body system chapter.

ICD-10-CM

Official
Guidelines for
Coding and
Reporting (2012)

Please refer to the companion Evolve website for the most current guidelines.

2012
Narrative changes appear in bold text
Items <u>underlined</u> have been moved within the guidelines since the 2011 version
***Italics* are used to indicate revisions to heading changes**

The Centers for Medicare and Medicaid Services (CMS) and the National Center for Health Statistics (NCHS), two departments within the U.S. Federal Government's Department of Health and Human Services (DHHS) provide the following guidelines for coding and reporting using the International Classification of Diseases, 10th Revision, Clinical Modification (ICD-10-CM). These guidelines should be used as a companion document to the official version of the ICD-10-CM as published on the NCHS website. The ICD-10-CM is a morbidity classification published by the United States for classifying diagnoses and reason for visits in all health care settings. The ICD-10-CM is based on the ICD-10, the statistical classification of disease published by the World Health Organization (WHO).

These guidelines have been approved by the four organizations that make up the Cooperating Parties for the ICD-10-CM: the American Hospital Association (AHA), the American Health Information Management Association (AHIMA), CMS, and NCHS.

These guidelines are a set of rules that have been developed to accompany and complement the official conventions and instructions provided within the ICD-10-CM itself. The instructions and conventions of the classification take precedence over guidelines. These guidelines are based on the coding and sequencing instructions in the Tabular List and Alphabetic Index of ICD-10-CM, but provide additional instruction. Adherence to these guidelines when assigning ICD-10-CM diagnosis codes is required under the Health Insurance Portability and Accountability Act (HIPAA). The diagnosis codes (Tabular List and Alphabetic Index) have been adopted under HIPAA for all healthcare settings. A joint effort between the healthcare provider and the coder is essential to achieve complete and accurate documentation, code assignment, and reporting of diagnoses and procedures. These guidelines have been developed to assist both the healthcare provider and the coder in identifying those diagnoses and procedures that are to be reported. The importance of consistent, complete documentation in the medical record cannot be overemphasized. Without such documentation accurate coding cannot be achieved. The entire record should be reviewed to determine the specific reason for the encounter and the conditions treated.

The term encounter is used for all settings, including hospital admissions. In the context of these guidelines, the term provider is used throughout the guidelines to mean physician or any qualified health care practitioner who is legally accountable for establishing the patient's diagnosis. Only this set of guidelines, approved by the Cooperating Parties, is official.

The guidelines are organized into sections. Section I includes the structure and conventions of the classification and general guidelines that apply to the entire classification, and chapter-specific guidelines that correspond to the chapters as they are arranged in the classification. Section II includes guidelines for selection of principal diagnosis for non-outpatient settings. Section III includes guidelines for reporting additional diagnoses in non-outpatient settings. Section IV is for outpatient coding and reporting. It is necessary to review all sections of the guidelines to fully understand all of the rules and instructions needed to code properly.

GENERAL CODING GUIDELINES

General coding guidelines apply to all healthcare settings and to the entire ICD-10-CM classification system.

In the Alphabetic Index of ICD-10-CM a dash (-) is used to indicate that there are further digits that need to be assigned for a valid code. In Figures 5-1 and 5-2, note that C50.91 would be an invalid code. A sixth digit is necessary to identify left, right, or unspecified breast. All codes must be assigned to the final level of subdivision. A valid code is at least three characters, but could be four, five, six, or seven characters.

> **Disease, diseased** (*Continued*)
> breast (*see also* Disorder, breast) N64.9
>   cystic (chronic) – *see* Mastopathy,
>   cystic
>   fibrocystic – *see* Mastopathy, cystic
>   Paget's
>   female, unspecified side C50.91-
>   male, unspecified side C50.92-
>   specified NEC N64.89
> Breda's – *see* Yaws
> Bretonneau's (diphtheritic malignant
>   angina) A36.0

FIGURE 5-1. Alphabetic Index entry for Paget's disease, female breast.

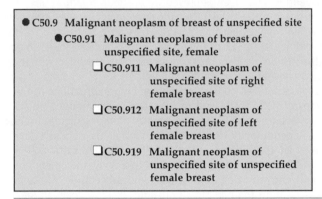

FIGURE 5-2. Tabular List entry for Paget's disease, female breast.

Section I. Conventions, general coding guidelines and chapter specific guidelines
The conventions, general guidelines and chapter-specific guidelines are applicable to all health care settings unless otherwise indicated. The conventions and instructions of the classification take precedence over guidelines.

B. General Coding Guidelines
  1. Locating a code in the ICD-10-CM
    To select a code in the classification that corresponds to a diagnosis or reason for visit documented in a medical record, first locate the term in the Alphabetic Index, and then verify the code in the Tabular List. Read and be guided by instructional notations that appear in both the Alphabetic Index and the Tabular List.

    It is essential to use both the Alphabetic Index and Tabular List when locating and assigning a code. The Alphabetic Index does not always provide the full code. Selection of the full code, including laterality and any applicable 7th character can only be done in the Tabular List. A dash (-) at the end of an Alphabetic Index entry indicates that additional characters are required. Even if a dash is not included at the Alphabetic Index entry, it is necessary to refer to the Tabular List to verify that no 7th character is required.

  2. Level of Detail in Coding
    Diagnosis codes are to be used and reported at their highest number of characters available.

    ICD-10-CM diagnosis codes are composed of codes with 3, 4, 5, 6 or 7 characters. Codes with three characters are included in ICD-10-CM as the heading of a category of codes that may be further subdivided by the use of fourth and/or fifth characters and/or sixth characters, which provide greater detail.

    A three-character code is to be used only if it is not further subdivided. A code is invalid if it has not been coded to the full number of characters required for that code, including the 7th character, if applicable.

EXERCISE 5-1

Using the Alphabetic Index and the Tabular List, assign the appropriate code(s).

1. Ankylosis right ankle

   Code from Alphabetic Index _____

   Code following verification in Tabular List _____

2. Hairy cell leukemia in remission

   Code from Alphabetic Index _____

   Code following verification in Tabular List _____

3. Traumatic spiral fracture shaft of left humerus

   Code from Alphabetic Index _____

   Code following verification in Tabular List _____

4. Bilateral carpal tunnel syndrome

   Code from Alphabetic Index _____

   Code following verification in Tabular List _____

3. **Code or codes from A00.0 through T88.9, Z00-Z99.8**

   The appropriate code or codes from A00.0 through T88.9, Z00-Z99.8 must be used to identify diagnoses, symptoms, conditions, problems, complaints or other reason(s) for the encounter/visit.

4. **Signs and symptoms**

   Codes that describe symptoms and signs, as opposed to diagnoses, are acceptable for reporting purposes when a related definitive diagnosis has not been established (confirmed) by the provider. Chapter 18 of ICD-10-CM, Symptoms, Signs, and Abnormal Clinical and Laboratory Findings, Not Elsewhere Classified (codes R00.0-R99) contains many, but not all codes for symptoms.

EXAMPLE   Pyrexia of unknown origin, R50.9.

5. **Conditions that are an integral part of a disease process**

   Signs and symptoms that are associated routinely with a disease process should not be assigned as additional codes, unless otherwise instructed by the classification.

6. **Conditions that are not an integral part of a disease process**

   Additional signs and symptoms that may not be associated routinely with a disease process should be coded when present.

EXAMPLE   Hematuria due to calculus of kidney, N20.0.

EXAMPLE   Ascites due to cirrhosis of the liver, K74.60, R18.8.

Chapter 18 of ICD-10-CM contains most but not all codes used to identify signs and symptoms.

Signs and symptoms codes are acceptable to code:

- When no definitive diagnosis has been established
- When they are not an integral part of the disease process
- When directed by the classification to assign an additional code

It is not acceptable to code signs or symptoms:
- When a definitive diagnosis has been established
- When they are an integral part of the disease process

EXERCISE 5-2

Answer the following questions.

1. List two common symptoms of gallstones. _____

2. List the symptom most commonly associated with costochondritis. _____

3. List two common symptoms of urinary tract infection. _____

4. A patient has osteoarthritis and anemia. The anemia is integral to the osteoarthritis.
   A. True
   B. False

5. A patient has dyspnea caused by congestive heart failure. Dyspnea should be assigned as an additional code.
   A. True
   B. False

Assign codes to the following conditions.

6. Nocturia due to benign prostatic hypertrophy _____

7. Anorexia due to acute appendicitis _____

8. Seizure due to glioblastoma multiforme right temporal lobe _____

9. Fever due to pneumonia _____

10. Headaches of undetermined etiology _____

7. Multiple coding for a single condition

In addition to the etiology/manifestation convention that requires two codes to fully describe a single condition that affects multiple body systems, there are other single conditions that also require more than one code. "Use additional code" notes are found in the Tabular List at codes that are not part of an etiology/manifestation pair where a secondary code is useful to fully describe a condition. The sequencing rule is the same as the etiology/manifestation pair, "use additional code" indicates that a secondary code should be added.

For example, for bacterial infections that are not included in chapter 1, a secondary code from category B95, Streptococcus, Staphylococcus, and Enterococcus, as the cause of diseases classified elsewhere, or B96, Other bacterial agents as the cause of diseases classified elsewhere, may be required to identify the bacterial organism causing the infection. A "use additional code" note will normally be found at the infectious disease code, indicating a need for the organism code to be added as a secondary code (Figure 5-3).

"Code first" notes are also under certain codes that are not specifically manifestation codes but may be due to an underlying cause. When there is a "code first" note and an underlying condition is present, the underlying condition should be sequenced first (Figure 5-4).

"Code, if applicable, any causal condition first", notes indicate that this code may be assigned as a principal diagnosis when the causal condition is unknown or not applicable. If a causal condition is known, then the code for that condition should be sequenced as the principal or first-listed diagnosis.

N10 **Acute tubulo-interstitial nephritis** 🔖
      Acute infectious interstitial nephritis
      Acute pyelitis
      Acute pyelonephritis
      Hemoglobin nephrosis
      Myoglobin nephrosis

      Use additional code (B95-B97), to identify infectious agent ←——————

FIGURE 5-3. Instruction to use additional code.

● H28 *Cataract in diseases classified elsewhere*
       Code first underlying disease, such as: ←——————
          hypoparathyroidism (E20.-)
          myotonia (G71.1-)
          myxedema (E03.-)
          protein-calorie malnutrition (E40-E46)
       Excludes1 cataract in diabetes mellitus (E08.33, E09.33,
                      E10.33, E11.33, E13.33)

FIGURE 5-4. Code first note.

Multiple codes may be needed for **sequela**, complication codes and obstetric codes to more fully describe a condition. See the specific guidelines for these conditions for further instruction.

EXAMPLE   Acute pyelonephritis due to *Escherichia coli (E. coli)*, N10, B96.20.

EXERCISE 5-3

Assign codes to the following conditions.

1. Dementia due to Parkinson's disease   _____
2. Hypertensive retinopathy, bilateral   _____
3. Cellulitis of left lower leg due to group A *streptococcus*   _____
4. Acute prostatitis due to *Escherichia coli*   _____
5. Anemia due to chronic kidney disease, stage 3   _____

8. Acute and Chronic Conditions

If the same condition is described as both acute (subacute) and chronic, and separate subentries exist in the Alphabetic Index at the same indentation level, code both and sequence the acute (subacute) code first (Figure 5-5).

EXAMPLE   Acute and chronic pancreatitis, K85.9, K86.1.

EXAMPLE   Acute and chronic cholecystitis, K81.2.
Separate subterms are included for "acute" and "chronic," but a subterm for "acute and chronic" is also provided.

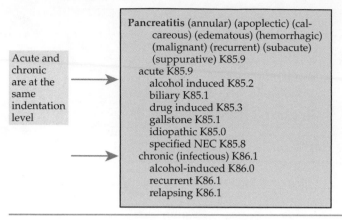

Acute and chronic are at the same indentation level

Pancreatitis (annular) (apoplectic) (calcareous) (edematous) (hemorrhagic) (malignant) (recurrent) (subacute) (suppurative) K85.9
  acute K85.9
    alcohol induced K85.2
    biliary K85.1
    drug induced K85.3
    gallstone K85.1
    idiopathic K85.0
    specified NEC K85.8
  chronic (infectious) K86.1
    alcohol-induced K86.0
    recurrent K86.1
    relapsing K86.1

FIGURE 5-5. Subterms for acute and chronic.

EXAMPLE

Acute and chronic otitis media, H66.90.
Separate subterms are provided for "acute" and "chronic," but they use the same code.

EXERCISE 5-4

Assign and sequence codes to the following conditions.

1. Subacute and chronic appendicitis   _____
2. Acute and chronic bronchitis   _____
3. Acute and chronic pyelonephritis   _____
4. Acute on chronic renal failure   _____
5. Acute on chronic respiratory failure   _____

9. Combination Code

A combination code is a single code used to classify:
Two diagnoses, or
A diagnosis with an associated secondary process (manifestation)
A diagnosis with an associated complication

Combination codes are identified by referring to subterm entries in the Alphabetic Index and by reading the inclusion and exclusion notes in the Tabular List.

Assign only the combination code when that code fully identifies the diagnostic conditions involved or when the Alphabetic Index so directs. Multiple coding should not be used when the classification provides a combination code that clearly identifies all of the elements documented in the diagnosis. When the combination code lacks necessary specificity in describing the manifestation or complication, an additional code should be used as a secondary code.

EXAMPLE

Chronic pyelonephritis due to vesicoureteral reflux, N11.0.

EXAMPLE

Pseudomonas pneumonia, J15.1.
The combination code includes the infection and the organism responsible for the infection (*Pseudomonas*). It would be incorrect to assign separate codes such as J18.9 for pneumonia and B96.5 to identify the *Pseudomonas* organism.

EXERCISE 5-5

Assign codes to the following conditions.

1. Urinary tract infection due to candidiasis   _____
2. Streptococcal group A pneumonia   _____
3. Food poisoning due to *Salmonella*   _____

---

10. *Sequela* **(Late Effects)**

A **sequela** is the residual effect (condition produced) after the acute phase of an illness or injury has terminated. There is no time limit on when a **sequela** code can be used. The residual may be apparent early, such as in cerebral infarction, or it may occur months or years later, such as that due to a previous injury. Coding of **sequela** generally requires two codes sequenced in the following order: The condition or nature of the **sequela** is sequenced first. The **sequela** code is sequenced second.

An exception to the above guidelines are those instances where the code for **the sequela** is followed by a manifestation code identified in the Tabular List and title, or the **sequela** code has been expanded (at the fourth, fifth or sixth character levels) to include the manifestation(s). The code for the acute phase of an illness or injury that led to the **sequela** is never used with a code for the late effect.

See Section I.C.9. Sequelae of cerebrovascular disease
See Section I.C.15. Sequelae of complication of pregnancy, childbirth and the puerperium
See Section I.C.19. **Application of 7ᵗʰ characters for Chapter 19**

EXERCISE 5-6

Write the term(s) that represent the sequela and its cause in the following cases on the lines provided, and assign the appropriate codes.

1. Keloid scar left right forearm, resulting from second-degree burns; injury occurred 1 year ago

Sequela: _____   Code: _____

Cause: _____   Code: _____

2. Traumatic arthritis in the right ankle joint due to previous nondisplaced lateral malleolar fracture

Sequela: _____   Code: _____

Cause: _____   Code: _____

3. Oropharyngeal phase dysphagia due to CVA 3 months ago

Sequela: _____   Code: _____

Cause: _____   Code: _____

---

11. **Impending or Threatened Condition**

Code any condition described at the time of discharge as "impending" or "threatened" as follows:

If it did occur, code as confirmed diagnosis.

If it did not occur, reference the Alphabetic Index to determine if the condition has a subentry term for "impending" or "threatened" and also reference main term entries for "Impending" and for "Threatened."

If the subterms are listed, assign the given code.

If the subterms are not listed, code the existing underlying condition(s) and not the condition described as impending or threatened.

Occasionally, conditions will be treated and documented as impending conditions. According to the guidelines, if the diagnosis has been confirmed, it should be coded as an active and current condition. If it is impending or threatened rather than active and current, check the Alphabetic Index to see whether a code is available that describes the impending condition. If no code is available, code the existing underlying condition(s).

EXAMPLE

Impending myocardial infarction, I20.0.

EXAMPLE

Impending fracture of the humerus due to multiple myeloma, C90.00.

12. Reporting Same Diagnosis Code More than Once
Each unique ICD-10-CM diagnosis code may be reported only once for an encounter. This applies to bilateral conditions when there are no distinct codes identifying laterality or two different conditions classified to the same ICD-10-CM diagnosis code.

13. Laterality
For bilateral sites, the final character of the codes in the ICD-10-CM indicates laterality. An unspecified side code is also provided should the side not be identified in the medical record. If no bilateral code is provided and the condition is bilateral, assign separate codes for both the left and right side.

EXAMPLE

Primary osteoarthritis both hips, M16.0.

14. Documentation for BMI and Pressure Ulcer Stages
For the Body Mass Index (BMI) and pressure ulcer stage codes, code assignment may be based on medical record documentation from clinicians who are not the patient's provider (i.e., physician or other qualified healthcare practitioner legally accountable for establishing the patient's diagnosis), since this information is typically documented by other clinicians involved in the care of the patient (e.g., a dietitian often documents the BMI and nurses often documents the pressure ulcer stages). However, the associated diagnosis (such as overweight, obesity, or pressure ulcer) must be documented by the patient's provider. If there is conflicting medical record documentation, either from the same clinician or different clinicians, the patient's attending provider should be queried for clarification.

The BMI codes should only be reported as secondary diagnoses. As with all other secondary diagnosis codes, the BMI codes should only be assigned when they meet the definition of a reportable additional diagnosis (see Section III, Reporting Additional Diagnoses).

EXAMPLE

The dietitian documents a BMI of 32. The physician documents obesity, E66.9, Z68.32.

15. Syndromes
Follow the Alphabetic Index guidance when coding syndromes. In the absence of Alphabetic Index guidance, assign codes for the documented manifestations of the syndrome.

EXAMPLE

Patient with Noonan's syndrome with undescended testicles, von Willebrand's, and mild intellectual disability, Q87.1, Q53.20, D68.0, F70.

16. **Documentation of Complications of Care**
    Code assignment is based on the provider's documentation of the relationship between the condition and the care or procedure. The guideline extends to any complications of care, regardless of the chapter the code is located in. It is important to note that not all conditions that occur during or following medical care or surgery are classified as complications. There must be a cause-and-effect relationship between the care provided and the condition, and an indication in the documentation that it is a complication. Query the provider for clarification, if the complication is not clearly documented.

EXAMPLE

Patient is seen in the clinic for routine post-surgical aftercare. Patient had appendectomy 5 days ago. Patient was treated for a UTI, Z48.815, Z90.49, N39.0.

There is no documentation that indicates that the urinary tract infection is a complication of the patient's recent surgery.

EXAMPLE

Patient was seen in the ER for dehiscence of external abdominal wound following appendectomy, T81.31×A, Y83.6, Z90.49.

EXERCISE 5-7

Assign codes to the following conditions.

1. Impending delirium tremens _____
2. Threatened miscarriage _____
3. Impending myocardial infarction _____
4. Impending fracture of femur due to severe osteoporosis _____
5. Impending stroke. Patient presented with dysarthria. _____
6. Physician documents sacral pressure ulcer. Nursing documentation indicates stage 3. _____
7. Patient is being treated for blackheads and cystic acne. _____
8. Patient has bilateral radial fractures. _____
9. Patient was admitted for physical therapy following a stroke with residual left-sided hemiparesis (non-dominant). _____
10. Physician documents that the patient (adult) is overweight. BMI is documented as 29.0 by dietitian. _____

SELECTION OF PRINCIPAL DIAGNOSIS

Section II. Selection of Principal Diagnosis
The circumstances of inpatient admission always govern the selection of principal diagnosis. The principal diagnosis is defined in the Uniform Hospital Discharge Data Set (UHDDS) as "that condition established after study to be chiefly responsible for occasioning the admission of the patient to the hospital for care."

The UHDDS definitions are used by hospitals to report inpatient data elements in a standardized manner. These data elements and their definitions can be found in the July 31, 1985, Federal Register (Vol. 50, No, 147), pp. 31038-40.

Since that time the application of the UHDDS definitions has been expanded to include all non-outpatient settings (acute care, short term, long term care and psychiatric hospitals; home health agencies; rehab facilities; nursing homes, etc).

In determining principal diagnosis the coding conventions in the ICD-10-CM, the Tabular List and Alphabetic Index take precedence over these official coding guidelines.
(See Section I.A., Conventions for the ICD-10-CM)

The importance of consistent, complete documentation in the medical record cannot be overemphasized. Without such documentation the application of all coding guidelines is a difficult, if not impossible, task.

A. Codes for symptoms, signs, and ill-defined conditions

Codes for symptoms, signs, and ill-defined conditions from Chapter 18 are not to be used as principal diagnosis when a related definitive diagnosis has been established.

EXAMPLE | Right lower quadrant abdominal pain due to acute appendicitis. The code for the abdominal pain is R10.31 (from Chapter 18), and it is due to acute appendicitis. The only code necessary is K35.80, for acute appendicitis.

B. Two or more interrelated conditions, each potentially meeting the definition for principal diagnosis.

When there are two or more interrelated conditions (such as diseases in the same ICD-10-CM chapter or manifestations characteristically associated with a certain disease) potentially meeting the definition of principal diagnosis, either condition may be sequenced first, unless the circumstances of the admission, the therapy provided, the Tabular List, or the Alphabetic Index indicate otherwise.

EXAMPLE | The patient had severe dehydration and hypokalemia that were treated with IV fluids and IV potassium supplements, E86.0, E87.6, or E87.6, E86.0.

C. Two or more diagnoses that equally meet the definition for principal diagnosis

In the unusual instance when two or more diagnoses equally meet the criteria for principal diagnosis as determined by the circumstances of admission, diagnostic workup and/or therapy provided, and the Alphabetic Index, Tabular List, or another coding guidelines does not provide sequencing direction, any one of the diagnoses may be sequenced first.

EXAMPLE | The patient was admitted with an exacerbation of her chronic obstructive pulmonary disease and decompensation of her congestive heart failure. Either J44.1 or I50.9 could be selected for the principal diagnosis, and the other code would be a secondary diagnosis code.

D. Two or more comparative or contrasting conditions.

In those rare instances when two or more contrasting or comparative diagnoses are documented as "either/or" (or similar terminology), they are coded as if the diagnoses were confirmed and the diagnoses are sequenced according to the circumstances of the admission. If no further determination can be made as to which diagnosis should be principal, either diagnosis may be sequenced first.

EXAMPLE | Peptic ulcer disease versus cholecystitis, K27.9, K81.9, or K81.9, K27.9.

E. A symptom(s) followed by contrasting/comparative diagnoses

When a symptom(s) is followed by contrasting/comparative diagnoses, the symptom code is sequenced first. All the contrasting/comparative diagnoses should be coded as additional diagnoses.

EXAMPLE | Abdominal pain due to peptic ulcer disease versus cholecystitis, R10.9, K27.9, K81.9.

F. Original treatment plan not carried out
Sequence as the principal diagnosis the condition, which after study occasioned the admission to the hospital, even though treatment may not have been carried out due to unforeseen circumstances.

EXAMPLE | The patient was admitted for cholecystectomy because of cholelithiasis. The patient was noted to be having an exacerbation of congestive heart failure (CHF), so the surgery was canceled and IV Lasix was administered to treat the CHF, K80.20, I50.9, Z53.09. No procedure code would be assigned because the procedure was canceled before it was started.

G. Complications of surgery and other medical care
When the admission is for treatment of a complication resulting from surgery or other medical care, the complication code is sequenced as the principal diagnosis. If the complication is classified to the T80-T88 series and the code lacks the necessary specificity in describing the complication, an additional code for the specific complication should be assigned.

EXAMPLE | The patient was admitted for dehiscence of external abdominal incision, T81.31xA, Y83.9.

H. Uncertain Diagnosis
If the diagnosis documented at the time of discharge is qualified as "probable", "suspected", "likely", "questionable", "possible", or "still to be ruled out", or other similar terms indicating uncertainty, code the condition as if it existed or was established. The bases for these guidelines are the diagnostic workup, arrangements for further workup or observation, and initial therapeutic approach that correspond most closely with the established diagnosis.
Note: This guideline is applicable only to inpatient admissions to short-term, acute, long-term care and psychiatric hospitals.

EXAMPLE | Possible adenovirus meningitis, A87.1.

In the chapter specific guidelines, there are three exceptions to the uncertain diagnosis guideline.
- Code B20 AIDS should only be assigned for confirmed cases
- Code J09.X- Avian influenza should only be assigned for confirmed cases
- Code J09.X- H1N1 influenza should only be assigned for confirmed cases

I. Admission from Observation Unit
1. Admission Following Medical Observation
When a patient is admitted to an observation unit for a medical condition, which either worsens or does not improve, and is subsequently admitted as an inpatient of the same hospital for this same medical condition, the principal diagnosis would be the medical condition which led to the hospital admission.

EXAMPLE | The patient was admitted for medical observation because of chest pain. After further investigation and testing, it was determined that the patient had a NSTEMI, and the patient was admitted for inpatient care, I21.4.

2. Admission Following Post-Operative Observation

When a patient is admitted to an observation unit to monitor a condition (or complication) that develops following outpatient surgery, and then is subsequently admitted as an inpatient of the same hospital, hospitals should apply the Uniform Hospital Discharge Data Set (UHDDS) definition of principal diagnosis as "that condition established after study to be chiefly responsible for occasioning the admission of the patient to the hospital for care."

J. Admission from Outpatient Surgery

When a patient receives surgery in the hospital's outpatient surgery department and is subsequently admitted for continuing inpatient care at the same hospital, the following guidelines should be followed in selecting the principal diagnosis for the inpatient admission:

- If the reason for the inpatient admission is a complication, assign the complication as the principal diagnosis.
- If no complication, or other condition, is documented as the reason for the inpatient admission, assign the reason for the outpatient surgery as the principal diagnosis.
- If the reason for the inpatient admission is another condition unrelated to the surgery, assign the unrelated condition as the principal diagnosis.

EXAMPLE The patient was admitted following an outpatient esophagogastroduodenoscopy for gastroesophageal reflux. The patient went into atrial fibrillation in the recovery room and was admitted, I97.191, I48.91, K21.9, Y83.8, Y92.238, 0DJ08ZZ.

REPORTING ADDITIONAL DIAGNOSES

Section III. Reporting Additional Diagnoses

GENERAL RULES FOR OTHER (ADDITIONAL) DIAGNOSES

For reporting purposes the definition for "other diagnoses" is interpreted as additional conditions that affect patient care in terms of requiring:

clinical evaluation; or

therapeutic treatment; or

diagnostic procedures; or

extended length of hospital stay; or

increased nursing care and/or monitoring.

The UHDDS item #11-b defines Other Diagnoses as "all conditions that coexist at the time of admission, that develop subsequently, or that affect the treatment received and/or the length of stay. Diagnoses that relate to an earlier episode which have no bearing on the current hospital stay are to be excluded." UHDDS definitions apply to inpatients in acute care, short-term, long term care and psychiatric hospital setting. The UHDDS definitions are used by acute care short-term hospitals to report inpatient data elements in a standardized manner. These data elements and their definitions can be found in the July 31, 1985, Federal Register (Vol. 50, No, 147), pp. 31038-40.

Since that time the application of the UHDDS definitions has been expanded to include all non-outpatient settings (acute care, short term, long term care and psychiatric hospitals; home health agencies; rehab facilities; nursing homes, etc).

The following guidelines are to be applied in designating "other diagnoses" when neither the Alphabetic Index nor the Tabular List in ICD-10-CM provide direction. The listing of the diagnoses in the patient record is the responsibility of the attending provider.

A. Previous conditions

If the provider has included a diagnosis in the final diagnostic statement, such as the discharge summary or the face sheet, it should ordinarily be coded. Some providers include in the diagnostic statement resolved conditions or diagnoses and status-post procedures from previous admission that have no bearing on the current stay. Such conditions are not to be reported and are coded only if required by hospital policy.

However, history codes (categories Z80-Z87) may be used as secondary codes if the historical condition or family history has an impact on current care or influences treatment.

EXAMPLE

> The patient is being treated for congestive heart failure and has a history of allergy to shellfish. A code is available for history of shellfish allergy, but it would not be necessary to assign this code unless facility policy directs the coder to do so. Some physicians list allergies and previous surgeries as diagnoses, I50.9.

EXAMPLE

> The patient is being treated for prostate cancer. A significant family history of prostate cancer has been reported, C61, Z80.42.

B. Abnormal findings

Abnormal findings (laboratory, x-ray, pathologic, and other diagnostic results) are not coded and reported unless the provider indicates their clinical significance. If the findings are outside the normal range and the attending provider has ordered other tests to evaluate the condition or prescribed treatment, it is appropriate to ask the provider whether the abnormal finding should be added.

Please note: This differs from the coding practices in the outpatient setting for coding encounters for diagnostic tests that have been interpreted by a provider.

EXAMPLE

> Potassium is noted to be low on laboratory testing. Potassium 20 mEq was ordered. Query the physician regarding the significance of the abnormal lab value and subsequent treatment.

C. Uncertain Diagnosis

If the diagnosis documented at the time of discharge is qualified as "probable", "suspected", "likely", "questionable", "possible", or "still to be ruled out" or other similar terms indicating uncertainty, code the condition as if it existed or was established. The bases for these guidelines are the diagnostic workup, arrangements for further workup or observation, and initial therapeutic approach that correspond most closely with the established diagnosis.

Note: This guideline is applicable only to inpatient admissions to short-term, acute, long-term care and psychiatric hospitals.

EXAMPLE

> Suspected aspiration pneumonitis, J69.0.

CHAPTER REVIEW EXERCISE

Select the correct answer for each of the following:

1. Conditions that are integral to a disease or condition should be coded as additional diagnoses.
   A. True
   B. False

2. When separate codes are used to identify acute and chronic conditions, the chronic code is sequenced first.
   A. True
   B. False

3. Reliance on only the Alphabetic Index or only the Tabular List can lead to errors in code assignments and less specificity in code selection in ICD-10-CM.
   A. True
   B. False

4. A patient has anemia due to chronic renal failure. The anemia is integral to the chronic renal failure.
   A. True
   B. False

5. A patient has right lower quadrant abdominal pain due to acute appendicitis. The abdominal pain should be assigned as an additional code.
   A. True
   B. False

6. In the inpatient setting, it is acceptable to code diagnoses that have not yet been confirmed but that are questionable or suspected at the time of discharge.
   A. True
   B. False

7. If the discharge diagnosis was abdominal pain due to acute appendicitis, abdominal pain would be coded as the principal diagnosis.
   A. True
   B. False

Assign codes to the following conditions.

8. Cerebral infarction due to thrombosis right carotid artery

   Code from Alphabetic Index   _____

   Code following verification in Tabular List   _____

9. Supervision of high risk pregnancy (second trimester) due to history of stillbirth

   Code from Alphabetic Index   _____

   Code following verification in Tabular List   _____

10. Spastic hemiplegia affecting right dominant side

    Code from Alphabetic Index   _____

    Code following verification in Tabular List   _____

Identify integral and nonintegral conditions by answering the following questions.

11. List two common symptoms of kidney stones.   _____

12. List two common symptoms associated with rheumatoid arthritis.   _____

13. List two common symptoms of acute renal failure.   _____

Assign and sequence codes to the following conditions.

14. Acute and chronic cystitis   _____

15. Acute on chronic oophoritis   _____

16. Dementia due to Alzheimer's   _____

17. Viral gastroenteritis with diarrhea and vomiting   _____

18. Fever and headache due to viral meningitis   _____

19. Constrictive pericarditis due to old tuberculosis infection of the heart   _____

20. Mild intellectual disability due to previous acute poliomyelitis   _____

CHAPTER GLOSSARY

This chapter is unique in that the glossary definitions are not provided within the chapter. These terms are used within the guidelines without definition. The glossary definitions are provided in this section for quick reference.

Acute: a short and relatively severe course.

Asymptomatic: without any symptoms.

Chronic: persistent over a long period.

Combination code: a single code used to classify two diagnoses; or a diagnosis with an associated secondary process (manifestation); or a diagnosis with an associated complication.

Conventions: general rules for use in classification that must be followed for accurate coding.

Etiology: cause or origin of a disease or condition.

Manifestation: symptom or condition that is the result of a disease.

Residual condition or effect: when the acute phase of an illness or injury has passed, but a residual condition or health problem remains.

Sequelae: residual conditions or effects; time when the acute phase of an illness or injury has passed, but residual conditions or health problems remain.

Sign: objective evidence of a disease or of a patient's condition as perceived by the patient's examining physician.

Subacute: somewhat acute; between chronic and acute.

Symptom: subjective evidence of a disease or of a patient's condition as perceived by the patient.

6

General Coding Guidelines for Medical and Surgical Procedures

LEARNING OBJECTIVES

1. Define principal procedure
2. Define significant procedures
3. Explain the surgical hierarchy
4. Assign codes for canceled, converted to open procedures, and bilateral procedures
5. Explain the purpose of a facility policy for procedure coding
6. Discuss the differences between ICD-9-CM, Volume 3, and ICD-10-PCS
7. Explain the use of the General Equivalence Mappings
8. Identify the format of ICD-10-PCS, Alphabetic Index, and PCS Tables
9. Define the root operations for the medical and surgical section of ICD-10-PCS

10. Define the approaches that are used in the medical and surgical section of ICD-10-PCS

11. Apply and assign the correct ICD-10-PCS codes in accordance with the conventions and ICD-10-PCS Coding Guidelines

ABBREVIATIONS/ ACRONYMS

BMI body mass index

CAS computer assisted surgery

CMS Centers for Medicare and Medicaid Services

COPD chronic obstructive pulmonary disease

CPT *Current Procedural Terminology*

ECMO extracorporeal membrane oxygenation

ER Emergency Room

GEMS General Equivalence Mappings

HCPCS Healthcare Common Procedure Coding System

ICD-9-CM *International Classification of Diseases, 9th Revision, Clinical Modification*

ICD-10-CM *International Classification of Diseases, 10th Revision, Clinical Modification*

ICD-10-PCS *International Classification of Diseases, 10th Revision, Procedure Coding System*

ICU intensive care unit

MCE Medicare Code Editor

MS-DRG Medicare Severity diagnosis-related group

NCHS National Center for Health Statistics

NEC not elsewhere classifiable

NOS not otherwise specified

NPI National Provider Identifier

OB obstetrics

OR Operating Room

PPN peripheral parenteral nutrition

PTCA percutaneous transluminal coronary angioplasty

UHDDS Uniform Hospital Discharge Data Set

VAD vascular access device

UHDDS DEFINITIONS

Uniform Hospital Discharge Data Set (UHDDS) definitions are used by acute care, short-term hospitals to report inpatient data elements in a standardized manner. Definitions that pertain to the assignment of procedure codes are presented in the following sections.

Principal Procedure

A **principal procedure** is one that was performed for definitive treatment rather than for diagnostic or exploratory purposes, or one necessary to take care of a complication. If two procedures appear to meet this definition, then the one most closely related to the principal diagnosis should be selected as the principal procedure.

Significant Procedure

To qualify as a **significant procedure**, one of the following criteria must be met:
- Is surgical in nature
- Carries a procedural risk
- Carries an anesthetic risk
- Requires specialized training

It should be noted that a significant procedure does not have to be performed in an OR. Procedures can be done in the Emergency Room (ER) before admission, at the patient's bedside, in a treatment room, or in an interventional radiology department. These procedures can be easily missed because an operative report describing the procedure may not have been completed. Often, these procedures are documented with a brief, handwritten note on the ER record or in a progress note. Consent for treatment may assist the coder in attempting to verify a procedure, but not all procedures require consent forms. Also, a signed consent form does not confirm that the procedure was actually performed. A complete review of the entire health record is necessary to ensure that all completed procedures have been coded.

Other UHDDS data elements that must be coded include the date of the procedure and the NPI (National Provider Identifier) of the person who performed the procedure. It may be the coder's responsibility to abstract these data elements.

PROCEDURE CODES THAT SHOULD BE REPORTED

Any procedures that affect payment or reimbursement must be reported. Other procedures may be reported at a hospital's discretion or in accordance with hospital policy. Encoders (coding software) may also have special popup notices that alert the coder about noncovered or limited coverage OR procedures.

After assigning procedure codes, the coder should review the diagnosis codes to ensure the assignment of diagnosis codes that support the performance of a procedure.

EXAMPLE

If it was determined that lysis of peritoneal adhesions was sufficient to warrant a procedure code in this male patient, it would make sense that a diagnosis code should be assigned to identify the peritoneal adhesions.
   Procedure: Lysis of peritoneal adhesions, 0DNW0ZZ.
   Diagnosis: Peritoneal adhesions, K66.0.

The Centers for Medicare and Medicaid Services (CMS) has categorized procedures into different classifications through the Medicare Code Editor (MCE). In some code books, these procedures may be highlighted to facilitate assignment of procedure codes. The **Medicare Code Editor** is software that detects errors in coding on Medicare claims. For example, it would identify a male-only procedure coded on a female patient's record.

During a patient's hospitalization, it may be necessary for a procedure to be performed at an outside facility. This could be for reasons such as the service may not be offered at the admitting hospital or equipment may malfunction. The patient may be transported by ambulance to this outside facility, and after the procedure, returns for continued care at the admitting hospital. In these cases, the admitting hospital may assign procedure codes for services performed at the outside facility. The admitting hospital also would include these charges on the hospital bill, and the admitting hospital would reimburse the outside facility for the procedure.

Valid OR Procedure

A **valid OR procedure** is a procedure that may affect MS-DRG assignment.

EXAMPLE

Vaginal hysterectomy is designated as a valid OR procedure, 0UT97ZZ.

Designation of a procedure as a valid OR procedure does not mean that it must be performed in the inpatient setting. Many surgical procedures can be safely performed on an outpatient basis, and many third party payers and/or insurance companies require that certain surgical procedures be performed in an outpatient setting. Repair of direct inguinal hernia is designated as a valid OR procedure, but this procedure is usually performed and billed as an outpatient procedure.

Non-OR Procedure Affecting MS-DRG Assignment

A procedure designated as a "**non-OR procedure affecting MS-DRG assignment**" is a procedure that may affect MS-DRG assignment, even though the procedure is not routinely performed in the OR.

EXAMPLE   Insertion of a totally implantable vascular access device (VAD), chest (percutaneous approach), 0JH63XZ. VADs may be used in patients who require long-term vascular access for chemotherapy, drug administration, or hemodialysis.

In some cases, the procedure code will make a difference in MS-DRG assignment; in other cases, it will not.

EXAMPLE   The patient was admitted with progressive chronic renal failure, stage 5. An abdominal VAD was implanted (percutaneously) for future hemodialysis, N18.5, 0JH83XZ.

In this case, the codes group to a surgical MS-DRG: MS-DRG 675, Other Kidney & Urinary Tract Procedures without CC/MCC.

EXAMPLE   The patient was admitted with primary liver cancer. It was decided to implant (percutaneous) a VAD in the chest for future chemotherapy, C22.8, 0JH63XZ.

In this case, the codes group to a medical MS-DRG: MS-DRG 437, Malignancy of Hepatobiliary System or Pancreas without CC/MCC.

Noncovered OR Procedure

Noncovered OR procedure codes are identified by the Medicare Code Editor as procedures for which Medicare does not provide reimbursement.

EXAMPLE   Vasectomy (excision of bilateral vas deferens, percutaneous) is identified as a noncovered OR procedure, Z30.2, 0VBQ3ZZ.

Sterilization procedures are usually not covered by Medicare. It is possible to assign an MS-DRG, but that does not guarantee payment.

Limited Coverage

Limited coverage procedures are identified by the Medicare Code Editor as procedures covered under limited circumstances.

EXAMPLE   Patient with cystic fibrosis had a bilateral lung transplantation (allogeneic), E84.0, 0BYM0Z0.

For a transplant facility to obtain Medicare coverage for organ transplantation, it must meet preapproved guidelines. Criteria are set forth and updated in *Federal Register* notices.

SURGICAL HIERARCHY

The **MS-DRG grouper** software (computer program that assigns an MS-DRG), using diagnosis and procedure codes, identifies whether a particular patient falls into a medical MS-DRG or a surgical MS-DRG. The MS-DRG grouper is able to determine which procedure is the most resource intensive and assigns the procedure to that particular surgical MS-DRG.

A patient has an open breast biopsy during the same operative episode as a modified radical mastectomy. The patient also has Crohn's disease. The pathology report confirms that the patient has cancer of the right upper outer quadrant.
  CODE ASSIGNMENTS: C50.411, K50.90, 0HTT0ZZ, 0HBT0ZX.
  (The codes were put into the MS-DRG grouper in this order.)
  MS-DRG: 582, MASTECTOMY FOR MALIGNANCY W CC/MCC

In this case, the patient was admitted and after study was determined to have breast cancer of the right upper outer quadrant. She also has a comorbidity of Crohn's disease. The principal procedure is one that is performed for definitive treatment; in this case, that would be the modified radical mastectomy. The mastectomy is more resource intensive than a breast biopsy. It is appropriate to code the diagnostic breast biopsy as an additional procedure code.

CODE ASSIGNMENTS: C50.411, K50.90, 0HBT0ZX, 0HTT0ZZ.
  MS-DRG: 582, MASTECTOMY FOR MALIGNANCY W CC/MCC

In this case, all the codes are the same, but the breast biopsy is incorrectly sequenced as the principal procedure instead of the mastectomy. Because of the surgical hierarchy within the grouper, it groups to the mastectomy MS-DRG, so the reimbursement and MS-DRG assignment would be correct. Even if the grouper will automatically arrange the codes to fit the surgical hierarchy, the code should be sequenced as the principal procedure on the basis of the UHDDS definition.

CODE ASSIGNMENTS: K50.90, C50.411, 0HTT0ZZ, 0HBT0ZX.
  MS-DRG: 983, EXTENSIVE OR PROCEDURE UNRELATED TO PRINCIPAL DIAGNOSIS W/O CC/MCC

In this case, a data entry error was made, and Crohn's disease was incorrectly sequenced as the principal diagnosis, resulting in a 983 MS-DRG assignment. Although MS-DRG 983 may be the correct assignment in some cases, it is not appropriate in this case, and the coder should review the entered codes.

In this case, the principal diagnosis combined with the procedure codes resulted in the MS-DRG assignment. If the data entry error had not been corrected before billing, the facility would have been incorrectly reimbursed.

CLOSED SURGICAL PROCEDURES AND CONVERSION TO OPEN PROCEDURES

As technology has advanced, procedures are increasingly being performed through scopes, which are less invasive than open procedures. This has resulted in quicker recoveries, shorter hospital stays, and fewer complications.

Common closed surgical approaches include laparoscopic, thoracoscopic, and arthroscopic procedures. The **laparoscopic approach** involves use of a laparoscope to examine and perform closed procedures within the abdomen. With a **thoracoscopic approach**, a thoracoscope is used to examine and perform closed procedures within the thorax. The **arthroscopic approach** requires the use of an arthroscope to examine and perform closed procedures within a joint. Closed procedures may be diagnostic and/or therapeutic in nature.

A surgical procedure may start with an endoscopic approach that may need to be converted to an open procedure. Some reasons for conversion to an open procedure include adhesions, bleeding, technical difficulties due to anatomic body structure and/or inflammatory changes, and injury to an organ. The reason for converting to an open procedure should be coded. According to ICD-10-PCS guidelines, two procedure codes are necessary: one for the endoscopic procedure and one for the open procedure. The root operation for the endoscopic procedure code may be inspection.

EXAMPLE
> A patient was admitted for a laparoscopic cholecystectomy for chronic cholecystitis with cholelithiasis. Because of excessive bleeding from the liver bed, the procedure was converted to an open cholecystectomy and the bleeding was controlled, K80.10, K91.61, Y83.6, Y92.234, 0FT40ZZ, 0FJ44ZZ.

PLANNED AND CANCELED PROCEDURES

When patients are admitted to the hospital for a scheduled procedure(s), under some circumstances, the procedure(s) may be canceled or not completed. If a patient's procedure is canceled prior to the time that he or she presents to the hospital, no code will be required because no services were provided, no bill was generated, and there is no health record. On some occasions, a patient presents to have a procedure performed, but for whatever reason the procedure has to be canceled. The principal diagnosis in this case is the reason why the patient was going to have the procedure performed. If a complication arose that resulted in the cancellation, a diagnosis code for that condition would be assigned as a secondary diagnosis. Also, Z codes describe the reason for the cancellation. They can be located in the Index under the main term, procedure (surgical) not done.

Z53.01	Procedure and treatment not carried out due to patient smoking
Z53.09	Procedure and treatment not carried out because of other contraindication
Z53.1	Procedure and treatment not carried out because of patient's decision for reasons of belief and group pressure
Z53.20	Procedure and treatment not carried out because of patient's decision for unspecified reasons
Z53.21	Procedure and treatment not carried out due to patient leaving prior to being seen by health care provider
Z52.29	Procedure and treatment not carried out because of patient's decision for other reasons
Z53.8	Procedure and treatment not carried out for other reasons
Z53.9	Procedure and treatment not carried out, unspecified reason

EXAMPLE
> A patient was admitted for hysterectomy because of uterine fibroids. Shortly after admission, the patient told the nurse that she was having second thoughts and had decided not to go through with the procedure; the patient was discharged, D25.9, Z53.29. No procedure code is assigned because the procedure was never started.

EXAMPLE
> A patient was admitted for coronary artery bypass grafting because of coronary atherosclerosis of the native arteries. The cardiac surgeon became ill, and the surgery was rescheduled. The patient was discharged, I25.10, Z53.8.

EXAMPLE
> A patient was admitted for laparoscopic cholecystectomy for cholelithiasis of gallbladder. It was noted that the patient was having an acute exacerbation of his COPD. The patient was treated with steroids and nebulizer treatments and was discharged. The cholecystectomy was rescheduled for next week, K80.20, J44.1, Z53.09.

Occasionally, a surgical procedure will be started that for whatever reason cannot be completed. The surgical procedure should be coded to the extent that it was performed. These circumstances are different from those surrounding a procedure that is canceled, in that the patient received anesthesia and surgery was begun.

EXAMPLE | A patient was admitted for colon resection because of cancer of the descending colon. A laparotomy incision through subcutaneous tissue and fascia was made, and the patient became unstable with atrial fibrillation. It was decided that the procedure should be terminated and the patient transferred to the ICU for further management. The incision was closed before any definitive surgery could be performed, C18.6, I97.791, I48.91, Y83.8, Y92.234, 0JJTXZZ.

BILATERAL PROCEDURES

A **bilateral procedure** occurs when the same procedure is performed on paired anatomic organs or tissues (i.e., eyes, ears, joints such as shoulder or knee). According to ICD-10-PCS guidelines, if the identical procedure is performed on contralateral body parts, and a bilateral body part value exists for that body part, a single procedure code using the bilateral body part value is assigned. If no bilateral body part value exists, each procedure is coded separately.

As procedures become less invasive, more bilateral procedures may be performed during the same operative episode.

EXAMPLE | Open repair of bilateral direct and indirect inguinal hernia with synthetic prosthesis, K40.20, 0YUA0JZ.

EXAMPLE | Primary osteoarthritis knees for bilateral total knee synthetic substitute replacement, M17.0, 0SRC0JZ, 0SRD0JZ.

FACILITY POLICY

Each facility should have its own written policy regarding the assignment of ICD-10 procedure codes. This policy should consider reimbursement, but it should also take into account other uses of a procedure database and how that information can be extracted. It may be necessary to determine what types of procedures are being performed for physician profiles and credentialing. Research is an important aspect of data collection.

As has been stated previously, because not all procedures are performed in the operating room, it may be difficult to locate documentation of all procedures performed. Procedures that are easy to overlook include mechanical ventilation, debridement, lumbar puncture, suturing, ECMO (extracorporeal membrane oxygenation), and procedures performed by interventional radiology.

HISTORY OF ICD-10-PCS

In 1992, the Centers for Medicare and Medicaid Services (CMS) funded a project to replace Volume 3 of ICD-9-CM, which was outdated and could not be expanded to classify procedures with more specific detail. 3M Health Information Systems was awarded a contract to develop a new system for procedural coding, ICD-10-PCS (Procedure Coding System). ICD-10-PCS was initially released in 1998. Since that time, it has been updated to incorporate changes that were made to ICD-9-CM, Volume 3. CMS is responsible for the maintenance of ICD-10-PCS. (Information about ICD-10-PCS is available on the CMS website.)

According to the National Center for Health Statistics (NCHS), the proposed implementation date for ICD-10-PCS is October 1, 2014.

The ICD-10 Procedure Coding System was developed with four characteristics in mind:
1. Completeness—Each procedure should have its own code.
2. Expandability—New procedure codes should be easily added (unlimited number of codes).

3. Multiaxial—Each code character should have the same meaning across and within body systems.
4. Standardized terminology—ICD-10-PCS will include definitions for terminology used, and multiple meanings will not be associated with the same term.

Other principles followed in the development of ICD-10-PCS include:

- Diagnostic information is not included in the procedure description.
- A "not otherwise specified" (NOS) option is *not* available.
- The "not elsewhere classifiable" (NEC) option is limited.
- All procedures are defined to a high level of specificity.

Differences Between ICD-9-CM and ICD-10-PCS

ICD-9-CM	ICD-10-PCS
Structure is similar to ICD-9 diagnosis codes	Structure is different with the use of tables
Limited number of codes	Expandable with unlimited number of codes
Codes are three to four digits with a decimal	All codes are seven characters, with no decimal after the second digit
Codes are numeric	Codes are alphanumeric
10 different values can be used for each digit, 0 through 9	34 different values can be used for each character, for numbers 0 through 9, and A through Z except for the letters I and O
Combination codes (e.g., tonsillectomy with adenoidectomy)	Separate procedures performed at the same time are coded separately

Mapping

Because of the drastic changes in structure and specificity, it is difficult to provide an accurate cross-reference between ICD-9-CM and ICD-10-PCS. As with ICD-10-CM, two sets of procedure code General Equivalence Mappings (GEMs) have been developed. These mappings are a way to find corresponding procedure codes in the two code sets. The GEM files are located on the CMS website, and the two filenames appear below:

1. ICD-9-CM to ICD-10-PCS (forward mapping; Figure 6-1)
2. ICD-10-PCS to ICD-9-CM (backward mapping; Figure 6-2)

ICD-9-CM	ICD-10-PCS	Flag
4701	0DTJ4ZZ	10000
4709	0DTJ0ZZ	10000
4709	0DTJ7ZZ	10000
4709	0DTJ8ZZ	10000
4711	0DTJ4ZZ	10000
4719	0DTJ0ZZ	10000
4719	0DTJ7ZZ	10000
4719	0DTJ8ZZ	10000

FIGURE 6-1. GEMs mapping file for ICD-9-CM to ICD-10-PCS.

ICD-10-PCS	ICD-9-CM	Flag
0DTJ0ZZ	4709	10000
0DTJ4ZZ	4701	10000
0DTJ7ZZ	4709	10000
0DTJ8ZZ	4709	10000
0DTK0ZZ	4579	10000
0DTK4ZZ	1739	10000
0DTK7ZZ	4579	10000
0DTK8ZZ	4579	10000

FIGURE 6-2. GEMs mapping file for ICD-10-PCS to ICD-9-CM.

EXERCISE 6-1

Using the ICD-9-CM to ICD-10-PCS and ICD-10-PCS to ICD-9-CM GEMs files on the CMS website (see Figures 6-1 and 6-2), map the following procedure codes.

1. 45.76   _____
2. 51.23   _____
3. 69.02   _____
4. 0W9B3ZZ   _____
5. 0DJ68ZZ   _____
6. 0YQ50ZZ   _____

Answer the following questions.

7. ICD-10-PCS is proposed for full implementation on this date.
   A. October 1, 2012
   B. October 31, 2013
   C. October 1, 2013
   D. October 1, 2014

8. Who is responsible for the maintenance of ICD-10-PCS?
   A. AHIMA
   B. AMA
   C. NCHS
   D. CMS

9. The terminology used in ICD-10-PCS is such that multiple meanings can be used for the same term.
   A. True
   B. False

10. ICD-10-PCS is expandable with an unlimited number of codes.
    A. True
    B. False

ORGANIZATION OF ICD-10-PCS

All ICD-10-PCS codes are seven characters (no decimal points are used), with each character representing a particular aspect of the procedure. Each character is represented by a letter or a number and is referred to as a "value." ICD-10-PCS codes are alphanumeric, so there are 34 possible values for each character, the numbers 0-9 and letters A-H, J-N, and P-Z. The letters I and O are not used in ICD-10-PCS.

Alphabetic Index and Tables

The ICD-10-PCS code book contains the Alphabetic Index and PCS Tables. Once you have become familiar with the table structure, it may not be necessary to even use the index, which is structured in a way that follows the organization of the tables but may only identify the first three or four characters of the procedure code. The two types of main terms that are listed in the Alphabetic Index are:

- Based on the root operation or general type of procedure
- Common procedure terms

No eponyms or acronyms are used in the Alphabetic Index. The index is used to assist with the location of the appropriate table that has the information necessary to construct a seven-character procedure code.

Appendectomy
see Excision, Appendix **0DBJ**
see Resection, Appendix **0DTJ**
Appendicolysis *see* Release, Appendix **0DNJ**
Appendicotomy *see* Drainage, Appendix **0D9J**

FIGURE 6-3. Alphabetic Index entry for appendectomy.

EXAMPLE

Alphabetic Index Entry for Appendectomy (Figure 6-3).
In this example, there are two possible tables, 0DBJ and 0DTJ. The root operation, excision or resection, needs to be determined to find the right table and to assign characters 4 through 7 for the appropriate code.

The PCS Tables are divided into 16 sections that classify the type of procedure within each section. The first character of an ICD-10-PCS code identifies the section that describes the category where the code is located. Sections 1 through 9 are medical- and surgical-related sections. Sections B through D and F through H represent ancillary sections of ICD-10-PCS. The largest section is the Medical and Surgical section and has a first character value of 0. The 16 sections and the corresponding section value are as follows:

SECTION	SECTION VALUE/FIRST CHARACTER
Medical and Surgical	0
Obstetrics	1
Placement	2
Administration	3
Measurement and Monitoring	4
Extracorporeal Assistance and Performance	5
Extracorporeal Therapies	6
Osteopathic	7
Other Procedures	8
Chiropractic	9
Imaging	B
Nuclear Medicine	C
Radiation Oncology	D
Physical Rehabilitation and Diagnostic Audiology	F
Mental Health	G
Substance Abuse Treatment	H

The Alphabetic Index assists with identifying the first three or four characters of a procedure code. Each table is identified by the first three characters of a procedure. In the Medical and Surgical section the first three characters identify the value for the following:
- Section
- Body System
- Operation

Each table contains four columns and a varying number of rows (Figure 6-4). Each column identifies the allowable values for characters 4-7. Each row identifies the valid combinations of values. For example, for the body parts anal sphincter (R), Greater Omentum (S), and Lesser Omentum (T), the only two valid approaches are open (0) and percutaneous endoscopic (4). Operative approach values 7 and 8 do not apply because they are not included in that row. The tables must always be used to assign a valid procedure code.

Section	0 Medical and Surgical
Body System	D Gastrointestinal System
Operation	T Resection: Cutting out or off, without replacement, all of a body part

Body Part	Approach	Device	Qualifier	
1 Esophagus, Upper 2 Esophagus, Middle 3 Esophagus, Lower 4 Esophagogastric Junction 5 Esophagus 6 Stomach 7 Stomach, Pylorus 8 Small Intestine 9 Duodenum A Jejunum B Ileum C Ileocecal Valve E Large Intestine F Large Intestine, Right G Large Intestine, Left H Cecum J Appendix K Ascending Colon L Transverse Colon M Descending Colon N Sigmoid Colon P Rectum Q Anus	0 Open 4 Percutaneous Endoscopic 7 Via Natural or Artificial Opening 8 Via Natural or Artificial Opening Endoscopic	Z No Device	Z No Qualifier	Row 1
R Anal Sphincter S Greater Omentum T Lesser Omentum	0 Open 4 Percutaneous Endoscopic	Z No Device	Z No Qualifier	Row 2
Column 1	Column 2	Column 3	Column 4	

FIGURE 6-4. Table ODT for resection of gastrointestinal system.

EXAMPLE

Appendectomy (the surgical removal of the appendix).

The root operation is resection, because all of the appendix is removed without replacement. In the Alphabetic Index, under *Resection,* go to Table ODT (see Figure 6-4) and assign Characters 4 through 7. Character 4 is *J,* for the appendix. Character 5 is *Open,* because no other approach was specified. Character 6 is *Z,* for no device, and Character 7 is *Z,* for no qualifier. Therefore, the ICD-10-PCS code for appendectomy *is ODTJ0ZZ.*

CHARACTER 1 SECTION	CHARACTER 2 BODY SYSTEM	CHARACTER 3 OPERATION	CHARACTER 4 BODY PART	CHARACTER 5 APPROACH	CHARACTER 6 DEVICE	CHARACTER 7 QUALIFIER
Medical and Surgical	Gastrointestinal System	Resection	Appendix	Open	No Device	No Qualifier
0	D	T	J	0	Z	Z

EXERCISE 6-2

Answer the following questions about the characters in an ICD-10-PCS code.

1. How many characters are in an ICD-10-PCS code? _____

2. Which character identifies the approach? _____

3. Which character identifies the body part? _____

Using the ICD-10-PCS, identify the section value for the following.

4. Radiation oncology _____

5. Administration _____

   6. Other procedure   _____

   7. Obstetrics   _____

   8. Mental health   _____

Using the Alphabetic Index only, identify the appropriate table for the following procedures.

   9. Cholecystectomy   _____

   10. Replacement, right knee   _____

   11. Tracheostomy   _____

   12. Psychiatric medication management   _____

   13. Transfusion of platelets via peripheral vein   _____

Using the table in Figure 6-4, answer the following questions.

   14. ODTR8ZZ is a valid code.
      A. True
      B. False

   15. ODT8OZZ is a valid code.
      A. True
      B. False

   16. A biopsy of the esophagus would be coded using Table ODT.
      A. True
      B. False

MEDICAL AND SURGICAL SECTION

Because the Medical and Surgical section is the largest section, and the section that is used the most, we will use this section to learn more about the structure and standardized definitions that are utilized by ICD-10-PCS. The character value for the Medical and Surgical section is 0 (the digit, not the letter *O*). All the codes from the tables in the Medical and Surgical section begin with a zero.

The meanings of the seven characters for codes from the Medical and Surgical section are as follows:

CHARACTER	REPRESENTS
1	Section
2	Body system
3	Root operation
4	Body part
5	Approach
6	Device
7	Qualifier

Body Systems

A **body system** defines an anatomic region or a general physiological system on which a procedure is performed. Some body systems may be further divided into multiple body systems. For example, the cardiovascular/circulatory system is divided into the following body systems:
- Heart and great vessels
- Upper arteries
- Lower arteries
- Upper veins
- Lower veins

The body systems or the second character for the Medical and Surgical section are as follows:

0	Central nervous system
1	Peripheral nervous system
2	Heart and great vessels
3	Upper arteries
4	Lower arteries
5	Upper veins
6	Lower veins
7	Lymphatic and hemic system
8	Eye
9	Ear, nose, sinus
B	Respiratory system
C	Mouth and throat
D	Gastrointestinal system
F	Hepatobiliary system and pancreas
G	Endocrine system
H	Skin and breast
J	Subcutaneous tissue and fascia
K	Muscles
L	Tendons
M	Bursae and ligaments
N	Head and facial bones
P	Upper bones
Q	Lower bones
R	Upper joints
S	Lower joints
T	Urinary system
U	Female reproductive system
V	Male reproductive system
W	Anatomical regions, general
X	Anatomical regions, upper extremities
Y	Anatomical regions, lower extremities

According to the guidelines, the procedure codes in the general anatomical regions body systems should only be used when the procedure is performed on an anatomical region rather than a specific body part. Also when body systems are designated as upper and lower, if the body part is located above the diaphragm it is upper, and if the body part is located below the diaphragm it is considered lower.

EXERCISE 6-3

Using reference material if necessary, answer the following questions about ICD-10-PCS.

1. The thoracic nerve is in what body system? _____

2. The lacrimal gland is in what body system? _____

3. The cystic duct is in what body system? _____

Root Operations

The root operation, or the third character, identifies the main objective of the procedure performed. There is a specific definition for each root operation. Although this is part of the standardization of terminology for ICD-10-PCS, it may not be the terminology used by physicians. According to the guidelines it is the coder's responsibility to determine what the documentation in the medical record equates to in the PCS definitions. Physicians are not expected to use terminology in the same way that has been defined by PCS. For example, a TURP (transurethral resection of the prostate) includes the word resection. In

PCS resection means the cutting out/off without replacement all of a body part. A TURP is not a resection of the whole body part (prostate) so it would be coded to an excision (cutting out/off without replacement some of a body) in PCS. It would be the coder's responsibility to determine this by reading the OR report and being knowledgeable about the surgical procedure. There are 31 root operations for the Medical and Surgical section. The character value for the root operation is in parentheses following the root operation term, and an example of a procedure that fits the root operation is in parentheses following the definition. The root operation character value is consistent throughout this section. There are no combination procedure codes in ICD-10-PCS. Each procedure performed during an operative episode with a distinct objective is coded separately (see guidelines for coding multiple procedures).

Root operations that remove some/all of a body part:

- **Destruction (5):** physical eradication of all or a portion of a body part by the direct use of energy, force, or a destructive agent (ablation of endometriosis)
- **Detachment (6):** cutting off all or a portion of the upper or lower extremities (above-knee amputation)
- **Excision (B):** cutting out or off, without replacement, a portion of a body part (partial nephrectomy)
- **Extraction (D):** pulling or stripping out or off all or a portion of a body part by the use of force (bone marrow biopsy)
- **Resection (T):** cutting out or off, without replacement, all of a body part (total lobectomy of lung)

Root operations that remove solid, fluids, or gases from a body part:

- **Drainage (9):** taking or letting out fluids and/or gases from a body part (paracentesis)
- **Extirpation (C):** taking or cutting out solid matter from a body part (thrombectomy)
- **Fragmentation (F):** breaking solid matter in a body part into pieces (extracorporeal shockwave lithotripsy)

Root operations that involve cutting or separation only:

- **Division (8):** cutting into a body part without draining fluids and/or gases from the body part in order to separate or transect a body part (osteotomy)
- **Release (N):** freeing a body part from an abnormal physical constraint (lysis of adhesions)

Root operations that put in, put back, or move some or all of a body part:

- **Reattachment (M):** putting back in or on all or a portion of a separated body part to its normal location or other suitable location (reattachment of finger)
- **Reposition (S):** moving to its normal location, or other suitable location, all or a portion of a body part (fracture reduction)
- **Transfer (X):** moving, without taking out, all or a portion of a body part to another location to take over the function of all or a portion of a body part (pedicle skin flap)
- **Transplantation (Y):** putting in or on all or a portion of a living body part taken from another individual or animal to physically take the place and/or function of all or a portion of a similar body part (kidney transplant)

Root operations that alter the diameter/route of a tubular body part:

- **Bypass (1):** altering the route of passage of the contents of a tubular body part (CABG)
- **Dilation (7):** expanding an orifice or the lumen of a tubular body part (PTCA)
- **Occlusion (L):** completely closing an orifice or lumen of a tubular body part (tubal ligation)
- **Restriction (V):** partially closing an orifice or lumen of a tubular body part (Nissen fundoplication)

Root operations that always involve a device:

- **Change (2):** taking out or off a device from a body part and putting back an identical or similar device in or on the same body part without cutting or puncturing the skin or a mucous membrane (changing a gastrostomy tube)
- **Insertion (H):** putting in a nonbiological appliance that monitors, assists, performs, or prevents a physiological function but does not physically take the place of a body part (insertion of pacemaker lead)

- **Replacement (R):** putting in or on biological or synthetic material that physically takes the place and/or function of all or a portion of a body part (total knee replacement)
- **Removal (P):** taking out or off a device from a body part (removing a chest tube)
- **Revision (W):** correcting, to the extent possible, a malfunctioning or displaced device (adjustment of knee prosthesis)
- **Supplement (U):** putting in or on biological or synthetic material that physically reinforces and/or augments the function of a portion of a body part (herniorrhaphy with mesh)

Root operations that involve examination only:

- **Inspection (J):** visually and/or manually exploring a body part (diagnostic arthroscopy)
- **Map (K):** locating the route of passage of electrical impulses and/or locating functional areas in a body part (cardiac mapping)

Root operations that include other repair:

- **Control (3):** stopping, or attempting to stop, postprocedural bleeding (control of post-tonsillectomy hemorrhage)
- **Repair (Q):** restoring, to the extent possible, a body part to its normal anatomic structure and function (herniorrhaphy)

The root operation repair is used when the root operation for the procedure performed cannot be classified to a more specific root operation.

Root operations that include other objectives:

- **Alteration (0):** modifying the natural anatomic structure of a body part without affecting the function of the body part (breast augmentation)
- **Creation (4):** making a new structure that does not take over the place of a body part (creation of a vagina in males for sex reassignment)
- **Fusion (G):** joining together portions of an articular body part rendering the articular body part immobile (spinal fusion)

Terms such as *incision* or *anastomosis* are not root operations, as they are always integral to another procedure. The identification and determination of the correct root operation is vital to the selection of the appropriate table.

EXERCISE 6-4

Without using reference material, answer the following questions about ICD-10-PCS.

1. Modifying the natural anatomic structure of a body part without affecting the function of the body part is
   - **A.** alteration
   - **B.** fusion
   - **C.** creation
   - **D.** repair

2. Cutting off all or a portion of the upper or lower extremities is
   - **A.** destruction
   - **B.** fragmentation
   - **C.** detachment
   - **D.** resection

3. Completely closing an orifice or lumen of a tubular body part is
   - **A.** bypass
   - **B.** restriction
   - **C.** dilation
   - **D.** occlusion

4. Freeing a body part from an abnormal physical constraint is
   - **A.** reposition
   - **B.** division
   - **C.** release
   - **D.** transfer

5. Taking or letting out fluids and/or gases from a body part is
   A. extirpation
   B. fragmentation
   C. extraction
   D. drainage

6. Stopping, or attempting to stop, postprocedural bleeding is
   A. inspection
   B. control
   C. mapping
   D. alteration

7. Taking out or off a device from a body part is
   A. replacement
   B. removal
   C. revision
   D. change

8. Moving to its normal location or other suitable location all or a portion of a body part is
   A. reposition
   B. release
   C. transfer
   D. transplantation

9. Cutting out or off, without replacement, a portion of a body part is
   A. resection
   B. excision
   C. destruction
   D. extraction

10. Cutting into a body part without draining fluids and/or gases from the body part in order to separate or transect a body part is
    A. reattachment
    B. release
    C. transfer
    D. division

11. Putting in or on biological or synthetic material that physically reinforces and/or augments the function of a portion of a body part is
    A. restriction
    B. insertion
    C. supplementation
    D. revision

12. Visually and/or manually exploring a body part is
    A. creation
    B. fusion
    C. inspection
    D. mapping

Body Part

The body part, the fourth character, identifies the specific body part on which the procedure was performed. Each body system will have corresponding body parts. Look at the various tables to get an idea about the body parts that are body part values (Figure 6-5).

According to the guidelines, if a procedure is performed on a portion of a body part that does not have a separate body part value, code the body part value corresponding to the whole body part. If the prefix "peri" is combined with a body part to identify the site of a procedure, the procedure is coded to the body part names (e.g., perirenal is coded to kidney body part). When a specific branch of a body part does not have its own body part value in PCS, the body part is coded to the closest proximal branch that has a specific body

Section	0 Medical and Surgical
Body System	B Respiratory System
Operation	5 Destruction: Physical eradication of all or a portion of a body part by the direct use of energy, force, or a destructive agent

Body Part	Approach	Device	Qualifier
1 Trachea 2 Carina 3 Main Bronchus, Right 4 Upper Lobe Bronchus, Right 5 Middle Lobe Bronchus, Right 6 Lower Lobe Bronchus, Right 7 Main Bronchus, Left 8 Upper Lobe Bronchus, Left 9 Lingula Bronchus B Lower Lobe Bronchus, Left C Upper Lung Lobe, Right D Middle Lung Lobe, Right F Lower Lung Lobe, Right G Upper Lung Lobe, Left H Lung Lingula J Lower Lung Lobe, Left K Lung, Right L Lung, Left M Lungs, Bilateral	0 Open 3 Percutaneous 4 Percutaneous Endoscopic 7 Via Natural or Artificial Opening 8 Via Natural or Artificial Opening Endoscopic	Z No Device	Z No Qualifier
N Pleura, Right P Pleura, Left R Diaphragm, Right S Diaphragm, Left	0 Open 3 Percutaneous 4 Percutaneous Endoscopic	Z No Device	Z No Qualifier

FIGURE 6-5. Table for destruction of respiratory system.

part value. If an identical procedure is performed on bilateral body parts and a bilateral body part value exists for that body part, a single procedure code is assigned. If no bilateral body part value exists, each procedure is coded separately using the appropriate body part value.

Approaches

The approach, the fifth character, identifies the operative approach or the method used to reach the operative site. There is a specific definition for each approach. Although this is part of the standardization of terminology for ICD-10-PCS, it may not be the terminology used by physicians. There are seven approaches for the Medical and Surgical section (Figure 6-6). An example is included in parentheses following the definition. The character value and definition for the approaches are as follows:

0   **Open:** cutting through the skin, mucous membrane, and any other body layers necessary to expose the site of the procedure (abdominal hysterectomy)

3   **Percutaneous:** entry, by puncture or minor incision, of instrumentation through the skin, mucous membrane, and any other body layers necessary to reach the site of the procedure (needle biopsy liver)

4   **Percutaneous endoscopic:** entry, by puncture or minor incision, of instrumentation through the skin, mucous membrane, and any other body layers necessary to reach and visualize the site of the procedure (laparoscopic cholecystectomy)

7   **Via natural or artificial opening:** entry of instrumentation through a natural or artificial external opening to reach the site of the procedure (endotracheal intubation)

8   **Via natural or artificial opening endoscopic:** entry of instrumentation through a natural or artificial external opening to reach and visualize the site of the procedure (colonoscopy)

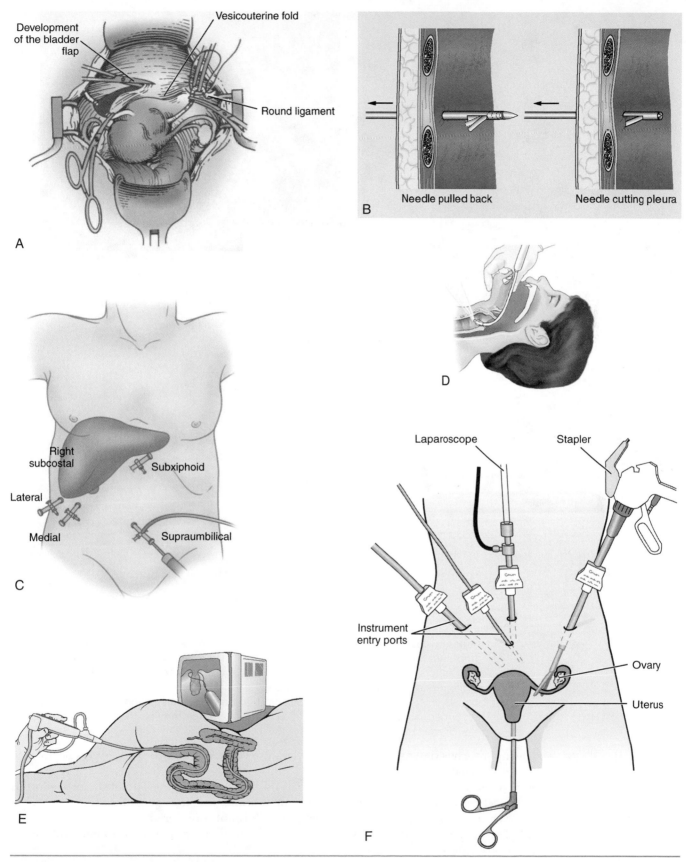

FIGURE 6-6. Surgical approaches.

Continued

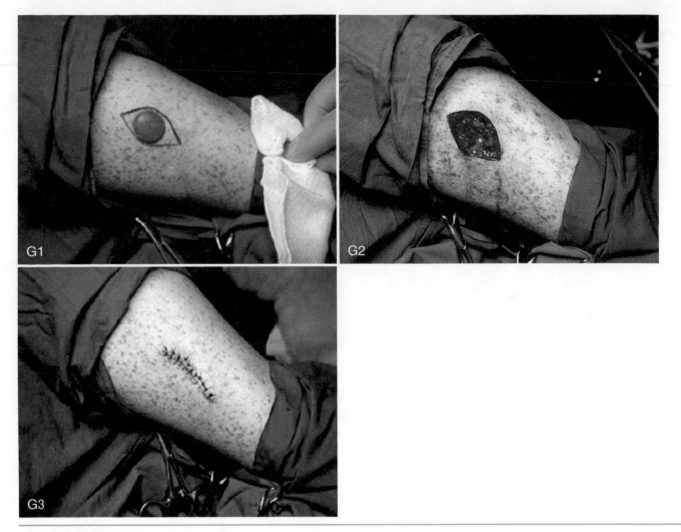

FIGURE 6-6, cont'd

F   **Via natural or artificial opening with percutaneous endoscopic assistance:** cutting through the skin, mucous membrane, and any other body layers necessary to expose the site of the procedure, and entry, by puncture or minor incision, of instrumentation through the skin, mucous membrane, and any other body layers necessary to aid in the performance of the procedure (laparoscopic-assisted vaginal hysterectomy)

X   **External:** procedures performed directly on the skin or mucous membrane and procedures performed indirectly by the application of external force through the skin or mucous membrane (tonsillectomy)

The approach is determined by the following three components for procedures performed on an internal body part:

■   Access location—specifies the external site through which the site of the procedure is reached, either through skin, mucous membrane, or external orifices

■   Method—specifies how the external access location is entered

■   Type of instrumentation—specifies the specialized equipment used to perform the procedure

According to the guidelines, procedures performed using an open approach with percutaneous endoscopic assistance are coded to open approach. External approach includes procedures performed within an orifice on structures that are visible without the aid of any instrumentation. Another example of an external approach is when a procedure is performed indirectly by using external force through the intervening body layers (e.g., closed reduction of a fracture). Procedures that are performed percutaneously via a device placed for the procedures are coded to percutaneous approach.

Computer and Robotic-Assisted Surgery

Advances in computer technologies have made it possible for computers to be utilized in the performance of diagnostic and therapeutic procedures. **Computer assisted surgery (CAS)** is an adjunct procedure that allows increased visualization and more precise navigation during surgery. CAS may be useful with surgical planning by using preoperative and intraoperative images. The computers identify particular landmarks and then establish spatial relationships between locations on the computer images with the actual corresponding anatomic locations on the patient. Navigation is real-time tracking of instruments during the procedure.

Robotic-assisted surgery is a minimally invasive technique that utilizes robotic arms to manipulate the surgical equipment and tools. A physician sits at a console and controls the joysticks that guide the robot in the performance of the surgical procedure. Unlike CAS, robotic-assisted procedures include the actual performance of the procedure. To identify that a procedure was assisted by computer or robotic technologies, an additional code from Table 8E0 is assigned (Figure 6-7).

| EXAMPLE | Patient with prostate cancer had a robotic-assisted laparoscopic radical prostatectomy including seminal vesicles with diagnostic pelvic lymphadenectomy (total of three nodes), C61, 0VT04ZZ, 0VT34ZZ, 07BC4ZX, 8E0W4CZ. |

EXERCISE 6-5

Without the use of reference material, answer the following questions about ICD-10-PCS.

1. Entry of instrumentation, by puncture or minor incision, through the skin, mucous membrane, and any other body layers necessary to reach the site of the procedure is
   A. open
   B. percutaneous
   C. percutaneous endoscopic
   D. open with percutaneous endoscopic assistance

2. Cutting through the skin, mucous membrane, and any other body layers necessary to expose the site of the procedure is
   A. open
   B. percutaneous
   C. percutaneous endoscopic
   D. open with percutaneous endoscopic assistance

3. Procedures performed directly on the skin or mucous membrane and procedures performed indirectly by the application of external force through the skin or mucous membrane are
   A. percutaneous
   B. open
   C. via natural or artificial opening
   D. external

SECTION: 8 OTHER PROCEDURES
BODY SYSTEM: E PHYSIOLOGICAL SYSTEMS AND ANATOMICAL REGIONS
OPERATION 0 OTHER PROCEDURES: *(on multiple pages)*

Methodologies which attempt to remediate or cure a disorder or disease

Body Region	Approach	Method	Qualifier
1 Nervous System	X External	6 Collection	J Cerebrospinal Fluid L Other Fluid
2 Circulatory System	X External	6 Collection	K Blood L Other Fluid
1 Nervous System U Female Reproductive System	X External	Y Other Method	7 Examination
2 Circulatory System	3 Percutaneous	D Near Infrared Spectroscopy	Z No Qualifier
9 Head and Neck Region W Trunk Region	0 Open 3 Percutaneous 4 Percutaneous Endoscopic 7 Via Natural or Artificial Opening 8 Via Natural or Artificial Opening Endoscopic	C Robotic Assisted Procedure ←	Z No Qualifier
9 Head and Neck Region W Trunk Region	X External →	B Computer Assisted Procedure	F With Fluoroscopy G With Computerized Tomography H With Magnetic Resonance Imaging Z No Qualifier
9 Head and Neck Region W Trunk Region	X External	C Robotic Assisted Procedure	Z No Qualifier
9 Head and Neck Region W Trunk Region	X External	Y Other Method	8 Suture Removal

FIGURE 6-7. Table 8E0, which shows computer and robotic assisted methods.

Device

The device, the sixth character, identifies a device that remains after the procedure is completed. There are four types of devices:

- Biological or synthetic material that takes the place of all or a portion of a body part
- Biological or synthetic material that assists or prevents a physiological function
- Therapeutic material that is not absorbed by, eliminated by, or incorporated into a body part
- Mechanical or electronic appliances used to assist, monitor, take the place of, or prevent a physiological function

The root operations change, insertion, removal, replacement, revision, and supplement always involve a device. Materials that are part of a procedure—such as clips, ligatures, and sutures—are not considered devices. There is a value for other devices (Y; Figure 6-8), which can be used until more specific devices are added to the ICD-10 coding procedural system.

Section	0 **Medical and Surgical**
Body System	0 **Central Nervous System**
Operation	2 **Change:** Taking out or off a device from a body part and putting back an identical or similar device in or on the same body part without cutting or puncturing the skin or a mucous membrane

Body Part	Approach	Device	Qualifier
0 Brain E Cranial Nerve U Spinal Canal	X External	0 Drainage Device Y Other Device ←	Z No Qualifier

FIGURE 6-8. Table for change in central nervous system.

EXERCISE 6-6

Without the use of reference material, answer the following questions about ICD-10-PCS.

1. Sutures are considered a device.
   A. True
   B. False

2. A device is left in place after completion of the procedure.
   A. True
   B. False

3. The root operation insertion always involves a device.
   A. True
   B. False

Qualifier

The qualifier, the seventh character, identifies a unique value for an individual procedure. A qualifier may indicate that a procedure was done for diagnostic purposes (Figure 6-9); in coronary artery bypass procedures, the qualifier identifies the origin of the bypass (Figure 6-10).

EXAMPLE Diagnostic thoracentesis, left pleura cavity (removal of fluid from pleural cavity).
The root operation is drainage, taking or letting out fluids and/or gases from a body part.
In the Alphabetic Index, under the term thoracentesis, it says to see Drainage, Anatomical Regions.
Under the term drainage, pleural cavity, go to Table 0W9 (Figure 6-11) and assign Characters 4 through 7. Character 4 is B for the pleural cavity, left. Character 5 is percutaneous because a thoracentesis is usually done percutaneously. Character 6 is Z, no device, and Character 7, is X because the procedure was diagnostic.

CHARACTER 1	CHARACTER 2	CHARACTER 3	CHARACTER 4	CHARACTER 5	CHARACTER 6	CHARACTER 7
0	W	9	B	3	Z	X

EXAMPLE Partial right laparoscopic nephrectomy for known malignant neoplasm.
The root operation is excision, cutting out or off, without replacement, a portion of a body part.
Under the term nephrectomy, excision, go to Table 0TB (Figure 6-12), and assign Characters 4 through 7. Character 4 is 0 for kidney, right. Character 5 is percutaneous endoscopic because the procedure was performed laparoscopically. Character 6 is Z, no device, and Character 7 is Z because the procedure was a definitive procedure for a known malignancy so it was not diagnostic.

CHARACTER 1	CHARACTER 2	CHARACTER 3	CHARACTER 4	CHARACTER 5	CHARACTER 6	CHARACTER 7
0	T	B	0	4	Z	Z

Section	**0 Medical and Surgical**			
Body System	**K Muscles**			
Operation	**B Excision:** Cutting out or off, without replacement, a portion of a body part			

Body Part	Approach	Device	Qualifier
0 Head Muscle **1** Facial Muscle **2** Neck Muscle, Right **3** Neck Muscle, Left **4** Tongue, Palate, Pharynx Muscle **5** Shoulder Muscle, Right **6** Shoulder Muscle, Left **7** Upper Arm Muscle, Right **8** Upper Arm Muscle, Left **9** Lower Arm and Wrist Muscle, Right **B** Lower Arm and Wrist Muscle, Left **C** Hand Muscle, Right **D** Hand Muscle, Left **F** Trunk Muscle, Right **G** Trunk Muscle, Left **H** Thorax Muscle, Right **J** Thorax Muscle, Left **K** Abdomen Muscle, Right **L** Abdomen Muscle, Left **M** Perineum Muscle **N** Hip Muscle, Right **P** Hip Muscle, Left **Q** Upper Leg Muscle, Right **R** Upper Leg Muscle, Left **S** Lower Leg Muscle, Right **T** Lower Leg Muscle, Left **V** Foot Muscle, Right **W** Foot Muscle, Left	**0** Open **3** Percutaneous **4** Percutaneous Endoscopic	**Z** No Device	**X** Diagnostic ◄ **Z** No Qualifier

FIGURE 6-9. Table for excision of muscles.

ICD-10-PCS CODING GUIDELINES

The ICD-10-PCS guidelines are available at the Centers for Medicare and Medicaid (CMS) website. The guidelines are divided into three parts:

A. Conventions
B. Medical and Surgical Section Guidelines
   • Body system
   • Root operation
   • Body part
   • Approach
   • Device
C. Obstetrics Section Guidelines

Please refer to the companion Evolve website for the most current guidelines.

There are many guidelines for ICD-10-PCS. Within the ICD-10-PCS guidelines, examples are given. Instead of providing the codes for those examples, you will be assigning the codes for most of the examples. This will give you practice with both coding and applying the guidelines. Practice is the best teacher. Assign only the ICD-10-PCS codes. Most of the guidelines deal with the root operation which is the main objective of the procedure.

Section	0 Medical and Surgical
Body System	2 Heart and Great Vessels
Operation	1 **Bypass**: Altering the route of passage of the contents of a tubular body part

Body Part	Approach	Device	Qualifier
0 Coronary Artery, One Site 1 Coronary Artery, Two Sites 2 Coronary Artery, Three Sites 3 Coronary Artery, Four or More Sites	0 Open	9 Autologous Venous Tissue A Autologous Arterial Tissue J Synthetic Substitute K Nonautologous Tissue Substitute	3 Coronary Artery 8 Internal Mammary, Right 9 Internal Mammary, Left C Thoracic Artery F Abdominal Artery W Aorta
0 Coronary Artery, One Site 1 Coronary Artery, Two Sites 2 Coronary Artery, Three Sites 3 Coronary Artery, Four or More Sites	0 Open	Z No Device	3 Coronary Artery 8 Internal Mammary, Right 9 Internal Mammary, Left C Thoracic Artery F Abdominal Artery
0 Coronary Artery, One Site 1 Coronary Artery, Two Sites 2 Coronary Artery, Three Sites 3 Coronary Artery, Four or More Sites	3 Percutaneous	4 Intraluminal Device, Drug-eluting D Intraluminal Device	4 Coronary Vein
0 Coronary Artery, One Site 1 Coronary Artery, Two Sites 2 Coronary Artery, Three Sites 3 Coronary Artery, Four or More Sites	4 Percutaneous Endoscopic	4 Intraluminal Device, Drug-eluting D Intraluminal Device	4 Coronary Vein
0 Coronary Artery, One Site 1 Coronary Artery, Two Sites 2 Coronary Artery, Three Sites 3 Coronary Artery, Four or More Sites	4 Percutaneous Endoscopic	9 Autologous Venous Tissue A Autologous Arterial Tissue J Synthetic Substitute K Nonautologous Tissue Substitute	3 Coronary Artery 8 Internal Mammary, Right 9 Internal Mammary, Left C Thoracic Artery F Abdominal Artery W Aorta
0 Coronary Artery, One Site 1 Coronary Artery, Two Sites 2 Coronary Artery, Three Sites 3 Coronary Artery, Four or More Sites	4 Percutaneous Endoscopic	Z No Device	3 Coronary Artery 8 Internal Mammary, Right 9 Internal Mammary, Left C Thoracic Artery F Abdominal Artery
6 Atrium, Right	0 Open 4 Percutaneous Endoscopic	9 Autologous Venous Tissue A Autologous Arterial Tissue J Synthetic Substitute K Nonautologous Tissue Substitute	P Pulmonary Trunk Q Pulmonary Artery, Right R Pulmonary Artery, Left

FIGURE 6-10. Table for bypass of heart and great vessels.

Section	0 Medical and Surgical
Body System	W Anatomical Regions, General
Operation	9 **Drainage**: Taking or letting out fluids and/or gases from a body part

Body Part	Approach	Device	Qualifier
0 Head 1 Cranial Cavity 2 Face 3 Oral Cavity and Throat 4 Upper Jaw 5 Lower Jaw 6 Neck 8 Chest Wall 9 Pleural Cavity, Right B Pleural Cavity, Left C Mediastinum D Pericardial Cavity F Abdominal Wall G Peritoneal Cavity H Retroperitoneum J Pelvic Cavity K Upper Back L Lower Back M Perineum, Male N Perineum, Female	0 Open 3 Percutaneous 4 Percutaneous Endoscopic	Z No Device	X Diagnostic Z No Qualifier

FIGURE 6-11. Table for drainage of anatomical region.

Section	0 **Medical and Surgical**
Body System	T **Urinary System**
Operation	B **Excision**: Cutting out or off, without replacement, a portion of a body part

Body Part	Approach	Device	Qualifier
0 Kidney, Right 1 Kidney, Left 3 Kidney Pelvis, Right 4 Kidney Pelvis, Left 6 Ureter, Right 7 Ureter, Left B Bladder C Bladder Neck	0 Open 3 Percutaneous 4 Percutaneous Endoscopic ←—————— 7 Via Natural or Artificial Opening 8 Via Natural or Artificial Opening Endoscopic	Z No Device ←———————	X Diagnostic Z No Qualifier
D Urethra	0 Open 3 Percutaneous 4 Percutaneous Endoscopic 7 Via Natural or Artificial Opening 8 Via Natural or Artificial Opening Endoscopic X External	Z No Device	X Diagnostic Z No Qualifier

FIGURE 6-12. Table for excision of urinary system.

ICD-10-PCS

Coding Guidelines
(2013)

See the CMS website at www.cms.gov for the Introduction to the ICD-10-PCS Coding Guidelines.

A. Conventions

A1. ICD-10-PCS codes are composed of seven characters. Each character is an axis of classification that specifies information about the procedure performed. Within a defined code range, a character specifies the same type of information in that axis of classification.
Example: The fifth axis of classification specifies the approach in sections 0 through 4 and 7 through 9 of the system.

A2. One of 34 possible values can be assigned to each axis of classification in the seven-character code: they are the numbers 0 through 9 and the alphabet (except I and O because they are easily confused with the numbers 1 and 0). The number of unique values used in an axis of classification differs as needed.
Example: Where the fifth axis of classification specifies the approach, seven different approach values are currently used to specify the approach.

A3. The valid values for an axis of classification can be added to as needed.
Example: If a significantly distinct type of device is used in a new procedure, a new device value can be added to the system.

A4. As with words in their context, the meaning of any single value is a combination of its axis of classification and any preceding values on which it may be dependent.
Example: The meaning of a body part value in the Medical and Surgical section is always dependent on the body system value. The body part value 0 in the Central Nervous body system specifies brain and the body part value 0 in the peripheral nervous body system specifies Cervical Plexus.

A5. As the system is expanded to become increasingly detailed, over time more values will depend on preceding values for their meaning.
Example: In the Lower Joints body system, the device value 3 in the root operation Insertion specifies Infusion Device and the device value 3 in the root operation Replacement specifies Ceramic Synthetic Substitute.

A6. The purpose of the alphabetic index is to locate the appropriate table that contains all information necessary to construct a procedure code. The PCS Tables should always be consulted to find the most appropriate valid code.

A7. It is not required to consult the index first before proceeding to the tables to complete the code. A valid code may be chosen directly from the tables.

A8. All seven characters must be specified to be a valid code. If the documentation is incomplete for coding purposes, the physician should be queried for the necessary information.

A9. Within a PCS table, valid codes include all combinations of choices in characters 4 through 7 contained in the same row of the table. In the example below, 0JHT3VZ is a valid code, and 0JHW3VZ is *not* a valid code.

Section: O Medical and Surgical
Body System: J Subcutaneous Tissue and Fascia
Operation: H Insertion: Putting in a nonbiological appliance that monitors, assists, performs, or prevents a physiological function but does not physically take the place of a body part

BODY PART	APPROACH	DEVICE	QUALIFIER
S Subcutaneous Tissue and Fascia, Head and Neck V Subcutaneous Tissue and Fascia, Upper Extremity W Subcutaneous Tissue and Fascia, Lower Extremity	0 Open 3 Percutaneous	1 Radioactive Element 3 Infusion Device	Z No Qualifier
T Subcutaneous Tissue and Fascia, Trunk	0 Open 3 Percutaneous	1 Radioactive Element 3 Infusion Device V Infusion Pump	Z No Qualifier

A10. "And," when used in a code description, means "and/or."
Example: Lower Arm and Wrist Muscle means lower arm and/or wrist muscle.

A11. Many of the terms used to construct PCS codes are defined within the system. It is the coder's responsibility to determine what the documentation in the medical record equates to in the PCS definitions. The physician is not expected to use the terms used in PCS code descriptions, nor is the coder required to query the physician when the correlation between the documentation and the defined PCS terms is clear.
Example: When the physician documents "partial resection" the coder can independently correlate "partial resection" to the root operation Excision without querying the physician for clarification.

B. *Medical and Surgical Section Guidelines (section O)*

B2. Body System
General guidelines

B2.1a. The procedure codes in the general anatomical regions body systems should only be used when the procedure is performed on an anatomical region rather than a specific body part (e.g., root operations Control and Detachment, drainage of a body cavity) or on the rare occasion when no information is available to support assignment of a code to a specific body part.
Example: Control of postoperative hemorrhage is coded to the root operation Control found in the general anatomical regions body systems.

B2.1b. Where the general body part values "upper" and "lower" are provided as an option in the Upper Arteries, Lower Arteries, Upper Veins, Lower Veins, Muscles and Tendons body systems, "upper" or "lower" specifies body parts located above or below the diaphragm respectively.
Example: Vein body parts above the diaphragm are found in the Upper Veins body system; vein body parts below the diaphragm are found in the Lower Veins body system.

B3. Root Operation
General guidelines

B3.1a. In order to determine the appropriate root operation, the full definition of the root operation as contained in the PCS Tables must be applied.

B3.1b. Components of a procedure specified in the root operation definition and explanation are not coded separately. Procedural steps necessary to reach the operative site and close the operative site, including anastomosis of a tubular body part, are also not coded separately.
Example: Resection of a joint as part of a joint replacement procedure is included in the root operation definition of Replacement and is not coded separately. Laparotomy performed to reach the site of an open liver biopsy is not coded separately. In a resection of sigmoid colon with anastomosis of descending colon to rectum, the anastomosis in not coded separately.

1. Total right shoulder replacement with prosthesis   _____

2. Laparotomy with open liver biopsy   _____

Multiple procedures

B3.2.   During the same operative episode, multiple procedures are coded if:

    a. The same root operation is performed on different body parts as defined by distinct values of the body part character.

    Example: Diagnostic excision of liver and pancreas are coded separately.

3. Diagnostic excision of liver and pancreas   _____

    b. The same root operation is repeated at different body sites that are included in the same body part value.

    Example: Excision of the sartorius muscle and excision of the gracilis muscle are both included in the upper leg muscle body part value, and multiple procedures are coded.

4. Excision of the sartorius muscle and excision of the gracilis   _____ muscle right upper leg

    c. Multiple root operations with distinct objectives are performed on the same body part.

    Example: Destruction of sigmoid lesion and bypass of sigmoid colon are coded separately.

5. Destruction of sigmoid lesion and bypass of sigmoid colon   _____ to rectum

    d. The intended root operation is attempted using one approach, but is converted to a different approach.

    Example: Laparoscopic cholecystectomy converted to an open cholecystectomy is coded as percutaneous endoscopic Inspection and open Resection.

6. Laparoscopic cholecystectomy with conversion to open   _____ cholecystectomy

Discontinued procedures

B3.3.   If the intended procedure is discontinued, code the procedure to the root operation performed. If a procedure is discontinued before any other root operation is performed, code the root operation Inspection of the body part or anatomical region inspected.

    Example: A planned aortic valve replacement procedure is discontinued after the initial thoracotomy and before any incision is made in the heart muscle, when the patient becomes hemodynamically unstable. This procedure is coded as an open Inspection of the mediastinum.

7. Planned aortic valve replacement but procedure canceled   _____ after thoracotomy was performed

Biopsy followed by more definitive treatment

B3.4.   If a diagnostic Excision, Extraction, or Drainage procedure (biopsy) is followed by a more definitive procedure, such as Destruction, Excision or Resection at the same procedure site, both the biopsy and the more definitive treatment are coded.

    Example: Biopsy of breast followed by partial mastectomy at the same procedure site, both the biopsy and the partial mastectomy procedure are coded.

8. Open excisional biopsy of left breast with partial left   _____
mastectomy

> *Overlapping body layers*
> **B3.5.**   If the root operations Excision, Repair or Inspection are performed on overlapping layers of the musculoskeletal system, the body part specifying the deepest layer is coded.
> *Example*: Excisional debridement that includes skin and subcutaneous tissue and muscle is coded to the muscle body part.

9. Open debridement of the subcutaneous tissue and   _____
brachioradialis muscle, right

> *Bypass procedures*
> **B3.6a.**   Bypass procedures are coded by identifying the body part bypassed "from" and the body part bypassed "to." The fourth character body part specifies the body part bypassed from, and the qualifier specifies the body part bypassed to.
> *Example*: Bypass from stomach to jejunum, stomach is the body part and jejunum is the qualifier.

10. Bypass from stomach to jejunum   _____

> **B3.6b.**   Coronary arteries are classified by number of distinct sites treated, rather than number of coronary arteries or anatomic name of a coronary artery (e.g., left anterior descending). Coronary artery bypass procedures are coded differently than other bypass procedures as described in the previous guideline. Rather than identifying the body part bypassed from, the body part identifies the number of coronary artery sites bypassed to, and the qualifier specifies the vessel bypassed from.
> *Example*: Aortocoronary artery bypass of one site on the left anterior descending coronary artery and one site on the obtuse marginal coronary artery is classified in the body part axis of classification as two coronary artery sites and the qualifier specifies the aorta as the body part bypassed from.
> **B3.6c.**   If multiple coronary artery sites are bypassed, a separate procedure is coded for each coronary artery site that uses a different device and/or qualifier.
> *Example*: Aortocoronary artery bypass and internal mammary coronary artery bypass are coded separately.

11. CABG (left anterior descending and obtuse marginal   _____
coronary arteries) with excision of right greater saphenous
vein via percutaneous endoscopic approach (see Guideline
B3.9) and left internal mammary coronary artery bypass

> *Control vs. more definitive root operations*
> **B3.7.**   The root operation Control is defined as, "Stopping, or attempting to stop, postprocedural bleeding." If an attempt to stop postprocedural bleeding is initially unsuccessful, and to stop the bleeding requires performing any of the definitive root operations Bypass, Detachment, Excision, Extraction, Reposition, Replacement, or Resection, then that root operation is coded instead of Control.
> *Example*: Resection of spleen to stop postprocedural bleeding is coded to Resection instead of Control.

12. Resection of spleen to stop postprocedural bleeding   _____

Excision vs. Resection

B3.8. PCS contains specific body parts for anatomical subdivisions of a body part, such as lobes of the lungs or liver and regions of the intestine. Resection of the specific body part is coded whenever all of the body part is cut out or off, rather than coding Excision of a less specific body part.

Example: Left upper lung lobectomy is coded to Resection of Upper Lung Lobe, Left rather than Excision of Lung, Left.

13. Left upper lung lobectomy   _____

Excision for graft

B3.9. If an autograft is obtained from a different body part in order to complete the objective of the procedure, a separate procedure is coded.

Example: Coronary bypass with excision of saphenous vein graft, excision of saphenous vein is coded separately.

Fusion procedures of the spine

B3.10a. The body part coded for a spinal vertebral joint(s) rendered immobile by a spinal fusion procedure is classified by the level of the spine (e.g. thoracic). There are distinct body part values for a single vertebral joint and for multiple vertebral joints at each spinal level.

Example: Body part values specify Lumbar Vertebral Joint, Lumbar Vertebral Joints, 2 or More; and Lumbosacral Vertebral Joint.

14. Posterior spinal fusion with L1-3 with BAK interbody fusion   _____
device and morsellized bone graft from the operative site
(See Guideline B3.10c)

B3.10b. If multiple vertebral joints are fused, a separate procedure is coded for each vertebral joint that uses a different device and/or qualifier.

Example: Fusion of lumbar vertebral joint, posterior approach, anterior column and fusion of lumbar vertebral joint, posterior approach, posterior column are coded separately.

B3.10c. Combinations of devices and materials are often used on a vertebral joint to render the joint immobile. When combinations of devices are used on the same vertebral joint, the device value coded for the procedure is as follows:

- If an interbody fusion device is used to render the joint immobile (alone or containing other material like bone graft), the procedure is coded with the device value Interbody Fusion Device
- If bone graft is the *only* device used to render the joint immobile, the procedure is coded with the device value Nonautologous Tissue Substitute or Autologous Tissue Substitute
- If a mixture of autologous and nonautologous bone graft (with or without biological or synthetic extenders or binders) is used to render the joint immobile, code the procedure with the device value Autologous Tissue Substitute

Examples: Fusion of a vertebral joint using a cage style interbody fusion device containing morsellized bone graft is coded to the device Interbody Fusion Device. Fusion of a vertebral joint using a bone dowel interbody fusion device made of cadaver bone and packed with a mixture of local morsellized bone and demineralized bone matrix is coded to the device Interbody Fusion Device.

Fusion of a vertebral joint using both autologous bone graft and bone bank bone graft is coded to the device Autologous Tissue Substitute.

Inspection procedures

B3.11a. Inspection of a body part(s) performed in order to achieve the objective of a procedure is not coded separately.

Example: Fiberoptic bronchoscopy performed for irrigation of bronchus, only the irrigation procedure is coded.

15. Fiberoptic bronchoscopy for irrigation of bronchus   _____

> **B3.11b.** If multiple tubular body parts are inspected, the most distal body part inspected is coded. If multiple non-tubular body parts in a region are inspected, the body part that specifies the entire area inspected is coded.
> *Examples*: Cystoureteroscopy with inspection of bladder and ureters is coded to the ureter body part value.
>   Exploratory laparotomy with general inspection of abdominal contents is coded to the peritoneal cavity body part value.

16. Diagnostic cystourethroscopy of bladder   _____

17. Exploratory laparotomy   _____

> **B3.11c.** When both an Inspection procedure and another procedure are performed on the same body part during the same episode, if the Inspection procedure is performed using a different approach than the other procedure, the Inspection procedure is coded separately.
> *Example*: Endoscopic Inspection of the duodenum is coded separately when open Excision of the duodenum is performed during the same procedural episode.

18. Endoscopic inspection of duodenum with open excision of   _____
    duodenum

> *Occlusion vs. Restriction for vessel embolization procedures*
> **B3.12.** If the objective of an embolization procedure is to completely close a vessel, the root operation Occlusion is coded. If the objective of an embolization procedure is to narrow the lumen of a vessel, the root operation Restriction is coded.
> *Examples*: Tumor embolization is coded to the root operation Occlusion, because the objective of the procedure is to cut off the blood supply to the vessel.
>   Embolization of a cerebral aneurysm is coded to the root operation Restriction, because the objective of the procedure is not to close off the vessel entirely, but to narrow the lumen of the vessel at the site of the aneurysm where it is abnormally wide.

19. Preoperative embolization of right renal artery in patient   _____
    with renal cell carcinoma right kidney

20. Embolization of right internal carotid artery aneurysm   _____

> *Release procedures*
> **B3.13.** In the root operation Release, the body part value coded is the body part being freed and not the tissue being manipulated or cut to free the body part.
> *Example*: Lysis of intestinal adhesions is coded to the specific intestine body part value.

21. Laparoscopic lysis of adhesions small bowel   _____

> *Release vs. Division*
> **B3.14.** If the sole objective of the procedure is freeing a body part without cutting the body part, the root operation is Release. If the sole objective of the procedure is separating or transecting a body part, the root operation is Division.
> *Examples*: Freeing a nerve root from surrounding scar tissue to relieve pain is coded to the root operation Release. Severing a nerve root to relieve pain is coded to the root operation Division.

22. Release of carpal tunnel, percutaneous endoscopic approach   _____

23. Trigeminal rhizotomy   _____

> *Reposition for fracture treatment*
> **B3.15.** Reduction of a displaced fracture is coded to the root operation Reposition and the application of a cast or splint in conjunction with the Reposition procedure is not coded separately. Treatment of a nondisplaced fracture is coded to the procedure performed.
> *Examples*: Putting a pin in a nondisplaced fracture is coded to the root operation Insertion.
> Casting of a nondisplaced fracture is coded to the root operation Immobilization in the Placement section.

24. Percutaneous pinning of right nondisplaced distal radial fracture   _____

25. Casting of nondisplaced left distal radial fracture   _____

> *Transplantation vs. Administration*
> **B3.16.** Putting in a mature and functioning living body part taken from another individual or animal is coded to the root operation Transplantation. Putting in autologous or nonautologous cells is coded to the Administration section.
> *Example*: Putting in autologous or nonautologous bone marrow, pancreatic islet cells or stem cells is coded to the Administration section.

26. Transplant of pancreatic islet cells (nonautologous) via portal vein   _____

> **B4. Body Part**
> *General guidelines*
> **B4.1a.** If a procedure is performed on a portion of a body part that does not have a separate body part value, code the body part value corresponding to the whole body part.
> *Example*: A procedure performed on the alveolar process of the mandible is coded to the mandible body part.
> **B4.1b.** If the prefix "peri" is combined with a body part to identify the site of the procedure, the procedure is coded to the body part named.
> *Example*: A procedure site identified as perirenal is coded to the kidney body part.

27. Percutaneous drainage of a left perirenal abscess   _____

> *Branches of body parts*
> **B4.2.** Where a specific branch of a body part does not have its own body part value in PCS, the body part is coded to the closest proximal branch that has a specific body part value.
> *Example*: A procedure performed on the mandibular branch of the trigeminal nerve is coded to the trigeminal nerve body part value

28. Release of maxillary nerve   _____

Bilateral body part values

B4.3. Bilateral body part values are available for a limited number of body parts. If the identical procedure is performed on contralateral body parts, and a bilateral body part value exists for that body part, a single procedure is coded using the bilateral body part value. If no bilateral body part value exists, each procedure is coded separately using the appropriate body part value.

Example: The identical procedure performed on both fallopian tubes is coded once using the body part value Fallopian Tube, Bilateral. The identical procedure performed on both knee joints is coded twice using the body part values Knee Joint, Right and Knee Joint, Left.

29. Laparoscopic occlusion of bilateral fallopian tubes using _____ extraluminal clips

30. Bilateral knee replacement (synthetic prostheses) _____

Coronary arteries

B4.4. The coronary arteries are classified as a single body part that is further specified by number of sites treated and not by name or number of arteries. Separate body part values are used to specify the number of sites treated when the same procedure is performed on multiple sites in the coronary arteries.

Examples: Angioplasty of two distinct sites in the left anterior descending coronary artery with placement of two stents is coded as Dilation of Coronary Arteries, Two Sites, with Intraluminal Device.

Angioplasty of two distinct sites in the left anterior descending coronary artery, one with stent placed and one without, is coded separately as Dilation of Coronary Artery, One Site with Intraluminal Device, and Dilation of Coronary Artery, One Site with no device.

31. PTCA of two distinct sites of the left anterior descending _____ artery with placement of two drug-eluting stents

32. PTCA of two distinct sites of the left anterior descending _____ artery with placement of one nondrug-eluting stent

Tendons, ligaments, bursae and fascia near a joint

B4.5. Procedures performed on tendons, ligaments, bursae and fascia supporting a joint are coded to the body part in the respective body system that is the focus of the procedure. Procedures performed on joint structures themselves are coded to the body part in the joint body systems.

Example: Repair of the anterior cruciate ligament of the knee is coded to the knee bursae and ligament body part in the bursae and ligaments body system. Knee arthroscopy with shaving of articular cartilage is coded to the knee joint body part in the Lower Joints body system.

Skin, subcutaneous tissue and fascia overlying a joint

B4.6. If a procedure is performed on the skin, subcutaneous tissue or fascia overlying a joint, the procedure is coded to the following body part:
- Shoulder is coded to Upper Arm
- Elbow is coded to Lower Arm
- Wrist is coded to Lower Arm
- Hip is coded to Upper Leg
- Knee is coded to Lower Leg
- Ankle is coded to Foot

33. Suture of laceration to skin and subcutaneous tissue left _____ knee

Fingers and toes

B4.7. If a body system does not contain a separate body part value for fingers, procedures performed on the fingers are coded to the body part value for the hand. If a body system does not contain a separate body part value for toes, procedures performed on the toes are coded to the body part value for the foot.
Example: Excision of finger muscle is coded to one of the hand muscle body part values in the Muscles body system.

B4.8. In the Gastrointestinal body system, the general body part values Upper Intestinal Tract and Lower Intestinal Tract are provided as an option for the root operations Change, Inspection, Removal and Revision. Upper Intestinal Tract includes the portion of the gastrointestinal tract from the esophagus down to and including the duodenum, and Lower Intestinal Tract includes the portion of the gastrointestinal tract from the jejunum down to and including the rectum and anus.
Example: In the root operation Change table, change of a device in the jejunum is coded using the body part Lower Intestinal Tract.

34. Excision of hypothenar muscle, right _____

B5. Approach
Open approach with percutaneous endoscopic assistance
B5.2. Procedures performed using the open approach with percutaneous endoscopic assistance are coded to the approach Open.
Example: Laparoscopic-assisted sigmoidectomy is coded to the approach Open.

35. Laparoscopic-assisted sigmoidectomy _____

External approach
B5.3a. Procedures performed within an orifice on structures that are visible without the aid of any instrumentation are coded to the approach External.
Example: Resection of tonsils is coded to the approach External.

36. Resection of tonsils _____

B5.3b. Procedures performed indirectly by the application of external force through the intervening body layers are coded to the approach External.
Example: Closed reduction of fracture is coded to the approach External.

37. Closed reduction of left distal radius fracture _____

Percutaneous procedure via device
B5.4. Procedures performed percutaneously via a device placed for the procedure are coded to the approach Percutaneous.
Example: Fragmentation of kidney stone performed via percutaneous nephrostomy is coded to the approach Percutaneous.

38. Fragmentation of right kidney stone performed via percutaneous nephrostomy _____

B6. Device
General guidelines
B6.1a. A device is coded only if a device remains after the procedure is completed. If no device remains, the device value No Device is coded.

39. Percutaneous insertion of central venous line in right _____
    internal jugular vein

> **B6.1b.** Materials such as sutures, ligatures, radiological markers and temporary post-operative wound drains are considered integral to the performance of a procedure and are not coded as devices.
>
> **B6.1c.** Procedures performed on a device only and not on a body part are specified in the root operations Change, Irrigation, Removal and Revision, and are coded to the procedure performed.
> _Example_: Irrigation of percutaneous nephrostomy tube is coded to the root operation Irrigation of indwelling device in the Administration section.

40. Irrigation of left percutaneous nephrostomy tube _____

> _Drainage device_
> **B6.2.** A separate procedure to put in a drainage device is coded to the root operation Drainage with the device value Drainage Device.

41. Insertion of indwelling Foley catheter _____

> **_Obstetric Section Guidelines (section 1)_**
> **C. Obstetrics Section**
> _Products of conception_
> **C1.** Procedures performed on the products of conception are coded to the Obstetrics section. Procedures performed on the pregnant female other than the products of conception are coded to the appropriate root operation in the Medical and Surgical section.
> _Example_: Amniocentesis is coded to the products of conception body part in the Obstetrics section. Repair of obstetric urethral laceration is coded to the urethra body part in the Medical and Surgical section.
> _Procedures following delivery or abortion_
> **C2.** Procedures performed following a delivery or abortion for curettage of the endometrium or evacuation of retained products of conception are all coded in the Obstetrics section, to the root operation Extraction and the body part Products of Conception, Retained. Diagnostic or therapeutic dilation and curettage performed during times other than the postpartum or post-abortion period are all coded in the Medical and Surgical section, to the root operation Extraction and the body part Endometrium.

EXERCISE 6-7

With the use of reference material, answer the following questions about ICD-10-PCS.

1. It is acceptable to choose a valid code directly from the tables.
    A. True
    B. False

2. Procedures that are performed using an open approach with percutaneous endoscopic assistance are coded to an open approach.
    A. True
    B. False

3. Body systems designated as "upper" contain body parts above the heart.
    A. True
    B. False

4. When a patient is having a hip replacement, a code for the resection of a joint is assigned in addition to the joint replacement code.
   A. True
   B. False

5. Procedures performed on the distal end of the humerus are coded to the Arm body part value.
   A. True
   B. False

6. A closed reduction of a fracture is coded to the manipulation approach.
   A. True
   B. False

7. It is acceptable to choose a valid code directly from the index.
   A. True
   B. False

8. Body systems designated as "lower" contain body parts below the diaphragm.
   A. True
   B. False

9. If the intended procedure is discontinued, code to the root operation that was intended.
   A. True
   B. False

10. If the identical procedure is performed on contralateral body parts, and a bilateral body part value is available for that body part, a single code with the bilateral body part should be assigned.
    A. True
    B. False

11. When used in a code description, the term *and* means "and/or."
    A. True
    B. False

12. It is acceptable to use a general body part value when the specific body part cannot be determined.
    A. True
    B. False

13. The body site for perirenal is "peritoneum."
    A. True
    B. False

14. A temporary postoperative wound drain is considered a device when assigning a ICD-10-PCS code.
    A. True
    B. False

15. Exploration or inspection of a body part that is integral to the performance of the procedure is not coded separately.
    A. True
    B. False

16. A bone marrow transplant is coded to the root operation transplant.
    A. True
    B. False

17. The root operation to stop postprocedural bleeding is control.
    A. True
    B. False

18. Procedures performed on the skin are coded to the body part values in the body system Skin and breast.
    A. True
    B. False

19. A device is only coded if the device remains after the procedure is completed.
    A. True
    B. False

20. The resection of tonsils is coded to an open approach.
    A. True
    B. False

CHAPTER REVIEW EXERCISE

Complete the following review exercises.

1. It is not acceptable to choose a valid code directly from the tables.
   A. True
   B. False

2. The resection of tonsils is coded to an external approach.
   A. True
   B. False

3. The body site for perirenal is kidney.
   A. True
   B. False

4. When a patient is having a knee replacement, a code for the resection of a joint is not assigned but is coded to the joint replacement.
   A. True
   B. False

5. A device is only coded if the device remains after the procedure is completed.
   A. True
   B. False

6. The root operation replacement always involves a device.
   A. True
   B. False

7. The approach for a laparoscopic cholecystectomy is percutaneous endoscopic.
   A. True
   B. False

8. The entry by puncture or minor incision, of instrumentation through the skin, mucous membrane, and any other body layers necessary to reach the operative site is an open approach.
   A. True
   B. False

9. All ICD-10-PCS codes have six characters.
   A. True
   B. False

10. The AMA is responsible for the maintenance of ICD-10-PCS.
    A. True
    B. False

11. Full implementation of the ICD-10-PCS system is proposed for what date?
    A. October 31, 2013
    B. October 1, 2013
    C. October 1, 2014
    D. October 31, 2014

12. The mapping files that crosswalk ICD-9-CM to ICD-10-PCS are known as
    A. GEMs
    B. ACTs
    C. HIMs
    D. CMS

13. Which of the following is a characteristic of ICD-10-PCS?
    A. Codes have a decimal point.
    B. Codes are similar to ICD-10-CM codes.
    C. There are 34 possible values for a character.
    D. The number of codes is limited.

14. The first character of an ICD-10-PCS code represents
    A. Body part
    B. Approach
    C. Section
    D. Device

Locate the following terms in the Alphabetic Index, and identify the first three to four characters of the ICD-10-PCS code.

15. Brachytherapy, prostate   _____

16. Fragmentation, right ureteral stone   _____

17. Kidney transplant, left   _____

18. Resection, adrenal glands   _____

19. PPN   _____

With the use of the two GEMs files on the CMS website answer the following.

Map the following procedure codes.

20. 03.51   _____

21. 34.20   _____

22. 38.31   _____

Map the following procedure codes.

23. 0SB00ZZ   _____

24. 0FB00ZX   _____

Assign the appropriate ICD-10-PCS codes to the following procedures in accordance with the coding guidelines.

25. Endometrial ablation via natural opening, endoscopic   _____

26. Above-knee amputation, right mid-shaft femoral region   _____

27. Open partial nephrectomy, left   _____

28. Therapeutic thoracentesis, right pleural cavity _____

29. ESWL, right ureter   _____

30. Open lysis of adhesions, gallbladder   _____

31. Laparoscopic Nissen fundoplication   _____

32. Right inguinal herniorrhaphy with mesh, open   _____

33. Endoscopic dilatation, esophagus   _____

34. Total right hip replacement with metal on metal prosthesis   _____

35. Laparoscopic appendectomy converted to open appendectomy   _____

36. Diagnostic bronchoscopy   _____

37. Removal of mole, right upper arm, diagnostic   _____

38. Laparoscopically assisted vaginal hysterectomy _____

CHAPTER GLOSSARY   *It is important to note that most of these definitions are as defined by ICD-10-PCS.*

Alteration: modifying the natural anatomic structure of a body part without affecting the function of the body part (breast augmentation).

Arthroscopic approach: an arthroscope is used to examine and perform closed procedures within a joint.

Bilateral procedure: operative procedure performed on paired anatomic organs or tissues during the same operative session.

Body system: an anatomic region or a general physiological system on which a procedure is performed.

Bypass: altering the route of passage of the contents of a tubular body part (CABG).

Change: taking out or off a device from a body part and putting back an identical or similar device in or on the same body part without cutting or puncturing the skin or a mucous membrane (change gastrostomy tube).

Computer assisted surgery (CAS): adjunctive procedure that allows increased visualization and more precise navigation while remaining minimally invasive.

Control: stopping, or attempting to stop, postprocedural bleeding (control of post-tonsillectomy hemorrhage).

Creation: making a new structure that does not take the place of a body part (creation of a vagina in males for sex reassignment).

Destruction: physical eradication of all or a portion of a body part by the direct use of energy, force, or a destructive agent (ablation of endometriosis).

Detachment: cutting off all or a portion of the upper or lower extremities (above-knee amputation).

Dilation: expanding an orifice or the lumen of a tubular body part (PTCA).

Division: cutting into a body part without draining fluids and/or gases from the body part in order to separate or transect a body part (osteotomy).

Drainage: taking or letting out fluids and/or gases from a body part (paracentesis).

Excision: Cutting out or off, without replacement, a portion of a body part (partial nephrectomy).

External: procedures performed directly on the skin or mucous membrane and procedures performed indirectly by the application of external force through the skin or mucous membrane (tonsillectomy).

Extirpation: taking or cutting out solid matter from a body part (thrombectomy).

Extraction: pulling or stripping out or off all or a portion of a body part by the use of force (bone marrow biopsy).

Fragmentation: breaking solid matter in a body part into pieces (extracorporeal shockwave lithotripsy).

Fusion: joining together portions of an articular body part, rendering the articular body part immobile (spinal fusion).

Insertion: putting in a nonbiological appliance that monitors, assists, performs, or prevents a physiological function but does not physically take the place of a body part (insertion of pacemaker lead).

Inspection: visually and/or manually exploring a body part (diagnostic arthroscopy).

Laparoscopic approach: uses a laparoscope to examine and perform closed procedures within the abdomen.

Limited coverage: procedures that are identified by the Medicare Code Editor as procedures covered under limited circumstances.

Map: locating the route of passage of electrical impulses and/or locating functional areas in a body part (cardiac mapping).

Medicare Code Editor: software that detects errors in coding on Medicare claims.

MS-DRG grouper: software that assigns MS-DRG using diagnosis and procedure codes.

Noncovered OR procedure: procedure code categorized by the Medicare Code Editor as a noncovered operating room procedure for which Medicare does not provide reimbursement.

Non-OR procedure affecting MS-DRG assignment: procedure code recognized by the MS-DRG grouper as a non–operating room procedure that may affect MS-DRG assignment.

Occlusion: completely closing an orifice or lumen of a tubular body part (tubal ligation).

Open: cutting through the skin, mucous membrane, and any other body layers necessary to expose the site of the procedure (abdominal hysterectomy).

Open with percutaneous endoscopic assistance: cutting through the skin, mucous membrane, and any other body layers necessary to expose the site of the procedure, and entry, by puncture or minor incision, of instrumentation through the skin, mucous membrane, and any other body layers necessary to aid in the performance of the procedure (laparoscopic-assisted vaginal hysterectomy).

Percutaneous: entry, by puncture or minor incision, of instrumentation through the skin, mucous membrane, and any other body layers necessary to reach the site of the procedure (needle biopsy liver).

Percutaneous endoscopic: entry, by puncture or minor incision, of instrumentation through the skin, mucous membrane, and any other body layers necessary to reach and visualize the site of the procedure (laparoscopic cholecystectomy).

Principal procedure: procedure that is performed for definitive treatment, rather than for diagnostic or exploratory purposes, or one performed that was necessary to take care of a complication.

Reattachment: putting back in or on all or a portion of a separated body part to its normal location or other suitable location.

Release: to free a body part from an abnormal physical constraint (lysis of adhesions).

Removal: taking out or off a device from a body part (remove chest tube).

Repair: restoring, to the extent possible, a body part to its normal anatomic structure and function (herniorrhaphy).

Replacement: putting in or on biological or synthetic material that physically takes the place and/or performs the function of all or a portion of a body part (total knee replacement).

Reposition: moving to its normal location, or other suitable location, all or a portion of a body part (fracture reduction).

Resection: cutting out or off, without replacement, all of a body part (total lobectomy of lung).

Restriction: partially closing an orifice or lumen of a tubular body part (Nissen fundoplication).

Revision: correcting, to the extent possible, a malfunctioning or displaced device (adjustment of knee prosthesis).

Robotic-assisted surgery: minimally invasive technique that utilizes robotic arms to manipulate the surgical equipment and tools.

Significant procedure: a procedure is considered significant if it is surgical in nature, carries a procedural risk, carries an anesthetic risk, and/or requires specialized training.

Supplement: putting in or on biological or synthetic material that physically reinforces and/or augments the function of a portion of a body part (herniorrhaphy with mesh).

Thoracoscopic approach: a thoracoscope is used to examine and perform closed procedures within the thorax.

Transfer: moving, without taking out, all or a portion of a body part to another location to take over the function of all or a portion of a body part (pedicle skin flap).

Transplantation: putting in or on all or a portion of a living body part taken from another individual or animal to physically take the place and/or function of all or a portion of a similar body part (kidney transplant).

Valid OR procedure: a procedure that may affect MS-DRG assignment.

Via natural or artificial opening: entry of instrumentation through a natural or artificial external opening to reach the site of the procedure (endotracheal intubation).

Via natural or artificial opening endoscopic: entry of instrumentation through a natural or artificial external opening to reach and visualize the site of the procedure (colonoscopy).

General Coding Guidelines for Other Medical- and Surgical-Related Procedures and Ancillary Procedures

CHAPTER OUTLINE

ICD-10-PCS Coding Guidelines
Other Medical- and Surgical-Related Procedures
Ancillary Sections
Chapter Review Exercise
Chapter Glossary

LEARNING OBJECTIVES

1. Apply the conventions and ICD-10-PCS Coding Guidelines
2. Define the root operations/types for each section of ICD-10-PCS
3. Define the approaches for each section of ICD-10-PCS
4. Assign procedure codes using ICD-10-PCS

ABBREVIATIONS/ ACRONYMS

CT computerized tomography
ECMO extracorporeal membrane oxygenation
ECT electroconvulsive therapy

ICD-10-PCS *International Classification of Diseases, 10th Revision, Procedure Coding System*

MRI magnetic resonance imaging
PET positron emission tomography

ICD-10-PCS

Coding Guidelines (2013)

Please refer to the companion Evolve website for the most current guidelines.
Transplantation vs. Administration
B3.16 Putting in a mature and functioning living body part taken from another individual or animal is coded to the root operation Transplantation. Putting in autologous or nonautologous cells is coded to the Administration section.
Example: Putting in autologous or nonautologous bone marrow, pancreatic islet cells or stem cells is coded to the Administration section.

EXAMPLE

Nonautologous bone marrow transplant via central venous line in patient with multiple myeloma, C90.00, 30243G1.

> *Obstetric Section Guidelines (section 1)*
> **C. Obstetrics Section**
> *Products of conception*
> **C1** Procedures performed on the products of conception are coded to the Obstetrics section. Procedures performed on the pregnant female other than the products of conception are coded to the appropriate root operation in the Medical and Surgical section.
> *Example*: Amniocentesis is coded to the products of conception body part in the Obstetrics section. Repair of obstetric urethral laceration is coded to the urethra body part in the Medical and Surgical section.

EXAMPLE Amniocentesis was performed to screen for genetic and chromosomal abnormalities, Z13.79, 10903ZU.

> *Procedures following delivery or abortion*
> **C2** Procedures performed following a delivery or abortion for curettage of the endometrium or evacuation of retained products of conception are all coded in the Obstetrics section, to the root operation Extraction and the body part Products of Conception, Retained. Diagnostic or therapeutic dilation and curettage performed during times other than the postpartum or post-abortion period are all coded in the Medical and Surgical section, to the root operation Extraction and the body part Endometrium.

EXAMPLE D&C for retained products of conception following a spontaneous abortion at 8 weeks' gestation, O03.4, Z3A.08 10D17ZZ.

OTHER MEDICAL- AND SURGICAL-RELATED PROCEDURES

The other medical- and surgical-related procedure sections of ICD-10-PCS include the following sections:

SECTION VALUE	DESCRIPTION
1	Obstetrics
2	Placement
3	Administration
4	Measurement and monitoring
5	Extracorporeal assistance and performance
6	Extracorporeal therapies
7	Osteopathic
8	Other procedures
9	Chiropractic

Obstetrics

Obstetrics include only those procedures that are performed on the products of conception. The term "**products of conception**" refers to all physical components of a pregnancy, including the fetus, amnion, umbilical cord, and placenta, regardless of gestational age. Procedures performed on a pregnant female other than on the products of conception are coded in the Medical and Surgical section. All ICD-10-PCS codes are seven characters, each character representing a particular aspect of the procedure. The meanings of the obstetric procedure characters are as follows:

CHARACTER	REPRESENTS
1	Section
2	Body system
3	Root operation
4	Body part
5	Approach
6	Device
7	Qualifier

Obstetric codes are found in Section 1, so they have a first-character value of 1. The second-character value for body system is Pregnancy. The third character identifies the root operation. There are a total of 12 root operations in the Obstetrics section. Ten of these are taken from the Medical and Surgical section and that includes:

CHARACTER	REPRESENTS
2	Change
9	Drainage
D	Extraction
H	Insertion
J	Inspection
P	Removal
Q	Repair
S	Reposition
T	Resection
Y	Transplantation

This section includes two additional root operations:
- **Abortion (A):** artificially terminating a pregnancy
- **Delivery (E):** assisting the passage of the products of conception from the genital canal

The fourth character classifies the body part. Body part values in this section are:
- Products of conception
- Products of conception, retained
- Products of conception, ectopic

The fifth character identifies the approach; these are defined in the Medical and Surgical section. The sixth character is for the device. The seventh character identifies various qualifiers, such as type of extraction, type of cesarean section, and so on.

EXAMPLE

Manually assisted delivery, 10E0XZZ

CHARACTER 1 SECTION	CHARACTER 2 BODY SYSTEM	CHARACTER 3 OPERATION	CHARACTER 4 BODY PART	CHARACTER 5 APPROACH	CHARACTER 6 DEVICE	CHARACTER 7 QUALIFIER
Obstetrics	Pregnancy	Delivery	Products of Conception	External	No Device	No Qualifier
1	0	E	0	X	Z	Z

The root operation, Delivery, applies only to manually-assisted, vaginal delivery and is defined as assisting the passage of the products of conception from the genital canal. Cesarean deliveries are coded in this section to the root operation extraction.

EXERCISE 7-1

Without the use of reference material, answer the following questions about ICD-10-PCS.

1. Obstetric procedures are any procedure performed on a pregnant woman.
   A. True
   B. False

2. In ICD-10-PCS, "abortion" is defined as "the spontaneous termination of a pregnancy."
   A. True
   B. False

3. Low cervical cesarean section would be identified by the fifth character, the approach.
   A. True
   B. False

Placement

Placement codes include procedures for putting a device in or on a body region for the purpose of protection, immobilization, stretching, compression, or packing. All ICD-10-PCS codes are seven characters, each representing a particular aspect of the procedure. The meanings of the placement procedure characters are as follows:

CHARACTER	REPRESENTS
1	Section
2	Body system
3	Root operation
4	Body region
5	Approach
6	Device
7	Qualifier

Placement codes are found in Section 2, so they have a first-character value of 2. The second-character value, for body system, is either anatomical region or body orifice. The third character identifies the root operation. The root operations in the placement section include only those procedures performed without making an incision or a puncture. Two of these are taken from the Medical and Surgical section and that includes:

CHARACTER	REPRESENTS
0	Change
5	Removal

Section 2 includes five additional root operations:

- **Compression (1):** putting pressure on a body region
- **Dressing (2):** putting material on a body region for protection
- **Immobilization (3):** limiting or preventing motion of a body region
- **Packing (4):** putting material in a body region or orifice
- **Traction (6):** exerting a pulling force on a body region in a distal direction

The fourth-character value classifies body region or natural orifice. The fifth-character value identifies the approach; and because all placement procedures are performed directly on the skin or mucous membranes, or indirectly by applying external force, the approach value is always X, for external. The sixth-character value classifies device. The seventh character is for a qualifier, but it is not used in the Placement section at this time, so the value is always no qualifier(Z).

EXAMPLE

Cast to right lower arm, 2W3CX2Z

CHARACTER 1 SECTION	CHARACTER 2 BODY SYSTEM	CHARACTER 3 OPERATION	CHARACTER 4 BODY REGION	CHARACTER 5 APPROACH	CHARACTER 6 DEVICE	CHARACTER 7 QUALIFIER
Placement	Anatomical Region	Immobilization	Lower Arm, Right	External	Cast	No Qualifier
2	W	3	C	X	2	Z

Splints and braces that are placed in the inpatient setting are coded in this section. If a fitting for a device such as a splint or brace is performed in the rehabilitation setting, the codes from the F0D table are assigned.

Administration

Administration codes include procedures for putting in or on a therapeutic, prophylactic, protective, diagnostic, nutritional, or physiological substance. All ICD-10-PCS codes are seven characters, each representing a particular aspect of the procedure. The meanings of the administration procedure characters are as follows:

CHARACTER	REPRESENTS
1	Section
2	Body system
3	Root operation
4	Body system/region
5	Approach
6	Substance
7	Qualifier

Administration codes are found in Section 3, so they have a first-character value of 3. The second character has three values: physiological systems and anatomical regions, circulatory system, or indwelling device. The third-character value identifies the root operation. Section 3 has three root operations:

- **Introduction (0):** putting in or on a therapeutic, diagnostic, nutritional, physiological, or prophylactic substance except blood or blood products
- **Irrigation (1):** putting in or on a cleansing substance
- **Transfusion (2):** putting in blood or blood products

The fourth-character value classifies body system/region. This identifies the site where the substance is administered. The fifth-character value identifies the approach, and each approach is defined in the Medical and Surgical section. Percutaneous is the approach for procedures that are introduced intradermally, subcutaneously, and intramuscularly (e.g., injections). The sixth-character value specifies the substance introduced. The seventh character is for a qualifier that indicates whether the substance used was autologous or nonautologous or to further specify the substance. **Autologous** means originating from the recipient, rather than from a donor, or transferred from the same individual's body, (e.g., a skin graft is taken from one part of the body and transferred to another part of the body on the same individual).

EXAMPLE

Administration of RBCs, nonautologous, via central vein, 30243N1

CHARACTER 1 SECTION	CHARACTER 2 BODY SYSTEM	CHARACTER 3 OPERATION	CHARACTER 4 BODY SYSTEM/ REGION	CHARACTER 5 APPROACH	CHARACTER 6 SUBSTANCE	CHARACTER 7 QUALIFIER
Administration	Circulatory	Transfusion	Central Vein	Percutaneous	Red Blood Cells	Nonautologous
3	0	2	4	3	N	1

EXERCISE 7-2

Without the use of reference material, answer the following questions.

1. Irrigation is a root operation that is found in the Placement section.
   A. True
   B. False

2. Immobilization is limiting or preventing motion of a body region.
   A. True
   B. False

3. In the Administration section, Character 6 identifies the substance being introduced.
   A. True
   B. False

Measurement and Monitoring

Measurement and monitoring codes include procedures for determining the level of a physiological or physical function. All ICD-10-PCS codes are seven characters, each representing a particular aspect of the procedure. The meanings of the measuring and monitoring procedure characters are as follows:

CHARACTER	REPRESENTS
1	Section
2	Body system
3	Root operation
4	Body system
5	Approach
6	Function/Device
7	Qualifier

Measurement and monitoring codes are found in Section 4, so they have a first-character value of 4. The second character has two values, for either physiological systems or physiological devices. The third-character value identifies the root operation. Section 4 has two root operations:

- **Measurement (0):** determining the level of a physiological or physical function at a point in time
- **Monitoring (1):** determining the level of a physiological or physical function repetitively over a period of time

The fourth-character value identifies the body system being measured or monitored. The fifth-character value identifies the approach, and each is defined in the Medical and Surgical section. The sixth-character value specifies the physiological or physical function monitored. The seventh character is for a qualifier used to further specify the body part or a variation of the procedure performed.

EXAMPLE

Holter monitoring, 4A12X45

CHARACTER 1 SECTION	CHARACTER 2 BODY SYSTEM	CHARACTER 3 OPERATION	CHARACTER 4 BODY SYSTEM	CHARACTER 5 APPROACH	CHARACTER 6 FUNCTION/DEVICE	CHARACTER 7 QUALIFIER
Measurement/ Monitoring	Physiological Systems	Monitoring	Cardiac	External	Electrical Activity	Ambulatory
4	A	1	2	X	4	5

Extracorporeal Assistance and Performance

Extracorporeal assistance and performance codes are used when equipment outside of the body is used to assist or perform a physiological function. All ICD-10-PCS codes are seven characters, each representing a particular aspect of the procedure. The meanings of the extracorporeal assistance and performance procedure characters are as follows:

CHARACTER	REPRESENTS
1	Section
2	Body system
3	Root operation
4	Body system
5	Duration
6	Function
7	Qualifier

Extracorporeal assistance and performance codes are found in Section 5, so they have a first-character value of 5. The second-character value is for physiological systems. The third-character value identifies the root operation. The section has three root operations:

- **Assistance (0):** taking over a portion of a physiological function by extracorporeal means such as intra-aortic balloon pump to support cardiac output.

- **Performance (1):** completely taking over a physiological function by extracorporeal means such as total mechanical ventilation or cardiopulmonary bypass.
- **Restoration (2):** returning, or attempting to return, a physiological function to its original state by extracorporeal means

Restoration defines only external cardioversion and defibrillation procedures. Failed cardioversion procedures are also included in the definition of restoration and are coded the same as successful procedures.

The fourth-character value classifies the body system to which the extracorporeal assistance or performance is applied. The fifth-character value identifies the duration of the procedure. The sixth-character value specifies the physiological function assisted or performed during the procedure. The seventh character is a qualifier that specifies the type of equipment used, if any.

EXAMPLE

Mechanical ventilation, continuous for 48 hours, 5A1945Z

CHARACTER 1 SECTION	CHARACTER 2 BODY SYSTEM	CHARACTER 3 OPERATION	CHARACTER 4 BODY SYSTEM	CHARACTER 5 DURATION	CHARACTER 6 FUNCTION	CHARACTER 7 QUALIFIER
Extracorporeal Assistance or Performance	Physiological Systems	Performance	Respiratory	24-96 consecutive hours	Ventilation	No Qualifier
5	A	1	9	4	5	Z

Extracorporeal Therapies

Extracorporeal therapy codes are used when equipment outside of the body is used for a therapeutic purpose that does not involve the assistance or performance of a physiological function. All ICD-10-PCS codes are seven characters, each representing a particular aspect of the procedure. The meanings of the extracorporeal therapies procedure characters are as follows:

CHARACTER	REPRESENTS
1	Section
2	Body system
3	Root operation
4	Body system
5	Duration
6	Qualifier
7	Qualifier

Extracorporeal therapy codes are found in Section 6, so they have a first-character value of 6. The second-character value is for physiological systems. The third-character value identifies the root operation. Section 6 has ten root operations:

- **Atmospheric control (0):** extracorporeal control of atmospheric pressure and composition
- **Decompression (1):** extracorporeal elimination of undissolved gas from body fluids
- **Electromagnetic therapy (2):** extracorporeal treatment by electromagnetic rays
- **Hyperthermia (3):** extracorporeal raising of body temperature
- **Hypothermia (4):** extracorporeal lowering of body temperature
- **Pheresis (5):** extracorporeal separation of blood products
- **Phototherapy (6):** extracorporeal treatment by light rays
- **Shock wave therapy (9):** extracorporeal treatment by shock waves
- **Ultrasound therapy (7):** extracorporeal treatment by ultrasound
- **Ultraviolet light therapy (8):** extracorporeal treatment by ultraviolet light

Hyperthermia can be used to treat temperature imbalance as well as an adjunct radiation treatment for cancer. When performed to treat temperature imbalance, the procedure is coded to this section.

When performed for cancer treatment, whole-body hyperthermia is classified as a modality qualifier in the radiation oncology section.

The fourth character identifies the body system to which the extracorporeal therapy is performed. The fifth character identifies the duration of the procedure. The sixth-character value is not specified and always has the value no qualifier. The seventh character is a qualifier used for the root operations of pheresis and ultrasound therapy.

EXAMPLE

Plasmapheresis, therapeutic, single encounter, 6A550Z3

CHARACTER 1 SECTION	CHARACTER 2 BODY SYSTEM	CHARACTER 3 OPERATION	CHARACTER 4 BODY SYSTEM	CHARACTER 5 DURATION	CHARACTER 6 QUALIFIER	CHARACTER 7 QUALIFIER
Extracorporeal Therapies	Physiological Systems	Pheresis	Circulatory	Single	No Qualifier	Plasma
6	A	5	5	0	Z	3

EXERCISE 7-3

Without the use of reference material, answer the following questions about ICD-10-PCS.

1. Hypothermia procedure is a type of extracorporeal therapy.
    A. True
    B. False

2. Measurement is defined as determining the level of physiological or physical function repetitively over a period of time.
    A. True
    B. False

3. Extracorporeal therapy uses equipment outside the body for a therapeutic purpose that does not involve the assistance or performance of a physiological function.
    A. True
    B. False

4. In the extracorporeal assistance and performance section, the definition for "performance" is "completely taking over a physiological function by extracorporeal means."
    A. True
    B. False

5. When a fifth-character is used for extracorporeal therapies, this specifies the duration of the patient's hospital stay.
    A. True
    B. False

Osteopathic

Osteopathic codes are used for osteopathic procedures. All ICD-10-PCS codes are seven characters, each representing a particular aspect of the procedure. The meanings of the procedure characters for the Osteopathic section are as follows:

CHARACTER	REPRESENTS
1	Section
2	Body system
3	Root operation
4	Body region
5	Approach
6	Method
7	Qualifier

Osteopathic codes are found in Section 7, so they have a first-character value of 7. The second character is for anatomical regions, and the third character identifies the root operation.

Section 7 has only one root operation:

■ **Treatment (0):** manual treatment to eliminate or alleviate somatic dysfunction and related disorders

The fourth character identifies the body region on which the osteopathic treatments are performed. The fifth character identifies the approach, which is always external. The sixth character specifies the method by which the treatment is performed. The seventh character is for a qualifier, but it is not specified in the osteopathic section at this time, so the value is always None(Z).

EXAMPLE

Indirect osteopathic treatment to the lumbar region, 7W03X4Z

CHARACTER 1 SECTION	CHARACTER 2 BODY SYSTEM	CHARACTER 3 OPERATION	CHARACTER 4 BODY REGION	CHARACTER 5 APPROACH	CHARACTER 6 METHOD	CHARACTER 7 QUALIFIER
Osteopathic	Anatomical Regions	Treatment	Lumbar	External	Indirect	No Qualifier
7	W	0	3	X	4	Z

Other Procedures

Other procedure codes are used for a variety of other procedures (e.g., acupuncture, suture removal, and in vitro fertilization). All ICD-10-PCS codes are seven characters, each representing a particular aspect of the procedure. The meanings of the other procedure characters are as follows:

CHARACTER	REPRESENTS
1	Section
2	Body system
3	Root operation
4	Body region
5	Approach
6	Method
7	Qualifier

Other procedure codes are found in Section 8, so they have a first-character value of 8. The second character is for physiological systems and anatomical region, and the third character identifies the root operation.

The section has only one root operation:

■ **Other procedures (0):** methodologies that attempt to remediate or cure a disorder or disease

The fourth character specifies the body region on which the procedure is performed. The fifth character identifies the approach, and each is defined in the Medical and Surgical section. The sixth-character value specifies the method by which the procedure is performed. The seventh character is to identify various qualifiers necessary to provide more information about a specific procedure.

EXAMPLE

Suture removal, left calf, 8E0YXY8

CHARACTER 1 SECTION	CHARACTER 2 BODY SYSTEM	CHARACTER 3 OPERATION	CHARACTER 4 BODY REGION	CHARACTER 5 APPROACH	CHARACTER 6 METHOD	CHARACTER 7 QUALIFIER
Other Procedures	Anatomical Regions	Other Procedures	Lower Extremity	External	Other	Suture Removal
8	E	0	Y	X	Y	8

Chiropractic

All ICD-10-PCS codes for chiropractic procedures are seven characters, each representing a particular aspect of the procedure. The meanings of the chiropractic procedure characters are as follows:

CHARACTER	REPRESENTS
1	Section
2	Body system
3	Root operation
4	Body region
5	Approach
6	Method
7	Qualifier

Chiropractic codes are found in Section 9, so they have a first-character value of 9. The second character identifies anatomical regions, and the third character identifies the root operation.

Section 9 has only one root operation:

- **Manipulation (B):** manual procedures that involve a directed thrust to move a joint past the physiological range of motion without exceeding the anatomical limit

The fourth character specifies the body region on which the chiropractic manipulation is performed. The fifth character identifies the approach, which is always external. The sixth-character value specifies the method by which the manipulation is performed. The seventh character is for a qualifier, but it is not specified in the chiropractic section at this time, so the value is always None(Z).

EXAMPLE

Chiropractic treatment to cervical spine, short lever specific contact, 9WB1XHZ

CHARACTER 1 SECTION	CHARACTER 2 BODY SYSTEM	CHARACTER 3 OPERATION	CHARACTER 4 BODY REGION	CHARACTER 5 APPROACH	CHARACTER 6 METHOD	CHARACTER 7 QUALIFIER
Chiropractic	Anatomical Regions	Manipulation	Cervical	External	Short lever specific contact	None
9	W	B	1	X	H	Z

EXERCISE 7-4

Without using reference material, answer the following questions about ICD-10-PCS.

1. The approach for chiropractic manipulation is always external.
   A. True
   B. False

2. Acupuncture can be coded in the Other Procedures section of ICD-10-PCS.
   A. True
   B. False

3. Any root operation in the Medical and Surgical section can be used in the Osteopathic section.
   A. True
   B. False

4. The approach for an osteopathic treatment is always external.
   A. True
   B. False

ANCILLARY SECTIONS

The ancillary sections of ICD-10-PCS include the following:

SECTION VALUE	DESCRIPTION
B	Imaging
C	Nuclear medicine
D	Radiation oncology
F	Physical rehabilitation and diagnostic audiology
G	Mental health
H	Substance abuse treatment

Imaging

Imaging procedures include plain radiography, fluoroscopy, CT, MRI, and ultrasound. All ICD-10-PCS codes are seven characters, each representing a particular aspect of the procedure. The meanings of the imaging procedure characters are as follows:

CHARACTER	REPRESENTS
1	Section
2	Body system
3	Root type
4	Body part
5	Contrast
6	Qualifier
7	Qualifier

Imaging codes are found in Section B, so they have a first-character value of B. Similar to the Medical and Surgical section, the second-character value identifies the body system. Instead of root operation, the third character identifies the type of imaging procedure. The root types are as follows:

- **Plain Radiography (0):** planar display of an image developed from the capture of external ionizing radiation on photographic or photoconductive plate.
- **Fluoroscopy (1):** single-plane or bi-plane real-time display of an image developed from the capture of external ionizing radiation on a fluorescent screen. The image may also be stored by either digital or analog means.
- **Computerized tomography (CT scans) (2):** computer reformatted digital display of multiplanar images developed from the capture of multiple exposures of external ionizing radiation.
- **Magnetic resonance imaging (MRI) (3):** computer reformatted digital display of multiplanar images developed from the capture of radio-frequency signals emitted by nuclei in a body site excited within a magnetic field.
- **Ultrasonography (4):** real-time display of images of anatomy or flow information developed from the capture of reflected and attenuated high frequency sound waves.

The fourth character specifies the body part, and the fifth character identifies whether the contrast material used is high or low osmolar when applicable. The sixth and seventh characters identify various qualifiers necessary to provide more information about a specific imaging procedure.

EXAMPLE

CT abdomen and pelvis without contrast, BW21ZZZ

CHARACTER 1 SECTION	CHARACTER 2 BODY SYSTEM	CHARACTER 3 ROOT TYPE	CHARACTER 4 BODY PART	CHARACTER 5 CONTRAST	CHARACTER 6 QUALIFIER	CHARACTER 7 QUALIFIER
Imaging	Anatomical Region	CT	Abdomen and pelvis	None	None	None
B	W	2	1	Z	Z	Z

Nuclear Medicine

Nuclear medicine procedures include nuclear medicine scans and PET scans. Radiation therapy is not included in this section. All ICD-10-PCS codes are seven characters, each representing a particular aspect of the procedure. The meanings of the nuclear medicine procedure characters are as follows:

CHARACTER	REPRESENTS
1	Section
2	Body system
3	Root type
4	Body part
5	Radionuclide
6	Qualifier
7	Qualifier

Nuclear medicine codes are found in Section C, so they have a first-character value of C. Similar to the Medical and Surgical section, the second character here specifies the body system. Instead of root operation, the third character identifies the type of nuclear medicine procedure. The root types are as follows:

- **Planar nuclear medicine imaging (1):** introduction of radioactive materials into the body for single-plane display of images developed from the capture of radioactive emissions.
- **Tomographic nuclear medicine imaging (2):** introduction of radioactive materials into the body for three-dimensional display of images developed from the capture of radioactive emissions.
- **Positron emission tomography (PET) (3):** introduction of radioactive materials into the body for three-dimensional display of images developed from the simultaneous capture, 180 degrees apart, of radioactive emissions.
- **Nonimaging nuclear medicine uptake (4):** introduction of radioactive materials into the body for measurements of organ functions, from detection of radioactive emissions.
- **Nonimaging nuclear medicine probe (5):** introduction of radioactive materials into the body for the study of distribution and fate of certain substances by the detection of radioactive emissions from an external source.
- **Nonimaging nuclear medicine assay (6):** introduction of radioactive materials into the body for the study of body fluids and blood elements, by the detection of radioactive emissions.
- **Systemic nuclear medicine therapy (7):** introduction of unsealed radioactive materials into the body for treatment.

The fourth character specifies body part or body region. The fifth character value identifies the radionuclide or radiation source. The sixth and seventh characters are for qualifiers, but they are not used in the Nuclear Medicine section at this time, so the value is always None.

EXAMPLE

Whole body PET scan, CW3NYZZ

CHARACTER 1 SECTION	CHARACTER 2 BODY SYSTEM	CHARACTER 3 ROOT TYPE	CHARACTER 4 BODY PART	CHARACTER 5 RADIONUCLIDE	CHARACTER 6 QUALIFIER	CHARACTER 7 QUALIFIER
Nuclear Medicine	Anatomical Region	PET	Whole Body	Other Radionuclide	None	None
C	W	3	N	Y	Z	Z

Radiation Oncology

Radiation oncology includes procedures that introduce radioactive material for the treatment of cancer. All ICD-10-PCS codes used here are seven characters, each representing a particular aspect of the procedure. The meanings of the radiation oncology procedure characters are as follows:

CHARACTER	REPRESENTS
1	Section
2	Body system
3	Root type
4	Body part
5	Modality qualifier
6	Isotope
7	Qualifier

Radiation oncology codes are found in Section D, so they have a first-character value of D. Similar to the Medical and Surgical section, the second character specifies the body system. Instead of root operation, the third character identifies the general modality used (e.g., beam radiation, brachytherapy, or stereotactic radiosurgery). The fourth character value specifies the body part that is the focus of the radiation therapy. The fifth character value, the modality qualifier, specifies the radiation modality used (e.g., photons, electrons). The sixth character specifies the isotopes introduced during the procedure, if applicable. The seventh character is used for other qualifiers.

EXAMPLE

HDR Brachytherapy of prostate using Palladium 103, DV109BZ

CHARACTER 1 SECTION	CHARACTER 2 BODY SYSTEM	CHARACTER 3 MODALITY	CHARACTER 4 BODY PART	CHARACTER 5 MODALITY QUALIFIER	CHARACTER 6 ISOTOPE	CHARACTER 7 QUALIFIER
Radiation Oncology	Male Reproductive	Brachytherapy	Prostate	High Dose Rate	Pd-103	None
D	V	1	0	9	B	Z

EXERCISE 7-5

Without using reference material, answer the following questions about ICD-10-PCS.

1. MRI procedures are located in the Nuclear Medicine section.
   A. True
   B. False

2. Radionuclide is the fifth character in the Nuclear Medicine section.
   A. True
   B. False

3. The first-character value for an imaging procedure is B.
   A. True
   B. False

4. The fourth character in the radiation oncology section specifies the body part that is the focus of the radiation therapy.
   A. True
   B. False

5. Isotope is the seventh-character qualifier in the Radiation Oncology section.
   A. True
   B. False

Physical Rehabilitation and Diagnostic Audiology

Physical rehabilitation procedures include physical therapy, occupational therapy, and speech-language pathology. Diagnostic audiology is also included in this section. All ICD-10-PCS codes are seven characters, each representing a particular aspect of the procedure. The meanings of the physical rehabilitation and diagnostic audiology procedure characters are as follows:

CHARACTER	REPRESENTS
1	Section
2	Section qualifier
3	Root type
4	Body system and region
5	Type qualifier
6	Equipment
7	Qualifier

Physical rehabilitation and diagnostic audiology codes are found in Section E, so they have a first-character value of E. There is a change from body system to section qualifier for the second-character value (e.g., rehabilitation or diagnostic audiology). Instead of root operation, the third character identifies the type of physical rehabilitation and diagnostic audiology procedure. There are 14 different root values. The root values are as follows:

- **Speech assessment (0):** measurement of speech and related functions
- **Motor and/or nerve function assessment (1):** measurement of motor, nerve, and related functions.
- **Activities of daily living assessment (2):** measurement of functional level for activities of daily living.
- **Hearing assessment (3):** measurement of hearing and related functions.
- **Hearing aid assessment (4):** measurement of the appropriateness and/or effectiveness of a hearing device.
- **Vestibular assessment (5):** measurement of vestibular system and related functions.
- **Speech treatment (6):** application of techniques to improve, augment, or compensate for speech and related functional impairment.
- **Motor treatment (7):** exercise or activities to increase or facilitate motor function.
- **Activities of daily living treatment (8):** exercise or activities to facilitate functional competence for activities of daily living.
- **Hearing treatment (9):** application of techniques to improve, augment, or compensate for hearing and related functional impairment.
- **Hearing aid treatment (B):** application of techniques to improve the communication abilities of individuals with cochlear implants.
- **Vestibular treatment (C):** application of techniques to improve, augment, or compensate for vestibular and related functional impairment.
- **Device fitting (D):** fitting of a device designed to facilitate or support achievement of a higher level of function.
- **Caregiver training (F):** training in activities to support patient's optimal level of function.

Treatment procedures include swallowing dysfunction exercises, bathing and showering techniques, wound management, gait training, and a host of activities typically associated with rehabilitation. The assessments are further classified into more than 100 different tests or methods. The majority of these focus on hearing and speech, but others focus on various aspects of body function, such as muscle performance, neuromotor development, and reintegration skills.

The fourth character specifies body part and body region. The fifth character, or type qualifier, further specifies the procedure performed. The sixth character identifies specific equipment used. Character seven is for a qualifier, but it is not used in this section at this time, so the value is always None.

EXAMPLE

Bedside swallow assessment, F00ZHZZ

CHARACTER 1 SECTION	CHARACTER 2 SECTION QUALIFIER	CHARACTER 3 ROOT TYPE	CHARACTER 4 BODY SYSTEM/ REGION	CHARACTER 5 TYPE QUALIFIER	CHARACTER 6 EQUIPMENT	CHARACTER 7 QUALIFIER
Physical Rehab & Diagnostic Audiology	Rehab	Speech Assessment	None	Bedside Swallowing and Oral Function	None	None
F	0	0	Z	H	Z	Z

Mental Health

Mental health procedures are coded in this section. All ICD-10-PCS codes are seven characters, each representing a particular aspect of the procedure. The meanings of the mental health procedure characters are as follows:

CHARACTER	REPRESENTS
1	Section
2	Body system
3	Root type
4	Type qualifier
5	Qualifier
6	Qualifier
7	Qualifier

Mental health codes are found in Section G, so they have a first-character value of G. The second-character value, for body system, has a value of None in this section. And instead of root operation, the third character identifies the type of mental health procedure. The root types are as follows:

- Psychological tests (1)
- Crisis intervention (2)
- Medication management (3)
- Individual psychotherapy (5)
- Counseling (6)
- Family psychotherapy (7)
- ECT (B)
- Biofeedback (C)
- Hypnosis (F)
- Narcosynthesis (G)
- Group psychotherapy (H)
- Light therapy (J)

The fourth-character value is a type qualifier (e.g., educational or vocational counseling). Values for Characters 5, 6, and 7 are for qualifiers but are not used in the Mental Health section at this time, so the value is always None.

EXAMPLE

Family psychotherapy session, GZ72ZZZ

CHARACTER 1 SECTION	CHARACTER 2 BODY SYSTEM	CHARACTER 3 ROOT TYPE	CHARACTER 4 TYPE QUALIFIER	CHARACTER 5 QUALIFIER	CHARACTER 6 QUALIFIER	CHARACTER 7 QUALIFIER
Mental Health	None	Family Psychotherapy	Other Family Psychotherapy	None	None	None
G	Z	7	2	Z	Z	Z

Substance Abuse Treatment Section

Treatments for substance abuse are coded in this section. All ICD-10-PCS codes are seven characters, each representing a particular aspect of the procedure. The meanings of the substance abuse procedure characters are as follows:

CHARACTER	REPRESENTS
1	Section
2	Body system
3	Root type
4	Type qualifier
5	Qualifier
6	Qualifier
7	Qualifier

Substance abuse treatment codes are found in Section H, so they have a first-character value of H. The second-character value for body system has a value of None in this section. And instead of root operation, the third-character value identifies the type of substance abuse procedure. The root types are as follows:

- Detoxification services (2)
- Individual counseling (3)
- Group counseling (4)
- Individual psychotherapy (5)
- Family counseling (6)
- Medication management (8)
- Pharmacotherapy (9)

The fourth-character value is a type qualifier (e.g., cognitive behavioral, 12-step, interpersonal). Values for Characters 5, 6, and 7 are for qualifiers but are not used in the Substance Abuse section at this time, so the value is always None.

EXAMPLE

Medication management for methadone maintenance, HZ81ZZZ

CHARACTER 1 SECTION	CHARACTER 2 BODY SYSTEM	CHARACTER 3 ROOT TYPE	CHARACTER 4 TYPE QUALIFIER	CHARACTER 5 QUALIFIER	CHARACTER 6 QUALIFIER	CHARACTER 7 QUALIFIER
Substance Abuse Treatment	None	Medication Management	Methadone Maintenance	None	None	None
H	Z	8	1	Z	Z	Z

EXERCISE 7-6

Without using reference material, answer the following questions.

1. The seventh character in the Physical Rehabilitation and Diagnostic Audiology section identifies whether the procedure is a physical rehabilitation procedure or a diagnostic audiology procedure.
   - **A.** True
   - **B.** False

2. Equipment is the sixth character in the physical rehabilitation and diagnostic audiology section.
   - **A.** True
   - **B.** False

3. The first-character value for a physical rehabilitation or diagnostic audiology procedure is B.
   - **A.** True
   - **B.** False

4. Hypnosis is a procedure that can be coded in the Mental Health section.
   A. True
   B. False

5. In the Substance Abuse section, Characters 5, 6, and 7 are for qualifiers.
   A. True
   B. False

6. The first-character value for a mental health procedure is G.
   A. True
   B. False

CHAPTER REVIEW EXERCISE

Complete the following review exercises using ICD-10-PCS.

1. CT procedures are located in the Nuclear Medicine section.
   A. True
   B. False

2. Detoxification services can be coded in the Mental Health section.
   A. True
   B. False

3. Obstetric tables include procedures performed on the products of conception only.
   A. True
   B. False

4. In ICD-10-PCS, *abortion* is defined as "spontaneous termination of a pregnancy."
   A. True
   B. False

5. Irrigation is defined as "the putting in or on of a cleansing substance."
   A. True
   B. False

6. Monitoring is defined as "determining the level of physiological or physical function repetitively over a period of time."
   A. True
   B. False

7. Extracorporeal therapy uses equipment outside the body for a therapeutic purpose that does not involve the assistance or performance of a physiological function.
   A. True
   B. False

8. The approach for an osteopathic treatment is always external.
   A. True
   B. False

Assign the appropriate ICD-10-PCS codes to the following procedures in accordance with the coding guidelines.

9. Placement of nasal packing, right nare   _____

10. Packing wound, abdomen wall   _____

11. Nonautologous bone marrow transplant via central venous catheter   _____

12. Mechanical ventilation, less than 24 hours   _____

13. ECMO, circulatory, continuous oxygenation   _____

14. Robotic assisted laparoscopic abdominal hysterectomy   _____

15. Chiropractic treatment to cervical spine using short lever specific   _____
    contact

16. Phototherapy with Bili-Lite, single treatment   _____

17. MRI brain   _____

18. Proton radiation therapy for brain metastasis   _____

19. Physical therapy treatment to increase ROM, right shoulder   _____

20. Hypnosis   _____

21. Twelve-step group therapy for alcohol addiction   _____

CHAPTER GLOSSARY

It is important to note that most of these definitions are as defined by ICD-10-PCS.

Abortion: artificially terminating a pregnancy.

Activities of daily living assessment: measurement of functional level for activities of daily living.

Activities of daily living treatment: exercise or activities to facilitate functional competence for activities of daily living.

Assistance: taking over a portion of a physiological function by extracorporeal means.

Atmospheric control: extracorporeal control of atmospheric pressure and composition.

Autologous: originating from the recipient, rather than from a donor; tissue transferred from the same individual's body (e.g., a skin graft taken from one part of the body is transferred to another part of the body on the same individual).

Caregiver training: training in activities to support patient's optimal level of function.

Compression: putting pressure on a body region.

Computerized tomography (CT scans): computer reformatted digital display of multiplanar images developed from the capture of multiple exposures of external ionizing radiation.

Decompression: extracorporeal elimination of undissolved gas from body fluids.

Delivery: assisting the passage of the products of conception from the genital canal.

Device fitting: fitting of a device designed to facilitate or support achievement of a higher level of function.

Dressing: putting material on a body region for protection.

Electromagnetic therapy: extracorporeal treatment by electromagnetic rays.

Fluoroscopy: single-plane or bi-plane real-time display of an image developed from the capture of external ionizing radiation on a fluorescent screen. The image may also be stored by either digital or analog means.

Hearing aid assessment: measurement of the appropriateness and/or effectiveness of a hearing device.

Hearing aid treatment: application of techniques to improve the communication abilities of individuals with cochlear implants.

Hearing assessment: measurement of hearing and related functions.

Hearing treatment: application of techniques to improve, augment, or compensate for hearing and related functional impairment.

Hyperthermia: extracorporeal raising of body temperature.

Hypothermia: extracorporeal lowering of body temperature.

Immobilization: limiting or preventing motion of a body region.

Introduction: putting in or on a therapeutic, diagnostic, nutritional, physiological, or prophylactic substance except blood or blood products.

Irrigation: putting in or on a cleansing substance.

Magnetic resonance imaging (MRI): computer reformatted digital display of multiplanar images developed from the capture of radio-frequency signals emitted by nuclei in a body site excited within a magnetic field.

Manipulation: manual procedures that involve a directed thrust to move a joint past the physiological range of motion without exceeding the anatomical limit.

Measurement: determining the level of a physiological or physical function at a point in time.

Monitoring: determining the level of a physiological or physical function repetitively over a period of time.

Motor and/or nerve function assessment: measurement of motor, nerve, and related functions.

Motor treatment: exercise or activities to increase or facilitate motor function.

Nonimaging nuclear medicine assay: introduction of radioactive materials into the body for the study of body fluids and blood elements, by the detection of radioactive emissions.

Nonimaging nuclear medicine probe: introduction of radioactive materials into the body for the study of distribution and fate of certain substances by the detection of radioactive emissions from an external source.

Nonimaging nuclear medicine uptake: introduction of radioactive materials into the body for measurements of organ functions, from detection of radioactive emissions.

Other procedures: methodologies that attempt to remediate or cure a disorder or disease.

Packing: putting material in a body region or orifice.

Performance: completely taking over a physiological function by extracorporeal means.

Pheresis: extracorporeal separation of blood products.

Phototherapy: extracorporeal treatment by light rays.

Plain Radiography: planar display of an image developed from the capture of external ionizing radiation on photographic or photoconductive plate.

Planar nuclear medicine imaging: introduction of radioactive materials into the body for single-plane display of images developed from the capture of radioactive emissions.

Positron emission tomography (PET): introduction of radioactive materials into the body for three-dimensional display of images developed from the simultaneous capture, 180 degrees apart, of radioactive emissions.

Products of conception: all physical components of a pregnancy including the fetus, amnion, umbilical cord, and placenta, regardless of gestational age.

Restoration: returning, or attempting to return, a physiological function to its original state by extracorporeal means.

Shock wave therapy: extracorporeal treatment by shock waves.

Speech assessment: measurement of speech and related functions.

Speech treatment: application of techniques to improve, augment, or compensate for speech and related functional impairment.

Systemic nuclear medicine therapy: introduction of unsealed radioactive materials into the body for treatment.

Tomographic nuclear medicine imaging: introduction of radioactive materials into the body for three-dimensional display of images developed from the capture of radioactive emissions.

Traction: exerting a pulling force on a body region in a distal direction.

Transfusion: putting in blood or blood products.

Treatment: manual treatment to eliminate or alleviate somatic dysfunction and related disorders.

Ultrasound therapy: extracorporeal treatment by ultrasound.

Ultrasonography: real-time display of images of anatomy or flow information developed from the capture of reflected and attenuated high frequency sound waves.

Ultraviolet light therapy: extracorporeal treatment by ultraviolet light.

Vestibular assessment: measurement of vestibular system and related functions.

Vestibular treatment: application of techniques to improve, augment, or compensate for vestibular and related functional impairment.

8

Symptoms, Signs, and Abnormal Clinical and Laboratory Findings Not Elsewhere Classified, and Z Codes

(ICD-10-CM Chapters 18 and 21, Codes R00-R99, Z00-Z99)

LEARNING OBJECTIVES

1. Apply and assign the correct ICD-10-CM/PCS codes in accordance with Official Guidelines for Coding and Reporting
2. Identify major differences between ICD-10-CM and ICD-9-CM related to the signs and symptoms and Z codes
3. Determine when to assign signs and symptoms codes
4. Assign the correct Z codes
5. Explain the importance of documentation in relation to MS-DRGs for reimbursement

ABBREVIATIONS/ ACRONYMS

ASCUS atypical squamous cells of undetermined significance

BMI body mass index

CEA carcinoembryonic antigen

COPD chronic obstructive pulmonary disease

CT computerized tomography

CVA cerebrovascular accident

MS-DRG Medicare Severity diagnosis-related group

FUO fever of unknown origin

HGSIL high-grade squamous intraepithelial lesion

**ABBREVIATIONS/
ACRONYMS**—cont'd

HIV human immunodeficiency virus

ICD-9-CM *International Classification of Diseases, 9th Revision, Clinical Modification*

ICD-10-CM *International Classification of Diseases,*

10th Revision, Clinical Modification

ICD-10-PCS *International Classification of Diseases, 10th Revision, Procedure Coding System*

OR Operating Room

PSA prostate-specific antigen

RW relative weight

SIDS sudden infant death syndrome

UTI urinary tract infection

ICD-10-CM

Official Guidelines for Coding and Reporting

Please refer to the companion Evolve site for the most current guidelines.

18. Chapter 18: Symptoms, signs, and abnormal clinical and laboratory findings, not elsewhere classified (R00-R99)

Chapter 18 includes symptoms, signs, abnormal results of clinical or other investigative procedures, and ill-defined conditions regarding which no diagnosis classifiable elsewhere is recorded. Signs and symptoms that point to a specific diagnosis have been assigned to a category in other chapters of the classification.

a. Use of symptom codes

Codes that describe symptoms and signs are acceptable for reporting purposes when a related definitive diagnosis has not been established (confirmed) by the provider.

EXAMPLE   Fever of unknown origin, R50.9.

b. Use of a symptom code with a definitive diagnosis code

Codes for signs and symptoms may be reported in addition to a related definitive diagnosis when the sign or symptom is not routinely associated with that diagnosis, such as the various signs and symptoms associated with complex syndromes. The definitive diagnosis code should be sequenced before the symptom code.

Signs or symptoms that are associated routinely with a disease process should not be assigned as additional codes, unless otherwise instructed by the classification.

EXAMPLE   Hematuria due to calculus of kidney, N20.0.

EXAMPLE   Ascites due to cirrhosis of the liver, K74.60, R18.8.

c. Combination codes that include symptoms

ICD-10-CM contains a number of combination codes that identify both the definitive diagnosis and common symptoms of that diagnosis. When using one of these combination codes, an additional code should not be assigned for the symptom.

EXAMPLE   Acute cystitis with hematuria, N30.01.

d. Repeated falls

Code R29.6, Repeated falls, is for use for encounters when a patient has recently fallen and the reason for the fall is being investigated.

Code Z91.81, History of falling, is for use when a patient has fallen in the past and is at risk for future falls. When appropriate, both codes R29.6 and Z91.81 may be assigned together.

e. *Coma* scale

The coma scale codes (R40.2-) can be used in conjunction with traumatic brain injury codes, acute cerebrovascular disease or sequelae of cerebrovascular disease codes.

These codes are primarily for use by trauma registries, but they may be used in any setting where this information is collected. The coma scale codes should be sequenced after the diagnosis code**(s)**.

These codes, one from each subcategory, are needed to complete the scale. The 7th character indicates when the scale was recorded. The 7th character should match for all three codes.

At a minimum, report the initial score documented on presentation at your facility. This may be a score from the emergency medicine technician (EMT) or in the emergency department. If desired, a facility may choose to capture multiple Glasgow coma scale scores.

Assign code R40.24, Glasgow coma scale, total score, when only the total score is documented in the medical record and not the individual score(s).

EXAMPLE | Patient admitted in a coma (Glasgow coma score was 5) due to traumatic subdural hemorrhage. Patient expired without regaining consciousness, due to brain injury, S06.5x7A, R40.243, X58.xxxA.

f. Functional quadriplegia

Functional quadriplegia (code R53.2) is the lack of ability to use one's limbs or to ambulate due to extreme debility. It is not associated with neurologic deficit or injury, and code R53.2 should not be used for cases of neurologic quadriplegia. It should only be assigned if functional quadriplegia is specifically documented in the medical record.

g. SIRS due to Non-Infectious Process

The systemic inflammatory response syndrome (SIRS) can develop as a result of certain non-infectious disease processes, such as trauma, malignant neoplasm, or pancreatitis. When SIRS is documented with a noninfectious condition, and no subsequent infection is documented, the code for the underlying condition, such as an injury, should be assigned, followed by code R65.10, Systemic inflammatory response syndrome (SIRS) of non-infectious origin without acute organ dysfunction, or code R65.11, Systemic inflammatory response syndrome (SIRS) of non-infectious origin with acute organ dysfunction. If an associated acute organ dysfunction is documented, the appropriate code(s) for the specific type of organ dysfunction(s) should be assigned in addition to code R65.11. If acute organ dysfunction is documented, but it cannot be determined if the acute organ dysfunction is associated with SIRS or due to another condition (e.g., directly due to the trauma), the provider should be queried.

EXAMPLE | Patient was admitted with acute pancreatitis. Documentation by the physician indicated the patient met SIRS criteria, K85.9, R65.10.

h. Death NOS

Code R99, Ill-defined and unknown cause of mortality, is only for use in the very limited circumstance when a patient who has already died is brought into an emergency department or other healthcare facility and is pronounced dead upon arrival. It does not represent the discharge disposition of death.

Apply the General Coding Guidelines as found in Chapter 5 and the Procedural Coding Guidelines as found in Chapters 6 and 7.

MAJOR DIFFERENCES BETWEEN ICD-10-CM AND ICD-9-CM

■ A number of Excludes1 notes found in this chapter will be helpful in determining if a symptom code should be assigned. It would be inappropriate to assign R09.2, Respiratory arrest, along with a code I46.-, Cardiac arrest (Figure 8-1).

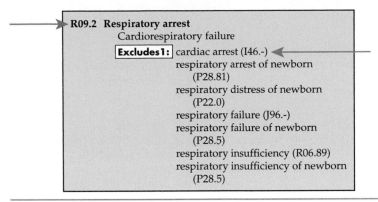

FIGURE 8-1. Excludes1 note in ICD-10-CM.

- There are ICD-10-CM codes to identify a patient's coma scale.
- SIRS due to noninfectious process is moved from Injury and Poisoning, Chapter 17 in ICD-9-CM, to ICD-10-CM Chapter 18, Symptoms, Signs, and Abnormal Clinical and Laboratory Findings, Not Elsewhere Classified.
- Repeated falls is assigned a V code in ICD-9-CM, but in ICD-10-CM repeated falls can be coded to a symptom code or a Z code for history of falling, or it may be appropriate to assign both codes.
- There are ICD-10-CM codes to identify a patient's blood type.

ANATOMY AND PHYSIOLOGY

Signs, symptoms, and abnormal clinical and laboratory findings, and Z codes can affect any of the body systems. The anatomy and physiology of these body systems are outlined in their respective chapters.

DISEASE CONDITIONS

Chapter 18 in the ICD-10-CM code book is divided into the following categories:

CATEGORY	SECTION TITLES
R00-R09	Symptoms and signs involving the circulatory and respiratory systems
R10-R19	Symptoms and signs involving the digestive system and abdomen
R20-R23	Symptoms and signs involving the skin and subcutaneous tissue
R25-R29	Symptoms and signs involving the nervous and musculoskeletal systems
R30-R39	Symptoms and signs involving the urinary system
R40-R46	Symptoms and signs involving cognition, perception, emotional state, and behavior
R47-R49	Symptoms and signs involving speech and voice
R50-R69	General symptoms and signs
R70-R79	Abnormal findings on examination of blood, without diagnosis
R80-R82	Abnormal findings on examination of urine, without diagnosis
R83-R89	Abnormal findings on examination of other bloody fluids, substances, and tissues, without diagnosis
R90-R94	Abnormal findings on diagnostic imaging and in function studies, without diagnosis
R97	Abnormal tumor markers
R99	Ill-defined and unknown cause of mortality

Chapter 21 (Z codes) in the ICD-10-CM code book is divided into the following blocks:

CATEGORY	SECTION TITLES
Z00-Z13	Persons encountering health services for examination and investigation
Z14-Z15	Genetic carrier and genetic susceptibility to disease
Z16	Infection with drug-resistant microorganisms
Z17	Estrogen receptor status
Z18	Retained foreign body fragments
Z20-Z28	Persons with potential health hazards related to communicable disease
Z30-Z39	Persons encountering health services in circumstances related to reproduction
Z40-Z53	Persons encountering health services for specific procedures and health care
Z55-Z65	Persons with potential health hazards related to socioeconomic and psychosocial circumstance
Z66	Do Not Resuscitate (DNR) status
Z67	Blood type
Z68	Body mass index (BMI)
Z69-Z76	Persons encountering health services in other circumstances
Z79-Z99	Persons with potential health hazards related to family and personal history and certain conditions influencing health status

See Figure 8-2 for details on an instructional note that appears at the very beginning of Chapter 18 of the Tabular List and applies to the entire chapter. This note provides information on the appropriate use of signs and symptoms codes.

A few Z code guidelines are explained within the various chapter guidelines; these will be addressed in those chapters. Some of them are repeated in the guidelines for Z codes and are reviewed in this chapter. These codes are addressed at the beginning of the book because they apply to all body systems. Z codes and signs and symptoms are common throughout this text.

Symptoms and Signs (R00-R69)

A **symptom** is subjective evidence of a disease or of a patient's condition as perceived by the patient.

Examples are fatigue, headache, and some types of pain. Symptoms may not be apparent to a physician on physical examination.

> **EXAMPLE** The patient presents to the ER complaining of a severe headache. The headache is an example of a symptom because it is a description of the patient's condition as perceived by the patient, R51.

A **sign** is objective evidence of a disease or of a patient's condition as perceived by the patient's examining physician.

Examples are elevated blood pressure, which can be measured or icterus and edema of the legs, which can be seen on physical examination.

> **EXAMPLE** The patient has a fever. This can be discerned by noting the patient's elevated temperature, R50.9.

It can be difficult to determine whether a sign or a symptom from Chapter 18 is routinely associated with the disease. It may be necessary to access resource books, such as *Merck's Manual*, or the Internet to find the most common symptoms of a disease or condition. As was previously stated in Chapter 5 of this text, signs and symptoms codes are acceptable to code:

- When no definitive diagnosis has been established
- When they are not an integral part of the disease process
- When directed by the classification to assign an additional code

CHAPTER 18

SYMPTOMS, SIGNS AND ABNORMAL CLINICAL AND LABORATORY FINDINGS, NOT ELSEWHERE CLASSIFIED (R00-R99)

Note: This chapter includes symptoms, signs, abnormal results of clinical or other investigative procedures, and ill-defined conditions regarding which no diagnosis classifiable elsewhere is recorded.

Signs and symptoms that point rather definitely to a given diagnosis have been assigned to a category in other chapters of the classification. In general, categories in this chapter include the less well-defined conditions and symptoms that, without the necessary study of the case to establish a final diagnosis, point perhaps equally to two or more diseases or to two or more systems of the body. Practically all categories in the chapter could be designated 'not otherwise specified', 'unknown etiology' or 'transient'. The Alphabetical Index should be consulted to determine which symptoms and signs are to be allocated here and which to other chapters. The residual subcategories, numbered .8, are generally provided for other relevant symptoms that cannot be allocated elsewhere in the classification.

The conditions and signs or symptoms included in categories R00-R94 consist of:
(a) cases for which no more specific diagnosis can be made even after all the facts bearing on the case have been investigated:
(b) signs or symptoms existing at the time of initial encounter that proved to be transient and whose causes could not be determined;
(c) provisional diagnosis in a patient who failed to return for further investigation or care;
(d) cases referred elsewhere for investigation or treatment before the diagnosis was made;
(e) cases in which a more precise diagnosis was not available for any other reason;
(f) certain symptoms, for which supplementary information is provided, that represent important problems in medical care in their own right.

Excludes2 abnormal findings on antenatal screening of mother (O28.-)
certain conditions originating in the perinatal period (P04-P96)
signs and symptoms classified in the body system chapters
signs and symptoms of breast (N63, N64.5)

FIGURE 8-2. Instructional note that appears at the beginning of Chapter 18.

It is not acceptable to code signs or symptoms:
- When a definitive diagnosis has been established
- When they are an integral part of the disease process

EXAMPLE Fever due to pneumonia, J18.9.
Fever is one of the symptoms of pneumonia that is integral to the disease process. Only the pneumonia should be coded.

EXAMPLE Dehydration due to pneumonia, J18.9, E86.0.
Although many patients who are admitted to the hospital may be dehydrated, not all patients who have pneumonia become dehydrated.

EXAMPLE Patient was admitted with right lower quadrant abdominal pain with nausea and vomiting. Patient has a low-grade fever. A diagnosis of acute appendicitis was confirmed upon removal of the patient's appendix in the Operating Room (OR), K35.80, 0DTJ0ZZ. The fever, abdominal pain, and nausea/vomiting are all symptoms of appendicitis and are not coded.

EXERCISE 8-1

Assign codes to the following conditions.

1. Alteration in mental status _____
2. Fever of unknown origin (FUO) _____
3. Right upper quadrant abdominal pain due to cholecystitis _____
   versus peptic ulcer disease
4. Ascites due to cirrhosis of liver _____
5. Oliguria _____
6. Palpitations _____
7. Change in bowel habits _____
8. Substernal chest pain _____
9. Loss of appetite _____
10. Ataxia _____
11. Generalized pain _____
12. Delirium _____

Abnormal Findings and Abnormal Tumor Markers (R70-R97)

Many times, an abnormality or elevation in a test result will lead to further investigation or repeat performance of certain tests. The patient may be without any signs or symptoms, and no definitive diagnosis may explain the abnormality. Some of the main terms that may be used to assist with location of these codes include "abnormal," "abnormality," "abnormalities," "elevation," and "findings, abnormal, inconclusive, without diagnosis." These abnormal findings must be documented by the physician to be coded. A coder should not code an abnormal finding on the basis of a review of laboratory results or reports of other diagnostic procedures.

EXAMPLE | Patient was seen by urologist because of an elevated PSA, R97.2.

EXAMPLE | Abnormal lung x-ray. Patient will be scheduled for a computerized tomography (CT) of the chest, R91.8.

EXERCISE 8-2

Assign codes to the following conditions.

1. Significant drop in hematocrit _____
2. Abnormal coagulation profile _____
3. Proteinuria _____
4. Abnormal Pap smear with atypical squamous cells of _____
   undetermined significance (ASCUS)
5. Abnormal mammogram _____
6. Bacteremia _____
7. Abnormal lead levels in blood _____
8. Positive Mantoux test _____
9. Elevated CA-125 _____
10. Transaminasemia _____

FACTORS INFLUENCING HEALTH STATUS AND CONTACT WITH HEALTH SERVICES (Z CODES Z00-Z99)

The Z codes are located in Chapter 21. According to the guidelines, ICD-10-CM provides codes that should be assigned to encounters for circumstances other than a disease or injury. The Z codes are provided to deal with occasions when circumstances other than a disease or injury are recorded as a diagnosis or problem.

Assignment of Z codes can be problematic because some can be used only as the principal diagnosis, others can be used as both principal and secondary diagnoses, and some can be used only as secondary diagnoses. It can be difficult to locate Z codes in the Alphabetic Index. Coders will often say, "I did not know there was a Z code for that." It is very important to be familiar with the different types and uses of Z codes. Because appropriate main terms are difficult to find in the Alphabetic Index, some common main terms are as follows:

Admission	Donor	Procedure (surgical)
Aftercare	Examination	Prophylactic
Attention to	Fitting of	Removal
Boarder	Healthy	Replacement
Care (of)	History	Screening
Carrier	Maintenance	Status
Checking	Maladjustment	Supervision (of)
Contraception	Observation	Test
Counseling	Problem	Transplant
Dialysis		Unavailability (of)
		Vaccination

Guidelines for Z codes provide a lot of detail and descriptions of the various sections of Z codes. It may be necessary to review these guidelines frequently; Z codes will also be addressed in most of the following chapters because some Z codes are specific to certain body systems.

Screening Z codes should be assigned only when the service fits the definition of a screening. A **screening examination** is one that occurs in the absence of any signs or symptoms. It consists of examination of an asymptomatic individual to detect a given disease, typically by means of an inexpensive diagnostic test. There are Z codes for prophylactic organ removal. A **prophylactic** measure is the use of medication or treatment to prevent a disease from occurring.

EXAMPLE   Screening mammogram for 45-year-old patient, Z12.31.

EXAMPLE   Screening mammogram in a 45-year-old patient with nipple discharge, N64.52.

In the second example, even though it was documented as a screening mammogram, it does not fit the definition because the nipple discharge is a symptom and a reason for the test. It would be inappropriate to assign the screening Z code.

Several Z codes identify the history of certain conditions. Documentation of a patient's medical and surgical history may be found within the History and Physical or the Admit Note. Sometimes, documentation in the health record may indicate a history of a particular disease or condition, and the disease or condition is actually a current or active problem. If any question arises as to whether a condition is currently an active problem, a physician query may be necessary.

Relevant family history is often documented. It may be important to code a family history of malignant neoplasm of the breast when a patient has been admitted with breast cancer and is having a mastectomy. In the Index under "History," "Family history" is a subterm, and it is found before the personal history Index entries (Figure 8-3).

Histoplasmosis *(Continued)*
  capsulati B39.4
    disseminated B39.3
    generalized B39.3
    pulmonary B39.2
      acute B39.0
      chronic B39.1
  Darling's B39.4
  duboisii B39.5
  lung NEC B39.2
History
  family (of) —*see also* History, personal
      (of)
    alcohol abuse Z81.1
    allergy NEC Z84.89
    anemia Z83.2
    arthritis Z82.61
    asthma Z82.5
    blindness Z82.1
    cardiac death (sudden) Z82.41
    carrier of genetic disease Z84.81
    chromosomal anomaly Z82.79
    chronic
      disabling disease NEC Z82.8
      lower respiratory disease
          Z82.5
    colonic polyps Z83.71
    congenital malformations and
        deformations Z82.79
      polycystic kidney Z82.71
    consanguinity Z84.3
    deafness Z82.2
    diabetes mellitus Z83.3
    disability NEC Z82.8
    disease or disorder (of)
      allergic NEC Z84.89
      behavioral NEC Z81.8
      blood and blood-forming organs
          Z83.2
      cardiovascular NEC Z82.49
      chronic disabling NEC Z82.8
      digestive Z83.79
      ear NEC Z83.52
      endocrine NEC Z83.49
      eye NEC Z83.518
        glaucoma Z83.511
      genitourinary NEC Z84.2
      glaucoma Z83.511
      hematological Z83.2
      immune mechanism Z83.2
      infectious NEC Z83.1
      ischemic heart Z82.49
      kidney Z84.1
      mental NEC Z81.8
      metabolic Z83.49
      musculoskeletal NEC Z82.69
      neurological NEC Z82.0
      nutritional Z83.49
      parasitic NEC Z83.1
      psychiatric NEC Z81.8
      respiratory NEC Z83.6
      skin and subcutaneous tissue NEC
          Z84.0
      specified NEC Z84.89
    drug abuse NEC Z81.3
    epilepsy Z82.0
    genetic disease carrier Z84.81
    glaucoma Z83.511
    hearing loss Z82.2
    human immunodeficiency virus
        (HIV) infection Z83.0
    Huntington's chorea Z82.0
    intellectual disability Z81.0
    leukemia Z80.6

History *(Continued)*
  family *(Continued)*
    malignant neoplasm (of) NOS
        Z80.9
      bladder Z80.52
      breast Z80.3
      bronchus Z80.1
      digestive organ Z80.0
      gastrointestinal tract Z80.0
      genital organ Z80.49
        ovary Z80.41
        prostate Z80.42
        specified organ NEC Z80.49
        testis Z80.43
      hematopoietic NEC Z80.7
      intrathoracic organ NEC Z80.2
      kidney Z80.51
      lung Z80.1
      lymphatic NEC Z80.7
      ovary Z80.41
      prostate Z80.42
      respiratory organ NEC Z80.2
      specified site NEC Z80.8
      testis Z80.43
      trachea Z80.1
      urinary organ or tract Z80.59
        bladder Z80.52
        kidney Z80.51
    mental
      disorder NEC Z81.8
    multiple endocrine neoplasia (MEN)
        syndrome Z83.41
    osteoporosis Z82.62
    polycystic kidney Z82.71
    polyps (colon) Z83.71
    psychiatric disorder Z81.8
    psychoactive substance abuse NEC
        Z81.3
    respiratory condition NEC Z83.6
      asthma and other lower
          respiratory conditions
          Z82.5
    self-harmful behavior Z81.8
    skin condition Z84.0
    specified condition NEC Z84.89
    stroke (cerebrovascular) Z82.3
    substance abuse NEC Z81.4
      alcohol Z81.1
      drug NEC Z81.3
      psychoactive NEC Z81.3
      tobacco Z81.2
    sudden cardiac death Z82.41
    tobacco abuse Z81.2
    violence, violent behavior Z81.8
    visual loss Z82.1
  personal (of) —*see also* History, family
      (of)
    abuse
      adult Z91.419
        physical and sexual Z91.410
        psychological Z91.411
      childhood Z62.819
        physical Z62.810
        psychological Z62.811
        sexual Z62.810
    alcohol dependence F10.21
    allergy (to) Z88.9
      analgesic agent NEC Z88.6
      anesthetic Z88.4
      antibiotic agent NEC Z88.1
      anti-infective agent NEC Z88.3
      contrast media Z91.041
      drugs, medicaments and biological
          substances Z88.9
        specified NEC Z88.8

Family history index entries → (annotation pointing to "family (of)")

Personal history index entries → (annotation pointing to "personal (of)")

FIGURE 8-3. Family and personal history Alphabetic Index entries.

EXAMPLE | Patient has a past history of chronic obstructive pulmonary disease (COPD). You would not assign a Z code to indicate a previous history of a respiratory condition but the code for the active disease. COPD is a chronic condition that cannot be cured, J44.9.

EXAMPLE | The patient has a history of urinary tract infections (UTIs). In this case, no documentation, such as antibiotic therapy, indicates that the patient currently has a UTI, so a history of UTI Z code is appropriate, Z87.440.

EXAMPLE | Family history of polycystic kidney disease, Z82.71.

EXAMPLE | Personal history of exposure to asbestos, Z77.090.

ICD-10-CM

Official Guidelines for Coding and Reporting

Please refer to the companion Evolve site for the most current guidelines.

21. **Chapter 21: Factors influencing health status and contact with health services (Z00-Z99)**
    Note: The chapter specific guidelines provide additional information about the use of Z codes for specified encounters.
    a. **Use of Z codes in any healthcare setting**
       Z codes are for use in any healthcare setting. Z codes may be used as either a first-listed (principal diagnosis code in the inpatient setting) or secondary code, depending on the circumstances of the encounter. Certain Z codes may only be used as first-listed or principal diagnosis.
    b. **Z Codes indicate a reason for an encounter**
       Z codes are not procedure codes. A corresponding procedure code must accompany a Z code to describe any procedure performed.

EXAMPLE | A female patient was admitted for elective sterilization and percutaneous endoscopic bilateral tubal occlusion with Falope ring was performed, Z30.2, 0UL74CZ.

    c. **Categories of Z Codes**
       1) **Contact/Exposure**
          Category Z20 indicates contact with, and suspected exposure to, communicable diseases. These codes are for patients who do not show any sign or symptom of a disease but are suspected to have been exposed to it by close personal contact with an infected individual or are in an area where a disease is epidemic.
          Category Z77, indicates contact with and suspected exposures hazardous to health.
          Contact/exposure codes may be used as a first-listed code to explain an encounter for testing, or, more commonly, as a secondary code to identify a potential risk.

EXAMPLE | Exposure to anthrax, Z20.810.

       2) **Inoculations and vaccinations**
          Code Z23 is for encounters for inoculations and vaccinations. It indicates that a patient is being seen to receive a prophylactic inoculation against a disease. Procedure codes are required to identify the actual administration of the injection and the type(s) of immunizations given. Code Z23 may be used as a secondary code if the inoculation is given as a routine part of preventive health care, such as a well-baby visit.

EXAMPLE | Vaccination for influenza, Z23, 3E0134Z.

3) Status

Status codes indicate that a patient is either a carrier of a disease or has the sequelae or residual of a past disease or condition. This includes such things as the presence of prosthetic or mechanical devices resulting from past treatment. A status code is informative, because the status may affect the course of treatment and its outcome. A status code is distinct from a history code. The history code indicates that the patient no longer has the condition.

A status code should not be used with a diagnosis code from one of the body system chapters, if the diagnosis code includes the information provided by the status code. For example, code Z94.1, Heart transplant status, should not be used with a code from subcategory T86.2, Complications of heart transplant. The status code does not provide additional information. The complication code indicates that the patient is a heart transplant patient.

For encounters for weaning from a mechanical ventilator, assign a code from subcategory J96.1, Chronic respiratory failure, followed by code Z99.11, Dependence on respirator [ventilator] status.

The status Z codes/categories are:

Z14   Genetic carrier

Genetic carrier status indicates that a person carries a gene, associated with a particular disease, which may be passed to offspring who may develop that disease. The person does not have the disease and is not at risk of developing the disease.

Z15   Genetic susceptibility to disease

Genetic susceptibility indicates that a person has a gene that increases the risk of that person developing the disease.

Codes from category Z15 should not be used as principal or first-listed codes. If the patient has the condition to which he/she is susceptible, and that condition is the reason for the encounter, the code for the current condition should be sequenced first. If the patient is being seen for follow-up after completed treatment for this condition, and the condition no longer exists, a follow-up code should be sequenced first, followed by the appropriate personal history and genetic susceptibility codes. If the purpose of the encounter is genetic counseling associated with procreative management, code Z31.5, Encounter for genetic counseling, should be assigned as the first-listed code, followed by a code from category Z15. Additional codes should be assigned for any applicable family or personal history.

Z16   <u>Resistance to antimicrobial drugs</u>

This code indicates that a patient has **a condition that** is resistant to **antimicrobial** drug treatment. Sequence the infection code first.

Z17   Estrogen receptor status

Z18   Retained foreign body fragments

Z21   Asymptomatic HIV infection status

This code indicates that a patient has tested positive for HIV but has manifested no signs or symptoms of the disease.

Z22   Carrier of infectious disease

Carrier status indicates that a person harbors the specific organisms of a disease without manifest symptoms and is capable of transmitting the infection.

Z28.3   Underimmunization status

Z33.1   Pregnant state, incidental

This code is a secondary code only for use when the pregnancy is in no way complicating the reason for visit. Otherwise, a code from the obstetric chapter is required.

Z66	Do not resuscitate
	This code may be used when it is documented by the provider that a patient is on do not resuscitate status at any time during the stay.
Z67	Blood type
Z68	Body mass index (BMI)
Z74.01	Bed confinement status
Z76.82	Awaiting organ transplant status
Z78	Other specified health status
	Code Z78.1, Physical restraint status, may be used when it is documented by the provider that a patient has been put in restraints during the current encounter. Please note that this code should not be reported when it is documented by the provider that a patient is temporarily restrained during a procedure.
Z79	Long-term (current) drug therapy
	Codes from this category indicate a patient's continuous use of a prescribed drug (including such things as aspirin therapy) for the long-term treatment of a condition or for prophylactic use. It is not for use for patients who have addictions to drugs. This subcategory is not for use of medications for detoxification or maintenance programs to prevent withdrawal symptoms in patients with drug dependence (e.g., methadone maintenance for opiate dependence). Assign the appropriate code for the drug dependence instead.
	Assign a code from Z79 if the patient is receiving a medication for an extended period as a prophylactic measure (such as for the prevention of deep vein thrombosis) or as treatment of a chronic condition (such as arthritis) or a disease requiring a lengthy course of treatment (such as cancer). Do not assign a code from category Z79 for medication being administered for a brief period of time to treat an acute illness or injury (such as a course of antibiotics to treat acute bronchitis).
Z88	Allergy status to drugs, medicaments and biological substances
	Except: Z88.9, Allergy status to unspecified drugs, medicaments and biological substances status
Z89	Acquired absence of limb
Z90	Acquired absence of organs, not elsewhere classified
Z91.0-	Allergy status, other than to drugs and biological substances
Z92.82	Status post administration of tPA (rtPA) in a different facility within the last 24 hours prior to admission to a current facility
	Assign code Z92.82, Status post administration of tPA (rtPA) in a different facility within the last 24 hours prior to admission to current facility, as a secondary diagnosis when a patient is received by transfer into a facility and documentation indicates they were administered tissue plasminogen activator (tPA) within the last 24 hours prior to admission to the current facility.
	This guideline applies even if the patient is still receiving the tPA at the time they are received into the current facility.
	The appropriate code for the condition for which the tPA was administered (such as cerebrovascular disease or myocardial infarction) should be assigned first.
	Code Z92.82 is only applicable to the receiving facility record and not to the transferring facility record.
Z93	Artificial opening status
Z94	Transplanted organ and tissue status
Z95	Presence of cardiac and vascular implants and grafts
Z96	Presence of other functional implants
Z97	Presence of other devices

Z98   Other postprocedural states
Assign code Z98.85, Transplanted organ removal status, to indicate that a transplanted organ has been previously removed. This code should not be assigned for the encounter in which the transplanted organ is removed. The complication necessitating removal of the transplant organ should be assigned for that encounter.
See section I.C19.g.3. for information on the coding of organ transplant complications.

Z99   Dependence on enabling machines and devices, not elsewhere classified
Note: Categories Z89-Z90 and Z93-Z99 are for use only if there are no complications or malfunctions of the organ or tissue replaced, the amputation site or the equipment on which the patient is dependent.

EXAMPLE

A patient was admitted for myocardial infarction. The patient is status post mitral valve replacement with porcine valve, I21.3, Z95.3.

Z79.- is assigned to identify the long-term use of a particular drug or medication. To locate these codes in the Alphabetic Index, the main term is "long-term drug therapy." These codes should not be used to identify drug abuse or dependence or to identify a medication that is used for a short period during an acute illness or injury. Drugs may be used to prevent a condition as a prophylactic measure or to treat a chronic condition. Sometimes a patient will need to have lab work to monitor the effectiveness of a particular medication or if the medication is causing any adverse effects. Code Z51.81 encounter for therapeutic drug monitoring would be assigned.

EXAMPLE

Patient has been taking Lipitor for hypercholesterolemia for one year. A hepatic function laboratory test was performed to assess any adverse effects on the patient's liver function. A fasting lipid profile was also done to assess the effectiveness of the Lipitor, Z51.81, Z79.899, E78.0.

In this example, the long-term use of Lipitor is identified with code Z51.81, long-term drug therapy of other medications, because the patient has been taking it for a year.

EXAMPLE

Patient was seen in the ER for acute bronchitis. The patient's family physician had seen the patient a couple of days ago and prescribed antibiotics. The patient was instructed to finish the antibiotics and follow-up with family physician, J20.9.

In this example the use of antibiotics is not assigned a Z code because it is only used for a short period of time to treat an acute illness.

4) History (of)
There are two types of history Z codes, personal and family. Personal history codes explain a patient's past medical condition that no longer exists and is not receiving any treatment, but that has the potential for recurrence, and therefore may require continued monitoring.

Family history codes are for use when a patient has a family member(s) who has had a particular disease that causes the patient to be at higher risk of also contracting the disease.

Personal history codes may be used in conjunction with follow-up codes and family history codes may be used in conjunction with screening codes to explain the need for a test or procedure. History codes are also acceptable on any medical record regardless of the reason for visit. A history of an illness, even if no longer present, is important information that may alter the type of treatment ordered.

The history Z code categories are:

Z80	Family history of primary malignant neoplasm
Z81	Family history of mental and behavioral disorders
Z82	Family history of certain disabilities and chronic diseases (leading to disablement)
Z83	Family history of other specific disorders
Z84	Family history of other conditions
Z85	Personal history of malignant neoplasm
Z86	Personal history of certain other diseases
Z87	Personal history of other diseases and conditions
Z91.4-	Personal history of psychological trauma, not elsewhere classified
Z91.5	Personal history of self-harm
Z91.8-	Other specified personal risk factors, not elsewhere classified
	Exception: Z91.83, Wandering in desease classified elsewhere
Z92	Personal history of medical treatment
	Except: Z92.0, Personal history of contraception
	Except: Z92.82, Status post administration of tPA (rtPA) in a different facility within the last 24 hours prior to admission to a current facility

EXAMPLE   A patient was admitted with congestive heart failure and coronary artery disease. The patient has a history of coronary artery bypass graft and a family history of coronary artery disease, I50.9, I25.10, Z95.1, Z82.49.

5) Screening

Screening is the testing for disease or disease precursors in seemingly well individuals so that early detection and treatment can be provided for those who test positive for the disease (e.g., screening mammogram).

The testing of a person to rule out or confirm a suspected diagnosis because the patient has some sign or symptom is a diagnostic examination, not a screening. In these cases, the sign or symptom is used to explain the reason for the test.

A screening code may be a first-listed code if the reason for the visit is specifically the screening exam. It may also be used as an additional code if the screening is done during an office visit for other health problems. A screening code is not necessary if the screening is inherent to a routine examination, such as a pap smear done during a routine pelvic examination.

Should a condition be discovered during the screening then the code for the condition may be assigned as an additional diagnosis.

The Z code indicates that a screening exam is planned. A procedure code is required to confirm that the screening was performed.

The screening Z codes/categories:

Z11	Encounter for screening for infectious and parasitic diseases
Z12	Encounter for screening for malignant neoplasms
Z13	Encounter for screening for other diseases and disorders
	Except: Z13.9, Encounter for screening, unspecified
Z36	Encounter for antenatal screening for mother

EXAMPLE   Screening for colon cancer, Z12.11.

6) Observation

There are two observation Z code categories. They are for use in very limited circumstances when a person is being observed for a suspected condition that is ruled out. The observation codes are not for use if an injury or illness or any signs or symptoms related to the suspected condition are present. In such cases the diagnosis/symptom code is used with the corresponding external cause code.

The observation codes are to be used as principal diagnosis only. Additional codes may be used in addition to the observation code but only if they are unrelated to the suspected condition being observed.

Codes from subcategory Z03.7, Encounter for suspected maternal and fetal conditions ruled out, may either be used as a first-listed or as an additional code assignment depending on the case. They are for use in very limited circumstances on a maternal record when an encounter is for a suspected maternal or fetal condition that is ruled out during that encounter (for example, a maternal or fetal condition may be suspected due to an abnormal test result). These codes should not be used when the condition is confirmed. In those cases, the confirmed condition should be coded. In addition, these codes are not for use if an illness or any signs or symptoms related to the suspected condition or problem are present. In such cases the diagnosis/symptom code is used.

Additional codes may be used in addition to the code from subcategory Z03.7, but only if they are unrelated to the suspected condition being evaluated.

Codes from subcategory Z03.7 may not be used for encounters for antenatal screening of mother. *See Section I.C.21.c.5, Screening.*

For encounters for suspected fetal condition that are inconclusive following testing and evaluation, assign the appropriate code from category O35, O36, O40 or O41.

The observation Z code categories:

Z03   Encounter for medical observation for suspected diseases and conditions ruled out

Z04   Encounter for examination and observation for other reasons
       Except: Z04.9, Encounter for examination and observation for unspecified reason

---

EXAMPLE   The driver of a car was admitted for observation after a rollover on the highway, Z04.1.

---

7) Aftercare

Aftercare visit codes cover situations when the initial treatment of a disease has been performed and the patient requires continued care during the healing or recovery phase, or for the long-term consequences of the disease. The aftercare Z code should not be used if treatment is directed at a current, acute disease. The diagnosis code is to be used in these cases. Exceptions to this rule are codes Z51.0, Encounter for antineoplastic radiation therapy, and codes from subcategory Z51.1, Encounter for antineoplastic chemotherapy and immunotherapy. These codes are to be first-listed, followed by the diagnosis code when a patient's encounter is solely to receive radiation therapy, chemotherapy, or immunotherapy for the treatment of a neoplasm. If the reason for the encounter is more than one type of antineoplastic therapy, code Z51.0 and a code from subcategory Z51.1 may be assigned together, in which case one of these codes would be reported as a secondary diagnosis.

The aftercare Z codes should also not be used for aftercare for injuries. For aftercare of an injury, assign the acute injury code with the appropriate 7th character (for subsequent encounter).

The aftercare codes are generally first-listed to explain the specific reason for the encounter. An aftercare code may be used as an additional code when some type of aftercare is provided in addition to the reason for admission and no diagnosis code is applicable. An example of this would be the closure of a colostomy during an encounter for treatment of another condition.

Aftercare codes should be used in conjunction with other aftercare codes or diagnosis codes to provide better detail on the specifics of an aftercare encounter visit, unless otherwise directed by the classification. Should a patient receive multiple types of antineoplastic therapy during the same encounter, code Z51.0, Encounter for antineoplastic radiation therapy, and codes from subcategory Z51.1, Encounter for antineoplastic chemotherapy and immunotherapy, may be used together on a record. The sequencing of multiple aftercare codes depends on the circumstances of the encounter.

Certain aftercare Z code categories need a secondary diagnosis code to describe the resolving condition or sequelae. For others, the condition is included in the code title.

Additional Z code aftercare category terms include fitting and adjustment, and attention to artificial openings.

EXAMPLE

A patient was admitted for takedown of a colostomy placed 3 months ago for diverticular disease. The descending colon was anastomosed to the rectum. Patient still has diverticulosis of the colon, Z43.3, K57.90, 0DQM0ZZ, 0WQFXZ2.

Status Z codes may be used with aftercare Z codes to indicate the nature of the aftercare. For example code Z95.1, Presence of aortocoronary bypass graft, may be used with code Z48.812, Encounter for surgical aftercare following surgery on the circulatory system, to indicate the surgery for which the aftercare is being performed. A status code should not be used when the aftercare code indicates the type of status, such as using Z43.0, Encounter for attention to tracheostomy, with Z93.0, Tracheostomy status.

The aftercare Z category/codes:

Z42	Encounter for plastic and reconstructive surgery following medical procedure or healed injury
Z43	Encounter for attention to artificial openings
Z44	Encounter for fitting and adjustment of external prosthetic device
Z45	Encounter for adjustment and management of implanted device
Z46	Encounter for fitting and adjustment of other devices
Z47	Orthopedic aftercare
Z48	Encounter for other postprocedural aftercare
Z49	Encounter for care involving renal dialysis
Z51	Encounter for other aftercare

Palliative care or comfort care is a specialized type of treatment that is given to patients that are terminal. The focus of the treatment is symptom management and pain control. Palliative care can be provided in a variety of healthcare settings including hospitals and hospice/home care. If a patient receives palliative care during an encounter it is appropriate to assign Z51.5, Encounter for palliative care. Z51.5 is not assigned as the reason for the encounter, but the terminal condition or underlying disease should be sequenced first.

EXAMPLE

Patient was admitted to hospice care for treatment of terminal ESRD, N18.6, Z51.5.

8) Follow-up

The follow-up codes are used to explain continuing surveillance following completed treatment of a disease, condition, or injury. They imply that the condition has been fully treated and no longer exists. They should not be confused with aftercare codes, or injury codes with a 7th character for subsequent encounter, that explain ongoing care of a healing condition or its sequelae. Follow-up codes may be used in conjunction with history codes to provide the full picture of the healed condition and its treatment. The follow-up code is sequenced first, followed by the history code.

A follow-up code may be used to explain multiple visits. Should a condition be found to have recurred on the follow-up visit, then the diagnosis code for the condition should be assigned in place of the follow-up code.

The follow-up Z code categories:

Z08	Encounter for follow-up examination after completed treatment for malignant neoplasm
Z09	Encounter for follow-up examination after completed treatment for conditions other than malignant neoplasm
Z39	Encounter for maternal postpartum care and examination

EXAMPLE Routine postpartum follow-up at 6 weeks. No problem or medical issues, Z39.2.

9) Donor

Codes in category Z52, Donors of organs and tissues, are used for living individuals who are donating blood or other body tissue. These codes are only for individuals donating for others, not for self-donations. They are not used to identify cadaveric donations.

EXAMPLE Patient is donating a kidney. A left laparoscopic nephrectomy was performed, Z52.4, 0TT14ZZ.

10) Counseling

Counseling Z codes are used when a patient or family member receives assistance in the aftermath of an illness or injury, or when support is required in coping with family or social problems. They are not used in conjunction with a diagnosis code when the counseling component of care is considered integral to standard treatment.

The counseling Z codes/categories:

Z30.0-	Encounter for general counseling and advice on contraception
Z31.5	Encounter for genetic counseling
Z31.6-	Encounter for general counseling and advice on procreation
Z32.2	Encounter for childbirth instruction
Z32.3	Encounter for childcare instruction
Z69	Encounter for mental health services for victim and perpetrator of abuse
Z70	Counseling related to sexual attitude, behavior and orientation
Z71	Persons encountering health services for other counseling and medical advice, not elsewhere classified
Z76.81	Expectant mother prebirth pediatrician visit

EXAMPLE Dietary counseling for diabetic diet, Z71.3, E11.9.

11) Encounters for Obstetrical and Reproductive Services

See Section I.C.15. Pregnancy, Childbirth, and the Puerperium, for further instruction on the use of these codes.

Z codes for pregnancy are for use in those circumstances when none of the problems or complications included in the codes from the Obstetrics chapter exist (a routine prenatal visit or postpartum care). Codes in category Z34, Encounter for supervision of normal pregnancy, are always first listed and are not to be used with any other code from the OB chapter.

Codes in category Z3A, Weeks of gestation, may be assigned to provide additional information about the pregnancy.

The outcome of delivery, category Z37, should be included on all maternal delivery records. It is always a secondary code. Codes in category Z37 should not be used on the newborn record.

Z codes for family planning (contraceptive) or procreative management and counseling should be included on an obstetric record either during the pregnancy or the postpartum stage, if applicable.

Z codes/categories for obstetrical and reproductive services:

Z30	Encounter for contraceptive management
Z31	Encounter for procreative management
Z32.2	Encounter for childbirth instruction
Z32.3	Encounter for childcare instruction
Z33	Pregnant state
Z34	Encounter for supervision of normal pregnancy
Z36	Encounter for antenatal screening of mother
Z3A	**Weeks of gestation**
Z37	Outcome of delivery
Z39	Encounter for maternal postpartum care and examination
Z76.81	Expectant mother prebirth pediatrician visit

EXAMPLE Obstetric patent admitted at 40 weeks. Vaginal delivery of a single female infant with no complications, O80, Z3A.40, Z37.0, 10E0XZZ.

12) Newborns and Infants

See Section I.C.16. Newborn (Perinatal) Guidelines, for further instruction on the use of these codes.

Newborn Z codes/categories:

Z76.1	Encounter for health supervision and care of foundling
Z00.1-	Encounter for routine child health examination
Z38	Liveborn infants according to place of birth and type of delivery

EXAMPLE Single liveborn female infant born via vaginal delivery, Z38.00

13) Routine and administrative examinations

The Z codes allow for the description of encounters for routine examinations, such as, a general check-up, or, examinations for administrative purposes, such as, a pre-employment physical. The codes are not to be used if the examination is for diagnosis of a suspected condition or for treatment purposes. In such cases the diagnosis code is used. During a routine exam, should a diagnosis or condition be discovered, it should be coded as an additional code. Pre-existing and chronic conditions and history codes may also be included as additional codes as long as the examination is for administrative purposes and not focused on any particular condition.

Some of the codes for routine health examinations distinguish between "with" and "without" abnormal findings. Code assignment depends on the information that is known at the time the encounter is being coded. For example, if no abnormal findings were found during the examination, but the encounter is being coded before test results are back, it is acceptable to assign the code for "without abnormal findings." When assigning a code for "with abnormal findings," additional code(s) should be assigned to identify the specific abnormal finding(s).

Pre-operative examination and pre-procedural laboratory examination Z codes are for use only in those situations when a patient is being cleared for a procedure or surgery and no treatment is given.

The Z codes/categories for routine and administrative examinations:

Z00	Encounter for general examination without complaint, suspected or reported diagnosis
Z01	Encounter for other special examination without complaint, suspected or reported diagnosis
Z02	Encounter for administrative examination Except: Z02.9, Encounter for administrative examinations, unspecified
Z32.0-	Encounter for pregnancy test

EXAMPLE   Preoperative examination for respiratory clearance for surgery. The patient has emphysema and is scheduled for cholecystectomy for cholelithiasis of the gallbladder, Z01.811, J43.9, K80.20.

14) **Miscellaneous Z codes**

The miscellaneous Z codes capture a number of other health care encounters that do not fall into one of the other categories. Certain of these codes identify the reason for the encounter; others are for use as additional codes that provide useful information on circumstances that may affect a patient's care and treatment.

Prophylactic Organ Removal

For encounters specifically for prophylactic removal of an organ (such as prophylactic removal of breasts due to a genetic susceptibility to cancer or a family history of cancer), the principal or first-listed code should be a code from category Z40, Encounter for prophylactic surgery, followed by the appropriate codes to identify the associated risk factor (such as genetic susceptibility or family history).

If the patient has a malignancy of one site and is having prophylactic removal at another site to prevent either a new primary malignancy or metastatic disease, a code for the malignancy should also be assigned in addition to a code from subcategory Z40.0, Encounter for prophylactic surgery for risk factors related to malignant neoplasms. A Z40.0 code should not be assigned if the patient is having organ removal for treatment of a malignancy, such as the removal of the testes for the treatment of prostate cancer.

Miscellaneous Z codes/categories:

Z28	Immunization not carried out Except: Z28.3, Underimmunization status
Z40	Encounter for prophylactic surgery
Z41	Encounter for procedures for purposes other than remedying health state Except: Z41.9, Encounter for procedure for purposes other than remedying health state, unspecified
Z53	Persons encountering health services for specific procedures and treatment, not carried out
Z55	Problems related to education and literacy
Z56	Problems related to employment and unemployment
Z57	Occupational exposure to risk factors
Z58	Problems related to physical environment
Z59	Problems related to housing and economic circumstances
Z60	Problems related to social environment
Z62	Problems related to upbringing
Z63	Other problems related to primary support group, including family circumstances

Z64	Problems related to certain psychosocial circumstances
Z65	Problems related to other psychosocial circumstances
Z72	Problems related to lifestyle
Z73	Problems related to life management difficulty
Z74	Problems related to care provider dependency
	Except: Z74.01, Bed confinement status
Z75	Problems related to medical facilities and other health care
Z76.0	Encounter for issue of repeat prescription
Z76.3	Healthy person accompanying sick person
Z76.4	Other boarder to healthcare facility
Z76.5	Malingerer [conscious simulation]
Z76.89	Persons encountering health services in other specified circumstances
Z91.1-	Patient's noncompliance with medical treatment and regimen
Z91.83	**Wandering in diseases classified elsewhere**
Z91.89	Other specified personal risk factors, not elsewhere classified

EXAMPLE   A patient was admitted for cosmetic surgery (bilateral silicone breast implants), Z41.1, 0H0V0JZ.

15) Nonspecific Z codes

Certain Z codes are so non-specific, or potentially redundant with other codes in the classification, that there can be little justification for their use in the inpatient setting. Their use in the outpatient setting should be limited to those instances when there is no further documentation to permit more precise coding. Otherwise, any sign or symptom or any other reason for visit that is captured in another code should be used.

Nonspecific Z codes/categories:

Z02.9	Encounter for administrative examinations, unspecified
Z04.9	Encounter for examination and observation for unspecified reason
Z13.9	Encounter for screening, unspecified
Z41.9	Encounter for procedure for purposes other than remedying health state, unspecified
Z52.9	Donor of unspecified organ or tissue
Z86.59	Personal history of other mental and behavioral disorders
Z88.9	Allergy status to unspecified drugs, medicaments and biological substances status
Z92.0	Personal history of contraception

16) Z Codes That May Only be Principal/First-Listed Diagnosis

The following Z codes/categories may only be reported as the principal/first-listed diagnosis, except when there are multiple encounters on the same day and the medical records for the encounters are combined:

Z00	Encounter for general examination without complaint, suspected or reported diagnosis
Z01	Encounter for other special examination without complaint, suspected or reported diagnosis
Z02	Encounter for administrative examination
Z03	Encounter for medical observation for suspected diseases and conditions ruled out
Z04	Encounter for examination and observation for other reasons
Z33.2	Encounter for elective termination of pregnancy
Z31.81	Encounter for male factor infertility in female patient
Z31.82	Encounter for Rh incompatibility status
Z31.83	Encounter for assisted reproductive fertility procedure cycle
Z31.84	Encounter for fertility preservation procedure
Z34	Encounter for supervision of normal pregnancy
Z39	Encounter for maternal postpartum care and examination

Z38	Liveborn infants according to place of birth and type of delivery
Z42	Encounter for plastic and reconstructive surgery following medical procedure or healed injury
Z51.0	Encounter for antineoplastic radiation therapy
Z51.1-	Encounter for antineoplastic chemotherapy and immunotherapy
Z52	Donors of organs and tissues Except: Z52.9, Donor of unspecified organ or tissue
Z76.1	Encounter for health supervision and care of foundling
Z76.2	Encounter for health supervision and care of other healthy infant and child
Z99.12	Encounter for respirator [ventilator] dependence during power failure

EXAMPLE   Single liveborn infant delivered by Cesarean section, Z38.01.

EXERCISE 8-3

Assign codes to the following conditions.

1. Patient receives long-term oxygen therapy for emphysema; _____
   patient has a history of tobacco abuse

2. Dietary counseling for morbid obesity in an adult patient; _____
   body mass index (BMI) is 41

3. Screening for prostate cancer; patient has no signs or _____
   symptoms

4. Family history of ischemic heart disease _____

5. Personal history of malaria _____

6. History of urinary calculi _____

7. Personal history of diabetes mellitus, type II; patient _____
   currently takes insulin for diabetes

8. Awaiting liver transplant for end-stage liver disease _____

9. Patient on Coumadin (anticoagulant) because of mechanical _____
   heart valve

10. Patient is noncompliant with diet and medications _____

Using the Z code guideline for principal/first-listed diagnosis, select the correct answer.

11. Z44.109 Fitting and adjustment of artificial leg
    A. First diagnosis only
    B. First and/or additional diagnosis

12. Z42.1 Encounter for breast reconstruction following mastectomy
    A. First diagnosis only
    B. First and/or additional diagnosis

13. Z41.2 Routine or ritual male circumcision
    A. First diagnosis only
    B. First and/or additional diagnosis

14. Z43.3 Attention to colostomy
    A. First diagnosis only
    B. First and/or additional diagnosis

15. Z34.01 Supervision of normal first pregnancy, first trimester
    A. First diagnosis only
    B. First and/or additional diagnosis

PROCEDURES

Procedures can be taken from any of the tables in ICD-10-PCS. When a Z code is used as a diagnosis for a given procedure or a reason for the encounter, a procedure code is still necessary to identify that the procedure was performed. It can be confusing when a Z code seems to describe a procedure.

Remember that ICD-10-PCS procedure codes only need to be assigned on inpatient encounters.

EXAMPLE Patient was admitted for sterilization. A laparoscopic ligation of the fallopian tubes was performed, Z30.2, 0UL74ZZ.

EXAMPLE Patient is donating a kidney. A left laparoscopic nephrectomy was performed, Z52.4, 0TT14ZZ.

EXERCISE 8-4

Assign codes for all diagnoses and procedures.

1. Encounter for hemodialysis due to end-stage renal disease _____
2. Admission for chemotherapy (via central vein) for ovarian cancer _____
3. Admission for replacement of tracheostomy tube _____
4. Admission following delivery in ambulance _____
5. Encounter for removal of internal fixation device, right femoral shaft _____

DOCUMENTATION/REIMBURSEMENT/MS-DRGs

Often, coding difficulties are due to lack of documentation. Signs and symptoms are often not correlated with a definitive diagnosis in the health record. Sometimes, pathology and other test results are not available at the time of discharge, or when the physician is dictating the discharge summary or reporting the final diagnoses. As a general rule, MS-DRGs that are assigned and have a principal diagnosis from Chapter 18 may have lower reimbursement than an MS-DRG that has a principal diagnosis of a definitive condition or disease.

Frequently missed complications/comorbidities from this chapter include the following:
- Coma
- Shock
- Febrile convulsion
- Hemoptysis
- Ascites, including malignant ascites
- Cachexia
- Z codes for organ replacement/transplant
- Suicidal ideation
- BMI less than 19 or greater than 40 (adult)

Symptoms That Are Integral to a Disease Process

EXAMPLE Patient was admitted with chest pain due to costochondritis, M94.0.

DIAGNOSES	CODES	MS-DRG	RW
Costochondritis	M94.0	206	0.7565
Chest pain due to costochondritis	R07.9, M94.0	313	0.5434

In this case, the symptom (chest pain) is due to a specific cause, and the chest pain is an integral part of costochondritis, so to assign a code for the chest pain would be incorrect, and would not be in accordance with the coding guidelines. The hospital would receive less reimbursement.

MS-DRG With and Without MCC/CC

EXAMPLE

Patient was admitted with abdominal pain. The patient has end-stage renal disease on dialysis. No cause was determined for the abdominal pain.

DIAGNOSES	CODES	MS-DRG	RW
Abd pain	R10.9	392	0.7241
Abd pain		391	1.1844
ESRD	R10.9, N18.6, Z99.2		

In this case, the patient has a chronic condition of ESRD so it should be reported as a secondary diagnosis. No cause was determined for the patient's abdominal pain, so assignment of R10.9 symptom code is correct for the principal diagnosis. The hospital receives less reimbursement than it deserves if the N18.6 code for the comorbidity is not assigned.

CHAPTER REVIEW EXERCISE

Assign codes for all diagnoses and procedures.

1. Paresthesia _____

2. Abnormal Pap smear with high-grade squamous intraepithelial lesion (HGSIL) _____

3. History of cardiac arrest _____

4. Anasarca _____

5. Chest pain due to unstable angina _____

6. Adult failure to thrive _____

7. Insulin pump training for Type I diabetic _____

8. Complex febrile seizure _____

9. Cachexia _____

10. Physical restraints were ordered by the physician _____

11. Debility _____

12. Patient has a gastrostomy tube and receives tube feedings _____

13. Headache due to migraine _____

14. Absence of kidney due to surgical removal _____

15. History of falls _____

16. Fussy baby _____

17. Elevated blood pressure _____

18. Screening mammogram in a high-risk patient with family history of breast cancer _____

19. Anemia with drop in hematocrit _____

20. Elevated carcinoembryonic antigen (CEA) _____

21. Admission for elective circumcision _____

22. Occult blood in stool _____

23. Screening for bladder cancer in patient with gross hematuria _____

24. Renal colic due to kidney stone _____

25. Abnormal liver function lab tests _____

26. Changing of gastrostomy tube in patient with dysphagia _____

27. Diarrhea due to gastroenteritis _____

28. Intramuscular vaccination for influenza _____

29. Patient has type I diabetes mellitus and has an insulin pump _____

30. Prophylactic removal of both ovaries due to strong family history _____
of ovarian cancer and genetic susceptibility. A bilateral salpingo-
oophorectomy was performed

31. Respiratory arrest _____

32. Sudden infant death syndrome (SIDS) _____

33. Decreased libido _____

34. Hypoxia _____

35. Nervousness _____

CHAPTER GLOSSARY   **Prophylactic:** medication or treatment used to prevent a disease from occurring.

Screening examination: one that occurs in the absence of any signs or symptoms. It involves examination of an asymptomatic individual to detect a given disease, typically by means of an inexpensive diagnostic test.

Sign: objective evidence of a disease or of a patient's condition as perceived by the patient's examining physician.

Symptom: subjective evidence of a disease or of a patient's condition as perceived by the patient.

9

Certain Infectious and Parasitic Diseases

(ICD-10-CM Chapter 1, Codes A00-B99)

LEARNING OBJECTIVES

1. Apply and assign the correct ICD-10-CM/PCS codes in accordance with Official Guidelines for Coding and Reporting

2. Identify major differences between ICD-10-CM and ICD-9-CM related to infectious and parasitic diseases

3. Recognize infectious and parasitic diseases

4. Assign the correct Z codes and procedure codes related to infectious and parasitic diseases
5. Identify common treatments, medications, laboratory values, and diagnostic tests
6. Explain the importance of documentation as it relates to MS-DRGs for reimbursement

ABBREVIATIONS/ ACRONYMS

AIDS acquired immunodeficiency syndrome

BCG Bacille Calmette Guerin vaccine

C. DIFF *Clostridium difficile*

CD4 Cluster of differentiation 4

CDC Centers for Disease Control and Prevention

DMAC disseminated *Mycobacterium avium-intracellulare* complex

EGD esophogastroduodenoscopy

HAART highly active antiretroviral therapy

HFMD hand, foot, and mouth disease

HIV human immunodeficiency virus

HIVAN HIV-associated nephropathy

HPV Human papilloma virus

HSV herpes simplex virus

ICD-9-CM *International Classification of Diseases, 9th Revision, Clinical Modification*

ICD-10-CM *International Classification of Diseases, 10th Revision, Clinical Modification*

ICD-10-PCS *International Classification of Diseases, 10th Revision, Procedure Coding System*

IVDU intravenous drug use

MAC *Mycobacterium avium-intracellulare* complex

MAI *Mycobacterium avium-intracellulare*

MOD multiple organ dysfunction

MRSA methicillin-resistant *Staphylococcus aureus*

MSSA methicillin-sensitive *Staphylococcus aureus*

PCP *Pneumocystis carinii* pneumonia

RPR rapid plasma reagin

SARS severe acute respiratory syndrome

SIRS systemic inflammatory response syndrome

STD sexually transmitted disease

STEC Shiga toxin-producing *E. coli*

TB tuberculosis

UTI urinary tract infection

VDRL Venereal Disease Research Laboratory

VRE vancomycin-resistant enterococcus

WBC white blood cells

ICD-10-CM

Official Guidelines for Coding and Reporting

Please refer to the companion Evolve website for the most current guidelines.

1. Chapter 1: Certain Infectious and Parasitic Diseases (A00-B99)
  a. Human Immunodeficiency Virus (HIV) Infections
    1) Code only confirmed cases
      Code only confirmed cases of HIV infection/illness. This is an exception to the hospital inpatient guideline Section II, H.

      In this context, "confirmation" does not require documentation of positive serology or culture for HIV; the provider's diagnostic statement that the patient is HIV positive, or has an HIV-related illness is sufficient.

EXAMPLE

Patient with possible human immunodeficiency virus (HIV). Even though in the inpatient setting it is acceptable to code diagnoses that are possible or suspected, in the case of possible HIV, you would not assign B20. You would have to query the physician regarding the patient's exact HIV status. This is one of the only exceptions to coding a diagnosis as if it exists when it is documented as possible or probable.

---

    2) Selection and sequencing of HIV codes
      (a) Patient admitted for HIV-related condition
        If a patient is admitted for an HIV-related condition, the principal diagnosis should be B20, **Human immunodeficiency virus [HIV] disease** followed by additional diagnosis codes for all reported HIV-related conditions.

EXAMPLE   The patient was admitted for treatment of Kaposi's sarcoma of the skin. The patient's HIV has been symptomatic for the past year, B20, C46.0.

(b) Patient with HIV disease admitted for unrelated condition
If a patient with HIV disease is admitted for an unrelated condition (such as a traumatic injury), the code for the unrelated condition (e.g., the nature of injury code) should be the principal diagnosis. Other diagnoses would be B20 followed by additional diagnosis codes for all reported HIV-related conditions.

EXAMPLE   Initial encounter for traumatic closed-fracture of the left femur in a patient who has acquired immunodeficiency syndrome (AIDS), S72.92xA, B20, W58.xxxA.

(c) Whether the patient is newly diagnosed
Whether the patient is newly diagnosed or has had previous admissions/encounters for HIV conditions is irrelevant to the sequencing decision.

(d) Asymptomatic human immunodeficiency virus
Z21, Asymptomatic human immunodeficiency virus [HIV] infection status, is to be applied when the patient without any documentation of symptoms is listed as being "HIV positive," "known HIV," "HIV test positive," or similar terminology. Do not use this code if the term "AIDS" is used or if the patient is treated for any HIV-related illness or is described as having any condition(s) resulting from his/her HIV positive status; use B20 in these cases.

EXAMPLE   The patient's HIV test last week was positive; the patient is asymptomatic, Z21.

(e) Patients with inconclusive HIV serology
Patients with inconclusive HIV serology, but no definitive diagnosis or manifestations of the illness, may be assigned code R75, Inconclusive laboratory evidence of human immunodeficiency virus [HIV].

(f) Previously diagnosed HIV-related illness
Patients with any known prior diagnosis of an HIV-related illness should be coded to B20. Once a patient has developed an HIV-related illness, the patient should always be assigned code B20 on every subsequent admission/encounter. Patients previously diagnosed with any HIV illness (B20) should never be assigned to R75 or Z21, Asymptomatic human immunodeficiency virus [HIV] infection status.

EXAMPLE   HIV patient with prior history of *Pneumocystis carinii* pneumonia (PCP), B20. PCP is an opportunistic lung infection that has been identified as an AIDS-defining illness.

(g) HIV Infection in Pregnancy, Childbirth and the Puerperium
During pregnancy, childbirth or the puerperium, a patient admitted (or presenting for a health care encounter) because of an HIV-related illness should receive a principal diagnosis code of O98.7-, Human immunodeficiency [HIV] disease complicating pregnancy, childbirth and the puerperium, followed by B20 and the code(s) for the HIV-related illness(es). Codes from Chapter 15 always take sequencing priority.

Patients with asymptomatic HIV infection status admitted (or presenting for a health care encounter) during pregnancy, childbirth, or the puerperium should receive codes of O98.7- and Z21.

EXAMPLE | The patient is 20 weeks pregnant and is admitted for treatment of esophageal candidiasis due to AIDS, O98.712, B20, B37.81.

EXAMPLE | A patient at 39 weeks delivered liveborn twins vaginally during her hospital stay. The mother's HIV has remained asymptomatic, O30.003, O98.72, Z21, Z37.2, 10E0XZZ.

(h) Encounters for testing for HIV

If a patient is being seen to determine his/her HIV status, use code Z11.4, Encounter for screening for human immunodeficiency virus [HIV]. Use additional codes for any associated high risk behavior.

If a patient with signs or symptoms is being seen for HIV testing, code the signs and symptoms. An additional counseling code Z71.7, Human immunodeficiency virus [HIV] counseling, may be used if counseling is provided during the encounter for the test.

When a patient returns to be informed of his/her HIV test results and the test result is negative, use code Z71.7, Human immunodeficiency virus [HIV] counseling.

If the results are positive, see previous guidelines and assign codes as appropriate.

EXAMPLE | Because of high-risk homosexual behavior, the patient is seen in the clinic for HIV screening, Z11.4, Z72.52.

EXAMPLE | The patient returns for test results that are negative and is counseled regarding HIV prevention, Z71.7.

EXAMPLE | The patient returns for test results that are positive and is asymptomatic. She is instructed regarding symptoms to watch for and means of prevention, Z21, Z71.7.

b. Infectious agents as the cause of diseases classified to other chapters

Certain infections are classified in chapters other than Chapter 1 and no organism is identified as part of the infection code. In these instances, it is necessary to use an additional code from Chapter 1 to identify the organism. A code from category B95, Streptococcus, Staphylococcus, and Enterococcus as the cause of diseases classified to other chapters, B96, Other bacterial agents as the cause of diseases classified to other chapters, or B97, Viral agents as the cause of diseases classified to other chapters, is to be used as an additional code to identify the organism. An instructional note will be found at the infection code advising that an additional organism code is required.

EXAMPLE | Patient is admitted to the hospital with pneumonia due to bacteriodes fragilis, J15.8, B96.6.

c. Infections resistant to antibiotics

Many bacterial infections are resistant to current antibiotics. It is necessary to identify all infections documented as antibiotic resistant. Assign a code **from category** Z16, **Resistance to antimicrobial drugs**, following the infection code **only if the infection code does not identify drug resistance.**

EXAMPLE | Patient is admitted to the hospital with pneumonia due to MRSA, J15.212.

EXAMPLE | VRE acute endocarditis, I33.0, B95.2, Z16.21.

d. Sepsis, Severe Sepsis, and Septic Shock
   1) Coding of Sepsis and Severe Sepsis
      (a) Sepsis
         For a diagnosis of sepsis, assign the appropriate code for the underlying systemic infection. If the type of infection or causal organism is not further specified, assign code A41.9, Sepsis, unspecified **organism.**

         A code from subcategory R65.2, Severe sepsis, should not be assigned unless severe sepsis or an associated acute organ dysfunction is documented.

EXAMPLE   Patient presents with sepsis. After study the attending physician documents sepsis secondary to staph aureus found in the blood cultures. The patient also has staph aureus pneumonia, A41.01, J15.211.

         (i) Negative or inconclusive blood cultures and sepsis
            Negative or inconclusive blood cultures do not preclude a diagnosis of sepsis in patients with clinical evidence of the condition, however, the provider should be queried.

EXAMPLE   Patient presents to the ER with shaking chills, temperature of 104°F, and WBC of 14,000. Physician suspects sepsis and takes blood cultures. Blood cultures are negative for bacteria. Physician documents on discharge summary that the patient has sepsis, A41.9.

         (ii) Urosepsis
            The term urosepsis is a nonspecific term. It is not to be considered synonymous with sepsis. It has no default code in the Alphabetic Index. Should a provider use this term, he/she must be queried for clarification.

EXAMPLE   Patient presents to the ER with fever and painful urination. The physician documents urosepsis and admits the patient to the hospital for IV antibiotics. Physician must be queried for clarification as to the condition as there is no ICD-10-CM code for this terminology.

         (iii) Sepsis with organ dysfunction
            If a patient has sepsis and associated acute organ dysfunction or multiple organ dysfunction (MOD), follow the instructions for coding severe sepsis.

EXAMPLE   Patient is admitted to the hospital with sepsis and acute renal failure secondary to sepsis, A41.9, R65.9, N17.9.

         (iv) Acute organ dysfunction that is not clearly associated with the sepsis
            If a patient has sepsis and an acute organ dysfunction, but the medical record documentation indicates that the acute organ dysfunction is related to a medical condition other than the sepsis, do not assign a code from subcategory R65.2, Severe sepsis. An acute organ dysfunction must be associated with the sepsis in order to assign the severe sepsis code. If the documentation is not clear as to whether an acute organ dysfunction is related to the sepsis or another medical condition, query the provider.

EXAMPLE Patient is admitted to the hospital with sepsis, pneumonia, and acute respiratory failure, A41.9, J18.9, J96.0. It would be a good idea to query the provider to see if the acute respiratory failure is related to the sepsis.

(b) Severe sepsis

The coding of severe sepsis requires a minimum of 2 codes: first a code for the underlying systemic infection, followed by a code from subcategory R65.2, Severe sepsis. If the causal organism is not documented, assign code A41.9, Sepsis, unspecified **organism**, for the infection. Additional code(s) for the associated acute organ dysfunction are also required.

Due to the complex nature of severe sepsis, some cases may require querying the provider prior to assignment of the codes.

2) Septic shock

(a) Septic shock **generally refers to** circulatory failure associated with severe sepsis, and therefore, it represents a type of acute organ dysfunction.

For cases of septic shock, the code for the systemic infection should be sequenced first, followed by code R65.21, Severe sepsis with septic shock or **code T81.12, Postprocedural septic shock**. Any additional codes for the other acute organ dysfunctions should also be assigned. **As noted in the sequencing instructions in the Tabular List, the code for septic shock cannot be assigned as a principal diagnosis.**

EXAMPLE The patient was admitted with septic shock and acute renal failure caused by a UTI due to *E. coli*. Discharge summary states sepsis due to *E. coli*, A41.51, N39.0, R65.21, N17.9.

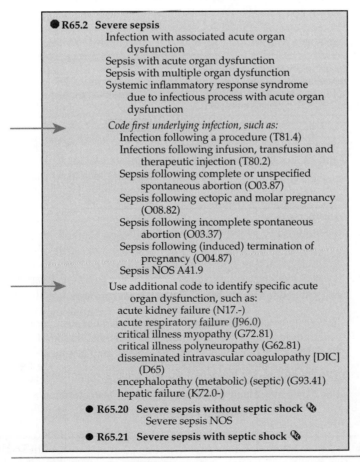

FIGURE 9-1. Severe Sepsis.

3) Sequencing of severe sepsis

If severe sepsis is present on admission, and meets the definition of principal diagnosis, the underlying systemic infection should be assigned as principal diagnosis followed by the appropriate code from subcategory R65.2 as required by the sequencing rules in the Tabular List. A code from subcategory R65.2 can never be assigned as a principal diagnosis.

When severe sepsis develops during an encounter (it was not present on admission) the underlying systemic infection and the appropriate code from subcategory R65.2 should be assigned as secondary diagnoses.

Severe sepsis may be present on admission but the diagnosis may not be confirmed until sometime after admission. If the documentation is not clear whether severe sepsis was present on admission, the provider should be queried.

EXAMPLE The patient was admitted with pneumonia due to *Staphylococcus aureus*. Several days after admission, the patient developed septic shock due to staph aureus sepsis, J15.211, A41.01, R65.21.

4) Sepsis and severe sepsis with a localized infection

If the reason for admission is both sepsis or severe sepsis and a localized infection, such as pneumonia or cellulitis, a code(s) for the underlying systemic infection should be assigned first and the code for the localized infection should be assigned as a secondary diagnosis. If the patient has severe sepsis, a code from subcategory R65.2 should also be assigned as a secondary diagnosis. If the patient is admitted with a localized infection, such as pneumonia, and sepsis/severe sepsis doesn't develop until after admission, the localized infection should be assigned first, followed by the appropriate sepsis/severe sepsis codes.

EXAMPLE The patient was admitted in acute respiratory failure due to *Staphylococcus aureus* pneumonia. The patient also presented with sepsis due to staph aureus infection associated with respiratory failure, A41.01, J15.211, J96.00, R65.20.

5) Sepsis due to a postprocedural infection
   (a) Documentation of causal relationship
      As with all postprocedural complications, code assignment is based on the provider's documentation of the relationship between the infection and the procedure.
   (b) Sepsis due to a postprocedural infection
      For such cases, the postprocedural infection code, such as, T80.2, Infections following infusion, transfusion, and therapeutic injection, T81.4, Infection following a procedure, T88.0, Infection following immunization, or O86.0, Infection of obstetric surgical wound, should be coded first, followed by the code for the specific infection. If the patient has severe sepsis the appropriate code from subcategory R65.2 should also be assigned with the additional code(s) for any acute organ dysfunction.
   (c) Postprocedural infection and postprocedural septic shock
      In cases where a postprocedural infection has occurred and has resulted in severe sepsis and postprocedural septic shock, the code for the precipitating complication such as code T81.4, Infection following a procedure, or O86.0, Infection of obstetrical surgical wound should be coded first followed by code R65.21, Severe sepsis with septic shock and a code for the systemic infection.

EXAMPLE Patient is admitted through the ER with an infection of her operative wound. The patient is septic. Two weeks ago she had an open appendectomy, T81.4xxA, A41.9, Y83.6.

6) Sepsis and severe sepsis associated with a noninfectious process (condition)

In some cases a noninfectious process (condition), such as trauma, may lead to an infection which can result in sepsis or severe sepsis. If sepsis or severe sepsis is documented as associated with a noninfectious condition, such as a burn or serious injury, and this condition meets the definition for principal diagnosis, the code for the noninfectious condition should be sequenced first, followed by the code for the resulting infection. If severe sepsis, is present a code from subcategory R65.2 should also be assigned with any associated organ dysfunction(s) codes. It is not necessary to assign a code from subcategory R65.1, Systemic inflammatory response syndrome (SIRS) of non-infectious origin, for these cases.

If the infection meets the definition of principal diagnosis it should be sequenced before the non-infectious condition. When both the associated non-infectious condition and the infection meet the definition of principal diagnosis either may be assigned as principal diagnosis.

Only one code from category R65, Symptoms and signs specifically associated with systemic inflammation and infection, should be assigned. Therefore, when a non-infectious condition leads to an infection resulting in severe sepsis, assign the appropriate code from subcategory R65.2, Severe sepsis. Do not additionally assign a code from subcategory R65.1, Systemic inflammatory response syndrome (SIRS) of non-infectious origin.

See Section I.C.18. SIRS due to non-infectious process

EXAMPLE Patient is admitted to the hospital with severe sepsis secondary to advanced lung cancer. IV antibiotics are administered and the patient is discharged on day 5, A41.9, R65.2, C34.90.

---

7) Sepsis and septic shock complicating abortion, pregnancy, childbirth, and the puerperium

See Section I.C.15. Sepsis and septic shock complicating abortion, pregnancy, childbirth and the puerperium

8) Newborn sepsis

See Section I.C.16. Newborn sepsis

e. Methicillin Resistant *Staphylococcus aureus* (MRSA) Conditions

1) Selection and sequencing of MRSA codes

(a) Combination codes for MRSA infection

When a patient is diagnosed with an infection that is due to methicillin resistant *Staphylococcus aureus* (MRSA), and that infection has a combination code that includes the causal organism (e.g., sepsis, pneumonia) assign the appropriate combination code for the condition (e.g., code A41.02, Sepsis due to Methicillin resistant Staphylococcus aureus or code J15.212, Pneumonia due to Methicillin resistant Staphylococcus aureus). Do not assign code B95.62, Methicillin resistant Staphylococcus aureus infection as the cause of diseases classified elsewhere, as an additional code because the combination code includes the type of infection and the MRSA organism. Do not assign a code from subcategory Z16.11, Resistance to penicillins, as an additional diagnosis.

*See Section C.1. for instructions on coding and sequencing of **sepsis and severe sepsis**.*

(b) Other codes for MRSA infection

When there is documentation of a current infection (e.g., wound infection, stitch abscess, urinary tract infection) due to MRSA, and that infection does not have a combination code that includes the causal organism, assign the appropriate code to identify the condition along with code B95.62, Methicillin resistant Staphylococcus aureus infection as the cause of diseases classified elsewhere for the MRSA infection. Do not assign a code from subcategory Z16.11, Resistance to penicillins.

(c) Methicillin susceptible Staphylococcus aureus (MSSA) and MRSA colonization

The condition or state of being colonized or carrying MSSA or MRSA is called colonization or carriage, while an individual person is described as being colonized or being a carrier. Colonization means that MSSA or MSRA is present on or in the body without necessarily causing illness. A positive MRSA colonization test might be documented by the provider as "MRSA screen positive" or "MRSA nasal swab positive". Assign code Z22.322, Carrier or suspected carrier of Methicillin resistant Staphylococcus aureus, for patients documented as having MRSA colonization. Assign code Z22.321, Carrier or suspected carrier of Methicillin susceptible Staphylococcus aureus, for patient documented as having MSSA colonization. Colonization is not necessarily indicative of a disease process or as the cause of a specific condition the patient may have unless documented as such by the provider.

(d) MRSA colonization and infection

If a patient is documented as having both MRSA colonization and infection during a hospital admission, code Z22.322, Carrier or suspected carrier of Methicillin resistant Staphylococcus aureus, and a code for the MRSA infection may both be assigned.

EXAMPLE   Pneumonia due to MRSA, J15.212.

EXAMPLE   UTI due to MRSA, N39.0, B95.62.

EXAMPLE   Patient is nasal swab positive for MRSA, Z33.322.

Apply the General Coding Guidelines as found in Chapter 5 and the Procedural Coding Guidelines as found in Chapters 6 and 7.

MAJOR DIFFERENCES BETWEEN ICD-10-CM AND ICD-9-CM

- Streptococcal sore throat in ICD-10-CM has been reclassified to Diseases of the Respiratory System.
- There is a new category in ICD-10-CM for infections with a predominantly sexual mode of transmission. Many codes from other chapters have been moved to this section.
- In ICD-10-CM, a note under the code for smallpox states the disease has been officially eradicated, but the code is maintained for surveillance purposes.
- In ICD-10-CM, the term *SIRS* is no longer assigned a separate code when due to an infectious process.
- Septicemia and bacteremia are coded to R78.81 in the chapter on symptoms.
- In ICD-10-CM, urosepsis is not assigned a default code. The use of this term requires a query to the provider.

ANATOMY AND PHYSIOLOGY

This chapter focuses on diseases that are **communicable** (easily spread from one to another) and **parasitic** (organism taking nourishment from another organism) and the organisms that are responsible for the disease conditions. Many times, two codes are required. If a condition is not considered communicable, it will be found in a body system chapter; in this case, an additional code from category B95-B97 may be assigned to identify causative organisms or infectious agents.

EXAMPLE   Acute *Staphylococcus* vaginitis, N76.0, B95.8.
To locate the code for *Staphylococcus*, the coder can look under the main term, "Infection," and then under the subterm "*Staphylococcus*." Sometimes, the organism and the disease condition have a combination code; this is the case for many of the pneumonia codes.
Klebsiella pneumonia, J15.0.

There is no one body system that causes or is affected by infectious disease. These organisms can be found in any or all of the body systems.

DISEASE CONDITIONS

Certain Infectious and Parasitic Diseases (A00-B99), Chapter 1 in the ICD-10-CM code book, is divided into the following categories:

CATEGORY	SECTION TITLE
A00-A09	Intestinal infectious diseases
A15-A19	Tuberculosis
A20-A28	Certain zoonotic bacterial diseases
A30-A49	Other bacterial diseases
A50-A64	Infections with a predominantly sexual mode of transmission
A65-A69	Other spirochetal diseases
A70-A74	Other diseases caused by *Chlamydiae*
A75-A79	Rickettsioses
A80-A89	Viral infections of the central nervous system
A90-A99	Arthropod-borne viral fevers and viral hemorrhagic fevers
B00-B09	Viral infections characterized by skin and mucous membrane lesions
B10	Other human herpesviruses
B15-B19	Viral hepatitis
B20-	Human immunodeficiency virus (HIV) disease
B25-B34	Other viral diseases
B35-B49	Mycoses
B50-B64	Protozoal diseases
B65-B83	Helminthiases
B85-B89	Pediculosis, acariasis, and other infestations
B90-B94	Sequelae of infectious and parasitic diseases
B95-B97	Bacterial, viral, and other infectious agents
B99	Other infectious diseases

Intestinal Infectious Diseases (A00-A09)

Clostridium difficile

Clostridium difficile, which is also known as *C. diff,* is a leading cause of pseudomembranous colitis. It can be found in the Index under "Enteritis, clostridium *difficile.*"

C. diff is one of the most common **nosocomial** infections (hospital acquired). In the hospital setting, it may be spread from healthcare worker to patient. Spores associated with this disease can survive up to 70 days. It can also be caused by antibiotic use. This disease is characterized by watery diarrhea and abdominal cramping. The intestinal tract has usually been altered in some way to allow *C. diff* bacteria to flourish.

If a physician suspects *C. diff* (often seen in elderly hospitalized patients), a stool specimen is tested for *C. diff* toxins (cytotoxicity assay). The test results can take between 24 and 48 hours to complete. Treatment depends on the severity of infection. Often, antibiotics are changed or discontinued; however, in severe cases, a patient is treated with metronidazole (Flagyl). Patients with *C. diff* are usually placed on isolation protocol.

EXAMPLE   *Clostridium difficile* colitis, A04.7.

Gastroenteritis

Gastroenteritis is the inflammation of the stomach, small intestine, and large intestine. Infectious gastroenteritis is the most common cause. It can be caused by viruses, bacteria, or parasites. In the United States viruses are most often the cause of gastroenteritis, with norovirus and rotavirus being the most common. Bacterial gastroenteritis is less common than viral gastroenteritis. It is most often caused by salmonella, campylobacter, shigella, and *E. coli.* The most common parasites causing gastroenteritis are giardia or cryptosporidium.

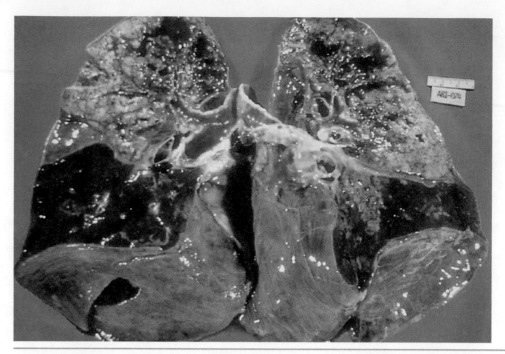

FIGURE 9-2. Tuberculosis.

Gastroenteritis may be treated with fluid replacement to treat any hypotension and fluid depletion. Vomiting and diarrhea can cause metabolic acidosis or alkalosis as well as renal failure, hyponatremia, and hypokalemia. Antibiotics may be used in some cases.

EXAMPLE   Patient is diagnosed with gastroenteritis due to salmonella, A02.0.

Tuberculosis (A15-A19)

Tuberculosis (TB) is an infection caused by *Mycobacterium tuberculosis* (Figure 9-2). These bacteria can attack any part of the body but most often attack the lungs. TB was the leading cause of death in the United States prior to the discovery of medicines to treat the disease. TB was almost eradicated but made a resurgence in the late 1980s.

TB is spread through the air via coughing or sneezing. TB of the lung is the only infectious form of TB. If TB occurs in the bones or kidney, it is not likely to be contagious. TB can be infectious only if it is an active disease. It may be necessary to isolate a patient who is suspected of having this condition, pending confirmation. A form of TB called "latent TB" occurs when a person breathes the bacteria but the immune system fights them off, and they remain alive in the body but are inactive. Latent TB can become active TB. Persons with latent TB usually have a positive TB test result.

Active TB usually occurs in the population whose immune systems are too weak to fight off this disease. This group would include individuals with human immunodeficiency virus (HIV), leukemia, substance abusers, young children, and organ transplant recipients.

EXAMPLE   Patient admitted for pneumonia due to tuberculosis, A15.0.

EXERCISE 9-1

Assign codes to the following conditions.

1. Pyelonephritis caused by tuberculosis   _____

2. Acute miliary tuberculosis   _____

3. Interstitial keratitis caused by tuberculosis; bacterial culture performed, results unknown. _____

4. Cavitation of the lung caused by tuberculosis _____

5. *Salmonella* sepsis _____

6. Food poisoning caused by *Salmonella* resulting in gastroenteritis _____

7. Enteritis caused by the rotavirus _____

8. Norwalk virus _____

9. Dysentery _____

10. Giardiasis _____

Certain Zoonotic Bacterial Diseases (A20-A28)

Anthrax

Anthrax is a bacterial infection that is usually found in wild or domestic animals. It is most common in agricultural regions of Central America, Africa, Asia, and the Caribbean. Anthrax occurs in three forms: cutaneous, inhalation, and gastrointestinal. The most serious form is the inhalation type, which causes severe breathing problems that are most often fatal. Since the 9/11 attack on the United States and threats of anthrax attacks, a code was developed for contact or exposure to anthrax.

EXAMPLE | Contact with or exposure to anthrax, Z20.810.

This code can be used for anyone who has been exposed to anthrax, or who is closely linked to persons with known exposure.

EXAMPLE | Patient is admitted to hospital with possible inhalation anthrax, A22.1.

Other Bacterial Diseases (A30-A49)

Mycobacterium Avium *Complex*

Mycobacterium avium complex (MAC) or *Mycobacterium avium-intercellulare* (MAI) is a bacterium which attacks immunocompromised individuals. This bacterium is found in soil and water; an individual who is not immunocompromised does not succumb to the disease. This has been classified as an acquired immunodeficiency syndrome (AIDS)–defining illness. Tests that show high blood levels of the liver enzyme alkaline phosphatase may indicate MAC. Symptoms of this disease include night sweats, weight loss, and diarrhea. Prior to the advent of highly active antiretroviral therapy (**HAART**), which is a group of drugs given to patients with AIDS for prophylaxis, a high incidence of this condition was reported. It generally affects individuals whose T4 cell count is under 50. A variety of antibiotics are used to treat patients with this disease. Individuals with advanced AIDS often develop disseminated *Mycobacterium avium-intracellulare* complex (DMAC). A unique presentation of patients with DMAC is severe anemia.

EXAMPLE | Infection from *Mycobacterium avium*, A31.0.

Meningococcal Infection

Meningococcal infections are caused by the bacterium meningococcus (Figure 9-3). These bacteria may be found in around 10% of the population (in the nose or throat) and cause

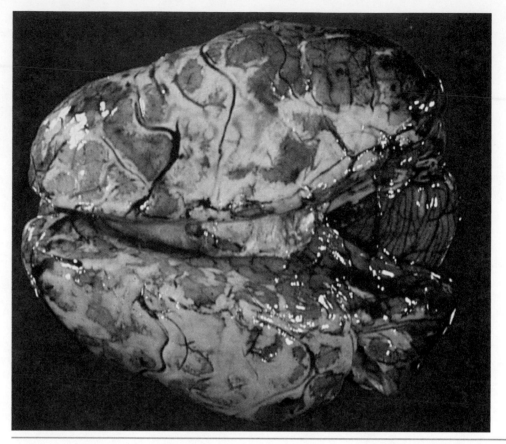

FIGURE 9-3. Bacterial meningitis. The surface of the brain is covered with pus.

no ill effects. These people are known as asymptomatic carriers. This bacterium can cause **meningitis**, which is an infection in the fluid of a person's spinal cord and brain. It also can cause septicemia (blood infection), which is known as meningococcal septicemia.

EXAMPLE	Meningococcal meningitis, A39.0.

EXAMPLE	Meningococcemia, A39.4.

Sepsis

Sepsis is a medical condition in which the immune system goes into overdrive, releasing chemicals that trigger widespread inflammation into the blood to combat infection. Four different levels of sepsis have been established by the American College of Chest Physicians and the Society of Critical Care Medicine.

1. Systemic inflammatory response syndrome (SIRS); there is no confirmed infectious process in SIRS
   - Hypothermia (temperature lower than 36° C/97° F) or fever (higher than 38° C/100° F)
   - Tachycardia (heart rate greater than 100 beats per minute)
   - Tachypnea (more than 20 breaths per minute)
   - Hypocapnia (arterial CO_2 less than 32 mm Hg)
2. Sepsis: SIRS in response to a confirmed infectious process
3. Severe sepsis: sepsis plus organ dysfunction
4. Septic shock

When coding sepsis in ICD-10-CM it is appropriate to assign the code for the underlying systemic infection. If the causal organism or type of infection is not further specified, assign code A41.9.

Some patients may have sepsis without positive blood cultures. If a physician documents urosepsis a query must be initiated for clarification. There is no Alphabetic Index term for this condition. If a patient has acute organ dysfunction and sepsis and the organ dysfunction is not directly attributed to the sepsis and there is no other underlying cause documented, a query should be initiated. Acute organ dysfunction attributable to sepsis should be assigned a code for severe sepsis. Septic shock represents a type of acute organ dysfunction and therefore should have a code for severe sepsis assigned.

Sequencing of the codes for *sepsis with a localized infection* (i.e., pneumonia, cellulitis) meeting the definition of principal diagnosis should be assigned in the following order:

- Assign the code for the underlying systemic infection
- Assign the code for the localized infection
- Assign the code for severe sepsis, if applicable
- Assign a code for any applicable acute organ dysfunction

Sequencing of codes for *sepsis due to a postprocedural infection*, which is an infection due to a complication of medical care, should be assigned in the following order:

- Assign the postprocedural infection code first (codes T80.2-, T81.4-, T88.0- O86.0).
- Assign code for the specific infection
- Assign a code for severe sepsis, if applicable
- Assign a code for any applicable acute organ dysfunction

Sepsis due to a noninfectious process (such as trauma, surgery, or burn) that meets the definition of principal diagnosis should have codes assigned in the following order:

- Assign the code for the noninfectious condition
- Assign the code for the resulting infection
- Assign a code for any applicable acute organ dysfunction
- Do not assign a code for SIRS of noninfectious origin (R65.1)

When a patient is admitted with a noninfectious condition and an infectious condition that both meet the definition of principal diagnosis, either may be sequenced first. Do not use a code from SIRS of noninfectious origin if the noninfectious condition leads to an infection resulting in severe sepsis.

EXAMPLE Patient admitted with pneumonia, fever, and tachycardia. Physician suspects sepsis and orders blood cultures. Two days after admittance, cultures are positive for pneumococcal bacteria and physician confirms pneumococcal sepsis, A40.3, J18.9.

EXERCISE 9-2

Assign codes to the following conditions.

1. Respiratory anthrax _____
2. Cutaneous anthrax _____
3. *Mycobacterium kansasii* _____
4. MAI _____
5. DMAC _____
6. Whooping cough _____
7. Patient has MAC and is on HAART. What other disease could you query for? _____
8. Meningococcal infection in the heart muscle _____
9. Sepsis due to meningococcal bacteria _____
10. Urosepsis _____
11. Gonococcal sepsis _____

12. Severe sepsis with acute respiratory failure _____
13. Sepsis of the newborn _____
14. Patient presents with fever, chills, and hypotension. _____
    The physician orders blood cultures for suspected sepsis.
    Results are negative. The discharge summary lists sepsis
    due to *Escherichia coli*.
15. Patient with sepsis secondary to pneumonia _____

Infections With a Predominantly Sexual Mode of Transmission (A50-A64)

Syphilis

Syphilis is a sexually transmitted disease (STD) that is caused by bacteria. Syphilis is passed through direct contact with syphilis sores. Sores occur in the vagina, penis, anus, or rectum. They can also occur on the lips and in the mouth. Syphilis can be passed on to babies through pregnant women. Syphilis occurs in three stages: primary, secondary, and late.

Primary syphilis is revealed by sores called "**chancres**" (Figure 9-4). These sores can last for 3 to 6 weeks. Treatment with a single injection of penicillin can cure the patient at this stage of the disease.

Secondary syphilis, which usually presents as a rash on the palms of the hands and feet, may be accompanied by fever, sore throat, headache, and fatigue. Lesions also may appear in the mouth, vagina, or penis. Sometimes, warty patches called "**condylomata** lata" may appear on the genitalia. These secondary signs eventually disappear even without treatment, but the infection then progresses to late stages.

Late syphilis is the hidden stage of the disease. No signs or symptoms are noted until it begins to damage internal organs, which may occur years later.

A blood test is performed to test for syphilis. This test is called VDRL (Venereal Disease Research Laboratory), or RPR (rapid plasma reagin).

EXAMPLE | Late neurosyphilis with ataxia, A52.11.

EXAMPLE | Two-year-old presents with syphilitic pemphigus, A50.06.

EXAMPLE | Genital chancre, A51.0.

Gonorrhea

Gonorrhea is caused by a bacterium and transmitted by sexual contact. Women may have no symptoms, but men usually report burning while urinating and discharge from the penis. Gonorrhea is treated with an antibiotic. If gonorrhea is not treated, complications usually occur.

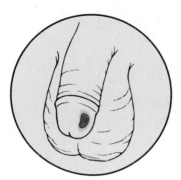

FIGURE 9-4. Chancre of primary syphilis.

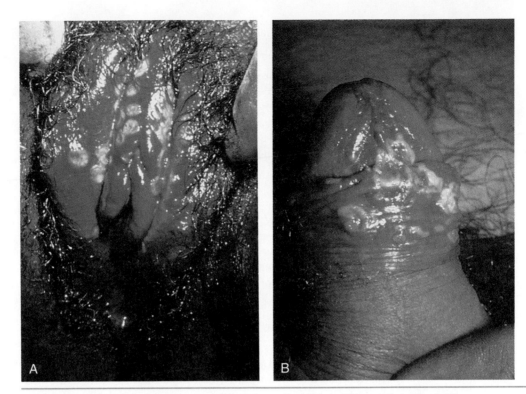

FIGURE 9-5. Genital herpes in the female patient **(A)** and the male patient **(B)**.

EXAMPLE | Female patient presents with acute gonococcal cervicitis, A54.03.

EXAMPLE | Male patient presents with chronic prostatitis due to gonorrhea, A54.22.

Herpes Simplex I and II

Herpes simplex virus is another name for a cold sore or fever blister, also known as HSV type I. The disease manifests as small fluid-filled blisters. It usually occurs on the face but occasionally is noted in the genital area. People usually acquire HSV I during infancy or childhood from people who kiss them or share towels or eating utensils. In type II or genital herpes, sores appear on the vagina, penis, or buttocks (Figure 9-5). Type II is transmitted via sexual intercourse. Antiviral medications are being used to suppress recurrences of herpes.

Genital herpes is considered an STD. It is highly unlikely that the virus is spread through contact with toilet seats or hot tubs. Herpes remains in the nerve cells of the body for life and can become active at any given time. There is no cure for herpes, but there are medicines such as acyclovir (Zovirax), Famciclovir (Famvir), and valacyclovir (Valtrex). Valtrex is also used as a preventive medicine.

EXAMPLE | Patient presents to physician's office with complaints of blisters on penis. Physician makes diagnosis of herpes infection of the penis, A60.01.

EXERCISE 9-3

Assign codes to the following conditions.

1. Patient has a chancre on the penis. _____
2. Patient presents with condyloma latum. _____

3. Latent syphilis with unknown date of infection   _____

4. Dementia due to syphilis   _____

5. Early congenital syphilis   _____

6. Exposure to gonorrhea   _____

7. Suspected carrier of gonorrhea   _____

8. Herpes simplex vaginitis   _____

9. Gonococcal conjunctivitis   _____

10. Pelvic inflammatory disease due to chlamydia   _____

Other Spirochetal Diseases (A65-A69)

Lyme disease, also known as borreliosis, is an inflammatory disease caused by bacteria carried by ticks. Ticks acquire this bacterium through biting deer that are infected. It was first reported in the Northeast United States but now has spread throughout the Midwest, as well as the Pacific Coast. The symptoms of this disease resemble the flu and include headache, fever, and muscle aches. Sometimes, a bull's-eye rash appears at the site of the tick bite.

A blood test can be performed to look for antibodies to the bacteria that cause Lyme disease. Treatment for Lyme disease consists of antibiotics and anti-inflammatory medicines. If this disease is left untreated, complications such as Lyme arthritis, heart problems, or neurologic disorders can occur.

EXAMPLE A patient presents with severe joint pain. Blood work reveals Lyme disease. The physician documents that the patient has arthritis due to Lyme disease, A69.23.

Viral and Prion Infections of the Central Nervous System (A80-A89)

Poliomyelitis (polio) is a viral disease that affects the nerves and is caused by the poliovirus. It is also known as infantile paralysis. This disease has been nearly eradicated in the United States as the result of mandatory vaccination.

If people are unvaccinated, this disease may be contracted through direct contact with infected persons. The virus usually enters the body through the mouth or nose. Symptoms can resemble the flu, and a person may or may not become paralyzed. Treatment consists of alleviating the symptoms and letting the virus run its course. Essentially three types of polio infection may occur: subclinical infection, nonparalytic, and paralytic. If the spinal cord or the brain is not affected (which is the case 90% of the time), then complete recovery can occur.

EXAMPLE A patient presents to the hospital with headache, muscle weakness, fever, and muscle spasms of the neck. After a battery of testing, it is determined that the patient has type I acute poliomyelitis, A80.9.

Viral meningitis, also known as aseptic meningitis, is an infection of the fluid in the spinal cord and the fluid around the brain. Viral meningitis is far less serious than bacterial meningitis and is rarely fatal.

No treatment is available for viral meningitis other than relieving the symptoms, which usually consist of headache, stiff neck, and photophobia. Many different viruses may cause meningitis, but most cases are caused by the enteroviruses, and these viruses may be associated with other diseases. Meningitis also may be transmitted via mosquito bites.

EXAMPLE | A patient presents to the hospital with severe headache and stiff neck. A lumbar puncture is performed, and it is determined that the patient has meningitis due to Echo virus, A87.0, 009U3ZX.

Arthropod-Borne Viral Fevers and Viral Hemorrhagic Fevers (A90-A99)

Dengue Fever

Dengue fever is a virus transmitted by an infected mosquito. It is not spread from person to person. Although very few cases have been reported in the United States, it is endemic to Puerto Rico and many tourist destinations in the Caribbean and Central America. According to the CDC there are 100 million cases worldwide each year. The symptoms of this disease include high fever, severe headache, and mild bleeding of the nose or gums. The more severe form of the disease, dengue hemorrhagic fever, includes severe abdominal pain and vomiting and capillary permeability, which can lead to ascites, pleural effusion, and shock. There is no vaccine or specific medicine to treat this disease.

West Nile

West Nile virus is a disease that is spread to individuals by a mosquito bite. People with healthy immune systems may be infected with this disease and have only mild symptoms such as fever or headache. Those people with weakened immune systems and the elderly may experience complications.

EXAMPLE | West Nile virus, A92.30.

EXAMPLE | West Nile encephalitis, A92.31.

Viral Infections Characterized by Skin and Mucous Membrane Lesions (B00-B09)

Hand, Foot, and Mouth Disease

Hand, foot, and mouth disease (HFMD) is a common viral illness of children. The symptoms include eruptions of blisters in the mouth and a rash usually found on the hands and feet. This is an infectious disease that is spread usually from infected hands. There is no specific treatment except to treat the symptoms. It is important to note that this disease is not the same as foot and mouth disease, which rarely occurs in humans.

EXAMPLE | Child is seen by pediatrician and is diagnosed with HFMD, B08.4.

Herpes Zoster

Herpes zoster, or shingles, is a disease that is caused by the same virus that causes chickenpox. Once a person has contracted chickenpox, the virus remains dormant in the body in certain nerves. Shingles usually occurs in people over 50 years of age but sometimes is reported in younger people. It is caused by conditions that weaken the body's immune system such as cancer, aging, and stress.

Shingles starts as a rash that turns into fluid-filled blisters that may become very painful. Sometimes, a case of shingles results in long-term pain, known as "postherpetic neuralgia."

EXAMPLE | Shingles with blepharitis, B02.39.

EXAMPLE | Trigeminal neuralgia as a result of shingles, B02.22.

EXERCISE 9-4

Assign codes to the following conditions.

1. Shingles
2. Stomatitis due to herpes simplex
3. Acute polio
4. West Nile virus
5. Ebola virus
6. Chickenpox
7. Monkeypox
8. German measles with pneumonia
9. Verruca plantaris
10. Molluscum contagiosum
11. Fifth disease

Viral Hepatitis (B15-B19)

Hepatitis

Hepatitis is inflammation of the liver and can be caused by, among other things, several different viruses, namely, A, B, C, D, and E. All of these strains of hepatitis cause acute viral hepatitis. Only B, C, and D viruses cause chronic hepatitis. In chronic hepatitis, the infection may last a lifetime. Symptoms of hepatitis include fatigue, jaundice, nausea and vomiting, headache, diarrhea, and fever.

Hepatitis A is most commonly spread via food or water that has been contaminated by feces from an infected person. International travelers are at risk for this disease. A vaccine is available. If contracted, this disease usually resolves on its own.

Hepatitis B is spread through contact with infected blood, via sex with an infected person, or during childbirth. A hepatitis B vaccine is available. In the past, this disease may have been acquired during a blood transfusion, but in 1992, testing was instituted to control infection transmitted through the blood supply. Acute hepatitis B usually resolves on its own, but chronic cases require drug treatment. Hepatitis B may cause cirrhosis of the liver, liver failure, and liver cancer. About 10% of those infected with the B virus may become carriers. A carrier will have B virus in his or her blood for 6 months or longer after the original infection subsides.

Hepatitis C is spread through infected blood, sexual contact, and childbirth. No vaccine is available for this disease; the only way to prevent it is through avoidance of risky behaviors such as needle sharing. Patients with chronic hepatitis C are treated with medications.

Hepatitis D is spread through infected blood. To acquire hepatitis D, a patient must already have hepatitis B infection. Those with chronic hepatitis D are treated with medications. This form was formerly known as delta.

Hepatitis E is spread through food or water that has been contaminated by feces from an infected person; it is unusual in the United Sates. No vaccine is available, and an outbreak usually resolves on its own.

EXAMPLE | Patient admitted is jaundiced and has chronic hepatitis B, B18.1.

EXAMPLE | Patient has elevated liver function tests and was diagnosed with alcoholic hepatitis. Patient drinks alcohol on a daily basis, K70.10, I10.20.

Codes are also available for carriers of viral hepatitis B, C, or D. These people have no symptoms, but the condition is identified by laboratory testing.

EXAMPLE   Hepatitis B carrier, Z22.51.

Human Immunodeficiency Virus (HIV) Disease (B20)

It is important to note that codes within this section are used only when the diagnosis has been confirmed. This is an exception to the hospital inpatient guideline that allows the coding of possible, probable, or suspected diagnoses. This rule is very important as once a person is diagnosed with AIDS there can be ramifications that could include psychological, social, and legal issues.

AIDS is an incurable disease of the immune system caused by the human immunodeficiency (**HIV**) virus and it is the final stage of HIV disease. It first appeared in the United States in 1981. In the beginning this virus was seen in the homosexual and intravenous drug user (IVDU) population and later spread to the heterosexual population. The virus is found in and transmitted by blood, semen, vaginal secretions, and breast milk. Transmission occurs through sexual contact, blood transfusions, needle sharing, or breastfeeding.

People who are infected with the HIV virus may not have any symptoms for up to 10 years. Once the immune system becomes weakened, they become susceptible to opportunistic infections. When HIV infects a person it most commonly attacks the CD4 cells, which are a type of lymphocyte (white blood cell). Over time in a person infected with HIV the number of CD4 cells decreases, which means the immune system is weakened. Normal CD4 counts are between 500 and 1600. When a CD4 count falls below 200 in an HIV-positive individual it is a sign of AIDS. Often CD4 percentages are used as a basis for determining AIDS. These are the percentages of total lymphocytes. When a CD4 percentage falls below 14%, a patient would be considered to have AIDS. Once a CD4 count goes below 350 cells/mL a patient may be at risk to develop herpes, TB, thrush, Kaposi's sarcoma, or non-Hodgkin's lymphoma. When the count goes below 50 a patient may develop *Mycobacterium avium* or cytomegalovirus (CMV).

AIDS may be treated with HAART (highly active antiretroviral therapy). Sometimes drugs are given on a prophylactic basis to prevent opportunistic infections. With the use of today's drugs, a patient's CD4 count can rebound above 200. However, this does not change the fact that they have AIDS and should be coded as B20. For example, it may be documented that a patient's CD4 nadir is 150. **Nadir** means the lowest level this patient's CD4 count has ever been. A patient with a nadir of 150 would be considered to have AIDS.

Once a patient develops AIDS, from then on he or she is always assigned code B20. When a patient is admitted for treatment of an HIV-related condition, the principal diagnosis should always be B20.

EXAMPLE   Patient admitted with Kaposi's sarcoma of subcutaneous tissue. Code first B20, AIDS; then, code C46.1, Kaposi's sarcoma.

If a patient is admitted with an AIDS-defining illness (Box 9-1), the principal diagnosis is B20. Likewise, if a patient is admitted with an HIV-related condition, the principal diagnosis is B20.

EXAMPLE   A patient presents with severely elevated blood pressure and known hypertension and HIVAN (HIV-associated nephropathy). The patient has ESRD and is currently on dialysis. The principal diagnosis in this case is B20.

When a patient is admitted with a condition unrelated to AIDS, then the code for the unrelated condition is the principal diagnosis.

BOX 9-1 LIST OF AIDS-DEFINING CONDITIONS[1]

The Centers for Disease Control and Prevention (CDC) considers a patient to have acquired immunodeficiency syndrome (AIDS) if a CD4+ T-cell count is below 200 cells/μl (or a CD4+ T-cell percentage of total lymphocytes is less than 14%), or if the patient has one of the following defining illnesses:

    Conditions included in the 1993 AIDS surveillance case definition

- Candidiasis of bronchi, trachea, or lungs
- Candidiasis, esophageal
- Cervical cancer, invasive
- Coccidioidomycosis, disseminated or extrapulmonary
- Cryptococcosis, extrapulmonary
- Cryptosporidiosis, chronic intestinal (longer than 1 month duration)
- Cytomegalovirus disease (other than liver, spleen, or nodes)
- Cytomegalovirus retinitis (with loss of vision)
- Encephalopathy, human immunodeficiency virus (HIV)-related
- Herpes simplex: chronic ulcer(s) (longer than 1 month duration); or bronchitis, pneumonitis, or esophagitis
- Histoplasmosis, disseminated or extrapulmonary
- Isosporiasis, chronic intestinal (longer than 1 month duration)
- Kaposi's sarcoma
- Lymphoma, Burkitt's (or equivalent term)
- Lymphoma, immunoblastic (or equivalent term)
- Lymphoma, primary, of brain
- *Mycobacterium avium* complex or *Mycobacterium kansasii,* disseminated or extrapulmonary
- *Mycobacterium tuberculosis,* any site (pulmonary or extrapulmonary)
- *Mycobacterium,* other species or unidentified species, disseminated or extrapulmonary
- *Pneumocystis carinii* pneumonia
- Pneumonia, recurrent
- Progressive multifocal leukoencephalopathy
- *Salmonella* septicemia, recurrent
- Toxoplasmosis of brain
- Wasting syndrome due to HIV

EXAMPLE | A patient with a history of AIDS is admitted in alcohol withdrawal, F10.239, B20.

Sometimes, patients test HIV positive but have no symptoms. Z21 is the code that should be used for these patients. Tests may have inconclusive results; then, the code R75 should be assigned, nonspecific serologic evidence of HIV. This code can be found in the Alphabetic Index under Human immunodeficiency virus disease, laboratory evidence.

EXAMPLE | Patient is being treated for thrush and is HIV positive, B37.0, Z21.

AIDS and Pregnancy

If a woman has AIDS and is pregnant, code O98.7- should be used, along with B20. Codes from Chapter 15 in the code book always take precedence.

Encounters for Testing for HIV

- Encounter for determining HIV status, Z11.4, Screening for other specified viral disease
- Encounter for counseling for an HIV-negative patient, Z71.7
- Encounter for an HIV-positive patient who is asymptomatic, Z21; counseling code may also be used
- Encounter for HIV-positive patient who is symptomatic, B20; counseling code may also be used

EXERCISE 9-5

Assign codes to the following conditions.

1. Patient with HIV and CD4 nadir of 100 _____

2. Patient has HIV and a history of invasive cervical cancer. _____

3. Patient is admitted with *Pneumocystis* pneumonia (PCP) and has a history of AIDS. _____

4. Patient is admitted with dehydration and has AIDS. _____

5. Patient is tested for AIDS in the physician's office, and the results are inconclusive. _____

6. Patient is in the first trimester of pregnancy and is positive for AIDS. _____

7. Patient is admitted with bacteremia and is an AIDS patient. _____

8. Patient is admitted with tuberculosis and has AIDS. _____

9. Patient is admitted with *E. coli* sepsis and a CD4 count of 32, with known HIV. _____

10. Patient is admitted with difficulty swallowing; after an esophagogastroduodenoscopy (EGD) was performed, it was discovered that the patient had candidal esophagitis and a history of being HIV positive. _____

11. Acute hepatitis B with hepatitis delta _____

12. Patient has chronic hepatitis C. _____

Other Viral Diseases (B25-B34)

Infectious Mononucleosis

Infectious mononucleosis is often caused by the Epstein Barr virus. This virus is often called the kissing disease as it is spread through saliva. It can occur at any age but most often occurs during the teenage years. Symptoms include fever, sore throat, and swollen glands. A blood test can confirm a diagnosis and treatment consists of treating the symptoms.

EXAMPLE   Patient is seen in doctor's office complaining of sore throat and swollen glands. Testing is done and confirms infectious mono, B27.90.

Mycoses (B35-B49)

Candidiasis

Candidiasis is caused by *Candida* fungi. These fungi often live harmlessly within the body until a patient's immune system becomes weak, or until he or she is taking medications that reduce the native bacteria that control this fungus. Usual spots in which *Candida* infections are found include the following:

Mouth—Thrush is found as white plaques on lips, cheeks, or tongue. It can be seen in babies, people with cancer, and diabetics.

Esophagus—often found in patients with AIDS and those on chemotherapy

Cutaneous—found in warm, moist areas that receive little ventilation, such as diaper areas, buttocks, and skin folds of the abdomen or breasts

Vaginal yeast infections are often caused by birth control pills, pregnancy, or frequent douching. Candidal infections are treated according to the area infected. Patients with thrush are generally treated with nystatin swish and swallow while those with candidal esophagitis are treated with fluconazole. Patients with vaginal yeast infection are treated with antifungals such as Monistat, nystatin, or Vagistat.

EXAMPLE Patient is being treated for candidal intertrigo under breast, B37.2.

Histoplasmosis

Histoplasmosis is a fungal disease that primarily affects the lungs. If it affects other organs, it is termed "disseminated histoplasmosis." The fungus causing this disorder is found in soil and material that is contaminated with bat and/or bird droppings. It is treated with antifungals, and mild forms of this disease can resolve on their own.

Protozoal Diseases (B50-B64)

Toxoplasmosis

Toxoplasmosis is caused by a parasite. Many people have the parasite but the majority do not get sick. If a person is immunocompromised, they are more likely to contract the disease. Pregnant women are at risk for this disease and if it is passed on to the baby there can be severe consequences either at birth or later in life. Symptoms can include headache, confusion, seizures, or lung problems. The disease can be transmitted from the waste of an infected cat, contaminated or raw meat, cutting boards that have been in contact with raw meat, or blood transfusions. This condition is treated with Pyrimethamine, an antimalarial medication, and Sulfadiazine, an antibiotic.

Helminthiases (B65-B83)

Helminthiases

Helminthiases is another word for diseases caused by parasitic worms. The most common parasitic worms are tapeworms, pin worms, round worms, and hook worms, and all are acquired in a variety of ways. Worms live in the intestines.

Tapeworms are acquired by eating undercooked meat or fish that have tapeworms. They can cause stomach aches, diarrhea, and loss of appetite. They can grow to 15-30 feet in length and can live for 20 years. When an invasive infection occurs, the larvae migrate to tissues or organs in the body and can cause other disorders such as seizures, hydrocephalus, or dementia.

Pinworms are a type of roundworm and the eggs are usually spread under the fingernails and then contaminate food, dishes, or play things. They are threadlike and found in the rectum and colon.

Roundworms are a type of worm that resemble an earthworm. They can be transmitted by eggs in human waste used as fertilizer or by pets. Hook worms are usually caused by unsanitary conditions. They can be transmitted through infected soil and walking barefoot.

EXAMPLE Child is in pediatrician's office with complaints of anal itching. The doctor diagnoses pinworms, B80.

EXAMPLE Patient had been working in Guatemala and acquired an infection with a pork tapeworm, B68.1.

Pediculosis, Acariasis, and Other Infestations (B85-B89)

Maggots can infest humans in areas of open sores or open body cavities. The condition is termed myiasis, and it occurs when flies lay eggs in areas of the body.

Contagious dermatitis caused by mites is known as **scabies**. The mite burrows under the skin and lays eggs (Figure 9-6). It causes a skin rash and intense itching, usually at night. Scabies is spread rapidly from skin to skin contact. Outbreaks often occur in institutions such as nursing homes and child care facilities. Scabies is treated with a scabicide, which is a form of pesticide.

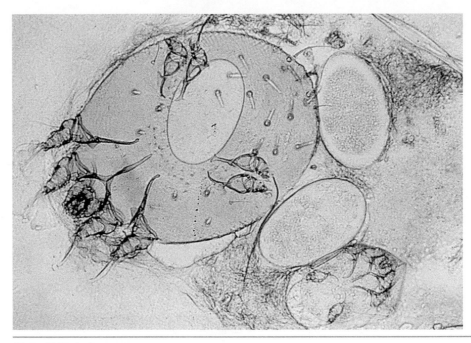

FIGURE 9-6. Scabies mite.

EXAMPLE A homeless man presented to the ER with diabetic ulcers of the right calf of the leg that are infested with maggots, E116.22, L972.19, B87.1.

Sequelae of Infectious and Parasitic Diseases (B90-B94)

Some infections result in **sequelae** or late effects of an acute disease or that may be due to an inactive condition. Hemoptysis can be a late effect of tuberculosis caused by residual cavitation of the lung. Codes in this category(B90-B94) are used for late effects of conditions from categories A00-B89. Sequelae are residuals of diseases from A00-B89. These codes are to be used for chronic current infections. When coding sequelae, two codes are required. The first code would be the condition resulting from the infectious or parasitic disease, and then the sequelae code would be second.

EXAMPLE Patient is seen for chronic uveitis of the right eye, which is a late effect of leprosy, H20.11, B92.

EXAMPLE Patient with left-sided hemiplegia following acute poliomyelitis, G81.94, B91.

Bacterial and Viral Infectious Agents (B95-B97)

The codes in these categories are supplementary codes. They should be used to identify infectious agents in diseases that are classified elsewhere (Figure 9-7). There will be an instructional note found at the infection code advising the coder that an additional code, if known, should be assigned to identify the organism. Practitioners sometimes define organisms as resistant to certain antibiotics. MRSA is methicillin-resistant *Staphyloccus aureus*. If a patient has pneumonia caused by *Staphylococcus aureus* and the organism is resistant to methicillin it would be coded as J15.212. Likewise, practitioners may identify organisms that are sensitive to antibiotics, such as MSSA, which is methicillin-sensitive *Staphylococcus aureus*. If a patient has pneumonia caused by *Staphylococcus aureus* that is susceptible to methicillin, it would be coded to J15.211.

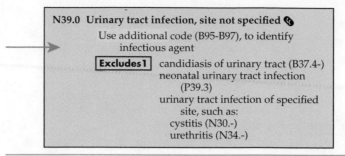

FIGURE 9-7. Use additional code to identify infectious agent.

EXAMPLE	Patient with UTI. Physician documents urine culture positive for *E. coli,* N39.0, B96.20.

EXAMPLE	UTI due to strep group D resistant to vancomycin, N39.0, B95.2, Z16.21.

EXERCISE 9-6

Assign codes to the following conditions.

1. Patient has jock itch. _____

2. Patient with known AIDS has thrush. _____

3. Patient with COPD presents to the physician's office with hemoptysis. Diagnosis is determined to be aspergillosis of the lung. _____

4. Patient with a history of being HIV positive is admitted to the hospital and diagnosed with *Pneumocystis carinii* pneumonia. _____

5. A patient was recently working in Ecuador and returns with a diagnosis of river blindness. _____

6. A child presents to the pediatrician with an itchy scalp. She is diagnosed with head lice. _____

7. Croup caused by RSV _____

8. Patient is seen by physician for chronic pulmonary histoplasmosis. _____

9. Patient is admitted to the hospital with severe abdominal pain. Discharge diagnosis is intestinal myiasis. _____

10. Patient has impetigo due to *Staphylococcus aureus.* _____

FACTORS INFLUENCING HEALTH STATUS AND CONTACT WITH HEALTH SERVICES (Z CODES)

As was discussed in Chapter 8, it may be difficult to locate Z codes in the Index. Coders often say, "I did not know there was a Z code for that." Refer to Chapter 8 for a listing of common main terms to locate Z codes.

A review of the Tabular reveals that some Z codes pertain to infectious and parasitic diseases:

CHAPTER 9: INFECTIOUS AND PARASITIC DISEASES

Z03.810	Encounter for observation for suspected exposure to anthrax ruled out
Z11.0	Encounter for screening for intestinal infectious diseases
Z11.1	Encounter for screening for respiratory tuberculosis
Z11.2	Encounter for screening for other bacterial diseases
Z11.3	Encounter for screening for infections with a predominantly sexual mode of transmission

Z11.4	Encounter for screening for human immunodeficiency virus [HIV]
Z11.5	Encounter for screening for other viral diseases
Z11.6	Encounter for screening for other protozoal diseases and helminthiases
Z11.8	Encounter for screening for other infectious and parasitic diseases
Z11.9	Encounter for screening for infectious and parasitic diseases, unspecified
Z16.10	Resistance to unspecified beta lactam antibiotics
Z16.11	Resistance to penicillins Resistance to amoxicillin Resistance to ampicillin
Z16.12	Extended spectrum beta lactamase (ESBL) resistance
Z16.19	Resistance to other specified beta lactam antibiotics Resistance to cephalosporins
Z16.20	Resistance to unspecified antibiotic Resistance to antibiotics NOS
Z16.21	Resistance to vancomycin
Z16.22	Resistance to vancomycin related antibiotics
Z16.23	Resistance to quinolones and fluoroquinolones
Z16.24	Resistance to multiple antibiotics
Z16.29	Resistance to other single specified antibiotic Resistance to aminoglycosides Resistance to macrolides Resistance to sulfonamides Resistance to tetracyclines
Z16.30	Resistance to unspecified antimicrobial drugs Drug resistance NOS
Z16.31	Resistance to antiparasitic drug(s) Resistance to quinine and related compounds
Z16.32	Resistance to antifungal drug(s)
Z16.33	Resistance to antiviral drug(s)
Z16.34	Resistance to antimycobacterial drug(s) Resistance to tuberculostatics
Z16.341	Resistance to single antimycobacterial drug Resistance to antimycobacterial drug NOS
Z16.342	Resistance to multiple antimycobacterial drugs
Z16.35	Resistance to multiple antimicrobial drugs Excludes1: Resistance to multiple antibiotics only (Z16.24)
Z16.39	Resistance to other specified antimicrobial drug
Z20.01	Contact with and (suspected) exposure to intestinal infectious diseases due to *Escherichia coli* (*E. coli*)
Z20.09	Contact with and (suspected) exposure to other intestinal infectious diseases
Z20.1	Contact with and (suspected) exposure to tuberculosis
Z20.2	Contact with and (suspected) exposure to infections with a predominantly sexual mode of transmission
Z20.3	Contact with and (suspected) exposure to rabies
Z20.4	Contact with and (suspected) exposure to rubella
Z20.5	Contact with and (suspected) exposure to viral hepatitis
Z20.6	Contact with and (suspected) exposure to human immunodeficiency virus [HIV]
Z20.7	Contact with and (suspected) exposure to pediculosis, acariasis, and other infestations
Z20.810	Contact with and (suspected) exposure to anthrax
Z20.811	Contact with and (suspected) exposure to meningococcus
Z20.818	Contact with and (suspected) exposure to other bacterial communicable diseases
Z20.820	Contact with and (suspected) exposure to varicella
Z20.828	Contact with and (suspected) exposure to other viral communicable diseases
Z20.89	Contact with and (suspected) exposure to other communicable diseases

Z20.9	Contact with and (suspected) exposure to unspecified communicable disease
Z21	Asymptomatic human immunodeficiency virus [HIV] infection status
Z22.0	Carrier of typhoid
Z22.1	Carrier of other intestinal infectious diseases
Z22.2	Carrier of diphtheria
Z22.31	Carrier of bacterial disease due to meningococci
Z22.32	Carrier of bacterial disease due to staphylococci
Z22.330	Carrier of Group B streptococcus
Z22.338	Carrier of other streptococcus
Z22.39	Carrier of other specified bacterial diseases
Z22.4	Carrier of infections with a predominantly sexual mode of transmission
Z22.50	Carrier of unspecified viral hepatitis
Z22.51	Carrier of viral hepatitis B
Z22.52	Carrier of viral hepatitis C
Z22.59	Carrier of other viral hepatitis
Z22.6	Carrier of human T-lymphotropic virus type 1 [HTLV-1]
Z22.8	Carrier of other infectious diseases
Z22.9	Carrier of infectious disease, unspecified
Z71.7	Human immunodeficiency virus [HIV] counseling
Z83.0	Family history of human immunodeficiency virus [HIV] disease
Z83.1	Family history of other infectious and parasitic diseases
Z86.11	Personal history of tuberculosis
Z86.12	Personal history of poliomyelitis
Z86.13	Personal history of malaria
Z86.19	Personal history of other infectious and parasitic diseases

EXAMPLE   Student presents to health clinic after exposure to meningitis, Z20.811.

EXAMPLE   Patient is seen in doctor's office after handling a package in a mail facility suspected to be contaminated by anthrax—exposure to anthrax was ruled out, Z03.810.

EXERCISE 9-7

Assign codes to the following condition.

1. History of malaria   _____

2. Exposure to chickenpox at daycare   _____

3. Patient returning from China; was exposed to SARS   _____

4. Patient needs vaccination for cholera   _____

5. Influenza vaccination not administered because   _____
   patient is hospitalized with pneumonia

COMMON TREATMENTS

See Table 9-1 for drugs commonly used to treat infectious diseases.

PROCEDURES

There are multiple therapeutic and diagnostic procedures that can be performed for infectious and parasitic diseases. There are no specific procedure tables for infectious and parasitic diseases.

TABLE 9-1 **DRUGS FOR INFECTIOUS DISEASES**[2]

Drug Category	Drug Action	Examples	Side Effects	Comments
Antibiotics	Destroy or inhibit the growth of bacterial strains or microorganisms but have not been found to be effective for viral infections	Penicillin V Potassium (Pen-V-K) Tetracycline (Sumycin) Amoxicillin (Amoxil) Cephalosporins (Keflex, Ceclor) Ciprofloxacin (Cipro) Metronidazole (Flagyl) Azithromycin (Zithromax)	Common side effects of any are nausea, GI upset, urticaria	Caution must be used when administering penicillin IM regarding observation after infection for potential of anaphylaxis Cipro: acute infections and prophylactic postanthrax exposure
Antifungals	Inhibit and kill fungal growth	Griseofulvin (Grisactin) Ketoconazole (Nizoral) Clotrimazole (Lotrimin) Fluconazole (Diflucan)	Nausea, vomiting, abdominal, pain, itching, urticaria	Some are available in oral form for systemic treatment, others are available in topical form
Antivirals	Inhibit viral growth	Acyclovir (Zovirax) Zidovudine (Retrovir) Amantadine (Symmetrel)	GI disturbances, headache, malaise, insomnia, dizziness	Should be taken at first sign of onset of viral attack for best relief of symptoms
Antiretrovirals	Treat infection by retroviruses	NRTIs (Retrovir, AZT, Epivir, Abacavir) NNRTIs (Sustiva, Viramunde) Protease inhibitors (Kaletra, Norvir)	Often have severe side effects; side effects are many and varied and can include anemia, GI problems, wasting, acidosis, bone problems	These drugs are given in combination
Antiprotozoals	Inhibit protozoal infections	Chloroquine HCl (Aralen HCl)	Headache, pruritus, GI disturbances, tinnitus	Also known as antimalarials
Antipyretics	Reduce fever	Acetaminophen (Tylenol) Acetylsalicylic acid (aspirin) Ibuprofen (Motrin)	Toxic doses of acetaminophen may cause irreversible and fatal liver damage	Caution must be exercised when administering Tylenol drops and syrup to infants and children; check dosage for either before administering
Antitubercular	Suppress mycobacterium causing tuberculosis	Isoniazid (INH) Ethambutol (Myambutol)	GI disturbances and hepatic disturbances	These drugs usually are given in combination

DOCUMENTATION/REIMBURSEMENT/MS-DRGs

Often, coding difficulties are due to lack of documentation. Sometimes pathology and other test results are not available at the time of discharge or when the physician is dictating the discharge summary or is reporting the final diagnoses.

Frequently missed complications and comorbidities from the Infectious and Parasitic Diseases chapter include the following:

- Sepsis
- Food poisoning
- Intestinal infections
- Herpes
- Post-herpetic conditions
- Viral hepatitis
- Lyme disease
- Candidiasis
- Tuberculosis
- Histoplasmosis

Causative Organism

When coding meningitis, the record should be reviewed for the causative organism.

EXAMPLE

DIAGNOSES	CODE	MS-DRG	RW
Viral meningitis	A87.9	076	0.9050
Salmonella meningitis	A02.21	096	1.9247

AIDS and AIDS Manifestations

Coding AIDS, HIV, and any manifestations correctly is very important to MS-DRG assignment.

EXAMPLE

DIAGNOSES	CODE	MS-DRG	RW
AIDS	B20	977	1.0486
AIDS with candidal esophagitis	B20, B37.81	976	0.8975
AIDS with candidal esophagitis and acute respiratory failure	S18.81, B20, B37.81, J96.00	974	2.5849

For reimbursement purposes, the coder must be aware of possible sepsis on admission. This condition may be suspected at the time of admission, and blood cultures may be taken. Results of the blood cultures may not become positive until several days into the patient's hospital stay. This does not mean that the condition was not present on admission.

CHAPTER REVIEW EXERCISE

Where applicable, assign codes for diagnoses and procedures.

1. Gastroenteritis due to *Salmonella* _____
2. Food poisoning, bacterial _____
3. UTI due to candidiasis _____
4. Diarrhea due to *Clostridium difficile* _____
5. Enteritis due to Rotavirus _____
6. Infectious colitis _____
7. Primary TB; patient in isolation _____
8. TB of the hip bone _____
9. Tuberculosis lichenoides _____
10. Bubonic plague _____
11. Gastrointestinal anthrax _____
12. Whooping cough with pneumonia _____
13. DMAC _____
14. Meningococcal endocarditis _____
15. MSSA sepsis _____
16. *Haemophilus influenzae* septicemia _____
17. Acute prostatitis due to *E. coli* _____
18. HIV positive _____
19. AIDS with Burkitt's lymphoma _____
20. Postherpetic syndrome _____

CHAPTER GLOSSARY

AIDS: Acquired Immunodeficiency Syndrome, an incurable disease of the immune system caused by a virus.

Anthrax: a bacterial infection usually found in wild or domestic animals.

Candidiasis: a fungal infection and is also known as a yeast infection.

Chancre: an ulcer that forms during the first stage of syphilis.

Clostridium difficile: microorganisms that are a leading cause of pseudomembranous colitis; also known as *C. diff.*

Communicable: easily spread from one person to another.

Condylomata: wart-type growth found usually in the genital or anal area.

Dengue fever: is a virus transmitted by an infected mosquito.

Gastroenteritis: is the inflammation of the stomach, small intestine and large intestine.

Gonorrhea: disease caused by a bacterium and transmitted by sexual contact.

HAART: highly active antiretroviral therapy, a group of drugs given to AIDS patients for prophylaxis.

Helminthiases: is another word for diseases caused by parasitic worms.

Hepatitis: an inflammation of the liver.

Herpes simplex: a virus also known as a *cold sore* or *fever blister.*

Herpes zoster: a disease caused by the same virus that causes chickenpox.

Histoplasmosis: is a fungal disease that primarily affects the lungs

HIV: Human Immunodeficiency Virus, is the virus that affects the immune system and can progress to AIDS.

Lyme disease: an inflammatory disease caused by bacteria carried by ticks.

Meningitis: an infection in the fluid of a person's spinal cord and brain.

Mycobacterium avium-intercellulare: a mycobacteria found in soil and water.

Nadir: the lowest level.

Nosocomial: hospital-acquired infection.

Parasitic: organism that lives on or takes nourishment from another organism.

Poliomyelitis: a viral disease that affects the nerves.

Scabies: is contagious dermatitis caused by mites.

Sepsis: is a medical condition in which the immune system goes into overdrive, releasing chemicals into the blood to combat infection that trigger widespread inflammation.

Septic shock: a condition caused by *infection* and *sepsis.* It can cause *multiple organ failure* and *death.*

Sequelae: late effect or residual of an acute disease.

SIRS: systemic inflammatory response syndrome, which can be caused by infection or trauma.

Syphilis: a sexually transmitted disease (STD) that is caused by bacteria.

Tuberculosis (TB): an infection caused by *Mycobacterium tuberculosis.*

Urosepsis: infection of urinary site.

Viral meningitis: a viral infection of the fluid in the spinal cord and around the brain.

West Nile: a viral disease that is spread to individuals by a mosquito bite.

REFERENCES

1. Castro KG, Ward JW, Slutsker L, Buehler JW, Jaffe HW, Berkelman RL (National Center for Infectious Diseases Division of HIV/AIDS). 1993 revised classification system for HIV infection and expanded surveillance: Case definition for AIDS among adolescents and adults. *Morb Mortal Wkly Rep,* December 18, 1992, 41(RR-17). Bethesda, MD, Centers for Disease Control and Prevention. Available at: http://www.cdc.gov/mmwr/preview/mmwrhtml/00018871.htm. Accessed April 4, 2008.

2. Modified from Frazier ME, Drzymkowki JW. Essentials of Human Diseases and Conditions, 3rd ed. St. Louis: Saunders, 2004, Appendix II, pp 766-767.

10

Neoplasms

(ICD-10-CM Chapter 2, Codes C00-D49)

LEARNING OBJECTIVES

1. Apply and assign the correct ICD-10-CM/PCS codes in accordance with Official Guidelines for Coding and Reporting

2. Identify major differences between ICD-10-CM and ICD-9-CM related to neoplasms

3. Identify pertinent anatomy and physiology for neoplasm

4. Identify neoplastic diseases

5. Assign the correct Z codes and procedure codes related to neoplasms
6. Identify common treatments, medications, laboratory values, and diagnostic tests
7. Explain the importance of documentation in relation to MS-DRGs for reimbursement

ABBREVIATIONS/ ACRONYMS

AIDS acquired immunodeficiency syndrome

ALL acute lymphocytic leukemia

BCC basal cell carcinoma

BMR biological response modifier

BMT bone marrow transplant

CC chief complaint

CDC Centers for Disease Control and Prevention

CLL chronic lymphocytic leukemia

CML chronic myelogenous leukemia

CNS central nervous system

DCIS ductal carcinoma in situ

FNA fine needle aspiration

HCC hepatocellular carcinoma

ICD-9-CM *International Classification of Diseases, 9th Revision, Clinical Modification*

ICD-10-CM *International Classification of Diseases, 10th Revision, Clinical Modification*

ICD-10-PCS *International Classification of Diseases, 10th Revision, Procedure Coding System*

KS Kaposi's sarcoma

MS-DRG Medicare severity diagnosis-related group

NHL non-Hodgkin's lymphoma

NSCLC non–small cell lung cancer

RCC renal cell carcinoma

SCLC small cell lung cancer

SCC squamous cell carcinoma

UHDDS Uniform Hospital Discharge Data Set

ICD-10-CM
Official Guidelines for Coding and Reporting

Please refer to the companion Evolve website for the most current guidelines.

2. Chapter 2: Neoplasms (C00-D49)

General guidelines

Chapter 2 of the ICD-10-CM contains the codes for most benign and all malignant neoplasms. Certain benign neoplasms, such as prostatic adenomas, may be found in the specific body system chapters. To properly code a neoplasm it is necessary to determine from the record if the neoplasm is benign, in-situ, malignant, or of uncertain histologic behavior. If malignant, any secondary (metastatic) sites should also be determined.

Primary malignant neoplasms overlapping site boundaries

A primary malignant neoplasm that overlaps two or more contiguous (next to each other) sites should be classified to the subcategory/code .8 ('overlapping lesion'), unless the combination is specifically indexed elsewhere. For multiple neoplasms of the same site that are not contiguous such as tumors in different quadrants of the same breast, codes for each site should be assigned.

Malignant neoplasm of ectopic tissue

Malignant neoplasms of ectopic tissue are to be coded to the site mentioned, e.g., ectopic pancreatic malignant neoplasms are coded to pancreas, unspecified (C25.9).

The neoplasm table in the Alphabetic Index should be referenced first. However, if the histological term is documented, that term should be referenced first, rather than going immediately to the Neoplasm Table, in order to determine which column in the Neoplasm Table is appropriate. For example, if the documentation indicates "adenoma," refer to the term in the Alphabetic Index to review the entries under this term and the instructional note to "see also neoplasm, by site, benign." The table provides the proper code based on the type of neoplasm and the site. It is important to select the proper column in the table that corresponds to the type of neoplasm. The Tabular List should then be referenced to verify that the correct code has been selected from the table and that a more specific site code does not exist.

See Section I.C.21. Factors influencing health status and contact with health services, Status, for information regarding Z15.0, codes for genetic susceptibility to cancer.

a. Treatment directed at the malignancy

If the treatment is directed at the malignancy, designate the malignancy as the principal diagnosis.

The only exception to this guideline is if a patient admission/encounter is solely for the administration of chemotherapy, immunotherapy or radiation therapy, assign the appropriate Z51.– code as the first-listed or principal diagnosis, and the diagnosis or problem for which the service is being performed as a secondary diagnosis.

EXAMPLE   The patient had a prostatectomy and a diagnostic bilateral pelvic lymphadenectomy (partial) for prostate acinar adenocarcinoma. Treatment is directed to the primary cancer of the prostate, C61, 0VT00ZZ, 07BC0ZX.

---

b. Treatment of secondary site

When a patient is admitted because of a primary neoplasm with metastasis and treatment is directed toward the secondary site only, the secondary neoplasm is designated as the principal diagnosis even though the primary malignancy is still present.

EXAMPLE   Three months ago, the patient was given a diagnosis of small cell lung carcinoma with metastasis to the liver. The patient's primary neoplasm is lung carcinoma; the secondary neoplasm is located in the liver. The patient underwent wedge resection for liver metastasis, C78.7, C34.90, 0FB00ZZ.

---

c. Coding and sequencing of complications

Coding and sequencing of complications associated with the malignancies or with the therapy thereof are subject to the following guidelines:

1) Anemia associated with malignancy

When admission/encounter is for management of an anemia associated with the malignancy, and the treatment is only for anemia, the appropriate code for the malignancy is sequenced as the principal or first-listed diagnosis followed by **the appropriate code for the anemia (such as** code D63.0, Anemia in neoplastic disease).

EXAMPLE   Anemia due to metastatic bone cancer. The patient has a history of primary breast cancer, which was treated with mastectomy 4 years ago. The patient was admitted for transfusion of packed red blood cells (percutaneous peripheral vein), C79.51, D63.0, Z85.3, Z90.10, 30233N1. ICD-10-CM instructs to code neoplasm first when anemia is due to neoplasm.

---

2) Anemia associated with chemotherapy, immunotherapy and radiation therapy

When the admission/encounter is for management of an anemia associated with an adverse effect **of the administration** of chemotherapy or immunotherapy and the only treatment is for the anemia, **the anemia code is sequenced first** followed by the appropriate codes for the neoplasm **and the adverse effect (T45.1X5, Adverse effect of antineoplastic and immunosuppressive drugs).**

When the admission/encounter is for management of an anemia associated with an adverse effect of radiotherapy, the anemia code should be sequenced first, followed by the appropriate neoplasm code and code Y84.2, Radiological procedure and radiotherapy as the cause of abnormal reaction of the patient, or of later complication, without mention of misadventure at the time of the procedure.

EXAMPLE   Aplastic anemia due to radiation. The patient is being treated for cancer of the brain. The patient was transfused with 2 units of packed red blood cells (percutaneous peripheral vein), D61.2, C71.9, Y84.2, 30233N1.

> **3) Management of dehydration due to the malignancy**
> When the admission/encounter is for management of dehydration due to the malignancy or the therapy, or a combination of both, and only the dehydration is being treated (intravenous rehydration), the dehydration is sequenced first, followed by the code(s) for the malignancy.

EXAMPLE

The patient underwent chemotherapy treatment a few days ago, and since that time has become severely dehydrated. The patient is receiving chemo for treatment of cancer of the colon, E86.0, C18.9.

> **4) Treatment of a complication resulting from a surgical procedure**
> When the admission/encounter is for treatment of a complication resulting from a surgical procedure, designate the complication as the principal or first-listed diagnosis if treatment is directed at resolving the complication.

EXAMPLE

Hernia of colostomy with repair of parastomal hernia. The colostomy was performed 1 year ago during colon cancer resection. The patient is no longer receiving treatment, and the cancer was completely resected, K43.5, Z85.038, 0WQFXZZ.

> **d. Primary malignancy previously excised**
> When a primary malignancy has been previously excised or eradicated from its site and there is no further treatment directed to that site and there is no evidence of any existing primary malignancy, a code from category Z85, Personal history of primary and secondary malignant neoplasm, should be used to indicate the former site of the malignancy. Any mention of extension, invasion, or metastasis to another site is coded as a secondary malignant neoplasm to that site. The secondary site may be the principal or first-listed with the Z85 code used as a secondary code.

EXAMPLE

The patient had a melanoma removed from his back 4 years ago. The patient is currently being treated for metastatic melanoma of the right lung, C78.01, Z85.820.

> **e. Admissions/Encounters involving chemotherapy, immunotherapy and radiation therapy**
> **1) Episode of care involves surgical removal of neoplasm**
> When an episode of care involves the surgical removal of a neoplasm, primary or secondary site, followed by adjunct chemotherapy or radiation treatment during the same episode of care, the code for the neoplasm should be assigned as principal or first-listed diagnosis.

EXAMPLE

The patient had a modified radical mastectomy for malignant neoplasm of the right (upper outer quadrant) breast with mets to right axillary nodes with adjunct chemotherapy (percutaneous central vein), C50.411, C77.3, 0HTT0ZZ, 07B50ZZ, 3E04305.

> **2) Patient admission/encounter solely for administration of chemotherapy, immunotherapy and radiation therapy**
> If a patient admission/encounter is solely for the administration of chemotherapy, immunotherapy or radiation therapy assign code Z51.0, Encounter for antineoplastic radiation therapy, or Z51.11, Encounter for antineoplastic chemotherapy, or Z51.12, Encounter for antineoplastic immunotherapy as the first-listed or principal diagnosis.

If a patient receives more than one of these therapies during the same admission more than one of these codes may be assigned, in any sequence.

The malignancy for which the therapy is being administered should be assigned as a secondary diagnosis.

EXAMPLE

The patient was admitted for chemotherapy (percutaneous central vein) treatment of acute lymphocytic leukemia (ALL), Z51.11, C91.00, 3E04305.

---

3) Patient admitted for radiation therapy, chemotherapy or immunotherapy and develops complications

When a patient is admitted for the purpose of radiotherapy, immunotherapy or chemotherapy and develops complications such as uncontrolled nausea and vomiting or dehydration, the principal or first-listed diagnosis is Z51.0, Encounter for antineoplastic radiation therapy, or Z51.11, Encounter for antineoplastic chemotherapy, or Z51.12, Encounter for antineoplastic immunotherapy followed by any codes for the complications.

EXAMPLE

The patient was admitted for chemotherapy (percutaneous peripheral artery) for lymphoma. Because of nausea and severe vomiting due to the chemotherapy, the patient was also treated for dehydration with IV fluids, Z51.11, C85.90, E86.0, T45.1x5A, R11.2, 3E05305.

---

f. Admission/encounter to determine extent of malignancy

When the reason for admission/encounter is to determine the extent of the malignancy, or for a procedure such as paracentesis or thoracentesis, the primary malignancy or appropriate metastatic site is designated as the principal or first-listed diagnosis, even though chemotherapy or radiotherapy is administered.

EXAMPLE

Patient has known carcinoma of the left kidney and left pleural effusion. Patient is admitted to determine if the renal cancer has spread and a thoracentesis is done, which confirms metastasis to the pleura with malignant pleural effusion, C78.2, J91.0, C64.2, 0W9B3ZX.

---

g. Symptoms, signs, and abnormal findings listed in Chapter 18 associated with neoplasms

Symptoms, signs, and ill-defined conditions listed in Chapter 18 characteristic of, or associated with, an existing primary or secondary site malignancy cannot be used to replace the malignancy as principal or first-listed diagnosis, regardless of the number of admissions or encounters for treatment and care of the neoplasm.

See section I.C.21. Factors influencing health status and contact with health services, Encounter for prophylactic organ removal.

EXAMPLE

The patient was admitted with a first time seizure due to brain cancer. The code R56.9 for seizure can be found in Chapter 18, so the brain cancer code would be sequenced as the principal diagnosis, C71.9, R56.9. Not all patients with brain cancer develop seizures, so it is appropriate to code the seizure code as a secondary diagnosis.

> h. **Admission/encounter for pain control/management**
> *See Section I.C.6. for information on coding admission/encounter for pain control/ management.*
> i. **Malignancy in two or more noncontiguous sites**
> A patient may have more than one malignant tumor in the same organ. These tumors may represent different primaries or metastatic disease, depending on the site. Should the documentation be unclear, the provider should be queried as to the status of each tumor so that the correct codes can be assigned.

EXAMPLE | Primary cancer of right lung with metastasis to the left lung, C34.91, C78.02.

> j. **Disseminated malignant neoplasm, unspecified**
> Code C80.0, Disseminated malignant neoplasm, unspecified, is for use only in those cases where the patient has advanced metastatic disease and no known primary or secondary sites are specified. It should not be used in place of assigning codes for the primary site and all known secondary sites.
> k. **Malignant neoplasm without specification of site**
> Code C80.1, Malignant neoplasm, unspecified, equates to Cancer, unspecified. This code should only be used when no determination can be made as to the primary site of a malignancy. This code should rarely be used in the inpatient setting.
> l. **Sequencing of neoplasm codes**
> 1) **Encounter for treatment of primary malignancy**
> If the reason for the encounter is for treatment of a primary malignancy, assign the malignancy as the principal/first listed diagnosis. The primary site is to be sequenced first, followed by any metastatic sites.

EXAMPLE | Patient has papillary thyroid cancer that has spread to the cervical lymph nodes, C73, C77.0.

> 2) **Encounter for treatment of secondary malignancy**
> When an encounter is for a primary malignancy with metastasis and treatment is directed toward the metastatic (secondary) site(s) only, the metastatic site(s) is designated as the principal/first listed diagnosis. The primary malignancy is coded as an additional code.

EXAMPLE | Patient is admitted for wedge resection of metastatic liver cancer.
Patient had a colorectal cancer removed 3 months ago and is undergoing treatment, C78.7, C19, 0FB00ZZ.

> 3) **Malignant neoplasm in a pregnant patient**
> When a pregnant woman has a malignant neoplasm, a code from subcategory O9A.1-, Malignant neoplasm complicating pregnancy, childbirth, and the puerperium, should be sequenced first, followed by the appropriate code from Chapter 2 to indicate the type of neoplasm.

EXAMPLE | Patient is in her second trimester and was found to have follicular thyroid cancer, O9A.112, Z3A.00, C73.

4) Encounter for complication associated with a neoplasm

When an encounter is for management of a complication associated with a neoplasm, such as dehydration, and the treatment is only for the complication, the complication is coded first, followed by the appropriate code(s) for the neoplasm.

The exception to this guideline is anemia. When the admission/encounter is for management of an anemia associated with the malignancy, and the treatment is only for anemia, the appropriate code for the malignancy is sequenced as the principal or first-listed diagnosis followed by code D63.0, Anemia in neoplastic disease.

EXAMPLE   Patient admitted for treatment of anemia due to gastric cancer with 2 units of packed red cells (percutaneously into peripheral vein), C16.9, D63.0, 30233N1.

EXAMPLE   Patient has become extremely dehydrated following last chemotherapy session for breast cancer. She is admitted for IV fluids, E86.0, C50.919.

5) Complication from surgical procedure for treatment of a neoplasm

When an encounter is for treatment of a complication resulting from a surgical procedure performed for the treatment of the neoplasm, designate the complication as the principal/first-listed diagnosis. See guideline regarding the coding of a current malignancy versus personal history to determine if the code for the neoplasm should also be assigned.

EXAMPLE   Patient developed an abdominal wall wound infection following surgery for colon cancer. Cellulitis was present. Cultures were negative. The patient is scheduled to begin chemo next week, T81.4xxA, L03.311, C18.9.

6) Pathologic fracture due to a neoplasm

When an encounter is for a pathological fracture due to a neoplasm, **and** the focus of treatment is the fracture, a code from subcategory M84.5, Pathological fracture in neoplastic disease, should be sequenced first, followed by the code for the neoplasm.

If the focus of treatment is the neoplasm with an associated pathological fracture, the neoplasm code should be sequenced first, followed by a code from M84.5 for the pathological fracture. The "code also" note at M84.5 provides this sequencing instruction.

EXAMPLE   The patient is being treated for pathologic vertebral fractures due to multiple myeloma, M84.58xA, C90.00.

m. Current malignancy versus personal history of malignancy

When a primary malignancy has been excised but further treatment, such as an additional surgery for the malignancy, radiation therapy or chemotherapy is directed to that site, the primary malignancy code should be used until treatment is completed.

When a primary malignancy has been previously excised or eradicated from its site, there is no further treatment (of the malignancy) directed to that site, and there is no evidence of any existing primary malignancy, a code from category Z85, Personal history of primary and secondary malignant neoplasm, should be used to indicate the former site of the malignancy.

See Section I.C.21. Factors influencing health status and contact with health services, History (of)

EXAMPLE

> Patient had a lobectomy for lung cancer 6 months ago. The patient will receive the fifth cycle of chemotherapy next week, C34.90, Z90.2.

EXAMPLE

> Patient had a mastectomy 5 years ago for breast cancer. She is not being actively treated, Z85.3, Z90.10.

n. Leukemia, Multiple Myeloma, and Malignant Plasma Cell Neoplasms in remission versus personal history
The categories for leukemia, and category C90, Multiple myeloma and malignant plasma cell neoplasms, have codes **indicating whether or not the leukemia has achieved** remission. There are also codes Z85.6, Personal history of leukemia, and Z85.79, Personal history of other malignant neoplasms of lymphoid, hematopoietic and related tissues. If the documentation is unclear, as to whether the **leukemia has achieved** remission, the provider should be queried.
> *See Section I.C.21. Factors influencing health status and contact with health services, History (of)*

EXAMPLE

> The patient's acute myeloid leukemia is in remission, C92.01.

o. Aftercare following surgery for neoplasm
See Section I.C.21. Factors influencing health status and contact with health services, Aftercare
p. Follow-up care for completed treatment of a malignancy
See Section I.C.21. Factors influencing health status and contact with health services, Follow-up

There are Z code categories for aftercare following surgery for a neoplasm and follow-up care after treatment of a malignancy. Many of these services are performed in the outpatient setting. Aftercare codes are generally listed first and explain the reason for the encounter. Aftercare codes are used following the initial treatment of a disease when the patient requires continued care during the healing and recovery stages or because of the long-term effects of the disease.

EXAMPLE

> Patient admitted to a long-term care facility to recover from major surgery for colon cancer. Patient will undergo chemotherapy after discharge, Z48.3, C18.9.

Even after a patient has been successfully treated for a malignancy, periodic, routine follow-up examinations may be necessary to determine if there has been any recurrence of the cancer. When there is no evidence of any type of recurrence, a code from the Z08 follow-up examination should be assigned. A Z code to identify the history of a neoplasm should also be assigned to show the reason for the follow-up examination. There is an instructional note to identify any acquired absence of organs. If there is any evidence of recurrence at the primary site and/or metastasis to a secondary site, the appropriate neoplasm code(s) are assigned.

EXAMPLE

> Patient had a surveillance cystoscopy done because of previous bladder cancer that was surgically removed. No evidence of recurrence was found. The patient will follow-up in 3 months, Z08, Z85.51, OTJB8ZZ.

q. **Prophylactic organ removal for prevention of malignancy**
   See Section I.C. 21, Factors influencing health status and contact with health services, Prophylactic organ removal

r. **Malignant neoplasm associated with transplanted organ**
   A malignant neoplasm of a transplanted organ should be coded as a transplant complication. Assign first the appropriate code from category T86.-, Complications of transplanted organs and tissue, followed by code C80.2, Malignant neoplasm associated with transplanted organ. Use an additional code for the specific malignancy.

EXAMPLE | Patient was diagnosed with hepatocellular carcinoma. Patient had a liver transplant 2 years ago, T86.49, C80.2, C22.0, Y83.0.

6. Chapter 6: Diseases of Nervous System and Sense Organs (G00-G99)
5) Neoplasm Related Pain
   Code G89.3 is assigned to pain documented as being related, associated or due to cancer, primary or secondary malignancy, or tumor. This code is assigned regardless of whether the pain is acute or chronic.

   This code may be assigned as the principal or first-listed code when the stated reason for the admission/encounter is documented as pain control/pain management. The underlying neoplasm should be reported as an additional diagnosis.

   When the reason for the admission/encounter is management of the neoplasm and the pain associated with the neoplasm is also documented, code G89.3 may be assigned as an additional diagnosis. It is not necessary to assign an additional code for the site of the pain.

   See Section I.C.2 for instructions on the sequencing of neoplasms for all other stated reasons for the admission/encounter (except for pain control/pain management).

When a patient has pain due to a previously identified neoplasm, code G89.3 is assigned. This code can be assigned as either principal or secondary, depending on the circumstances of the admission.

   If a patient is admitted for pain management or pain control, the G89.3 code is assigned as the principal diagnosis, and the malignancy code(s) is assigned as a secondary code(s).

EXAMPLE | Patient was admitted for control of back pain due to vertebral metastasis. Patient has a history of prostate cancer. After pain medications were adjusted and pain was controlled, he was discharged to hospice care, G89.3, C79.51, Z85.46.

   If a patient is admitted for management of the malignancy and the pain associated with the malignancy, the malignancy code is assigned as the principal diagnosis with the G89.3 pain code assigned as a secondary diagnosis.

EXAMPLE | Patient was admitted for back pain due to vertebral metastasis. An MRI indicates that the disease has progressed. Patient has a history of prostate cancer. Beam radiation with heavy particles was administered, C79.51, G89.3, Z85.46, DP0C4ZZ.

   Apply the General Coding Guidelines as found in Chapter 5 and the Procedural Coding Guidelines as found in Chapters 6 and 7.

MAJOR DIFFERENCES BETWEEN ICD-10-CM AND ICD-9-CM

- In ICD-10-CM, when an encounter is for the management of anemia associated with malignancy, the malignancy is sequenced as the principal or first-listed diagnosis because of an instructional note, and there is a guideline that addresses this situation.
- There is a change in terminology for neoplasm codes that could be identified with regard to remission status. The terminology in ICD-9-CM is "without mention of remission," but in ICD-10-CM, "not in remission" is used.
- There are ICD-10-CM guidelines related to sequencing of neoplasm codes.

ANATOMY AND PHYSIOLOGY

Neoplasms can affect any of the body systems. The anatomy and physiology of these body systems are outlined in their respective chapters. It is important to understand some of the terminology that is specific to neoplasms and their behavior. According to the National Cancer Institute, the most common cancers in the United States include the following:

- Bladder
- Breast
- Colon and rectal
- Endometrial
- Kidney (renal cell)
- Leukemia
- Lung
- Melanoma
- Non-Hodgkin's lymphoma
- Pancreatic
- Prostate
- Skin (nonmelanoma)
- Thyroid

A **neoplasm** is an abnormal tissue that grows by cellular proliferation more rapidly than normal tissue. Neoplasms show partial or complete lack of structural organization and functional coordination with normal tissue, and they usually form a distinct mass of tissue that may be benign (benign tumor) or malignant (cancer) (Figure 10-1). Both benign and malignant neoplasms are classified according to the type of tissue in which they are found. **Benign** neoplasms are tumors that are not malignant. **Malignancy** is a neoplasm that has the ability to invade adjacent structures and spread to distant sites. **Fibromas** are benign neoplasms of fibrous connective tissue, and **melanomas** are malignant changes of melanin

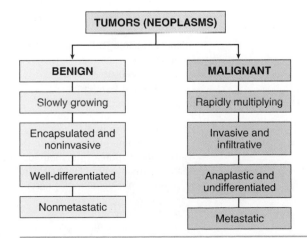

FIGURE 10-1. Differences between benign and malignant neoplasms.

cells. Malignant tumors originating from epithelial tissue (e.g., skin, bronchi, stomach) are called **carcinomas** (Table 10-1). Malignancies of epithelial glandular tissue such as those found in the breast, prostate, and colon are known as **adenocarcinomas**. Malignant growths of connective tissue (e.g., muscle, cartilage, bone) are called **sarcomas** (Table 10-2). **Lymphomas** form in lymphatic tissue, and **leukemias** are malignancies that arise from white blood cells. A **myeloma** originates within the bone marrow.

The **primary site** is the location at which the neoplasm begins, or originates. It is important for the treating physician to identify the site of origin so that the best treatment course and prognosis can be determined. **Metastasis** is the spread of cancer from one part of the body to another, as is seen when neoplasms occur in parts of the body separate from the site of the primary tumor. Metastasis occurs through dissemination of tumor cells by the lymphatics or blood vessels, or by direct extension through serous cavities or other spaces.

Grading involves pathologic examination of tumor cells. The degree of abnormality of cells determines the grade of cancer (Table 10-3). When the level of cell abnormality is greater, the cancer is of higher grade. Cells that are **well-differentiated** closely resemble mature, specialized cells. Tumor cells that are **undifferentiated** are highly abnormal (i.e., immature and primitive).

Cancerous tissue is classified according to degree of malignancy, from grade 1—barely malignant—to grade 4—highly malignant. In practice, it is not always possible for the pathologist to determine the degree of malignancy, and sometimes it may be difficult even to determine whether a particular tumor tissue is benign or malignant.

TABLE 10-1 CARCINOMA AND THE EPITHELIAL TISSUES FROM WHICH THEY DERIVE[1]

Types of Epithelial Tissue	Malignant Tumor (Carcinoma)
Gastrointestinal Tract	
Colon	Adenocarcinoma of the colon
Esophagus	Esophageal carcinoma
Liver	Hepatocellular carcinoma (hepatoma)
Stomach	Gastric adenocarcinoma
Glandular Tissue	
Adrenal glands	Carcinoma of the adrenals
Breast	Carcinoma of the breast
Pancreas	Carcinoma of the pancreas (pancreatic adenocarcinoma)
Prostate	Carcinoma of the prostate
Thyroid	Carcinoma of the thyroid
Kidney and Bladder	
	Renal cell carcinoma (hypernephroma)
	Transitional cell carcinoma of the bladder
Lung	
	Adenocarcinoma (bronchioloalveolar)
	Large cell carcinoma
	Small (oat) cell carcinoma
	Squamous cell (epidermoid)
Reproductive Organs	
	Adenocarcinoma of the uterus
	Carcinoma of the penis
	Choriocarcinoma of the uterus or testes
	Cystadenocarcinoma (mucinous or serous) of the ovaries
	Seminoma and embryonal cell carcinoma (testes)
	Squamous cell (epidermoid) carcinoma of the vagina or cervix
Skin	
Basal cell layer	Basal cell carcinoma
Melanocyte	Malignant melanoma
Squamous cell layer	Squamous cell carcinoma

TABLE 10-2 SARCOMAS AND THE CONNECTIVE TISSUES FROM WHICH THEY DERIVE[2]

Types of Connective Tissue	Malignant Tumor
Bone	
	Osteosarcoma (osteogenic sarcoma)
	Ewing's sarcoma
Muscle	
Smooth (visceral) muscle	Leiomyosarcoma
Striated (skeletal) muscle	Rhabdomyosarcoma
Cartilage	
	Chondrosarcoma
Fat	
	Liposarcoma
Fibrous Tissue	
	Fibrosarcoma
Blood Vessel Tissue	
	Angiosarcoma
Blood-Forming Tissue	
All leukocytes	Leukemias
Lymphocytes	Hodgkin's disease
Plasma cells	Non-Hodgkin's lymphoma
	Burkitt's lymphoma
	Multiple myeloma
Nerve Tissue	
Embryonic nerve tissue	Neuroblastoma
Glial tissue	Astrocytoma (tumors of glial cells, called "astrocytes")
	Glioblastoma multiforme

TABLE 10-3 GRADES OF NEOPLASMS

Grade 1	Cells slightly abnormal and well-differentiated
Grade 2	Cells more abnormal and moderately differentiated
Grade 3	Cells very abnormal and poorly differentiated
Grade 4	Cells immature and undifferentiated

Staging, a means of categorizing a particular cancer, helps the clinician to determine a particular patient's treatment plan and the need for further therapy. Each type of cancer is staged according to specific characteristics:

- In situ cancers have been diagnosed at the earliest possible stage.
- Stage I or "local" cancers have been diagnosed early and have not spread.
- Stage II has spread into surrounding tissues but not beyond the location of origin.
- Stage III or "regional" cancer has spread to nearby lymph nodes.
- Stage IV or "distant" cancers have spread to other parts of the body and are the most difficult to treat.

See Table 10-4 for an example of how the TNM (tumor-node-metastasis) staging system would be used to classify a lung cancer.

Neoplasm Table

The coding of most neoplasms requires an extra step, which involves use of the Neoplasm Table (Figure 10-2). The main term for the type of neoplasm is located in the Alphabetic Index. All subterms must be reviewed to facilitate assignment of proper codes. One must

TABLE 10-4 INTERNATIONAL TNM STAGING SYSTEMS FOR LUNG CANCER[3]

Stage	TNM Description	5-Year Survival, %
I	T1-T2, N0, M0	60-80
II	T1-T2, N1, M0	25-50
IIIA	T3, N0-N1, M0	25-40
IIIB	T1-T3, N2, M0	10-30
IV	Any T4 or N3, M0	<5
	Any M1	<5
Primary Tumor (T)		
T1	Tumor <3 cm in diameter	
T2	Tumor <3 cm in diameter or with associated atelectasis–obstructive pneumonitis extending to the hilar region	
T3	Tumor with direct extension into the chest wall, diaphragm, mediastinum, pleura, or pericardium	
T4	Tumor invades the mediastinum, or presence of a malignant pleural effusion	
Regional Lymph Nodes (N)		
N0	No node involvement	
N1	Metastasis to lymph nodes in the peribronchial and ipsilateral (same side as the primary tumor) hilar regions	
N2	Metastasis to ipsilateral hilar and subcarinal (under the bifurcation of the trachea into the lungs) lymph nodes	
N3	Metastasis to contralateral mediastinal or hilar nodes or any nodes new to the clavicular (collar) bone	
Distance Metastasis (M)		
M0	No known metastasis	
M1	Distant metastasis present with site specified (e.g., brain, tumor)	

follow all instructions, such as *see* Neoplasm, by site, benign, or *see* Neoplasm, by site, malignant. It is important to follow all steps to ensure correct code assignment. The temptation to go directly to the Neoplasm Table should be avoided.

In the following examples, a step-by-step explanation will be given for coding of neoplasms.

EXAMPLE

Basal cell carcinoma left cheek (primary site) (Figure 10-3).
1. Look up "Carcinoma" in Alphabetic Index.
2. Review subterms; "basal cell" is a subterm.
3. Follow instructions to *see also* Neoplasm, skin, malignant.
4. Go to the Neoplasm Table.
5. Locate the site—skin—and review subterms under "skin."
6. Locate the subterm "cheek," and find the code under the appropriate column, which, in this case, is a primary malignancy of the cheek due to basal cell carcinoma.
7. Assign code C44.319.

EXAMPLE

Squamous cell in situ carcinoma of the endocervix, D06.0.
1. Look up carcinoma-in-situ in the Alphabetic Index.
2. Review subterms; "squamous cell" is a subterm.
3. Follow instructions, specified site—*see also* Neoplasm, by site, in situ.
4. Go to the Neoplasm Table.
5. Locate the site—cervix—and review subterms under "Cervix."
6. Locate the subterm "endocervix," and find the code under the appropriate column, which, in this case, is a carcinoma in situ of the endocervix.
7. Assign codes (in situ) D06.0.

ICD-10-CM TABLE of NEOPLASMS

The list below gives the code numbers for neoplasms by anatomical site. For each site there are six possible code numbers according to whether the neoplasm in question is malignant, benign, in situ, of uncertain behavior, or of unspecified nature. The description of the neoplasm will often indicate which of the six columns is appropriate; e.g., malignant melanoma of skin, benign fibroadenoma of breast, carcinoma in situ of cervix uteri.

Where such descriptors are not present, the remainder of the Index should be consulted where guidance is given to the appropriate column for each morphological (histological) variety listed; e.g., Mesonephroma — see Neoplasm, malignant; Embryoma — see also Neoplasm, uncertain behavior; Disease, Bowen's — see Neoplasm, skin, in situ. However, the guidance in the Index can be overridden if one of the descriptors mentioned above is present; e.g., malignant adenoma of colon is coded to C18.9 and not to D12.6 as the adjective "malignant" overrides the Index entry "Adenoma — see also Neoplasm, benign."

Codes listed with a dash -, following the code have a required additional character for laterality. The tabular must be reviewed for the complete code.

N

	Malignant Primary	Malignant Secondary	Ca in situ	Benign	Uncertain Behavior	Unspecified Behavior
N						
Neoplasm, neoplastic	C80.1	C79.9	D09.9	D36.9	D48.9	D49.9
abdomen, abdominal	C76.2	C79.8-	D09.8	D36.7	D48.7	D49.89
cavity	C76.2	C79.8-	D09.8	D36.7	D48.7	D49.89
organ	C76.2	C79.8-	D09.8	D36.7	D48.7	D49.89
viscera	C76.2	C79.8-	D09.8	D36.7	D48.7	D49.89
wall — see also Neoplasm, abdomen, wall, skin	C44.509	C79.2-	D04.5	D23.5	D48.5	D49.2
connective tissue	C49.4	C79.8-	—	D21.4	D48.1	D49.2
skin	C44.509					
basal cell carcinoma	C44.519	—	—	—	—	—
specified type NEC	C44.599	—	—	—	—	—
squamous cell carcinoma	C44.529	—	—	—	—	—
abdominopelvic	C76.8	C79.8-	—	D36.7	D48.7	D49.89
accessory sinus — see Neoplasm, sinus						
acoustic nerve	C72.4-	C79.49	—	D33.3	D43.3	D49.7

FIGURE 10-2. Excerpt from the Neoplasm Table.

EXERCISE 10-1

Assign codes to the following conditions.

1. Malignant melanoma, skin left foot _____
2. Leukemia _____
3. Adenoma of the prostate _____
4. Renal cell carcinoma, right _____

Primary and Secondary Neoplasms

Sometimes incomplete documentation makes it difficult to determine whether a neoplasm is primary or secondary. It is possible to have more than one primary cancer. At times, a secondary or metastatic cancer has been found, and the primary is unknown or has yet to be determined. Documentation in the health record may be incomplete and the terminology confusing.

Carcinoma (malignant) —*see also*
Neoplasm, by site, malignant
acidophil
specified site —*see* Neoplasm,
malignant, by site
unspecified site C75.1
acidophil-basophil, mixed
specified site —*see* Neoplasm,
malignant, by site
unspecified site C75.1
adnexal (skin) —*see* Neoplasm, skin,
malignant
adrenal cortical C74.0-
alveolar —*see* Neoplasm, lung,
malignant
cell —*see* Neoplasm, lung, malignant
ameloblastic C41.1
upper jaw (bone) C41.0
apocrine
breast —*see* Neoplasm, breast,
malignant
specified site NEC —*see* Neoplasm,
skin, malignant
unspecified site C44.99
basal cell (pigmented) (*see also*
Neoplasm, skin, malignant) C44.91
fibro-epithelial —*see* Neoplasm, skin,
malignant
morphea —*see* Neoplasm, skin,
malignant
multicentric —*see* Neoplasm, skin,
malignant
basaloid
basal-squamous cell, mixed —*see*
Neoplasm, skin, malignant
basophil
specified site —*see* Neoplasm,
malignant, by site
unspecified site C75.1
basophil-acidophil, mixed
specified site —*see* Neoplasm,
malignant, by site
unspecified site C75.1
basosquamous —*see* Neoplasm, skin,
malignant
bile duct
with hepatocellular, mixed C22.0
liver C22.1
specified site NEC —*see* Neoplasm,
malignant, by site
unspecified site C22.1
branchial or branchiogenic C10.4
bronchial or bronchogenic —*see*
Neoplasm, lung, malignant

Carcinoma (*Continued*)
bronchiolar —*see* Neoplasm, lung,
malignant
bronchioloalveolar —*see* Neoplasm,
lung, malignant
C cell
specified site —*see* Neoplasm,
malignant, by site
unspecified site C73
ceruminous C44.29-
cervix uteri
in situ D06.9
endocervix D06.0
exocervix D06.1
specified site NEC D06.7
chorionic
specified site —*see* Neoplasm,
malignant, by site
unspecified site
female C58
male C62.90
chromophobe
specified site —*see* Neoplasm,
malignant, by site
unspecified site C75.1
cloacogenic
specified site —*see* Neoplasm,
malignant, by site
unspecified site C21.2
diffuse type
specified site —*see* Neoplasm,
malignant, by site
unspecified site C16.9
duct (cell)
with Paget's disease —*see* Neoplasm,
breast, malignant
infiltrating
with lobular carcinoma (in situ)
specified site —*see* Neoplasm,
malignant, by site
unspecified site (female)
C50.91-
male C50.92-
specified site —*see* Neoplasm,
malignant, by site
unspecified site (female) C50.91-
male C50.92-
ductal
with lobular
specified site —*see* Neoplasm,
malignant, by site
unspecified site (female) C50.91-
male C50.92-
ductular, infiltrating
specified site —*see* Neoplasm,
malignant, by site
unspecified site (female) C50.91-
male C50.92-
embryonal
liver C22.7
endometrioid
specified site —*see* Neoplasm,
malignant, by site
unspecified site
female C56.9
male C61
eosinophil
specified site —*see* Neoplasm,
malignant, by site
unspecified site C75.1
epidermoid —*see also* Carcinoma,
squamous cell
in situ, Bowen's type —*see* Neoplasm,
skin, in situ

FIGURE 10-3. Index entry for main term "Carcinoma."

As was described previously, a metastatic neoplasm is a secondary neoplasm that has spread from the original or primary site. The site of the metastasis may be close to the original site (e.g., breast spread to axillary lymph nodes) or to distant sites (e.g., lung spread to the brain). Neoplasms can metastasize to more than one site. If this is the case, codes are assigned to each metastatic site. Terminology used to describe metastatic sites varies greatly, depending on the documenting physician. For example, if a patient has a non–small cell primary lung carcinoma with secondary malignancy of the brain, it may be documented in the health record as follows:

EXAMPLE | Lung cancer with metastasis to the brain, C34.90, C79.31.

The code that would be assigned is primary lung cancer with a secondary code assigned for the metastatic brain malignancy.

EXAMPLE | Lung cancer metastatic to the brain, C34.90, C79.31.

The codes assigned are the same as in the preceding example.

EXAMPLE | Brain cancer metastatic from the lung, C34.90, C79.31.

The codes assigned are the same as in the preceding example.

EXAMPLE | Non–small cell carcinoma of lung and brain, C34.90, C79.31.

Non–small cell carcinoma is a malignancy that originates in the lung, so the lung is primary. If a cancer that originates in the lung has spread to the brain, that is a metastasis.

EXAMPLE | Metastatic lung cancer, C34.90, C79.9.

If a morphology type is not stated, assign the site qualified as "metastatic" to the primary malignant code for that site. The code assigned is primary lung cancer (C34.90), with an unknown secondary malignancy site (C79.9) because the metastatic site was not documented in this example.

If the documentation in the health record only identifies one site and it is identified as metastatic, then a determination has to be made as to whether to code the site as a primary malignancy or secondary malignancy. The following steps are followed to make that determination:

1. If the morphology type is documented, refer to the morphology type in the Alphabetic Index and code to the primary condition of that site.

EXAMPLE | Metastatic islet cell carcinoma of the pancreas, C25.4, C79.9.

In the preceding example, the carcinoma is documented as metastatic. The first step is to locate the morphology type in the Alphabetic Index. There are subterms for islet cell of the pancreas with code C25.4, so that code should be assigned. If no specific site is listed as a subterm, assign the code for primary neoplasm of an unspecified site (C80.1). When a primary site has been determined, a code must be assigned to identify a secondary (metastatic) site. If no metastatic site is specified, then the code C79.9, unknown site, secondary, is assigned.

2. If the process in step 1 leads to code C80.0 or C80.1, or if the morphology is not stated, the site should be coded as a primary malignancy, unless it is included in the following list of exceptions.

Malignant neoplasms of the following sites are exceptions, and instead of coding to an unknown primary or to the morphology, the following sites are always coded as secondary neoplasms of that site:

- Bone
- Brain
- Diaphragm
- Heart
- Liver
- Lymph nodes
- Mediastinum
- Meninges
- Peritoneum
- Pleura
- Retroperitoneum
- Spinal cord
- Sites classifiable to C76

EXAMPLE Metastatic carcinoma of the breast, C50.919, C79.9.

In the preceding example, there is no subterm for breast or unspecified site. In the Neoplasm Table, unspecified site, primary is coded to C80.1. When code C80.1 is obtained, then a review of the exception list is performed. Because breast is not on the list, it is assigned as the primary site, C50.919, and the code C79.9 is used to identify the unknown secondary.

EXAMPLE Metastatic brain cancer (depending on the reason for the patient's admission) C80.1, C79.31 or C79.31, C80.1.

In this example, the brain is on the list of secondary neoplasms, and the morphology type is not stated; therefore the code (C79.31) is assigned for secondary neoplasm of the brain and (C80.1) for unknown primary. Sequencing of the primary and secondary neoplasms would depend on the focus of treatment.

EXAMPLE Renal cell carcinoma (RCC) with metastasis to the adrenal glands
    Primary neoplasm: Renal cell carcinoma (kidney)
    Secondary neoplasm: Adrenal glands

EXAMPLE Metastatic bone cancer
Primary neoplasm: Unknown primary site
Secondary neoplasm: Bones

Specific instructions are provided at the beginning of the "Neoplasm" chapter in the code book (Figure 10-4).

EXERCISE 10-2

Identify the following neoplasms in terms of primary or secondary, as in the earlier examples.

1. Colorectal adenocarcinoma with metastatic liver cancer
   Primary neoplasm _____
   Secondary neoplasm _____

2. Thyroid malignancy with mets to the lymph nodes of the neck
   Primary neoplasm _____
   Secondary neoplasm _____

3. Metastatic ovarian cancer
   Primary neoplasm _____
   Secondary neoplasm _____

4. Pancreatic cancer with extension into the liver
   Primary neoplasm _____
   Secondary neoplasm _____

5. Recurrence of cancer in the bladder
   Primary neoplasm _____
   Secondary neoplasm _____

6. Adenocarcinoma sigmoid colon with pericolic nodal involvement
   Primary neoplasm _____
   Secondary neoplasm _____

7. Inflammatory breast cancer with spread to the axillary lymph nodes
   Primary neoplasm _____
   Secondary neoplasm _____

8. Metastatic bone cancer from the prostate
   Primary neoplasm _____
   Secondary neoplasm _____

9. Endometrial adenocarcinoma with metastasis to the ovary
   Primary neoplasm _____
   Secondary neoplasm _____

10. Acinic cell carcinoma of the parotid gland
    Primary neoplasm _____
    Secondary neoplasm _____

Contiguous Sites

As is pointed out in the instructional note (see Figure 10-4), a neoplasm can overlap two or more subcategories, and determination of the exact point of origin may be difficult. These would be assigned to subcategory 8, "Other," unless the combination is specifically indexed elsewhere.

It is important to code any alterations to the functional activity of an organ caused by the neoplasm. Neoplasms of the endocrine glands or organs that secrete hormones are

CHAPTER 2

NEOPLASMS (C00-D49)

This chapter contains the following blocks:

C00-C14	Malignant neoplasms of lip, oral cavity and pharynx
C15-C26	Malignant neoplasms of digestive organs
C30-C39	Malignant neoplasms of respiratory and intrathoracic organs
C40-C41	Malignant neoplasms of bone and articular cartilage
C43-C44	Melanoma and other malignant neoplasms of skin
C45-C49	Malignant neoplasms of mesothelial and soft tissue
C50	Malignant neoplasms of breast
C51-C58	Malignant neoplasms of female genital organs
C60-C63	Malignant neoplasms of male genital organs
C64-C68	Malignant neoplasms of urinary tract
C69-C72	Malignant neoplasms of eye, brain and other parts of central nervous system
C73-C75	Malignant neoplasms of thyroid and other endocrine glands
C7A	Malignant neuroendocrine tumors
C7B	Secondary neuroendocrine tumors
C76-C80	Malignant neoplasms of ill-defined, other secondary and unspecified sites
C81-C96	Malignant neoplasms of lymphoid, hematopoietic and related tissue
D00-D09	In situ neoplasms
D10-D36	Benign neoplasms, except benign neuroendocrine tumors
D3A	Benign neuroendocrine tumors
D37-D48	Neoplasms of uncertain behavior, polycythemia vera and myelodysplastic syndromes
D49	Neoplasms of unspecified behavior

Notes: Functional activity

All neoplasms are classified in this chapter, whether they are functionally active or not. An additional code from Chapter 4 may be used, to identify functional activity associated with any neoplasm.

Morphology [Histology]

Chapter 2 classifies neoplasms primarily by site (topography), with broad groupings for behavior, malignant, in situ, benign, etc. The Table of Neoplasms should be used to identify the correct topography code. In a few cases, such as for malignant melanoma and certain neuroendocrine tumors, the morphology (histologic type) is included in the category and codes.

Primary malignant neoplasms overlapping site boundaries

A primary malignant neoplasm that overlaps two or more contiguous (next to each other) sites should be classified to the subcategory/code .8 ('overlapping lesion'), unless the combination is specifically indexed elsewhere. For multiple neoplasms of the same site that are not contiguous, such as tumors in different quadrants of the same breast, codes for each site should be assigned.

Malignant neoplasm of ectopic tissue

Malignant neoplasms of ectopic tissue are to be coded to the site mentioned, e.g., ectopic pancreatic malignant neoplasms are coded to pancreas, unspecified (C25.9).

FIGURE 10-4. Instructional notes at the beginning of the "Neoplasm" chapter in the Tabular List.

more likely to have disturbances in their functional activity because hormone production may increase or decrease because of the neoplasm.

EXAMPLE	Malignant neoplasm of the thyroid with hyperthyroidism, C73, E05.90.

DISEASE CONDITIONS

Chapter 2 in the ICD-10-CM code book is divided into the following categories:

CATEGORY	SECTION TITLE
C00-C14	Malignant neoplasm of lip, oral cavity, and pharynx
C15-C26	Malignant neoplasm of digestive organs
C30-C39	Malignant neoplasm of respiratory and intrathoracic organs
C40-C41	Malignant neoplasm of bone and articular cartilage
C43-C44	Melanoma and other malignant neoplasms of skin
C45-C49	Malignant neoplasm of mesothelial and soft tissue
C50	Malignant neoplasm of breast
C51-C58	Malignant neoplasm of female genital organs
C60-C63	Malignant neoplasm of male genital organs
C64-C68	Malignant neoplasm of urinary tract
C69-C72	Malignant neoplasm of eye, brain, and other parts of the central nervous system
C73-C75	Malignant neoplasm of thyroid and other endocrine glands
C76-C80	Malignant neoplasm of ill-defined, secondary, and unspecified sites
C81-C96	Malignant neoplasm of lymphoid, hematopoietic, and related tissue
D00-D09	In situ neoplasms
D10-D36	Benign neoplasms
D37-D48	Neoplasms of uncertain behavior
D49	Neoplasms of unspecified behavior

Malignant Neoplasm of Lip, Oral Cavity, and Pharynx (C00-C14)

Several types of oral cancers have been identified; 90% of these are squamous cell carcinomas. Cancers are often discovered after they have already spread, usually to the lymph nodes of the neck. Smoking has been associated with about 70% to 80% of oral cancers. Also, heavy alcohol adds to the risk. The lips and tongue are most commonly affected (Figure 10-5).

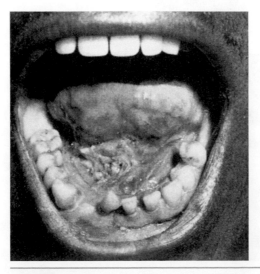

FIGURE 10-5. Squamous cell carcinoma of the mouth.

EXAMPLE	The patient is being treated for squamous cell carcinoma of the hypopharynx, C13.9.

EXERCISE 10-3

Assign codes to the following conditions.

1. Squamous cell carcinoma, base of tongue _____

2. Adenocarcinoma of parotid gland _____

3. Biopsy-proven squamous cell carcinoma, right tonsil _____

4. Cancer lower lip _____

Malignant Neoplasm of Digestive Organs (C15-C26)

According to the Centers for Disease Control and Prevention (CDC), colorectal cancer (Figure 10-6) primarily affects men and women aged 50 years or older. For men, colorectal cancer is the third most common cancer after prostate cancer and lung cancer. For women, colorectal cancer is the third most common cancer after breast cancer and lung cancer. The best prevention is regular screening.

Hepatocellular carcinoma is a primary neoplasm of the liver (Figure 10-7). Patients who develop primary liver cancer often have some type of chronic liver disease such as cirrhosis. The liver is also a common site for metastasis.

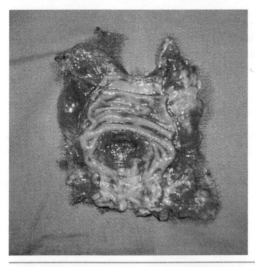

FIGURE 10-6. Adenocarcinoma distal rectum.

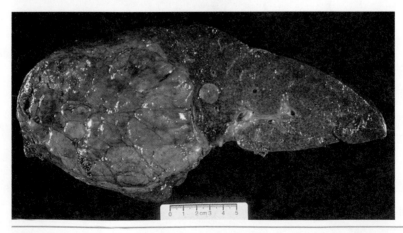

FIGURE 10-7. Hepatocellular carcinoma.

Malignant ascites is a condition in which excess fluid that contains malignant cells accumulates in the abdomen or peritoneum. A diagnostic paracentesis can be performed to determine if cancer cells are present. Patients with breast, ovarian, uterine, colon, stomach, intestinal, and pancreatic cancers are more likely to develop malignant ascites. Ascites can be very uncomfortable for the patient and a therapeutic paracentesis may be necessary to drain the fluid and provide relief. There is an instructional note in the code book to code the responsible neoplasm first. As the code for malignant ascites is a symptom code from Chapter 18, there is a guideline that states that a code from this chapter, when associated with an existing primary or secondary malignancy site, it cannot be used as a principal or first-listed diagnosis. In a patient with cancer and multiple metastatic sites, it may be necessary to query the physician as to which cancer site is causing the ascites.

EXAMPLE | Patient presented to the ER with shortness of breath due to extensive malignant ascites. She has inoperable ovarian cancer. A therapeutic percutaneous peritoneal cavity paracentesis was performed, C56.9, R18.0, 0W9G3ZZ.

EXAMPLE | The patient has adenocarcinoma of the rectosigmoid junction, C19.

EXERCISE 10-4

Assign codes to the following conditions.

1. Hepatocellular carcinoma _____
2. Adenocarcinoma, head of pancreas _____
3. Fibrosarcoma of spleen _____
4. Adenocarcinoma of the duodenum _____
5. Gastric adenocarcinoma _____
6. Cholangiocarcinoma of the extrahepatic bile ducts _____

Malignant Neoplasm of Respiratory and Intrathoracic Organs (C30-C39)

Lung cancer, which is one of the most common types of cancer, is classified into two main categories: small cell lung cancer (SCLC) and non–small cell lung cancer (NSCLC). More than 85% of lung cancers are caused by smoking. Bronchogenic carcinoma is the most common type of malignant lung cancer (Figure 10-8). The lung is frequently a site for metastasis. Benign tumors of the lung are rare.

Malignant pleural effusion is a condition in which fluid accumulates in the pleural space and contains malignant cells. Malignant pleural effusions can result from lymphomas, breast cancer, and small cell lung cancer. Pleural effusions can be very uncomfortable for the patient and a therapeutic thoracentesis may be necessary to drain the fluid and provide relief. There is an instructional note in the code book to code first malignant neoplasm, if known. In the past, malignant pleural effusions were coded to secondary neoplasm of the pleura, but metastasis to the pleura is not always present in a patient with malignant pleural effusions.

EXAMPLE | Patient presented to the ER with shortness of breath due to right-sided malignant pleural effusion due to right SCLC. A thoracentesis was performed, C34.91, J91.0, 0W993ZZ.

EXAMPLE | The patient was diagnosed with adenocarcinoma, right lower lobe of lung, C34.31.

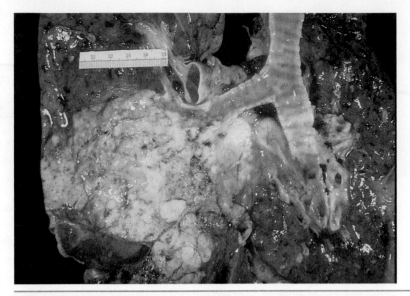

FIGURE 10-8. Bronchogenic carcinoma. The tumor, a squamous cell carcinoma, appears gray-white and infiltrates the lung tissue.

EXERCISE 10-5

Assign codes to the following conditions.

1. Malignancy of supraglottis   _____
2. Cancer of the larynx   _____
3. Oat cell cancer of right main bronchus   _____
4. Squamous cell carcinoma of thymus   _____
5. Cancer maxillary sinus   _____

Malignant Neoplasm of Bone, Articular Cartilage, and Skin (C40-C44)

Cancers of the connective tissue develop in the muscles, fat, blood and lymph vessels, and nerves. There are three main types of skin cancer:

■ **Basal cell carcinoma (BCC)** is the most common type of skin cancer. Most cases occur in areas of the body that have been exposed to the sun, such as the head and neck. Usually does not metastasize.

■ **Squamous cell carcinoma (SCC)** is the second most common type of skin cancer and also occurs in areas of the body that have been exposed to the sun. SCC of the lip and ears have high metastatic and recurrence rates.

■ **Malignant melanoma** is a malignant neoplasm of the melanocytes and the most common place of occurrence is the skin. Melanoma is the most dangerous skin cancer and is responsible for 75% of deaths due to skin cancer. Early signs of melanoma are summarized by "ABCDE":

• **A**symmetry
• **B**orders (irregular)
• **C**olor (variegated)
• **D**iameter (greater than 6 mm—about the size of a pencil eraser)
• **E**volving over time

Osteosarcoma is the most common primary malignant cancer of the bone and usually occurs in young people between the age of 10 and 30. These tumors develop most often in bones of the arms, legs, or pelvis.

| EXAMPLE | The patient is being seen for Ewing's sarcoma distal left femur, C40.22. |

EXERCISE 10-6

Assign codes to the following conditions.

1. Ewing's sarcoma 7th rib   _____
2. Basal cell carcinoma right ear   _____
3. Osteosarcoma left humerus   _____
4. Lentigo malignant melanoma sole of left foot   _____

Malignant Neoplasm of Mesothelial and Soft Tissue (C45-C49)

Malignant mesothelioma is a rare aggressive cancer that develops in the protective lining or mesothelium that surrounds and protects the internal organs. The most common site for occurrence is the pleura, which is the outer lining of the lungs. Other sites include the peritoneum, which is the lining of the abdominal cavity, the pericardium, which surrounds the heart, and the tunica vaginalis, which surrounds the testicles. The most common cause is exposure to asbestos. Symptoms will vary depending on the site of occurrence. Symptoms of pleural mesothelioma may include:

- Chest/rib pain
- Cough
- Shortness of breath
- Unusual nodules under the skin on chest
- Unexplained weight loss

| EXAMPLE | Patient is being treated for malignant mesothelioma of the pleura, C45.0. |

Kaposi's sarcoma (KS) is a cancer that develops from the lining of lymph or blood vessels. Purple, red, or brown blotches or lesions may form on the skin. Kaposi's can also occur in internal organs such as the lungs and gastrointestinal tract. Patients with HIV and those who have had organ transplants are at high risk for this malignancy. Both types of patients would be immunocompromised. KS may occur in more than one site. Each site should be coded separately and should be assigned codes for primary neoplasm instead of coding additional sites as a secondary neoplasm. If the Kaposi's sarcoma is due to HIV disease, B20 is coded first.

| EXAMPLE | Patient is seen in the clinic because of Kaposi's sarcoma lesions on the skin of the left leg. Patient has AIDS, B20, C46.0. |

EXERCISE 10-7

1. Kaposi's sarcoma palate in patient with HIV   _____
2. Mesothelioma of lung   _____
3. Fibrosarcoma, right tibia   _____
4. Malignant schwannoma, left sciatic nerve   _____

Malignant Neoplasm of Breast, Female and Male Genitourinary Organs (C50-C68)

One woman in eight has or will develop breast cancer in her lifetime (Figure 10-9). The 5-year survival rate exceeds 95% if detected early. Infiltrating or invasive ductal carcinoma is the most common type of breast cancer.

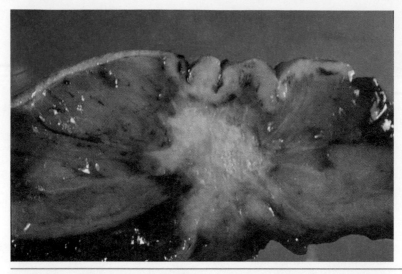

FIGURE 10-9. Breast carcinoma.

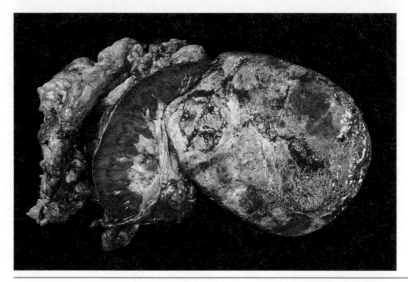

FIGURE 10-10. Renal cell carcinoma.

Malignancy can affect any organ in the genitourinary system. Many neoplasms are related to age; for example, Wilms' tumor is a common childhood tumor of the kidney. Testicular cancer usually affects young men, and the incidence of prostate cancer increases with age. Most kidney (Figure 10-10) and bladder (Figure 10-11) malignancies occur in adults between 60 and 70 years of age. As with many cancers, genetic, environmental, and behavioral risk factors may contribute to the cause.

EXAMPLE | The patient is being treated for a malignancy of his right testis (descended), C62.11.

EXERCISE 10-8

Assign codes to the following conditions.

1. Endometrial carcinoma _____

2. Renal cell carcinoma, left _____

3. Tubo-ovarian cancer _____

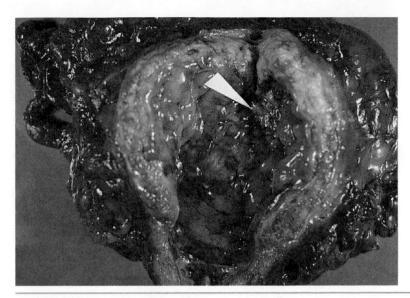

FIGURE 10-11. Bladder cancer.

4. Transitional cell carcinoma lower neck of bladder, causing _____
   urinary obstruction
5. Leiomyosarcoma of uterus _____
6. Upper outer quadrant malignancy right breast (female) _____
7. Malignant neoplasm left breast (male) _____

Malignant Neoplasm of Eye, Brain, and Other Parts of Central Nervous System (C69-C72) and Malignant Neoplasm of Thyroid and Other Endocrine Glands (C73-C75)

These sections contain a variety of neoplasms including those of the eye, brain, spinal cord, thyroid, and other endocrine glands. The most common type of primary malignant brain neoplasm is a **glioma**. This means that the malignancy has started in the glial cells of the central nervous system. Gliomas are classified into four grades. Grades I and II are low-grade and slow-growing while grade III grows at a moderate rate and grade IV is the most aggressive. There are different types of glial cells in which gliomas form. Some of these include:

- Pilocytic astrocytoma
- Diffuse astrocytoma
- Anaplastic astrocytoma
- Glioblastoma multiforme (GBM)
- Oligodendroglioma
- Ependymoma

EXAMPLE | Patient was seen in the clinic and the results of recent biopsy were discussed. The patient has a pilocytic astrocytoma of the cerebellum, C71.6.

There are four major types of thyroid cancer:

- Papillary
- Follicular
- Medullary
- Anaplastic

The most common types are papillary and follicular cancer. Prior irradiation to the head and neck may be a risk factor for the development of thyroid cancer. There is an instructional note under category C73, malignant neoplasm of the thyroid gland, to use an additional code to identify any functional activity.

EXAMPLE | Hypothyroidism due to malignancy of the thyroid gland, C73, E03.8.

EXERCISE 10-9

Assign codes to the following conditions.

1. Seizure due to carcinoma of parietal lobe of the brain _____
2. Glioblastoma multiforme brain _____
3. Left orbital rhabdomyosarcoma _____
4. Anaplastic astrocytoma spinal cord with metastasis to the _____
   vertebral bodies

Neuroendocrine Tumors

Code categories C7a and C7b include codes for primary and secondary malignant carcinoid neoplasms. Neuroendocrine tumors can be benign and/or malignant neoplasms that arise in the endocrine or neuroendocrine cells throughout the body. These neoplasms are usually slow growing. There are two groups of neuroendocrine neoplasms:
- Carcinoid
- Pancreatic endocrine

The most common sites for carcinoid neoplasms are the bronchi, stomach, small intestine, appendix, and rectum. They are classified according to the embryonic site of origin such as:
- **Foregut**—bronchi and stomach
- **Midgut**—small intestine and appendix
- **Hindgut**—colon and rectum

Malignant tumors are larger than benign tumors and do metastasize. The most common metastatic sites are lymph nodes, liver, lung, bone, and skin.

EXAMPLE | Malignant carcinoid neoplasm of the appendix, C7a.020.

EXERCISE 10-10

Assign codes to the following conditions.

1. Malignant carcinoid tumor foregut _____
2. Carcinoid neoplasm, small intestine, malignant _____
3. Neuroblastoma left adrenal gland _____
4. Teratocarcinoma pineal gland _____

Malignant Neoplasm of Ill-defined, Secondary, and Unspecified Sites (C76-C80)

This section is where secondary or metastatic neoplasm codes are located. The C77 category is used to identify the spread of cancer to the lymph nodes. In contrast, code C79.51 is the code assigned to metastasis to the bone and in this case specificity is not necessary for code assignment. It does not matter whether this is a vertebral bone, a pelvic bone, or the humerus.

EXAMPLE | The patient has metastatic lung cancer; no known primary, C78.00, C80.1 (sequencing will depend on reason for the encounter).

EXERCISE 10-11

1. Metastatic melanoma to the brain; melanoma skin lesion excised 5 years ago _____
2. Carcinomatosis _____
3. Metastasis to the mastectomy site; left mastectomy performed 1 year ago _____

Malignant Neoplasm of Lymphoid, Hematopoietic, and Related Tissue (C81-C96)

Lymphoma is cancer of the lymphatic system. Two main types have been identified: Hodgkin's disease (HD) (Figure 10-12) or **lymphoma**, and **non-Hodgkin's lymphoma** (NHL). The incidence of non-Hodgkin's is greater than that of Hodgkin's disease. The lymphatic system follows the blood vessels, and groups are located in areas of the neck, axillary, groin, abdomen, and pelvic regions. Some organs contain lymphatic tissue and may be affected. These organs include the spleen, thymus gland, bone marrow, tonsils, and adenoids. Although lymphoma may be present in different or multiple areas of the body, this is not considered metastatic. Lymphomas should not be confused with solid tumors (malignancies) that have metastasized to the lymph nodes.

If a patient is in remission, he or she is considered to have lymphoma. There are different classifications of remission. **Complete remission** means there are no signs or symptoms of the cancer. **Partial remission** means there are still a few signs and symptoms of the cancer and the cancer cells have significantly decreased.

Leukemia is cancer of the white blood cells that begins in the blood-forming cells of the bone marrow. As the disease progresses, leukemic cells invade other parts of the body,

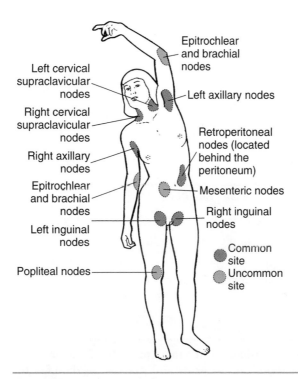

FIGURE 10-12. Lymph node sites for Hodgkin's disease.

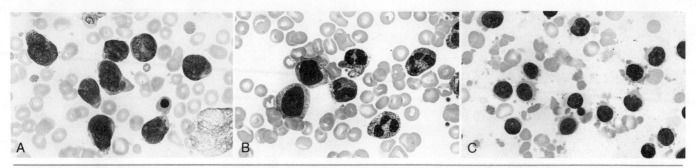

FIGURE 10-13. Peripheral blood smears. **A,** Acute lymphoblastic leukemia. **B,** Chronic myelogenous leukemia. **C,** Chronic lymphocytic leukemia.

such as the lymph nodes, spleen, liver, and central nervous system. Various types of leukemia have been identified (Figure 10-13). Some develop suddenly and are acute leukemias; others are of the chronic variety.

EXAMPLE The patient was diagnosed with nodular sclerosis Hodgkin's, C81.10.

EXERCISE 10-12

Assign codes to the following conditions.

1. Acute lymphocytic leukemia (ALL), relapsed   _____
2. Acute promyelocytic leukemia   _____
3. Chronic myelogenous leukemia (CML)   _____
4. Lymphoma ileum   _____
5. Burkitt's lymphoma in remission   _____

In Situ Neoplasms (D00-D09)

Carcinoma in situ consists of malignant cells that remain within the original site with no spread or invasion to neighboring tissues (Figure 10-14). Usually, the physician or the pathology report will confirm that the condition is "in situ." These tumors are usually curable because they are at the earliest stage of development.

EXAMPLE Patient has Bowen's disease, right thigh, D04.71.

EXERCISE 10-13

Assign codes to the following conditions.

1. Carcinoma in situ of the cervix   _____
2. Carcinoma in situ of the urinary bladder   _____
3. Cervical intraepithelial neoplasia III   _____
4. Ductal carcinoma in situ (DCIS) left breast   _____

Benign Neoplasms (D10-D36)

A benign neoplasm or tumor is not malignant. It will not metastasize to other parts of the body, but it could continue to grow and may cause damage to neighboring organs and structures. It may be necessary to remove a benign neoplasm. Benign neoplasms may recur.

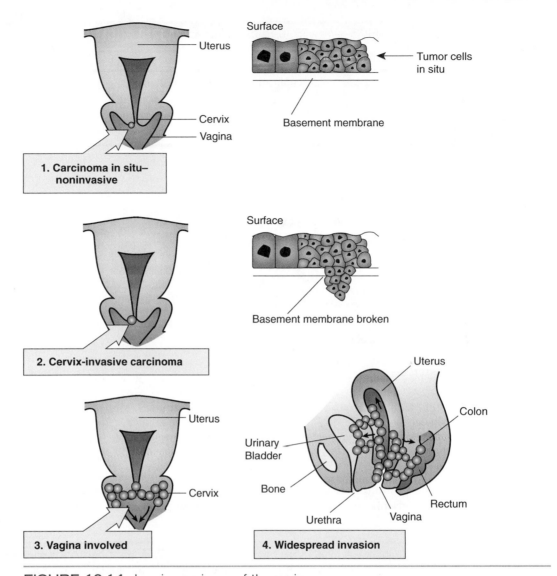

FIGURE 10-14. Invasive carcinoma of the cervix.

Lipoma is a growth of fat cells within a capsule that is usually found just below the skin. Lipomas are the most common benign soft tissue growths. For the most part, lipomas are small and movable, and they remain the same size and are not painful. It may be necessary to excise a lipoma if it becomes painful or infected, if it limits function or mobility, or if it increases in size.

Leiomyoma or uterine fibroids are tumors or growths within the walls of the uterus. These are the most common benign tumors in women of childbearing age. Not all fibroids cause symptoms. When fibroids become symptomatic, the following symptoms may be present:

- Heavy bleeding
- Painful periods
- Feeling of fullness in the pelvic region
- Urinary frequency
- Pain during sex
- Infertility, miscarriage, or early onset of labor

Treatment will depend on the severity of symptoms, the size and location of the fibroids, and the patient's age and desired fertility.

EXAMPLE	Patient is being seen because of a cavernous lymphangioma, D18.1.

EXAMPLE	Benign carcinoid neoplasm of the rectum, D3a.026.

EXERCISE 10-14

Assign codes to the following conditions.

1. Warthin's tumor _____
2. Adenoma of the pituitary gland _____
3. Chondromyxoid fibroma of the left tibia _____
4. Squamous papilloma soft palate _____
5. Osteoma proximal right femur _____
6. Enchondroma right fifth metacarpal _____
7. Lipoma spermatic cord _____
8. Rhabdomyoma left ventricle of heart _____
9. Hemangioma of liver _____
10. Submucosal uterine fibroid _____
11. Benign carcinoid tumor, rectum _____

Neoplasms of Uncertain Behavior and Unspecified Behavior (D37-D49)

Neoplasms that fall into the categories of uncertain behavior are neither malignant nor benign. On pathologic examination, the behavior cannot be determined or predicted. In some instances, progression to some type of malignancy may occur. For example, myelodysplastic syndrome has been known to progress to leukemia.

EXAMPLE	Patient was being seen in the clinic and the findings of her path were discussed. The path showed granulosa cell tumors of the right ovary (undetermined behavior), D39.11.

Terms such as "growth," "neoplasm," or "tumor" are used to describe a medical finding. At times, this condition may require further investigation and testing. Sometimes, these findings are not investigated because the patient is elderly and has other chronic conditions, and aggressive treatment would not be pursued.

On occasion, a physician will document a patient as having a mass with no further specification other than site or location of the mass. Usually, this occurs when no pathology report is available when the physician is documenting details in the health record. According to *Coding Clinic for ICD-9-CM* (2006:1Q:p4),[4] if the diagnosis is documented as "mass" or "lesion," it would be incorrect to select a code for neoplasm of unspecified behavior.

EXAMPLE	Mass of the liver, R16.0.

The *Coding Clinic for ICD-9-CM* states if there is no index entry for a specific site, go to the main term "disease." If terms such as lump or lesion are used, the same logic is applied. If a subterm cannot be found under "lump," "lesion," or "mass," go to the main term "disease."

EXAMPLE	Patient will need to follow up for definitive diagnosis of neoplasm sigmoid colon D49.0.

EXERCISE 10-15

Assign codes to the following conditions.

1. Intracranial tumor _____
2. Neoplasm bladder _____
3. Growth left ovary _____
4. Mass right lung _____
5. Right breast lump _____
6. Lesion brain was identified by MRI _____
7. Myelodysplastic syndrome (MDS) _____
8. Polycythemia vera _____
9. Refractory anemia _____
10. Paraganglioma of carotid body _____

Coding and Sequencing of Neoplasms

In addition to assigning neoplasm codes, it is important to know how these codes are sequenced in accordance with the guidelines. The principal diagnosis is determined according to the reason the patient is admitted and the treatment provided. Documentation by physicians may be confusing in determining the principal diagnosis. They often will document the cancer as the reason for admission. Physicians may document cancers that have been previously removed. Physicians are not trained to document in accordance with coding guidelines. They may document the reason for admission as the cancer when the patient is receiving treatment for a complication of the cancer or of the cancer treatments.

Malignancy as Principal Diagnosis

When a patient is admitted for determination of whether a malignancy is present and a malignancy is found, the code for the primary malignancy is the principal diagnosis.

EXAMPLE | Patient was admitted for total thyroidectomy. Fine needle aspiration biopsy on an outpatient basis was inconclusive. Total thyroidectomy was performed, and a diagnosis of anaplastic cancer was determined, C73, 0GTK0ZZ.

As in the previous example, during the course of determining whether a malignancy is present, a malignancy is found and a secondary malignancy is identified. The code for the primary neoplasm is the principal diagnosis, and the secondary malignancy is assigned as an additional code.

EXAMPLE | Patient has papillary thyroid cancer that has spread to the cervical lymph nodes, C73, C77.0.

Recurrence of Primary Malignancy

If a primary malignancy was previously excised or eradicated but has now recurred at the site of origin, the malignancy is coded to a primary malignant neoplasm.

EXAMPLE | Recurrence of transitional cell bladder cancer, posterior wall, C67.4.

Physicians may document a malignancy as recurrent at a site where a malignancy and the organ has been previously excised. This cannot be an actual recurrent neoplasm if the organ is no longer present. It may be necessary to query the physician to determine the metastatic site(s).

EXAMPLE   Recurrent ovarian cancer. Patient had hysterectomy and bilateral salpingo-oophorectomy 3 years ago, C79.9, Z85.43, Z90.722, Z90.710, Z90.79 (may need to query site of recurrence).

When a patient is admitted for removal of a known malignancy, the malignancy is the principal diagnosis. In some cases, a biopsy may have been performed previously that confirms the presence of a malignancy. The patient is readmitted for more definitive surgery. The pathology report following the surgery may report negative findings for malignancy. If the physician documents the malignancy as shown on the biopsy, the malignancy is assigned as the principal diagnosis for the definitive surgery even though no further evidence of malignancy is seen on the pathology report.

EXAMPLE   Patient has a fine needle aspiration biopsy that shows Hürthle carcinoma of the left lobe of the thyroid. Patient is admitted for a partial thyroidectomy with removal of the left lobe. The pathology report from the thyroidectomy shows no evidence of malignancy, C73, 0GTG0ZZ.

When a patient is admitted with a sign or symptom (which codes to Chapter 18) related to a known primary or secondary malignancy, the primary or secondary malignancy code is the principal diagnosis.

EXAMPLE   Convulsion due to glioblastoma multiforme temporal lobe of brain, C71.2, R56.9 (the convulsion is coded as an additional code because convulsions are not integral to the brain neoplasm).

When a patient is admitted with a primary neoplasm and a metastatic neoplasm, and treatment is directed to the metastatic neoplasm, the metastatic neoplasm is the principal diagnosis.

EXAMPLE   Patient is admitted for wedge resection of metastatic liver cancer.
Patient had a colorectal cancer removed 3 months ago and is undergoing treatment, C78.7, C19, 0FB00ZZ.

According to *Coding Clinic for ICD-9-CM* (1988:1Q:p4-5),[5] when a patient is admitted to the hospital for treatment by brachytherapy, the principal diagnosis is the malignancy that is being treated (which could be either a primary or a secondary malignancy).

EXAMPLE   Patient was admitted for implantation of brachytherapy (high dose rate Iridium 192) for cancer of cervix, C53.9, DU1198Z.

Complications as Principal Diagnosis

Often, complications are associated with malignancies or the treatment of malignancies. When the complication is the reason for admission or treatment, the complication is the principal diagnosis. The guidelines address some of the most common examples such as neutropenic fever and dehydration.

EXAMPLE   Patient has become extremely dehydrated following last chemotherapy session for breast cancer. Patient is admitted for IV fluids, E86.0, C50.919.

EXAMPLE | Neutropenic fever with neutropenia due to chemotherapy for acute lymphocytic leukemia, D70.2, R50.81, T45.1x5A, C91.00.

Principal Diagnosis for Encounters for Chemotherapy/Immunotherapy and Radiation

When a patient is admitted solely for the administration of chemotherapy, chemoembolization, immunotherapy, and/or radiation, the principal diagnosis will be a Z51.- code. In cases where chemotherapy, chemoembolization, immunotherapy, or radiation is performed in conjunction with surgical removal of a neoplasm, the primary or secondary neoplasm code is the principal diagnosis, and no Z51.- code is assigned.

If a patient is admitted for both radiation and chemotherapy during the same encounter, either Z code can be sequenced as the principal with the other Z code used as a secondary diagnosis code.

If complications occur during an encounter for chemotherapy/immunotherapy/radiation treatment, codes to identify the complications are assigned as secondary diagnosis codes.

EXAMPLE | Patient was admitted for chemotherapy (percutaneous central vein) for osteosarcoma of right humerus. Patient became dehydrated and was treated with additional IV fluids, Z51.11, C40.01, E86.0, 3E04305.

EXAMPLE | Patient is admitted for chemotherapy (percutaneous central vein) for Burkitt's lymphoma, Z51.11, C83.70, 3E04305.

EXAMPLE | Patient is admitted for radiation therapy (heavy particle) for prostate cancer, Z51.0, C61, DV004ZZ.

Coding of Previously Excised Malignancies

If a primary malignancy has been previously excised and is no longer being treated, it is assigned a Z code for history of personal malignancy.

EXAMPLE | Patient had a mastectomy 5 years ago for breast cancer. She is not being actively treated, Z85.3, Z90.10.

However, if a previously excised malignancy is still being treated actively, it is appropriate to assign the neoplasm code.

EXAMPLE | Patient had a lobectomy for lung cancer 6 months ago. The patient will receive the fifth cycle of chemotherapy next week, C34.90, Z90.2.

EXERCISE 10-16

Complete the following exercises.

1. If a patient is admitted and treated for dehydration due to a malignancy, the malignancy code is the principal diagnosis.
   A. True
   B. False

2. If a patient has a complication during an encounter for chemotherapy, the complication code is the principal diagnosis.
   A. True
   B. False

3. If a malignancy of the bladder has been previously excised and now there is a recurrence of a malignancy within the bladder, the recurrence is coded as a primary malignancy.
    A. True
    B. False

4. A personal history Z code is assigned for a history of a primary malignancy when it is no longer being treated.
    A. True
    B. False

5. The primary neoplasm is always principal even if the treatment is directed at the secondary neoplasm.
    A. True
    B. False

6. If a patient is admitted for treatment of dehydration due to a malignancy, the dehydration is the principal diagnosis.
    A. True
    B. False

7. When a patient is admitted for immunotherapy, the Z51.12 is assigned as the principal diagnosis.
    A. True
    B. False

8. When a patient is admitted for brachytherapy, the Z51.0 is assigned as the principal diagnosis.
    A. True
    B. False

FACTORS INFLUENCING HEALTH STATUS AND CONTACT WITH HEALTH SERVICES (Z CODES)

As was discussed in Chapter 8, it may be difficult to locate Z codes in the Index. Coders often say, "I did not know there was a Z code for that." Refer to Chapter 8 for a listing of common main terms used to locate Z codes.

The guidelines provide instructions for the use and sequencing of some important Z codes. If a patient is admitted solely for administration of chemotherapy, immunotherapy, or radiation therapy, a code from category Z51.- should be the principal diagnosis followed by codes for the malignancies being treated. If they are admitted for more than one type of therapy, either code can be principal.

Z codes that may be used with neoplasms include the following:

Z08	Encounter for follow-up examination after completed treatment for malignant neoplasm
Z12.0	Encounter for screening for malignant neoplasm of stomach
Z12.10	Encounter for screening for malignant neoplasm of intestinal tract, unspecified
Z12.11	Encounter for screening for malignant neoplasm of colon
Z12.12	Encounter for screening for malignant neoplasm of rectum
Z12.13	Encounter for screening for malignant neoplasm of small intestine
Z12.2	Encounter for screening for malignant neoplasm of respiratory organs
Z12.31	Encounter for screening mammogram for malignant neoplasm of breast
Z12.39	Encounter for other screening for malignant neoplasm of breast
Z12.4	Encounter for screening for malignant neoplasm of cervix
Z12.5	Encounter for screening for malignant neoplasm of prostate
Z12.6	Encounter for screening for malignant neoplasm of bladder
Z12.71	Encounter for screening for malignant neoplasm of testis
Z12.72	Encounter for screening for malignant neoplasm of vagina

Z12.73	Encounter for screening for malignant neoplasm of ovary
Z12.79	Encounter for screening for malignant neoplasm of other genitourinary organs
Z12.81	Encounter for screening for malignant neoplasm of oral cavity
Z12.82	Encounter for screening for malignant neoplasm of nervous system
Z12.83	Encounter for screening for malignant neoplasm of skin
Z12.89	Encounter for screening for malignant neoplasm of other sites
Z12.9	Encounter for screening for malignant neoplasm, site unspecified
Z15.01	Genetic susceptibility to malignant neoplasm of breast
Z15.02	Genetic susceptibility to malignant neoplasm of ovary
Z15.03	Genetic susceptibility to malignant neoplasm of prostate
Z15.04	Genetic susceptibility to malignant neoplasm of endometrium
Z15.09	Genetic susceptibility to other malignant neoplasm
Z17.0	Estrogen receptor positive status [ER+]
Z17.1	Estrogen receptor negative status [ER-]
Z40.00	Encounter for prophylactic removal of unspecified organ
Z40.01	Encounter for prophylactic removal of breast
Z40.02	Encounter for prophylactic removal of ovary
Z40.09	Encounter for prophylactic removal of other organ
Z42.1	Encounter for breast reconstruction following mastectomy
Z51.0	Encounter for antineoplastic radiation therapy
Z51.11	Encounter for antineoplastic chemotherapy
Z51.12	Encounter for antineoplastic immunotherapy
Z79.810	Long term (current) use of selective estrogen receptor modulators (SERMs)
Z79.811	Long-term (current) use of aromatase inhibitors
Z79.818	Long-term (current) use of other agents affecting estrogen receptors and estrogen levels
Z80.0	Family history of malignant neoplasm of digestive organs
Z80.1	Family history of malignant neoplasm of trachea, bronchus and lung
Z80.2	Family history of malignant neoplasm of other respiratory and intrathoracic organs
Z80.3	Family history of malignant neoplasm of breast
Z80.41	Family history of malignant neoplasm of ovary
Z80.42	Family history of malignant neoplasm of prostate
Z80.43	Family history of malignant neoplasm of testis
Z80.49	Family history of malignant neoplasm of other genital organs
Z80.51	Family history of malignant neoplasm of kidney
Z80.52	Family history of malignant neoplasm of bladder
Z80.59	Family history of malignant neoplasm of other urinary tract organ
Z80.6	Family history of leukemia
Z80.7	Family history of other malignant neoplasms of lymphoid, hematopoietic and related tissues
Z80.8	Family history of malignant neoplasm of other organs or systems
Z80.9	Family history of malignant neoplasm, unspecified
Z85.00	Personal history of malignant neoplasm of unspecified digestive organ
Z85.01	Personal history of malignant neoplasm of esophagus
Z85.020	Personal history of malignant carcinoid tumor of stomach
Z85.028	Personal history of other malignant neoplasm of stomach
Z85.030	Personal history of malignant carcinoid tumor of large intestine
Z85.038	Personal history of other malignant neoplasm of large intestine
Z85.040	Personal history of malignant carcinoid tumor of rectum
Z85.048	Personal history of other malignant neoplasm of rectum, rectosigmoid junction, and anus

Z85.05	Personal history of malignant neoplasm of liver
Z85.060	Personal history of malignant carcinoid tumor of small intestine
Z85.068	Personal history of other malignant neoplasm of small intestine
Z85.07	Personal history of malignant neoplasm of pancreas
Z85.09	Personal history of malignant neoplasm of other digestive organs
Z85.110	Personal history of malignant carcinoid tumor of bronchus and lung
Z85.118	Personal history of other malignant neoplasm of bronchus and lung
Z85.12	Personal history of malignant neoplasm of trachea
Z85.20	Personal history of malignant neoplasm of unspecified respiratory organ
Z85.21	Personal history of malignant neoplasm of larynx
Z85.22	Personal history of malignant neoplasm of nasal cavities, middle ear, and accessory sinuses
Z85.230	Personal history of malignant carcinoid tumor of thymus
Z85.238	Personal history of malignant neoplasm of thymus
Z85.29	Personal history of malignant neoplasm of other respiratory and intrathoracic organs
Z85.3	Personal history of malignant neoplasm of breast
Z85.40	Personal history of malignant neoplasm of unspecified female genital organ
Z85.41	Personal history of malignant neoplasm of cervix uteri
Z85.42	Personal history of malignant neoplasm of other parts of uterus
Z85.43	Personal history of malignant neoplasm of ovary
Z85.44	Personal history of malignant neoplasm of other female genital organs
Z85.45	Personal history of malignant neoplasm of unspecified male genital organ
Z85.46	Personal history of malignant neoplasm of prostate
Z85.47	Personal history of malignant neoplasm of testis
Z85.48	Personal history of malignant neoplasm of epididymis
Z85.49	Personal history of malignant neoplasm of other male genital organs
Z85.50	Personal history of malignant neoplasm of unspecified urinary tract organ
Z85.51	Personal history of malignant neoplasm of the bladder
Z85.520	Personal history of malignant carcinoid tumor of kidney
Z85.528	Personal history of other malignant neoplasm of kidney
Z85.53	Personal history of malignant neoplasm of renal pelvis
Z85.54	Personal history of malignant neoplasm of ureter
Z85.59	Personal history of malignant neoplasm of other urinary tract organ
Z85.6	Personal history of leukemia
Z85.71	Personal history of Hodgkin lymphoma
Z85.72	Personal history of non-Hodgkin lymphomas
Z85.79	Personal history of other malignant neoplasms of lymphoid, hematopoietic and related tissues
Z85.810	Personal history of malignant neoplasm of tongue
Z85.818	Personal history of malignant neoplasm of other sites of lip, oral cavity, and pharynx
Z85.819	Personal history of malignant neoplasm of unspecified site of lip, oral cavity, and pharynx
Z85.820	Personal history of malignant melanoma of skin
Z85.821	Personal history of Merkel cell carcinoma
Z85.828	Personal history of other malignant neoplasm of skin
Z85.830	Personal history of malignant neoplasm of bone
Z85.831	Personal history of malignant neoplasm of soft tissue
Z85.840	Personal history of malignant neoplasm of eye
Z85.841	Personal history of malignant neoplasm of brain
Z85.848	Personal history of malignant neoplasm of other parts of nervous tissue

Z85.850	Personal history of malignant neoplasm of thyroid
Z85.858	Personal history of malignant neoplasm of other endocrine glands
Z85.89	Personal history of malignant neoplasm of other organs and systems
Z85.9	Personal history of malignant neoplasm, unspecified
Z86.000	Personal history of in-situ neoplasm of breast
Z86.001	Personal history of in-situ neoplasm of cervix uteri
Z86.008	Personal history of in-situ neoplasm of other site
Z86.010	Personal history of colonic polyps
Z86.011	Personal history of benign neoplasm of the brain
Z86.012	Personal history of benign carcinoid tumor
Z86.018	Personal history of other benign neoplasm
Z86.03	Personal history of neoplasm of uncertain behavior
Z92.21	Personal history of antineoplastic chemotherapy
Z92.22	Personal history of monoclonal drug therapy
Z92.23	Personal history of estrogen therapy
Z92.3	Personal history of irradiation

There are some important Z code categories related to neoplasms and the treatment and follow-up of neoplasms. First, there are a number of screening codes and codes for family history of malignancies. A screening examination occurs in the absence of any signs or symptoms. The patient is asymptomatic.

EXAMPLE | Patient has no symptoms. Screening for prostate cancer, Z12.5.

EXAMPLE | Patient has a family history of leukemia, Z80.6.

EXERCISE 10-17

Assign codes to the following conditions.

1. History of adenocarcinoma of the prostate _____
2. Screening mammogram for patient with strong family history _____
   of breast cancer
3. Personal history of benign brain neoplasm previously removed _____
4. Admission for takedown of colostomy; previous colon _____
   resection for malignancy

COMMON TREATMENTS

Cancer is treated by various modalities (i.e., surgery, chemotherapy, radiation, immunotherapy, or other methods). The type of treatment will depend on the location, grading, and stage of the neoplasm and the health of the patient. Chemotherapy destroys cancer cells, but may also target fast-growing healthy tissue. Often chemotherapy drugs are used in combinations because the drugs work better together than separately. Immunotherapy agents stimulate the immune system's response against tumors. Radiation therapy uses ionizing radiation to destroy cancer cells and shrink tumors. It is administered externally by external beam therapy or internally via brachytherapy.

CONDITION	MEDICATION/TREATMENT
Malignancies	Chemotherapy drugs are often given in combination with other chemotherapy drugs or hormonal therapy. The treatment will depend on the type of cancer. Some common drugs include carboplatin (Paraplatin), cisplatin (Platinol), cyclophosphamide (Cytoxan, Neosar), docetaxel (Taxotere), doxorubicin (Adriamycin), erlotinib (Tarceva), etoposide (VePesid, Toposar, Etopophos), fluorouracil (5-FU), gemcitabine (Gemzar), ifosfamide (Ifex), imatinib mesylate (Gleevec), irinotecan (Camptosar), methotrexate (Folex, Mexate, Amethopterin), mitomycin (Mitomycin-C), paclitaxel (Taxol, Abraxane), rituximab (Rituxan), sorafenib (Nexavar), sunitinib (Sutent), topotecan (Hycantin), vinblastine (Velban), vincristine (Oncovin, Vincasar PFS).
Melanoma and kidney cancer	Immunotherapy with interleukin and interferon
Superficial bladder cancer	Intravesical Bacillus Calmette-Guerin (BCG) immunotherapy
Certain types of breast or colon cancer	Capecitabine (Xeloda)—interferes with cancer cell growth and reproduction
Certain types of breast cancer	Tamoxifen (Nolvadex)—interferes with estrogen activity
Advanced prostate cancer in men and uterine fibroid tumors in women	Leuprolide acetate for depot suspension (Lupron Depot)
Certain types of leukemia (CML) and certain gastrointestinal stromal tumors	Imatinib (Gleevec) prevents the growth of cancer cells
Neutropenia due to chemotherapy	Pegfilgrastim (Neulasta) or filgrastim (Neupogen) builds up or stimulates white cell counts
Anemia due to malignancy	Epoetin alfa (Procrit, Epogen), darbepoetin alfa (Aranesp)
Symptoms of malignancy and treatment	Pain medications (narcotics), antiemetics to suppress nausea and vomiting
Human papilloma virus	Vaccination for prevention

PROCEDURES

Neoplasms can affect any body system, so for ICD-10-PCS, any of the tables in the Medical and Surgical section may be used. There may also be procedures that can be located in the Radiation Oncology, Placement, and Administration sections.

Chemotherapy/Immunotherapy/Radiation

Operative procedures are often performed to biopsy and resect or excise areas or organs that are affected by neoplastic conditions. At times, a neoplasm is considered unresectable, and other treatments are necessary. Sometimes, patients will receive chemotherapy or radiation therapy to shrink the tumor before surgery is performed. **Chemotherapy** consists of administration of drugs or medications to treat disease. In cancer patients, antineoplastic drugs are used. These drugs can be given intravenously, orally, subcutaneously, intramuscularly, or intrathecally. The introduction of chemotherapy is found in the Administration section of ICD-10-PCS. **Chemoembolization** is the intra-arterial administration of chemotherapy with collagen particles to enhance the delivery of chemotherapy to the targeted area. This should be treated as an encounter for chemotherapy, and Z51.11 should be assigned as the principal diagnosis. An additional diagnosis code is assigned for the malignancy. **Radiation** treatment involves the use of high-energy radiation to treat patients with cancer. **Brachytherapy** is the placement of radioactive material directly into or near the cancer. The radiation is delivered by needles, wires, or catheters and may be in the form of seeds. When a patient is admitted for treatment of a malignancy by implantation or insertion of radioactive elements, the principal diagnosis is the neoplastic condition (malignancy) being treated with the radioactive element. Radiation and brachytherapy are found under the Radiation Oncology section of ICD-10-PCS. **Immunotherapy** is the administration of agents that stimulate the immune system's response against tumors. **Biological response modifiers (BRMs)** are a type of immunotherapy and are used to fight certain cancers and even conditions such as rheumatoid arthritis. They can destroy cancer cells, stimulate the immune system to destroy cancer cells, or change cancer cells to normal cells. Immunotherapy is found in the Administration section of ICD-10-PCS.

The Guidelines provide instructions for the use and sequencing of some important Z codes. If a patient is admitted solely for administration of chemotherapy, immunotherapy, or radiation therapy, a code from category Z51.- should be the principal diagnosis followed by codes for the malignancies being treated. If they are admitted for more than one type of therapy, either code can be principal.

EXAMPLE

> Patient was admitted for the administration of chemotherapy (percutaneous central vein) for osteosarcoma of upper end of the tibia, Z51.11, C40.20, 3E04305.

EXAMPLE

> Radioactive seeds were implanted within Iodine 125 at high dose rate for treatment of prostate cancer, C61, DV1099Z.

EXAMPLE

> Patient is admitted for chemoembolization of hepatocellular carcinoma, Z51.11, C22.0, 3E063GC.

Palliative procedures may be performed to correct a condition that is causing problems or pain for the patient. It is not meant to cure. Palliative surgery may be performed to relieve an obstruction caused by a tumor. Sometimes radiation is administered for palliative treatment.

Biopsy

Biopsy specimens can be obtained in several ways. The approach used varies with the location of the mass, the age of the patient, and the technology that is available. A **biopsy** consists of removal of a representative sample of a tumor mass for pathologic examination and diagnosis. A biopsy is a diagnostic procedure and the root operation for biopsy is excision.

- **Incisional biopsy:** This is the removal of a small piece of tumor.
- **Core biopsy:** This procedure is less invasive than surgical biopsy. A large needle is used to extract a core sample. Usually, a smaller sample of tissue is provided, and the cancerous tissue may be missed. Occasionally, a new sample must be obtained.
- **Fine needle aspiration (FNA):** This method, which requires use of a very small needle, works best for masses that are superficial or easily accessible. The specimen is small, and sometimes, findings are inconclusive.
- **Endoscopic biopsy:** This is a biopsy that is performed during an endoscopic examination. After a biopsy is performed, a more definitive surgical procedure may be necessary.

EXAMPLE

> Patient had an FNA biopsy of a thyroid mass last week; this confirmed papillary thyroid cancer. Patient underwent total thyroidectomy, C73, 0GTK0ZZ.

Occasionally, a biopsy will be performed during the same operative episode as a more definitive treatment. In these cases, sequencing of the procedures would follow the Uniform Hospital Discharge Data Set (UHDDS) guidelines for selection of a principal procedure, and the procedure that is performed for definitive treatment is the principal procedure.

EXAMPLE | Patient (female) was taken to the operating room for an open biopsy of a breast mass in the right upper outer quadrant. Frozen section showed invasive ductal carcinoma; a simple mastectomy with removal of three axillary lymph nodes was performed during the same operative episode. Nodes were negative for malignancy, C50.411, 0HTT0ZZ, 07B50ZX, 0HBT0ZX.

Surgery

Endoscopic procedures are minimally invasive procedures during which a scope is used to examine the inside of the body. It is also possible for the clinician to perform a biopsy, remove a small polyp or foreign body, or control bleeding with the use of an endoscope.

Preventive or prophylactic surgery is performed to remove tissue that has the potential to become cancerous. A woman may have a prophylactic mastectomy as the result of a strong family history of breast cancer and/or a positive breast cancer gene (*BRCA1* or *BRCA2*). The principal or first-listed diagnosis should be a code from subcategory Z40.-, prophylactic organ removal. The appropriate Z codes to identify the reason for the removal should also be assigned. If a patient has a malignancy of the breast and decides to have the other breast removed also as a prophylactic measure, the malignancy code should be assigned first with a Z40.01 code for the prophylactic removal of the other breast. **Staging surgeries** are performed to determine the extent of the disease and are generally more accurate than laboratory and imaging tests. **Debulking** procedures are performed when it is impossible to remove the tumor entirely. In many of these cases a number of organs may be involved and may also have to be removed. The tumor is removed to as great an extent as is possible, and adjunctive treatment such as chemotherapy or radiation may be used to treat the remaining disease. **Restorative or reconstructive** surgery is performed to restore function and enhance aesthetic appearance after surgery. Breast reconstruction is commonly performed after a mastectomy. Breast reconstruction procedures will be covered in Chapter 20.

EXAMPLE | Patient was admitted for prophylactic removal of ovaries due to genetic susceptibility and positive family history of ovarian cancer with laparoscopic removal, Z40.02, Z80.41, Z15.02, 0UT24ZZ.

EXERCISE 10-18

Assign codes for all diagnoses and procedures.

1. Refractory aplastic anemia with excess blasts (RAEB-2) for bone marrow transplant (BMT) via central vein; donor is the patient's sister _____

2. Transitional cell carcinoma of the bladder with transurethral resection of tumor _____

3. Renal cell cancer of the right kidney with right laparoscopic nephrectomy _____

4. Vaginal brachytherapy with high dose rate Iridium 192 for endometrial carcinoma _____

5. Acoustic neuroma with hearing loss; craniotomy for removal of tumor _____

6. Wide excision of melanoma right shoulder with skin grafting; _____
   split-thickness graft taken from left thigh

7. Diagnostic percutaneous biopsy of intrathoracic lymph node _____
   showed non-Hodgkin's lymphoma in patient who has had a
   kidney transplant

8. Admission for chemotherapy via central vein; patient has a _____
   malignancy of the esophagus

9. Wedge resection liver for HCC _____

10. Ascending colon cancer with right hemicolectomy (resection _____
    of ascending colon)

DOCUMENTATION/REIMBURSEMENT/MS-DRGs

Often, coding difficulties are due to lack of documentation. Sometimes pathology and other test results are not available at the time of discharge or when the physician is dictating the discharge summary or is reporting the final diagnoses.

The physician may document the cancer as if it is the principal diagnosis because it is the most serious and can be a life-threatening condition. However, the cancer may not fit the definition of a principal diagnosis or may not follow the neoplasm guidelines. Physicians will sometimes document metastatic breast carcinoma, and further into the record, it may be noted that the patient has had a mastectomy and has received a combination of chemotherapy and radiation therapy. In this case, it is most likely a primary breast cancer that has spread to an undocumented secondary site.

It is difficult to pinpoint any particular codes that may be frequently missed complications/comorbidities from this chapter. There are numerous primary and secondary neoplasms on the CC listing. There are no neoplasm codes on the MCC listing. It is important to code all current primary and secondary neoplasms, even when this is not the main reason for a patient's admission to the hospital.

Assign All Procedure Codes

It is very important to assign all procedure codes because this could make the difference between a medical MS-DRG and a surgical MS-DRG. Likewise, it is also important to follow the guidelines for selection of the appropriate principal diagnosis.

EXAMPLE

DIAGNOSES	CODES	MS-DRG	RW
Malignant neoplasm brain with craniotomy with excision of tumor	C71.9 00B00ZZ	027	2.1317
Malignant neoplasm brain with craniotomy with excision of tumor (in the body of the operative report is documentation of chemo wafers implanted on the brain)	C71.9 00B00ZZ 3E0Q705	023	5.3625

MS-DRG With and Without MCC/CC

EXAMPLE

DIAGNOSES	CODES	MS-DRG	RW
Hodgkin's lymphoma, multiple sites, patient is cachectic	C81.98 R64	841	1.6342
Hodgkin's lymphoma, multiple sites	C81.98	842	1.0133

The presence of a CC can make a difference in reimbursement depending on the principal diagnosis and the MS-DRG assigned. The code for cachexia (R64) is a CC.

CHAPTER REVIEW EXERCISE

Assign codes for all diagnoses and procedures.

1. Adenocarcinoma of the prostate with radical retropubic excision and regional pelvic lymph nodes _____

2. Adenocarcinoma of the distal esophagus; patient is status post-laparoscopic jejunostomy prior to radiation treatments _____

3. Chronic lymphocytic leukemia (CLL) _____

4. Splenectomy showed non-Hodgkin's lymphoma of the spleen _____

5. Von Recklinghausen's disease _____

6. Hydrocephalus due to malignant ependymoma fourth ventricle; the patient was admitted for ventriculoperitoneal shunt placement _____

7. Diagnostic percutaneous needle biopsy of the right adrenal gland; physician documented pheochromocytoma _____

8. Fibrosarcoma of the soft tissue of left thigh with mets to brain _____

9. Malignant melanoma left thigh previously excised; patient admitted for immunotherapy with high-dose interleukin-2 via central venous infusion because of spread to inguinal lymph nodes _____

10. Intraperitoneal metastatic carcinoma; unknown primary; treatment focused on determining primary source _____

11. Short-term memory loss due to tumor frontal lobe _____

12. Hodgkin's lymphoma in cervical lymph node. Admitted for chemotherapy _____

13. Admission for red blood cell transfusion (peripheral venous) due to anemia caused by renal cell carcinoma _____

14. Dehydration due to chemotherapy in patient with carcinoma of breast with metastasis to axillary lymph nodes _____

15. Recurrent seizures due to metastasis to brain from lung cancer _____

16. Cerebral meningioma _____

17. Right choroidal melanoma _____

18. Admission for chemoembolization of hepatocellular carcinoma (HCC) _____

19. Neutropenic fever in a patient who is undergoing treatment for leukemia; patient is anemic due to chemotherapy _____

20. Intestinal obstruction due to peritoneal metastasis from inoperable colorectal cancer _____

21. Impending hip fracture due to metastasis to bone; patient has a previous history of left breast cancer treated with mastectomy; internal fixation of upper right femur _____

22. Patient's myelodysplastic syndrome has progressed to acute myelogenous leukemia _____

23. Prophylactic removal of both breasts due to positive genetic susceptibility and positive family history of breast cancer; a bilateral modified radical mastectomy was performed _____

24. Chronic myeloproliferative disease _____

25. Falx cerebri meningioma surgically removed   _____

26. Basophil adenoma of the pituitary gland causing Cushing's   _____
    syndrome

27. Carcinoma of the breast in the right upper and lower quadrant   _____

28. Metastatic ovarian cancer admitted for pain control   _____

29. Cancer head of pancreas with spread to the liver   _____

30. Endometrial adenocarcinoma with mets to right ovary   _____

31. Parotidectomy (partial excision of gland) for Warthin's tumor of   _____
    the left parotid gland

32. Adenocarcinoma of the upper stomach with spread to the lower   _____
    esophagus and lungs

Write the correct answer(s) in the blank(s) provided.

33. If a hospital's base payment rate was $4,000.00, what would be   _____
    the hospital payment for MS-DRG 023?

34. At the hospital in #33, what would the payment rate be for   _____
    MS-DRG 027?

35. If a coder missed the procedure code for the chemo wafer, how   _____
    much reimbursement would be lost?

CHAPTER GLOSSARY

Adenocarcinomas: malignancies of epithelial glandular tissue such as those found in the breast, prostate, and colon.

Basal cell carcinoma (BCC): most common type of skin cancer.

Benign: neoplasm or tumor; means that it is not malignant.

Biological response modifier (BRM): immunotherapy that can destroy cancer cells, stimulate the immune system to destroy cancer cells, or change cancer cells to normal cells.

Biopsy: removal of a representative sample for pathologic examination and diagnosis.

Brachytherapy: placement of radioactive material directly into or near the cancer.

Carcinomas: malignant tumors originating from epithelial tissue (e.g., in the skin, bronchi, and stomach).

Carcinoma in situ: malignant cells that remain within the original site with no spread or invasion into neighboring tissue.

Chemoembolization: intra-arterial administration of chemotherapy with collagen particles to enhance the delivery of chemotherapy to the targeted area.

Chemotherapy: the use of drugs or medications to treat disease.

Complete remission: there are no signs or symptoms of the cancer.

Core biopsy: procedure in which a large needle is used to extract a core sample.

Debulking: procedures performed when it is impossible to remove the tumor entirely.

Endoscopic biopsy: biopsy that is performed during endoscopic examination.

Fibromas: neoplasms of fibrous connective tissue.

Fine needle aspiration: procedure in which a very small needle is used; works best for masses that are superficial or easily accessible.

Foregut: bronchi and stomach (sites of carcinoid neoplasms).

Glioma: a primary malignant brain neoplasm that starts in the glial cells of the central nervous system.

Grading: pathologic examination of tumor cells. Degree of cell abnormality determines the grade of cancer.

Hindgut: colon and rectum (sites of carcinoid neoplasms).

Histologic type: type of tissue or cell in which the neoplasm occurs.

Immunotherapy: administration of agents that stimulate the immune system's response against tumors.

Incisional biopsy: procedure in which a representative sample of a tumor mass is removed to permit pathologic examination.

Kaposi's sarcoma (KS): cancer that develops from the lining of lymph or blood vessels.

Leiomyoma: tumor or growth within the walls of the uterus. Also called *uterine fibroid.*

Leukemia: cancer of the white blood cells that begins in the blood-forming cells of the bone marrow.

Lipoma: growth of fat cells within a capsule that is usually found just below the skin.

Lymphoma: cancer of the lymphatic system.

Lymphoma: a type of cancer of the lymphatic system.

Malignancy: neoplasm that has the ability to invade adjacent structures and spread to distant sites.

Malignant ascites: excess fluid that contains malignant cells accumulates in the abdomen or peritoneum.

Malignant melanoma: malignant neoplasm of the melanocytes, and the most common place of occurrence is the skin.

Malignant mesothelioma: rare aggressive cancer that develops in the protective lining or mesothelium that surrounds and protects the internal organs.

Malignant pleural effusion: fluid accumulates in the pleural space and contains malignant cells.

Melanomas: malignant changes of melanin cells.

Metastasis: spread of a cancer from one part of the body to another, as in the appearance of neoplasms in parts of the body separate from the site of the primary tumor.

Midgut: small intestine and appendix (sites of carcinoid neoplasms).

Morphology codes (M codes): codes that identify the type of cell that has become neoplastic and its biological activity or behavior.

Myeloma: malignancy that originates in the bone marrow.

Neoplasm: abnormal growth.

Non-Hodgkin's lymphoma: a type of cancer of the lymphatic system.

Palliative: procedure performed to correct a condition that is causing problems for the patient.

Partial remission: there are still a few signs and symptoms of the cancer, and the cancer cells have significantly decreased.

Preventive or prophylactic surgery: procedure performed to remove tissue that has the potential to become cancerous.

Primary site: site at which the neoplasm begins or originates.

Radiation: use of high-energy radiation to treat cancer.

Restorative or reconstructive: surgery performed to restore function and enhance aesthetic appearance after surgery.

Sarcomas: malignant growths of connective tissue (e.g., muscle, cartilage, lymph tissue, and bone).

Staging: means of categorizing a particular cancer that assists in determination of a patient's treatment plan and the need for further therapy.

Staging surgeries: procedures performed to help the clinician determine the extent of disease; these are generally more accurate than laboratory and imaging tests.

Squamous cell carcinoma (SCC): second most common type of skin cancer that also occurs in areas of the body that have been exposed to the sun.

Undifferentiated: tumor cells that are highly abnormal (e.g., immature, primitive).

Well-differentiated: tumor cells that closely resemble mature, specialized cells.

REFERENCES

1. Chabner D. The Language of Medicine, 8th ed. St. Louis: Saunders, 2007, Table 19-2, p 776.
2. Chabner D. The Language of Medicine, 8th ed. St. Louis: Saunders, 2007, Table 19-3, p 777.
3. Modified from Harrison's Manual of Medicine, 15th ed. New York: McGraw-Hill Professional, 2002, p 284.
4. American Hospital Association. *Coding Clinic for ICD-9-CM* 2006:1Q:p4. Correct coding of mass or lesion.
5. American Hospital Association. *Coding Clinic for ICD-9-CM* 1988:1Q:p4-5. Implantation or insertion of radioactive elements.

11

Diseases of the Blood and Blood-Forming Organs and Certain Disorders Involving the Immune Mechanism

(ICD-10-CM Chapter 3, Codes D50-D89)

LEARNING OBJECTIVES

1. Apply and assign the correct ICD-10-CM/PCS codes in accordance with Official Guidelines for Coding and Reporting

2. Identify major differences between ICD-10-CM and ICD-9-CM related to the blood-forming organs and immune mechanism

3. Identify pertinent anatomy and physiology of the blood and blood-forming organs and immune mechanism

4. Identify diseases of the blood and blood-forming organs and immune mechanism

5. Assign the correct Z codes and procedure codes related to the blood-forming organs and immune mechanism

6. Identify laboratory values and diagnostic tests
7. Explain the importance of documentation in relation to MS-DRGs for reimbursement

ABBREVIATIONS/ACRONYMS

ASA aspirin

CBC complete blood count

DIC disseminated intravascular coagulation

ESRD end-stage renal disease

GVHD graft-versus-host disease

Hct hematocrit

Hgb hemoglobin

HIV human immunodeficiency virus

ICD-9-CM *International Classification of Diseases, 9th Revision, Clinical Modification*

ICD-10-CM *International Classification of Diseases, 10th Revision, Clinical Modification*

ICD-10-PCS *International Classification of Diseases, 10th Revision, Procedure Classification System*

ITP idiopathic thrombocytopenic purpura

MS-DRG Medicare Severity diagnosis-related group

PT prothrombin time

PTT partial thromboplastin time

SCID severe combined immunodeficiency

WBC white blood cell

ICD-10-CM

Official Guidelines for Coding and Reporting

Please refer to the companion Evolve website for the most current guidelines.
3. **Chapter 3: Disease of the blood and blood-forming organs and certain disorders involving the immune mechanism (D50-D89)**
Reserved for future guideline expansion.

Although there are no ICD-10-CM guidelines specifically for Chapter 3, there are a couple of guidelines that affect the coding and sequencing of anemia when it is associated with a malignancy or the treatment of a malignancy.

2. **Chapter 2: Neoplasms (C00-D49)**
c. **Coding and sequencing of complications**
Coding and sequencing of complications associated with the malignancies or with the therapy thereof are subject to the following guidelines:
1) **Anemia associated with malignancy**
When admission/encounter is for management of an anemia associated with the malignancy, and the treatment is only for anemia, the appropriate code for the malignancy is sequenced as the principal or first-listed diagnosis followed by **the appropriate code for the anemia (such as** code D63.0, Anemia in neoplastic disease).

EXAMPLE | Anemia due to metastatic bone cancer. The patient has a history of primary right breast cancer that was treated with mastectomy 4 years ago, C79.51, D63.0, Z85.3, Z90.11.

2) **Anemia associated with chemotherapy, immunotherapy and radiation therapy**
When the admission/encounter is for management of an anemia associated with an adverse effect **of the administration** of chemotherapy or immunotherapy and the only treatment is for the anemia, **the anemia code is sequenced first** followed by the appropriate codes for the neoplasm **and the adverse effect (T45.1X5, Adverse effect of antineoplastic and immunosuppressive drugs).**
    When the admission/encounter is for management of an anemia associated with an adverse effect of radiotherapy, the anemia code should be sequenced first, followed by the appropriate neoplasm code and code Y84.2, Radiological procedure and radiotherapy as the cause of abnormal reaction of the patient, or of later complication, without mention of misadventure at the time of the procedure.

EXAMPLE | Patient is being treated for anemia due to chemotherapy. The patient has primary rectal cancer, D64.81, T45.1x5A, C20.

Apply the General Coding Guidelines as found in Chapter 5 and the Procedural Coding Guidelines as found in Chapters 6 and 7.

MAJOR DIFFERENCES BETWEEN ICD-10-CM AND ICD-9-CM

Most of the codes from ICD-9-CM Chapter 4 are included in ICD-10-CM Chapter 3. In ICD-10-CM, there are some codes from ICD-9-CM, Chapter 1, Certain Infectious and Parasitic Diseases (e.g., D86 sarcoidosis), and Chapter 3, Endocrine, Nutritional, and Metabolic Diseases and Certain Disorders involving the Immune Mechanism.

- In ICD-10-CM, many conditions or diseases can be coded with greater specificity.
- In ICD-10-CM, under the D63 category, Anemia in chronic diseases classified elsewhere, there are instructional notations to code first the underlying disease.
- Procedural complications affecting the spleen are included in Chapter 3 of ICD-10-CM.

ANATOMY AND PHYSIOLOGY

Blood is a viscous fluid that circulates through the vessels of the circulatory system as a result of the pumping action of the heart. Blood has three major functions. First, it transports oxygen, nutrients, hormones, enzymes, waste products, and carbon dioxide to and from cells. Second, blood promotes homeostasis and regulates body temperature. **Homeostasis** means balance or equilibrium. It is the ability of an organism or cell to maintain internal equilibrium by adjusting its physiologic processes. Third, blood provides a protective mechanism that combats foreign materials and assists in the body's defense against disease. Blood loss is prevented by clotting mechanisms within the body.

Blood is composed of plasma and formed elements or corpuscles. Corpuscles include erythrocytes (red blood cells), leukocytes (white blood cells), and platelets or thrombocytes. All of these components differ in terms of appearance, structure and type, function, life span, numbers, and means of production. **Erythrocytes**, or red blood cells, are made within the marrow of the bones; their main responsibility is to carry oxygen throughout the body and remove carbon dioxide. These are the cells that give blood its red color. **Leukocytes**, or white blood cells, increase in number to battle infection, inflammation, and other diseases. Five different types of white blood cells have been identified, and each has a role in fighting infection. White cells are comprised of neutrophils, monocytes, lymphocytes, eosinophils, and basophils. **Platelets** or **thrombocytes** circulate in the blood and assist in the clotting process.

Complete blood count (CBC) is a blood test that is commonly used to evaluate a patient's overall health; it detects a variety of disorders such as anemia, infection, and leukemia. This test measures the following:

- Hemoglobin (Hgb), a protein in red blood cells that carries oxygen to body tissues
- Hematocrit (Hct), the percentage of blood volume made up of red blood cells
- White blood cells (WBCs), which fight infection
- Platelets, which are essential to blood clotting
  See Table 11-1 for normal values.

The **immune system,** the body's major defense mechanism, responds to invasion of the body by foreign substances. The immune system consists of lymphoid tissues such as thymus, bone marrow, tonsils, adenoids, spleen, and appendix. When the immune system malfunctions and homeostasis is interrupted, the response may be classified as one of the following:

- Hyperactive responses (such as allergies)
- Immunodeficiency in which the response is inadequate (such as acquired immunodeficiency syndrome [AIDS])
- Autoimmune disorders in which the immune response is misdirected (such as systemic lupus erythematosus)
- Attacks on beneficial foreign tissues (such as transplants or blood transfusion)

DISEASE CONDITIONS

Chapter 3 in ICD-10-CM focuses on Diseases of the Blood and Blood-Forming Organs and Certain Disorders Involving the Immune Mechanism (D50-D89). Of interest is an Excludes2 note that appears at the beginning of the chapter (Figure 11-1). This note applies to

TABLE 11-1	**NORMAL LABORATORY VALUES**[1]

WBC 5000-10,000 mm³ or µL

Differential:

Segs (polyps)	54%-62%
Lymphs	20%-40%
Eos	1%-3%
Baso	0%-1%
Mono	3%-7%
RBC	(M) 4.5-6.0 million per mm³ or µL
	(F) 4.0-5.5 million per mm³ or µL
Hct	(M) 40%-50%
	(F) 37%-47%
HGB	(M) 14-16 g/dL
	(F) 12-14 g/dL
Platelets	150,000-350,000/mm³ or µL

Baso, Basophils; *Eos*, eosinophils; *Hct*, hematocrit; *HGB*, hemoglobin; *Lymphs*, lymphocytes; *Mono*, monocytes; *RBC*, red blood cell; *Segs*, segments; *WBC*, white blood cell.

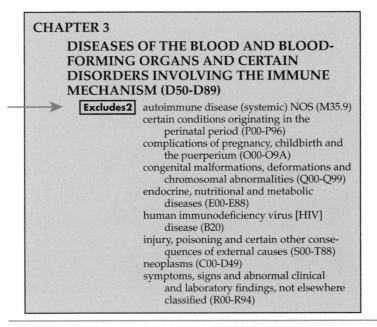

FIGURE 11-1. Excludes2 note that affects the entire chapter.

the entire chapter. An Excludes2 note means that these conditions are not coded within this chapter, but it is possible for a patient to have one of these conditions with a condition from this chapter. The Excludes1 note under category D58 is a pure Excludes note. This means codes from category P55.- cannot be assigned with any codes from category D58.- (Figure 11-2).

Diseases of the Blood and Blood-Forming Organs and Certain Disorders Involving the Immune Mechanism (D50-D89), Chapter 3 in the ICD-10-CM code book, is divided into the following categories:

CATEGORY	SECTION TITLES
D50-D53	Nutritional anemias
D55-D59	Hemolytic anemias
D60-D64	Aplastic and other anemias and other bone marrow failure syndromes
D65-D69	Coagulation defects, purpura, and other hemorrhagic conditions
D70-D77	Other disorders of blood and blood-forming organs
D78	Intraoperative and postprocedural complications of the spleen
D80-D89	Certain disorders involving the immune mechanism

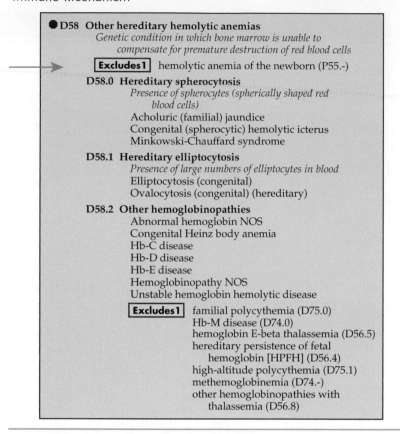

FIGURE 11-2. Excludes1 note that affects category D58.-.

Nutritional Anemias (D50-D53)

Anemia occurs when hemoglobin drops, which interrupts the transport of oxygen throughout the body. The most common type of anemia is iron deficiency anemia. In women, this condition is often due to heavy blood loss during menstrual periods. In older men and women, it may be an indication of gastrointestinal blood loss. Pregnant women and children need more iron, so a deficiency is likely due to insufficient iron in the diet. Testing may be necessary to determine a cause.

If a particular cause were determined, it would be appropriate to code the underlying condition. The sequencing of diagnoses would be determined by the coding guidelines and instructional notations in the tabular. Some of the reasons for iron deficiency include the following:

- Inadequate intake of iron in the diet
- Chronic blood loss
- Impaired absorption during digestion
- Liver disease
- Infection
- Cancers (neoplasms)

Numerous symptoms can indicate anemia; these include pallor, fatigue, lethargy, cold intolerance, irritability, stomatitis, headache, loss of appetite, numbness and tingling sensations, brittle hair, spoon-shaped and brittle nails, and edema, especially of the ankles. Severe anemia can result in tachycardia, palpitations, dyspnea (difficulty breathing), and syncope (fainting). Treatment depends on the cause, but the approach may be as simple as eating iron-rich foods or taking an iron supplement such as ferrous sulfate or ferrous gluconate. Blood transfusions may be necessary.

Look up the main term "Anemia" in the Index, and see the many subterms for the various types of anemia. "Deficiency" is also a subterm with many subterms, as is shown in Figure 11-3. At the subterm "in," entries are found for anemia in end-stage renal disease/

Anemia (*Continued*)
   deficiency (*Continued*) ——————— Subterm "deficiency"
      combined B12 and folate D53.1
      enzyme D55.9
         drug-induced (hemolytic) D59.2
         glucose-6-phosphate dehydroge-
            nase (G6PD) D55.0
         glycolytic D55.2
         nucleotide metabolism D55.3
         related to hexose monophosphate
            (HMP) shunt pathway NEC
            D55.1
      specified type NEC D55.8
      erythrocytic glutathione D55.1
      folate D52.9
         dietary D52.0
         drug-induced D52.1
      folic acid D52.9
         dietary D52.0
         drug-induced D52.1

FIGURE 11-3. Alphabetic Index entry for "anemia" and the subterm "deficiency."

Anemia (*Continued*)
   in (due to) (with)
      chronic kidney disease D63.1
      end stage renal disease D63.1
      failure, kidney (renal) D63.1
      neoplastic disease (*see also* Neoplasm)
         D63.0

FIGURE 11-4. Anemia due to certain chronic diseases.

chronic kidney disease and anemia in neoplastic disease (Figure 11-4). The term *chronic anemia* is not equated to "chronic simple anemia" or "anemia in chronic disease." Chronic anemia is coded to D64.9 because no specific subterm is available for chronic, so the default code for anemia code is assigned.

EXAMPLE   Patient is being treated as an outpatient for anemia due to inadequate dietary iron intake, D50.8.

EXAMPLE   Patient is being treated for folate deficiency anemia, D52.9.

EXERCISE 11-1

Assign codes to the following conditions.

1. Iron deficiency anemia due to chronic blood loss   _____
2. Vitamin B$_{12}$ deficiency anemia   _____
3. Megaloblastic anemia   _____

Hemolytic Anemias (D55-D59)

The hemolytic anemias are assigned to hereditary and acquired code categories (Figure 11-5). **Hemolytic anemia** results from abnormal or excessive destruction of red blood cells. **Sickle cell anemia** is one of the more common types of hereditary hemolytic anemia; it is found often in the African American population and among people living in Africa, the Mediterranean, Arabia, and South Asia. Red blood cells change from a disc shape to a crescent or "sickle" shape. This causes obstruction of the small blood vessels and eventual damage from thrombus formation, repeated organ infarctions, and tissue necrosis throughout the body. Varying degrees of disease severity and symptoms have been reported. Symptoms include severe anemia, hyperbilirubinemia or jaundice, splenomegaly, delayed and impaired growth and development, vascular occlusion, and infarctions, which can result in permanent damage, pain, frequent infection, and congestive heart failure. ICD-10-CM uses

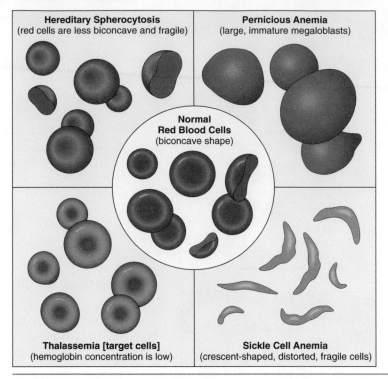

Hereditary Spherocytosis
(red cells are less biconcave and fragile)

Pernicious Anemia
(large, immature megaloblasts)

**Normal
Red Blood Cells**
(biconcave shape)

Thalassemia [target cells]
(hemoglobin concentration is low)

Sickle Cell Anemia
(crescent-shaped, distorted, fragile cells)

FIGURE 11-5. Normal red blood cells and red blood cells in several types of anemia.

combination code(s) that identifies the sickle cell crisis along with a manifestation such as acute chest syndrome or splenic sequestration. Most treatment is supportive in nature. A drug called Hydrea (hydroxyurea) has reduced the number of crises.

Code D57.3 for sickle cell trait is assigned when a patient is a carrier and the disease has remained asymptomatic. When both sickle cell trait and sickle cell anemia are present, only sickle cell anemia is coded.

EXAMPLE   Patient was admitted with sickle cell crisis with acute chest syndrome. Patient has Hb-SS disease, D57.01.

Another hereditary disease that is prevalent among people from Greece and Italy (Mediterranean countries), the Middle East, South Asia, and Africa is **thalassemia**. Similar to sickle cell anemia, the disease manifests in varying degrees. Cooley's anemia is another name that is used to describe the beta thalassemias. Frequent blood transfusions are administered, along with treatment with an iron chelation drug, which helps the body get rid of excess iron resulting from repeated transfusions. Occasionally, bone marrow transplant is performed, but this is a risky procedure, and a suitable donor is required.

EXAMPLE   Patient admitted with sickle cell thalassemia with vaso-occlusive pain crisis, D57.419.

EXERCISE 11-2

Assign codes to the following conditions.

1. Cooley's anemia   _____
2. Sickle cell trait with sickle cell anemia   _____
3. Acholuric jaundice   _____
4. Sickle cell Hb-C with vaso-occlusive crisis   _____
5. Sickle cell thalassemia crisis with splenic sequestration   _____

Aplastic and Other Anemias and Other Bone Marrow Failure Syndromes (D60-D64)

Aplastic anemia is characterized by a reduction in new blood cells due to impairment or failure of bone marrow function. Decreased production of erythrocytes (red blood cells), leukocytes (white blood cells), and thrombocytes (platelets), also defined as pancytopenia, can lead to many complications. In 50% of cases, the cause of aplastic anemia is unknown or **idiopathic** in nature. Some drugs, industrial agents, chemicals, or radiation can affect the function of the bone marrow. If the causative factor can be identified and eliminated, the bone marrow possibly can recover. Viruses such as hepatitis C may also cause aplastic anemia.

If a patient has the following three conditions—neutropenia, thrombocytopenia, and anemia, also known as **pancytopenia**—the code D61.81X would be assigned. According to *Coding Clinic for ICD-9-CM* (2005:3Q:p11-12),[2] an exception occurs when a patient is admitted with neutropenic fever and is also pancytopenic; in this case, it is acceptable to assign the neutropenia code D70.9 as the principal diagnosis, with an additional code D61.818 used to describe the pancytopenia and R50.81 for the fever. When a patient is admitted for neutropenic fever, investigations for any infectious source(s) are performed. Blood, sputum, and urine, and other sites may be cultured to try to identify an infection. The patient will be started on antibiotics, blood counts will be monitored, and neutropenic precautions will be implemented. If an infectious source is identified, treatment will be adjusted for that infection and the infection should be the principal diagnosis.

EXAMPLE | Patient was admitted with neutropenic fever. Patient is currently being treated for diffuse large B-cell lymphoma. Broad-spectrum antibiotics were started. The urine culture and chest x-ray were negative. The blood cultures from the Hickman catheter and peripheral vein site were positive for *Staphylococcus aureus*. Vancomycin therapy was increased to 1 g every 12 hours. Patient has an MSSA bacteremia due to central line infection, T80.211A, R78.81, C83.30, B95.61, Y84.8.

EXAMPLE | Patient has pancytopenia due to oral methotrexate which is taken for treatment of rheumatoid arthritis, initial encounter, D61.811, T45.1x5A, M06.9.

EXAMPLE | Infant was seen for follow up for congenital aplastic anemia, D61.09.

Category D62 includes acute posthemorrhagic anemia or anemia due to acute blood loss. Confusion arises regarding anemia related to blood loss and whether blood loss is acute or chronic and/or both. Sometimes, blood loss is well documented, but the resultant anemia may not be documented by the physician. Whenever doubt occurs, the coder should query the physician. If acute and chronic blood loss anemia is present, only a code for the acute blood loss anemia is assigned because of the Excludes1 notes for D62 and D50.0.

EXAMPLE | Patient treated for anemia due to acute blood loss, D62.

Category D63 includes codes that are assigned when anemia is due to neoplastic disease or malignancy, chronic kidney disease (CKD), or other chronic diseases that are classified elsewhere. In the ICD-10-CM Tabular, there are Instructional notes to code the chronic condition that is responsible for the anemia first (Figure 11-6). Sometimes a physician will document anemia due to chronic disease but will not specify which disease is responsible. A query may be necessary to identify the underlying disease.

EXAMPLE | Patient is seen in the clinic for anemia due to hypothyroidism, E03.9, D63.8.

EXAMPLE | Patient has anemia due to gastric cancer, C16.9, D63.0.

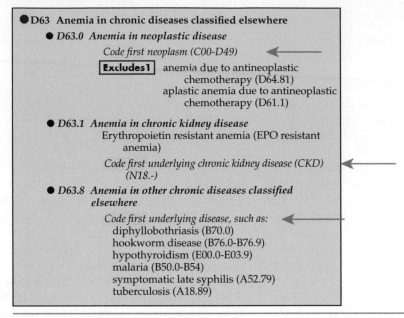

●D63 **Anemia in chronic diseases classified elsewhere**

  ● *D63.0 Anemia in neoplastic disease*

   Code first neoplasm (C00-D49)

   Excludes1 anemia due to antineoplastic chemotherapy (D64.81)
   aplastic anemia due to antineoplastic chemotherapy (D61.1)

  ● *D63.1 Anemia in chronic kidney disease*
   Erythropoietin resistant anemia (EPO resistant anemia)

   Code first underlying chronic kidney disease (CKD) (N18.-)

  ● *D63.8 Anemia in other chronic diseases classified elsewhere*

   Code first underlying disease, such as:
   diphyllobothriasis (B70.0)
   hookworm disease (B76.0-B76.9)
   hypothyroidism (E00.0-E03.9)
   malaria (B50.0-B54)
   symptomatic late syphilis (A52.79)
   tuberculosis (A18.89)

FIGURE 11-6. Tabular instructional notes for anemia in chronic diseases.

EXERCISE 11-3

Assign codes to the following conditions.

1. Aplastic anemia due to hepatitis C _____

2. Idiopathic aplastic anemia _____

3. Fanconi's anemia _____

4. Anemia due to end-stage renal disease (ESRD) _____

5. Normocytic anemia _____

6. Sideroblastic anemia _____

7. Anemia due to rheumatoid arthritis _____

8. Pancytopenia in patient with aplastic anemia _____

Coagulation Defects, Purpura, and Other Hemorrhagic Conditions (D65-D69)

Excessive bleeding that occurs after a minor injury may be a sign of a **coagulation defect**, which is a breakdown in the blood clotting process. Multiple reasons may account for excessive bleeding:

■ Acute viral infection in children
■ Autoimmune reactions in adults
■ End-stage renal failure
■ Ingestion of aspirin (acetylsalicylic acid [ASA])
■ Vitamin K deficiency
■ Liver disease
■ Inherited disorders
■ Hemorrhagic fever viruses

Multiple warning signs may indicate a coagulation defect; these include bleeding from gums or repeated nosebleeds, petechiae (Figure 11-7), ecchymoses (bruises), hemarthroses (bleeding into a joint), hemoptysis (coughing up blood), hematemesis (vomiting blood), melena (blood in feces), anemia, feeling faint and anxious, low blood pressure, and increased pulse. Blood tests that involve bleeding time, prothrombin time (PT), or partial thromboplastin time (PTT) can measure the coagulation of blood. Occasionally, patients who take anticoagulants such as warfarin (Coumadin) will have complications. Some

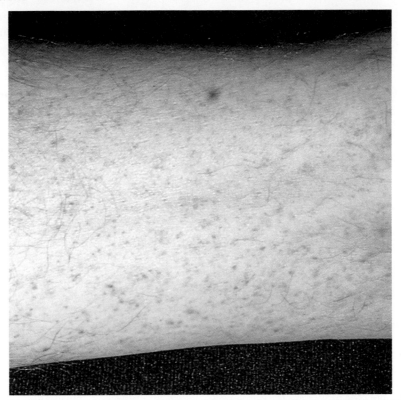

FIGURE 11-7. Petechiae.

common complications include gastrointestinal bleeding, epistaxis, hematuria, or hemorrhage from any tissue. Their coagulation laboratory test results may be abnormal, but this does not mean that they have a coagulopathy, and the condition should not be coded as such. It should be coded to abnormal coagulation profile, R79.1. It is a common mistake to assign code D68.9 (coagulopathy) when a patient is taking an anticoagulant. In fact, a physician may even document coagulopathy or coagulopathy due to Coumadin. Codes for coagulation defects are not appropriate for patients that are on anticoagulation therapy for some other type of medical condition. The Z code Z79.01 is assigned to identify the long-term use of anticoagulant medication such as Coumadin, which is located in the Alphabetic Index under the main term "Long-term drug therapy." A code may also be assigned for the diagnosis for which the patient is on anticoagulation therapy.

EXAMPLE   Patient is taking Coumadin for previous history of pulmonary embolism, Z86.711, Z79.01.

EXAMPLE   Patient was treated for coagulopathy due to chronic liver disease, D68.4, K76.9.

Disseminated intravascular coagulation (DIC) is a disorder that causes depletion of clotting factors in the blood. Risk factors include recent sepsis, severe injury or trauma, recent surgery and anesthesia, complications of labor and delivery, cancer, transfusion reaction, and liver disease. Treatment may include transfusion of coagulation factors with fresh frozen plasma; the underlying cause must be determined so the appropriate treatment can be provided.

Hemophilia is an inherited clotting disorder. **Hemophilia A**, the most common form, is a deficiency or abnormality of clotting factor VIII. **Hemophilia B** (Christmas disease) is the result of a deficiency of factor IX, and **Hemophilia C** is a mild form characterized by a decrease in factor XI. As with some of the other diseases of the blood, varying degrees of severity are reported. A common treatment consists of replacement therapy for factor VIII with cryoprecipitate. Unfortunately, transmission of viruses such as hepatitis and human immunodeficiency virus (HIV) has resulted from this treatment. Currently, blood products are treated in an effort to destroy known viruses, but risk of unknown infection or immune reaction is still present.

EXAMPLE

Patient has classical hemophilia, D66.

Purpura is characterized by ecchymoses or small hemorrhages in the skin, mucous membranes, or serosal surfaces that are due to blood disorders, vascular abnormalities, or trauma. A patient with idiopathic thrombocytopenic purpura (ITP) experiences a decrease in the number of platelets with no identifiable cause. Following laboratory testing, a bone marrow biopsy may be necessary. Treatments may include corticosteroids, immunosuppressive therapy, and possibly splenectomy.

Secondary thrombocytopenia is characterized by a decrease in the number of platelets; it is due to specific diseases such as congestive splenomegaly, Felty's syndrome, tuberculosis, sarcoidosis, lupus erythematosus, and chronic alcoholism. Some external causes include drugs, blood transfusions, and overhydration.

EXAMPLE

Thrombocytopenia due to chronic alcoholism, D69.59, F10.20.

EXAMPLE

Patient admitted with idiopathic thrombocytopenic purpura, D69.3.

EXERCISE 11-4

Assign codes to the following conditions.

1. Rosenthal's hemophilia _____
2. Hemophilia A _____
3. Christmas disease _____
4. DIC _____
5. von Willebrand's disease _____
6. Idiopathic nonthrombocytopenic purpura _____
7. Thrombocytopenia due to systemic lupus erythematosus _____
8. Schönlein-Henoch purpura _____
9. Low platelets _____
10. Factor V Leiden mutation _____

Other Disorders of Blood and Blood-Forming Organs (D70-D77)

Leukocytosis (neutrophilia or granulocytosis) is characterized by an increase in the number of white cells in the blood. Usually, no treatment is required. If leukocytosis persists, investigation to rule out a neoplastic process or infection may become necessary. Leukocytosis may also be related to certain drugs or may occur in response to stress. The most common white blood cell condition is agranulocytosis, or **neutropenia**, which is an abnormal decrease in granular leukocytes in the blood. Radiation therapy, drugs used for chemotherapy, and other chemicals may cause neutropenia. With severe neutropenia, a patient may become immunocompromised; his or her ability to fight infection may be hampered, and treatment often consists of antibiotics. Testing may be necessary to determine cause and select appropriate treatment.

| EXAMPLE | Infant is being treated for congenital agranulocytosis, D70.0. |

The spleen serves as a blood reservoir, filters the blood and removes old or defective blood cells, and serves as part of the immune system by helping to fight infection. The spleen can become enlarged (**splenomegaly**) due to infections or other diseases. A swollen spleen is at risk for rupturing, which could result in significant blood loss.

| EXAMPLE | Physician documents that the ultrasound exam showed that the patient has a splenic infarction, D73.5. |

EXERCISE 11-5

Assign codes to the following conditions.

1. Neutropenic fever   _____
2. Leukocytosis   _____
3. Eosinophilia   _____
4. Leukopenia   _____

Certain Disorders Involving the Immune Mechanism (D80-D89)

Disorders that are coded in this section include acquired hypogammaglobulinemia, selective immunoglobulin A deficiency, X-linked agammaglobulinemia, severe combined immunodeficiency (SCID), sarcoidosis, and thymic hypoplasia or DiGeorge's syndrome.

Patients may become immunocompromised by medications; this is seen when patients undergo transplantation and are taking antirejection drugs, or when a patient undergoes chemotherapy treatment for cancer. A patient may also be in an immunocompromised state that is associated with a disease process. According to *Coding Clinic for ICD-9-CM* (1992:3Q:p13-14),[3] an expected side effect for transplant patients or chemotherapy patients is a comprised immune system, and codes should not be assigned for the immunocompromised state. However, if the cause of that state is not identified, code D89.9, unspecified disorder of immune mechanism, should be assigned.

| EXAMPLE | Patient has a diagnosis of Wiskott-Aldrich syndrome, D82.0. |

Graft-versus-host disease (GVHD) is a common complication that can occur after a stem cell or bone marrow transplant in which the newly transplanted material attacks the transplant recipient's body. GVHD can sometimes occur following blood transfusion or any organ transplant where white blood cells are present. There is less risk of GVHD when the match between donor and recipient is optimal. The greater the mismatch, the greater the risk of GVHD.

There are two types of graft-versus-host disease:

- Acute—usually occurs during the first 3 months following a transplant.
- Chronic—usually occurs after the third month following a transplant.

It is possible to develop acute on chronic GVHD.

Symptoms in acute GVHD include:

- Abdominal pain and cramps
- Diarrhea
- Fever
- Jaundice
- Skin rash and/or desquamation
- Vomiting
- Weight loss

Symptoms in chronic GVHD include:

- Dry eye and dry mouth
- Hair loss
- IIepatitis
- Lung and digestive tract disorders
- Skin rash
- Skin thickening

In both acute and chronic GVHD, the patient is more susceptible to infections. Treatment includes corticosteroids, immunosuppressants, antibiotics, and immunoglobulins.

EXAMPLE | Patient was seen in the clinic for desquamation of skin. He had a bone marrow transplant 2 months ago. The physician is treating him for acute GVHD, T86.09, D89.810, R23.4.

EXERCISE 11-6

Assign codes to the following conditions.

1. Pulmonary sarcoidosis _____
2. Selective deficiency of IgA _____
3. Severe combined immunodeficiency disorder _____
4. Common variable immunodeficiency _____
5. Interstitial pneumonitis due to chronic GVHD in patient who is status post bone marrow transplant 8 months ago _____

FACTORS INFLUENCING HEALTH STATUS AND CONTACT WITH HEALTH SERVICES (Z CODES)

As was discussed in Chapter 8, it may be difficult to locate Z codes in the Index. Coders often say, "I did not know there was a Z code for that." Refer to Chapter 8 for a listing of common main terms used to locate Z codes.

A review of the Tabular reveals that some Z codes pertain diseases of the blood and blood-forming organs and immune mechanism:

Z01.83	Encounter for blood typing
Z13.0	Encounter for screening for diseases of the blood and blood-forming organs and certain disorders involving the immune mechanism
Z14.01	Asymptomatic hemophilia A carrier
Z14.02	Symptomatic hemophilia A carrier
Z52.000	Unspecified donor, whole blood
Z52.001	Unspecified donor, stem cells
Z52.008	Unspecified donor, other blood
Z52.010	Autologous donor, whole blood
Z52.011	Autologous donor, stem cells
Z52.018	Autologous donor, other blood
Z52.090	Other blood donor, whole blood
Z52.091	Other blood donor, stem cells
Z52.098	Other blood donor, other blood
Z52.3	Bone marrow donor
Z67.10	Type A blood, Rh positive
Z67.11	Type A blood, Rh negative

Z67.20	Type B blood, Rh positive
Z67.21	Type B blood, Rh negative
Z67.30	Type AB blood, Rh positive
Z67.31	Type AB blood, Rh negative
Z67.40	Type O blood, Rh positive
Z67.41	Type O blood, Rh negative
Z67.90	Unspecified blood type, Rh positive
Z67.91	Unspecified blood type, Rh negative
Z79.01	Long-term (current) use of anticoagulants
Z79.02	Long-term (current) use of antithrombotics/antiplatelets
Z79.82	Long-term (current) use of aspirin
Z83.2	Family history of diseases of the blood and blood-forming organs and certain disorders involving the immune mechanism
Z86.2	Personal history of diseases of the blood and blood-forming organs and certain disorders involving the immune mechanism
Z90.81	Acquired absence of spleen
Z94.81	Bone marrow transplant status
Z94.84	Stem cells transplant status

Some Z codes describe the long-term use of a particular type of medication such as anticoagulants or antiplatelets/antithrombotics. **Anticoagulants** are medications that are used to prevent venous thrombi. They can be administered parenterally with heparin, or warfarin (Coumadin) can be taken orally. **Parenteral** drug administration is when medications are administered other than through the digestive tract, such as by intravenous or intramuscular injections. **Antiplatelet** drugs are used to prevent clumping of platelets or formation of an arterial thrombus. Medications that are used as antiplatelet therapy include clopidogrel (Plavix), ticlopidine (Ticlid), dipyridamole (Persantine), and aspirin (ASA).

EXAMPLE   Screening for iron deficiency anemia, Z13.0.

EXAMPLE   Long-term use of ASA due to family history of stroke, Z79.82, Z82.3.

EXERCISE 11-7

Assign codes to the following conditions.

1. History of stem cell transplant   _____
2. Long-term use of Coumadin   _____
3. Screening for sickle cell disease   _____
4. Long-term use of Plavix   _____

COMMON TREATMENTS

CONDITION	MEDICATION/TREATMENT
Anemia	Treatment depends on the cause
Anemia due to chronic kidney disease	Epoetin alfa (Epogen, Procrit)
Iron deficiency anemia	Iron supplements, ferrous sulfate (FeoSol)
Pernicious anemia	B_{12} injections
Anemia of chronic disease	Treatment of the underlying cause/disease

CONDITION	MEDICATION/TREATMENT
Sickle cell anemia	Hydroxyurea (Droxia, Hydrea)
Hemophilia A	Desmopressin acetate (DDAVP), recombinant or plasma concentrate factor VIII, cryoprecipitate
Neutropenia	Filgrastim (Neupogen)

PROCEDURES

Procedures related to the blood and blood-forming organs in ICD-10-PCS can be located in the following tables:

072-07Y	Lymphatic and Hemic Systems
302-3EI	Administration
4A0-4B0	Measuring and Monitoring

Blood transfusion, which can be performed for many reasons, is the administration of donor blood cells into a patient. The root operation in ICD-10-PCS for transfusion is transfusion (putting in blood or blood products). The most common types of transfusions consist of red blood cells, plasma, and platelets. Sometimes, before undergoing an elective surgery, a patient will donate his or her own blood to be used in the event a transfusion is needed. This is known as an **autologous transfusion**.

Apheresis is a procedure that separates the different components of the blood and removes a certain part of the blood, such as occurs in leukapheresis, plateletpheresis, and plasmapheresis. A therapeutic plasmapheresis or plasma exchange occurs when the plasma is removed and is replaced with fresh plasma. The root operation in ICD-10-PCS for therapeutic plasmaphersis is pheresis (extracorporeal separation of blood products).

Bone marrow biopsy and/or aspiration are diagnostic procedures that can be used to identify types of blood disorders. The root operation in ICD-10-PCS for bone marrow biopsy is extraction (pulling or stripping out/off without replacement some or all of a body part). The root operation in ICD-10-PCS for bone marrow aspiration is drainage (taking or letting out fluids or gases). It may also be performed to evaluate the patient's response to treatment.

Peripheral stem cell and bone marrow transplants (Figure 11-8) are used to treat patients with certain leukemias and cancers, bone marrow failure syndromes, and genetic disease. Prior to transplant, the patient is prepared with radiation and/or chemotherapy to get rid of the defective or malignant cells and reduce the body's immunity so it will not reject the transplanted cells. According to the ICD-10-PCS Guidelines, the putting in of autologous or nonautologous bone marrow, pancreatic islet cells, or stem cells is coded in the Administration section.

EXERCISE 11-8

Assign codes for all diagnoses and procedures.

1. Patient with profound pancytopenia had a diagnostic percutaneous bone marrow biopsy iliac crest _____

2. Thrombocytopenia was treated with transfusion of platelets (nonautologous infusion in peripheral vein) _____

3. Therapeutic single plasmapheresis performed on patient with thrombotic thrombocytopenic purpura _____

4. DIC with transfusion of frozen plasma (percutaneous infusion, central vein, nonautologous) _____

5. Postoperative blood loss anemia with autologous transfusion of red blood cells _____

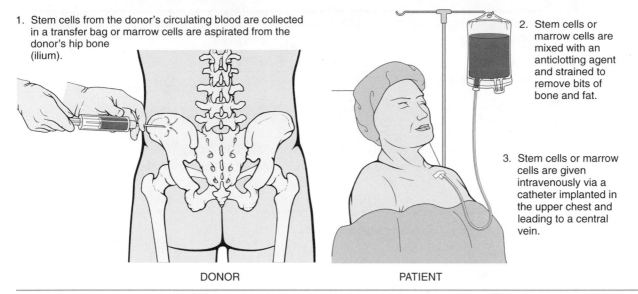

1. Stem cells from the donor's circulating blood are collected in a transfer bag or marrow cells are aspirated from the donor's hip bone (ilium).

2. Stem cells or marrow cells are mixed with an anticlotting agent and strained to remove bits of bone and fat.

3. Stem cells or marrow cells are given intravenously via a catheter implanted in the upper chest and leading to a central vein.

DONOR   PATIENT

FIGURE 11-8. Peripheral stem cell and bone marrow transplants.

DOCUMENTATION/REIMBURSEMENT/MS-DRGs

Often, coding difficulties are due to lack of documentation. Sometimes pathology and other test results are not available at the time of discharge or when the physician is dictating the discharge summary or is reporting the final diagnoses.

Documentation difficulties include lack of documentation regarding various types of anemia and the relationship of anemia to other chronic illnesses and diseases such as ESRD and neoplastic disease. Sometimes, acute and/or chronic blood loss is documented, but in the record, no mention of associated anemia is made by the physician.

Frequently missed complications/comorbidities from this chapter include:

- Acute post-hemorrhagic anemia
- Aplastic anemia
- DIC
- Pancytopenia

MS-DRG With and Without MCC/CC

EXAMPLE   A patient had a total abdominal hysterectomy for fibroid uterus. The patient was symptomatic with menorrhagia. Patient has von Willebrand's disease.

DIAGNOSES	CODES	MS-DRG	RW
Fibroid uterus with menorrhagia and von Willebrand's disease	D25.9, N92.0, D68.0 0UT90ZZ, 0UTC0ZZ	742	1.4262
Total abdominal hysterectomy			
Fibroid uterus with menorrhagia	D25.9, N92.0 0UT90ZZ, 0UTC0ZZ	743	0.9306
Total abdominal hysterectomy			

In this case, von Willebrand's disease is a CC, and by coding this chronic condition, the hospital will receive payment for a higher-weighted MS-DRG.

Correct Procedure Code

It is important to assign all procedure codes. A surgical MS-DRG is likely to have a higher relative weight than a medical MS-DRG. Reimbursement may be lost if the appropriate procedure codes are not assigned.

EXAMPLE

A patient is being admitted for a total splenectomy for treatment of idiopathic thrombocytopenic purpura (ITP).

DIAGNOSES	CODES	MS-DRG	RW
ITP with splenectomy	D69.3	801	1.5138
	07TP0ZZ		
ITP	D69.3	813	1.5098

In this case, the total splenectomy affects the MS-DRG assignment. An MS-DRG with a higher relative weight means better reimbursement for the hospital.

CHAPTER REVIEW EXERCISE

Assign codes for all diagnoses and procedures.

1. Bandemia _____

2. Pernicious anemia _____

3. Coagulopathy indicated by abnormal coagulation profile due to Coumadin taken for atrial fibrillation. Patient has been on Coumadin for 1 year. _____

4. Hemophilia A carrier _____

5. DiGeorge's syndrome _____

6. Polycythemia, benign _____

7. Severe congenital aplastic anemia treated with bone marrow transplant, allogeneic from related donor (percutaneous central vein) _____

8. Sickle cell Hb-SS disease with crisis _____

9. Anemia due to AIDS _____

10. Anemia due to acute and chronic blood loss treated with transfusion of 2 units of packed red blood cells (percutaneous peripheral vein, nonautologous) _____

11. Coagulopathy due to cirrhosis of the liver _____

12. History of bone marrow transplant _____

13. Chronic agranulocytosis _____

14. Sarcoidosis of skin _____

15. Neutropenic fever with no infections source found _____

16. Congestive splenomegaly _____

17. Vegan anemia _____

18. Lymphocytic leukemoid reaction _____

19. Lupus anticoagulant syndrome _____

20. Neutropenia due to infection _____

Write the correct answer(s) in the space(s) provided.

21. Which blood component is essential for clotting?

_____

22. Describe apheresis.

_____

23. List two warning signs of a coagulation disorder.

_____

24. Which cells fight infection, inflammation, and other diseases?

_____

25. Define idiopathic.

_____

CHAPTER GLOSSARY

Anemia: occurs when hemoglobin drops, which interrupts the transport of oxygen throughout the body.

Anticoagulant medications: medications that are used to prevent venous thrombi.

Antiplatelet medications: medications that are used to prevent clumping of platelets or formation of an arterial thrombus.

Apheresis: procedure that separates different components of blood and removes a certain part of the blood, such as occurs in leukapheresis, plateletpheresis, and plasmapheresis.

Aplastic anemia: reduction in new blood cells due to impairment or failure of bone marrow function.

Autologous transfusion: transfusion of a patient's own blood. Blood may have been donated prior to an elective procedure.

Blood: viscous fluid that circulates through the vessels of the circulatory system as a result of the pumping action of the heart.

Bone marrow biopsy: diagnostic procedure that is used to identify types of anemia and cell deficiencies and to detect leukemia.

Coagulation defect: breakdown in the clotting process of the blood.

Disseminated intravascular coagulation: disorder that results in depletion of clotting factors in the blood.

Erythrocytes: another name for red blood cells that are made in the marrow of bones; their main responsibility is to carry oxygen around the body and remove carbon dioxide. These are the cells that give blood its red color.

Graft-versus-host disease (GVHD): common complication that can occur after a stem cell or bone marrow transplant in which the newly transplanted material attacks the transplant recipient's body.

Hemolytic anemias: result from abnormal or excessive destruction of red blood cells.

Hemophilia A: most common type of hemophilia; deficiency or abnormality in clotting factor VIII.

Hemophilia B: another name for Christmas disease, which results from a deficiency of factor IX.

Hemophilia C: mild form of hemophilia with decreased factor XI.

Homeostasis: the ability of an organism or cell to maintain internal equilibrium by adjusting its physiologic processes.

Idiopathic: causative factor is unknown.

Immune system: includes the bone marrow, lymph nodes, thymus, and spleen. Its purpose is to protect the body from all types of infections, toxins, neoplastic cell growth, and foreign blood or tissues from another person.

Leukocytes: white blood cells increase in number to battle infection, inflammation, and other diseases.

Leukocytosis: increase in the number of white cells in the blood; it may be a sign of infection or may indicate stress on the body.

Neutropenia: abnormal decrease in granular leukocytes in the blood.

Pancytopenia: decrease in production of erythrocytes (red blood cells), leukocytes (white blood cells), and thrombocytes (platelets).

Parenteral: when medications are administered other than through the digestive tract, such as by intravenous or intramuscular injection.

Platelets: another name for thrombocytes. Platelets circulate in the blood and assist in the clotting process.

Purpura: ecchymoses or small hemorrhages in the skin, mucous membranes, or serosal surfaces due to blood disorders, vascular abnormalities, or trauma.

Secondary thrombocytopenia: decrease in the number of platelets due to specific diseases or external causes, such as drugs, blood transfusions, and overhydration.

Sickle cell anemia: one of the most common hemolytic anemias, in which the shape of the red blood cell changes from a disc to a crescent or "sickle," causing obstruction of small blood vessels and eventual damage throughout the body.

Splenomegaly: enlarged spleen.

Thalassemia: hereditary disease that is similar to sickle cell anemia and occurs in varying degrees.

Thrombocytes: another name for platelets. Thrombocytes circulate in the blood and assist in the clotting process.

REFERENCES

1. Chabner D. The Language of Medicine, 8th ed. St. Louis: Saunders, 2007, p 506.
2. American Hospital Association. *Coding Clinic for ICD-9-CM* 2005:3Q:p11-12. Neutropenic fever with pancytopenia.
3. American Hospital Association. *Coding Clinic for ICD-9-CM* 1992:3Q:p13-14. Immunocompromised state due to medication.

12

Endocrine, Nutritional, and Metabolic Diseases

(ICD-10-CM Chapter 4, Codes E00-E89)

LEARNING OBJECTIVES

1. Apply and assign the correct ICD-10-CM/PCS codes in accordance with Official Guidelines for Coding and Reporting
2. Identify major differences between ICD-10-CM and ICD-9-CM related to the endocrine, nutritional, and metabolic diseases
3. Identify pertinent anatomy and physiology of the endocrine, nutritional, and metabolic diseases
4. Identify endocrine, nutritional, and metabolic diseases
5. Assign the correct Z codes and procedure codes related to the endocrine, nutritional, and metabolic diseases
6. Identify common treatments, medications, laboratory values, and diagnostic tests
7. Explain the importance of documentation in relation to MS-DRGs for reimbursement

ABBREVIATIONS/ ACRONYMS

AIDS acquired immunodeficiency syndrome

AML acute myeloid leukemia

BMI body mass index

BPD biliopancreatic diversion

CC complication/comorbidity

CDC Centers for Disease Control and Prevention

CF cystic fibrosis

CKD chronic kidney disease

DI diabetes insipidus

DM diabetes mellitus

hGH human growth hormone

ICD-9-CM *International Classification of Diseases, 9th Revision, Clinical Modification*

ICD-10-CM *International Classification of Diseases, 10th Revision, Clinical Modification*

ICD-10-PCS *International Classification of Diseases, 10th Revision, Procedure Coding System*

IDDM insulin-dependent diabetes mellitus

IV intravenous

MEN multiple endocrine neoplasia

MS-DRG Medicare Severity diagnosis-related group

NIDDM non–insulin-dependent diabetes mellitus

OIG Office of the Inspector General

PKU phenylketonuria

PVD peripheral vascular disease

SIADH syndrome of inappropriate antidiuretic hormone secretion

TLS tumor lysis syndrome

TPN total parenteral nutrition

TSH thyroid-stimulating hormone

UTI urinary tract infection

VBG vertical banded gastroplasty

ICD-10-CM

Official Guidelines for Coding and Reporting

Please refer to the companion Evolve website for the most current guidelines.

4. Chapter 4: Endocrine, Nutritional, and Metabolic Diseases (E00-*E89*)

a. Diabetes mellitus

The diabetes mellitus codes are combination codes that include the type of diabetes mellitus, the body system affected, and the complications affecting that body system. As many codes within a particular category as are necessary to describe all of the complications of the disease may be used. They should be sequenced based on the reason for a particular encounter. Assign as many codes from categories E08-E13 as needed to identify all of the associated conditions that the patient has.

1) Type of diabetes

The age of a patient is not the sole determining factor, though most type 1 diabetics develop the condition before reaching puberty. For this reason type 1 diabetes mellitus is also referred to as juvenile diabetes.

EXAMPLE Juvenile diabetes, E10.9.

EXAMPLE The patient is a 16-year-old with obesity and diabetes mellitus, type 2, uncontrolled, E11.65, E66.9.

In ICD-10-CM, out of control and poorly controlled diabetes are coded to the type of diabetes with hyperglycemia per the Alphabetic Index.

---

2) Type of diabetes mellitus not documented

If the type of diabetes mellitus is not documented in the medical record the default is E11.-, Type 2 diabetes mellitus.

EXAMPLE The patient takes daily insulin for diabetes, E11.9, Z79.4.

---

3) Diabetes mellitus and the use of insulin

If the documentation in a medical record does not indicate the type of diabetes but does indicate that the patient uses insulin, code E11, Type 2 diabetes mellitus, should be assigned. Code Z79.4, Long-term (current) use of insulin, should also be assigned to indicate that the patient uses insulin. Code Z79.4 should not be assigned if insulin is given temporarily to bring a type 2 patient's blood sugar under control during an encounter.

EXAMPLE A patient with type 2 diabetes has been undergoing changes to daily insulin dosages. The patient's diabetes is uncontrolled, E11.65, Z79.4.

4) Diabetes mellitus in pregnancy and gestational diabetes
See Section I.C.15. Diabetes mellitus in pregnancy.
See Section I.C.15. Gestational (pregnancy induced) diabetes

5) Complications due to insulin pump malfunction

(a) Underdose of insulin due *to* insulin pump failure
An underdose of insulin due to an insulin pump failure should be assigned to a code from subcategory T85.6, Mechanical complication of other specified internal and external prosthetic devices, implants and grafts, that specifies the type of pump malfunction, as the principal or first-listed code, followed by code T38.3x6-, Underdosing of insulin and oral hypoglycemic [antidiabetic] drugs. Additional codes for the type of diabetes mellitus and any associated complications due to the underdosing should also be assigned.

(b) Overdose of insulin due to insulin pump failure
The principal or first-listed code for an encounter due to an insulin pump malfunction resulting in an overdose of insulin, should also be T85.6-, Mechanical complication of other specified internal and external prosthetic devices, implants and grafts, followed by code T38.3x1-, Poisoning by insulin and oral hypoglycemic [antidiabetic] drugs, accidental (unintentional).

EXAMPLE Patient has type 1 diabetes with hyperglycemia due to mechanical failure of insulin pump, which resulted in underdosing, T85.614A, T38.3x6A, E10.65.

EXAMPLE Patient has type 1 diabetes with hypoglycemia due to mechanical failure of insulin pump, which resulted in overdosing, T85.614A, T38.3x1A, E10.649.

6) Secondary *diabetes mellitus*
Codes under categories E08, Diabetes mellitus due to underlying condition, and E09, Drug or chemical induced diabetes mellitus, identify complications/manifestations associated with secondary diabetes mellitus. Secondary diabetes is always caused by another condition or event (e.g., cystic fibrosis, malignant neoplasm of pancreas, pancreatectomy, adverse effect of drug, or poisoning).

(a) Secondary diabetes mellitus and the use of insulin
For patients who routinely use insulin, code Z79.4, Long-term (current) use of insulin, should also be assigned. Code Z79.4 should not be assigned if insulin is given temporarily to bring a patient's blood sugar under control during an encounter.

(b) Assigning and sequencing secondary diabetes codes and its causes
The sequencing of the secondary diabetes codes in relationship to codes for the cause of the diabetes is based on the Tabular List instructions for categories E08 and E09. For example, for category E08, Diabetes mellitus due to underlying condition, code first the underlying condition; for category E09, Drug or chemical induced diabetes mellitus, code first the drug or chemical (T36-T65).

(i) Secondary diabetes mellitus due to pancreatectomy
For postpancreatectomy diabetes mellitus (lack of insulin due to the surgical removal of all or part of the pancreas), assign code E89.1, Postprocedural hypoinsulinemia. Assign a code from category E13 and a code from subcategory 290.41-, Acquired absence of pancreas, as additional codes.

(ii) Secondary diabetes due to drugs
Secondary diabetes may be caused by an adverse effect of correctly administered medications, poisoning or **sequela** of poisoning.
See section I.C.19.e for coding of adverse effects and poisoning, and section I.C.20 for external cause code reporting.

EXAMPLE	Uncontrolled diabetes mellitus due to Cushing's syndrome. Patient has been on insulin for the last year, E24.9, E08.65, Z79.4.

Apply the General Coding Guidelines as found in Chapter 5 and the Procedural Coding Guidelines as found in Chapters 6 and 7.

MAJOR DIFFERENCES BETWEEN ICD-10-CM AND ICD-9-CM

■ In ICD-10-CM, there are five category codes for diabetes mellitus:

E08	Diabetes mellitus due to underlying condition
E09	Drug or chemical induced diabetes mellitus
E10	Type 1 diabetes mellitus
E11	Type 2 diabetes mellitus
E13	Other specified diabetes mellitus

■ In ICD-10-CM, if a condition such as diabetes mellitus is drug induced, there is an instructional Code first (T36-T65) note to identify the drug or chemical involved.

■ In ICD-9-CM, there are fifth digits to identify whether a patient's diabetes is controlled, uncontrolled, or unspecified. In ICD-10-CM, out of control and poorly controlled diabetes are coded to the type of diabetes with hyperglycemia per the Alphabetic Index.

■ In ICD-9-CM there is no specific code to identify hyperglycemia with diabetes. In ICD-10-CM, there are codes to identify both hyperglycemia and hypoglycemia in a diabetic patient.

■ Procedural complications affecting the endocrine system and metabolic complications are included in Chapter 4 of ICD-10-CM. Some of the complications include:
  • Hypofunction of various endocrine glands following surgery
  • Postoperative hemorrhage and hematoma

ANATOMY AND PHYSIOLOGY

The **endocrine system** (Figure 12-1) works with the nervous system to maintain body functions, homeostasis, and to respond to stress. The endocrine system is composed of many glands that are located throughout the body. These glands secrete **hormones** that can regulate bodily functions such as urinary output, cellular metabolic rate, growth, and development.

Major endocrine glands include the following:
■ Anterior pituitary
■ Posterior pituitary
■ Thyroid
■ Parathyroid
■ Adrenal cortex
■ Adrenal medulla
■ Pancreas
■ Ovaries
■ Testes
■ Thymus
■ Pineal gland

See Table 12-1 for a listing of the glands, corresponding hormones, and expected hormonal response.

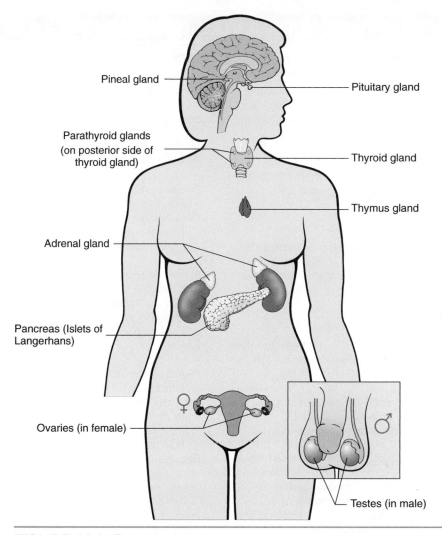

FIGURE 12-1. The endocrine system.

Endocrine diseases may result from an abnormal decrease or increase in hormone production. Changes in the size of a gland can alter hormone production. If the gland becomes larger, this is called **hyperplasia** and/or **hypertrophy**. If the gland becomes smaller, this is called **hypoplasia** and/or **atrophy**. Infection, inflammation, radiation, trauma, and surgical procedures can produce changes in the gland and hormonal dysfunction.

Some common mental and physical symptoms include the following:

- Growth abnormalities
- Emotional disturbances
- Skin, hair, and nail changes
- Edema
- Hypertension or hypotension
- Cardiac arrhythmias
- Changes in urine output
- Muscle weakness or atrophy
- Menstrual irregularities
- Impotence
- Changes in libido
- Infertility
- Fatigue

TABLE 12-1 MAJOR ENDOCRINE GLAND SECRETIONS AND FUNCTIONS[1]

Endocrine Gland	Hormone	Target Action
Anterior pituitary	Growth hormone (GH)	Promotes bone and tissue growth
	Thyrotropin (thyroid-stimulating hormone [TSH])	Stimulates thyroid gland and production of thyroxine
	Corticotropin (adrenocorticotropic hormone [ACTH])	Stimulates adrenal cortex to produce glucocorticoids
	Gonadotropin	Initiates growth of eggs in ovaries; stimulates spermatogenesis in testes
	Follicle-stimulating hormone (FSH)	
	Luteinizing hormone (LH)	Causes ovulation; stimulates ovaries to produce estrogen and progesterone; stimulates testosterone production
	Prolactin	Stimulates breast development and formation of milk during pregnancy and after delivery
	Melanocyte-stimulating hormone (MSH)	Regulates skin pigmentation
Posterior pituitary	Vasopressin (antidiuretic hormone [ADH])	Stimulates water resorption by renal tubules; has antidiuretic effect
	Oxytocin	Stimulates uterine contractions; stimulates ejection of milk in mammary glands; causes ejection of secretions in male prostate gland
Thyroid	Thyroxine (T_4) and triiodothyronine (T_3)—thyroid hormone (TH)	Regulates rate of cellular metabolism (catabolic phase)
	Calcitonin	Promotes retention of calcium and phosphorus in bone; opposes effect of parathyroid hormone
Parathyroid	Parathyroid hormone (parathormone, PTH)	Regulates metabolism of calcium; elevates serum calcium levels by drawing calcium from bones
Adrenal cortex	Mineralocorticoids (MCs), primarily aldosterone	Promote retention of sodium by kidneys; regulate electrolyte and fluid homeostasis
	Glucocorticoids (GCs): cortisol, corticosterone, cortisone	Regulate metabolism of carbohydrates, proteins, and fats in cells
	Gonadocorticoids: androgens, estrogens, progestins	Govern secondary sex characteristics and masculinization
Adrenal medulla	Catecholamines: epinephrine and norepinephrine	Produce quick-acting "fight or flight" response during stress; increase blood pressure, heart rate, and blood glucose level; dilate bronchioles
Pancreas	Insulin	Regulates metabolism of glucose in body cells; maintains proper blood glucose level
	Glucagon	Increases concentration of glucose in blood by causing conversion of glycogen to glucose
Ovaries	Estrogens	Cause development of female secondary sex characteristics
	Progesterone	Prepares and maintains endometrium for implantation and pregnancy
Testes	Testosterone	Stimulates and promotes growth of male secondary sex characteristics and is essential for erections
Thymus	Thymosin	Promotes development of immune cells (gland atrophies during adulthood)
Pineal gland	Melatonin	Regulates daily patterns of sleep and wakefulness; inhibits hormones that affect ovaries; other functions unknown

DISEASE CONDITIONS

Diseases of the endocrine system and nutritional and metabolic disorders (E00 to E89), covered in Chapter 4 of the ICD-10-CM code book, are divided into the following categories:

CATEGORY	SECTION TITLES
E00-E07	Disorders of the thyroid gland
E08-E13	Diabetes mellitus
E15-E16	Other disorders of glucose regulation and pancreatic internal secretion
E20-E35	Disorders of other endocrine glands
E36	Intraoperative complications of endocrine system
E40-E46	Malnutrition
E50-E64	Other nutritional deficiencies
E65-E68	Overweight, obesity, and other hyperalimentation
E70-E88	Metabolic disorders
E89	Postprocedural endocrine and metabolic complications and disorders, not elsewhere classified

Disorders of Thyroid Gland (E00-E07)

Goiter

Goiter is an enlargement of the thyroid gland (Figure 12-2). This enlargement may be uniform throughout the gland or diffuse. Enlargement may also occur in the form of nodules or nodular goiter. A goiter can cause difficulties in swallowing and/or breathing and may or may not be associated with hormonal disturbances. The most common cause is lack of iodine in the diet. Goiters due to iodine deficiency are rare in the United States since the introduction of iodized salt.

EXAMPLE Patient has a multinodular goiter, E04.2.

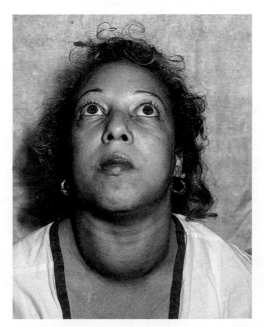

FIGURE 12-2. Goiter. Note the enlarged neck due to enlargement of the thyroid gland.

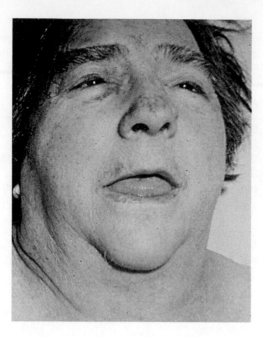

FIGURE 12-3. Myxedema.

Hypothyroidism

Hypothyroidism is diminished production of thyroid hormone, manifested by low metabolic rate, tendency toward weight gain, somnolence, and sometimes myxedema. **Myxedema** is a skin and tissue disorder that is usually due to severe, prolonged hypothyroidism (Figure 12-3). Symptoms include dull, puffy, yellowed skin; coarse, sparse hair; and periorbital edema and prominent tongue.

EXAMPLE | Patient has hypothyroidism, E03.9.

Hashimoto's disease is an inflammation of the thyroid gland that often results in hypothyroidism. It is most common in women and individuals who have a family history of thyroid disease. Onset of Hashimoto's is slow, and it may not be detected for years. The most common signs and symptoms of Hashimoto's disease include the following:

- Intolerance to cold
- Weight gain
- Fatigue
- Constipation
- Goiter
- Dry skin
- Hair loss
- Heavy or irregular menses
- Difficulty with concentration

EXAMPLE | Patient has constipation and fatigue due to autoimmune thyroiditis, E06.3, K59.00.

Hyperthyroidism/Graves' Disease

Hyperthyroidism (Figure 12-4) is an abnormality of the thyroid gland in which secretion of thyroid hormone is usually increased and is no longer under the regulatory control of hypothalamic-pituitary centers.

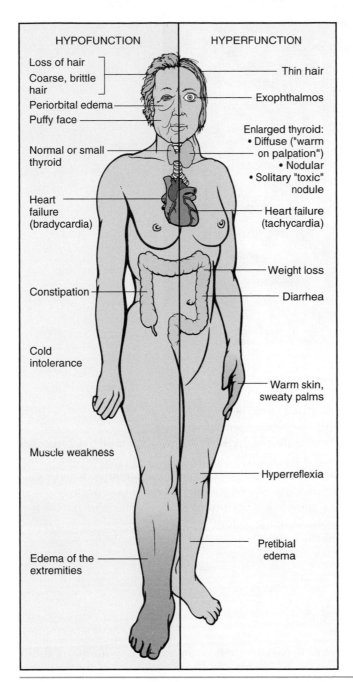

FIGURE 12-4. Comparison of hyperthyroidism and hypothyroidism.

Graves' disease, the most common form of hyperthyroidism, occurs as the result of an autoimmune response that attacks the thyroid gland, resulting in overproduction of the thyroid hormone thyroxine. Graves' disease is most common among women between 20 and 40 years of age. The most common signs and symptoms include the following:

■ Anxiety
■ Irritability
■ Difficulty sleeping
■ Rapid or irregular heartbeat
■ Tremor of hands or fingers
■ Increased perspiration
■ Sensitivity to heat
■ Weight loss

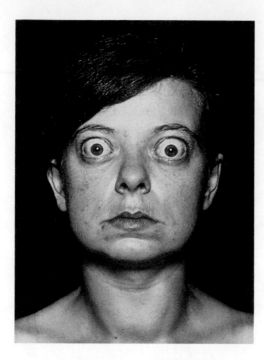

FIGURE 12-5. Exophthalmos in Graves' disease.

- Brittle hair
- Goiter
- Light menstrual periods
- Frequent bowel movements

Graves' ophthalmopathy is also fairly common and may result in **exophthalmos**, or bulging eyes (Figure 12-5). A complication of hyperthyroidism is **thyrotoxic crisis or storm**. This is a sudden intensification of symptoms combined with fever, rapid pulse, and delirium. Medical attention is required when a crisis episode occurs.

Common causes of a thyrotoxic storm or crisis include a medical illness or infection. Other causes include the following:

- Emotional stress
- Diabetic ketoacidosis
- Hypoglycemia
- Cerebrovascular accident
- Pulmonary embolism
- Bowel infarct
- Trauma
- Increase in thyroid hormone from surgery, radioiodine therapy, or iodinated contrast dye

EXAMPLE Weight loss due to Graves' disease, E05.00.

EXERCISE 12-1

Assign codes to the following conditions.

1. Thyroid nodule _____
2. Sick-euthyroid syndrome _____
3. Graves' disease with thyrotoxic crisis _____
4. Hashimoto's disease _____
5. Congenital hypothyroidism _____

Diabetes Mellitus (E08-E13) and Other Disorders of Glucose Regulation and Pancreatic Internal Secretion (E15-E16)

Diabetes Mellitus

Diabetes mellitus is a chronic syndrome of impaired carbohydrate, protein, and fat metabolism caused by insufficient production of insulin by the pancreas or faulty utilization of insulin by the cells. The coding of diabetes mellitus (DM) may be complicated because various manifestations are associated with the disease.

There are two major types of diabetes mellitus: type 1 and type 2. These types vary in origin, pathology, genetics, age of onset, and treatment (Table 12-2). Patients with type 1 diabetes are insulin dependent; this condition usually develops early in life. The pancreas produces insulin in very small amounts or not at all. Type 2 diabetes usually is of adult onset. The pancreas continues to produce insulin, but it is not properly metabolized. Occasionally, patients with type 2 diabetes must be treated with insulin so that acceptable glucose levels are maintained; the fact that they are taking insulin does not mean that they are dependent on insulin, or that they have type 1 diabetes. Type 2 diabetes is much more common than type 1; 90% to 95% of diabetic patients have type 2 diabetes. Type 2 diabetes in adolescents and children is a relatively new phenomenon, and statistics are still being collected. Sometimes, diabetes is documented as insulin-dependent diabetes mellitus (IDDM) or non–insulin-dependent diabetes mellitus (NIDDM). Documentation of insulin dependence does not determine the type of diabetes, because a patient with type 2 diabetes may be on insulin. If only IDDM is documented, and type 1 or type 2 is not specified, according to coding guidelines, the default is type 2 diabetes. There are also code categories for diabetes that is due to an underlying condition, due to a drug or chemical, or due to other specified conditions such as a genetic defect.

Two types of complications may occur with diabetes mellitus. One of these is the acute metabolic complication that is part of diabetes itself. The other is the complication or manifestation that occurs in another body system due to the diabetes (Figure 12-6).

EXAMPLE

> The patient is treated for diabetic ketoacidosis. Patient has type 1 DM, E10.10.
>   Acidosis would not be coded as an additional code in a diabetic patient with ketoacidosis, per the Excludes1 note under code E87.2.

Category E11.9, Diabetes mellitus without mention of complication, would have no additional diabetic codes or manifestation codes (Figure 12-7).

There are subcategories for metabolic complications that require no additional manifestation code (Figure 12-8). Subcategories are available for the following diabetic complications and manifestations (Figure 12-9).

TABLE 12-2 COMPARISON OF TYPE 1 AND TYPE 2 DIABETES MELLITUS[2]

	Type 1	Type 2
Features	Usually occurs before age 30	Usually occurs after age 30
	Abrupt, rapid onset	Gradual onset; asymptomatic
	Little or no insulin production	Insulin usually present
	Thin or normal body weight at onset	85% are obese
	Ketoacidosis often occurs	Ketoacidosis seldom occurs
Symptoms	Polyuria (glycosuria promotes loss of water)	Polyuria sometimes seen
	Polydipsia (dehydration causes thirst)	Polydipsia sometimes seen
	Polyphagia (tissue breakdown causes hunger)	Polyphagia sometimes seen
Treatment	Insulin	Diet; oral hypoglycemics or insulin

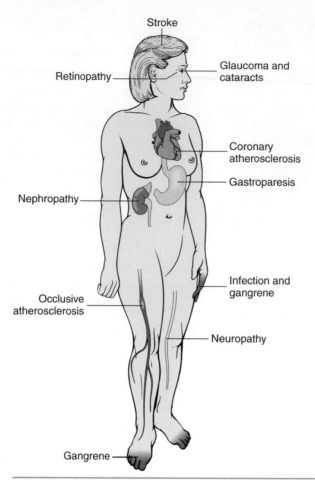

FIGURE 12-6. Possible manifestations/complications of diabetes mellitus.

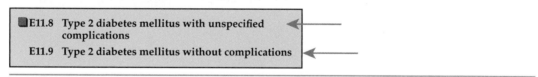

FIGURE 12-7. Type 2 diabetes mellitus without complications or unspecified.

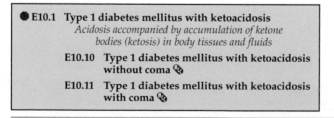

FIGURE 12-8. Diabetes type 1 with metabolic complication (ketoacidosis).

Subcategory E11.8 is reserved for diabetes with unspecified complication (Figure 12-7). It may be beneficial to query the physician for specific documentation regarding any diabetic complications and/or manifestations.

If a patient's diabetes is documented as being poorly controlled or out of control, the Alphabetic Index gives instructions to code the type of diabetes with hyperglycemia.

It is possible for a diabetic patient to have more than one complication and/or manifestation of diabetes, so it is necessary for the coder to use as many codes as necessary to

● **E11.2 Type 2 diabetes mellitus with kidney complications**

    E11.21 Type 2 diabetes mellitus with diabetic nephropathy
        Type 2 diabetes mellitus with intercapillary glomerulosclerosis
        Type 2 diabetes mellitus with intracapillary glomerulonephrosis
        Type 2 diabetes mellitus with Kimmelstiel-Wilson disease

    E11.22 Type 2 diabetes mellitus with diabetic chronic kidney disease
        Type 2 diabetes mellitus with chronic kidney disease due to conditions classified to .21 and .22
        Use additional code to identify stage of chronic kidney disease (N18.1-N18.6)

    E11.29 Type 2 diabetes mellitus with other diabetic kidney complication
        Type 2 diabetes mellitus with renal tubular degeneration

● **E11.3 Type 2 diabetes mellitus with ophthalmic complications**

    ● **E11.31 Type 2 diabetes mellitus with unspecified diabetic retinopathy**

        ■ **E11.311 Type 2 diabetes mellitus with unspecified diabetic retinopathy with macular edema**

        ■ **E11.319 Type 2 diabetes mellitus with unspecified diabetic retinopathy without macular edema**

    ● **E11.32 Type 2 diabetes mellitus with mild nonproliferative diabetic retinopathy**
        Type 2 diabetes mellitus with nonproliferative diabetic retinopathy NOS

        E11.321 Type 2 diabetes mellitus with mild nonproliferative diabetic retinopathy with macular edema

        E11.329 Type 2 diabetes mellitus with mild nonproliferative diabetic retinopathy without macular edema

FIGURE 12-9. Diabetes type 2 manifestations.

completely describe the patient's diabetic conditions. It is very important to follow the guidelines with regard to coding and sequencing of manifestation codes.

EXAMPLE A patient is admitted with diabetic gangrene of the left little toe. The toe was completely amputated. The patient has uncontrolled type 1 diabetes, E10.52, F10.65, 0Y6Y0Z0.

EXAMPLE Patient is admitted with diabetic ketoacidosis. Patient also has diabetic gastroparesis (type 1), E10.10, E10.43, K31.84.

Before a diagnosis can be coded as a diabetic manifestation, a direct cause-and-effect relationship must be established. The manifestation must be documented as diabetic, due to diabetes, or associated with diabetes. For a patient who has diabetes and a cataract, diabetic cataract may not be assigned without documentation linking the cataract to the diabetes.

EXAMPLE Patient has diabetes and senile cataracts bilaterally, E11.9, H25.9.

EXAMPLE Patient has cataracts due to diabetes, E11.36.

The most common body systems that are affected by diabetes include renal, ophthalmic, neurological, and the circulatory system. Other complications involve the joints and skin.

The fourth digit of the 5 diabetes mellitus categories are as follows:

- Kidney—fourth digit 2
- Ophthalmic—fourth digit 3
- Neurological—fourth digit 4
- Circulatory—fourth digit 5
- Other specified complications—fourth digit 6
- Unspecified complications—fourth digit 8
- Without complications—fourth digit 9

Renal or kidney complications are common in patients with diabetes and often result in chronic kidney disease (CKD). If diabetic CKD is present, there is an instructional note that states an additional code to identify the stage of the CKD (N18.1-N18.6) should be assigned. Notice that N18.9 is not included in the range of codes in the instructional note. N18.9 is the code for unspecified CKD so if the specific stage is not documented, no additional code is assigned. A physician query may be necessary to establish the stage of the chronic kidney disease. In patients that have diabetic chronic kidney disease and hypertension, three codes are required.

EXAMPLE	Patient with diabetic CKD, stage 4 and hypertension, E11.22, I12.9, N18.4.

Retinopathy is a common ophthalmic complication in diabetic patients. There are specific diabetic retinopathy codes that identify the type of retinopathy, if macular edema is present or not, and the severity of nonproliferative diabetic retinopathy.

Diabetic neuropathy is caused by damage to nerves throughout the body. This may affect the peripheral, cranial, and/or autonomic nervous systems. There are fifth digits to identify if the neuropathy is:

- Unspecified
- Mononeuropathy
- Polyneuropathy
- Autonomic (poly)neuropathy
- Amyotrophy
- Other neurological complication

Secondary Diabetes

Secondary diabetes mellitus is a form of the disease that develops as a result of another disease or condition. Secondary diabetes can be caused by any condition that damages or interferes with the function of the pancreas. Common conditions that may cause secondary diabetes include pancreatitis, tumor of the pancreas, cystic fibrosis, hemochromatosis, acromegaly, Cushing's syndrome, pheochromocytoma, and drug usage (e.g., corticosteroids). If the underlying cause can be successfully treated, insulin production may improve or return to normal.

The codes for secondary or drug-induced diabetes are similar to the Type 1 and Type 2 diabetes codes. There are subcategory codes for metabolic complications and manifestations.

EXAMPLE	Patient has uncontrolled diabetic nephropathy. Diabetes is due to chronic pancreatitis, K86.1, E08.21, E08.65.

Steroid-induced diabetes is a drug-induced diabetes that results from the use of steroids. Steroids enhance insulin resistance, making insulin less effective. If the pancreas cannot make enough insulin to keep blood glucose within a normal range and the patient is on steroids, this could be steroid-induced diabetes. Steroid-induced diabetes may go away when steroids are discontinued. If the patient has a condition that requires long-term treatment with steroids, diabetes may remain. An episode of steroid-induced diabetes may be an indicator that the patient is at risk for developing diabetes later in life.

EXAMPLE   Patient with steroid-induced diabetes due to long-term use of prednisone taken for rheumatoid arthritis, E09.9, T38.0x5S, M06.9.

Hypoglycemia

Hypoglycemia occurs when glucose or blood sugar becomes abnormally low. This is a relatively common occurrence in a diabetic patient. Hypoglycemia can also occur in patients who do not have diabetes mellitus. Normal fasting blood glucose levels range from 70 to 99 mg/dL.

EXAMPLE   Patient was seen in the ER with hypoglycemia, E16.2.

EXAMPLE   Patient who has type 2 diabetes with hypoglycemia, E11.649.

Hyperglycemia

Hyperglycemia occurs when glucose or blood sugar becomes abnormally high. This also is a relatively common occurrence in a diabetic patient. Patients who do not have diabetes may have episodes of hyperglycemia. Sometimes, medication such as steroids can cause hyperglycemia.

EXAMPLE   Patient with diabetes and hyperglycemia, E11.65.

EXAMPLE   Patient with hyperglycemia due to long-term use of prednisone taken for rheumatoid arthritis, R73.9, T38.0x5S, M06.9.

Gestational Diabetes

Gestational diabetes is discussed in Chapter 21, Complications of Pregnancy, Childbirth, and the Puerperium.

EXERCISE 12-2

Assign codes to the following conditions.

1. Diabetic with episode of hypoglycemia   _____
2. Diabetic retinopathy, DM type 2   _____
3. Diabetic hyperosmolar coma   _____
4. Zollinger-Ellison syndrome   _____
5. Diabetic gangrene, left big toe   _____
6. Diabetes type 2, uncontrolled. Patient also has peripheral   _____
   vascular disease
7. Steroid-induced diabetes (sequela of long term steroid use) in _____
   patient with Crohn's disease
8. Charcot's arthropathy right foot due to diabetes, type 1   _____
   uncontrolled
9. Hypoglycemic coma in type 1 diabetes   _____
10. Overactive bladder due to diabetes   _____
11. Diabetic patient with hyperglycemia treated with insulin.   _____
    Patient is normally on oral medication for diabetes.
12. Syncope caused by autonomic neuropathy due to diabetes   _____
    mellitus. The patient has type 2 diabetes.

Disorders of Other Endocrine Glands (E20-E35)

Hypoparathyroidism

Hypoparathyroidism is caused by an underactive parathyroid gland that results in decreased levels of circulating calcium. The primary manifestation is **tetany**, a continuous muscle spasm. Vitamin D and calcium supplements are often used to treat this condition.

EXAMPLE   The patient had tetany due to hypoparathyroidism. The patient is treated with calcium supplements, E20.9.

Hyperparathyroidism

Hyperparathyroidism results from an overactive parathyroid gland that secretes excessive parathyroid hormone, causing increased levels of circulating calcium due to loss of calcium in the bone.

Hyperparathyroidism may be primary or secondary. In most cases, primary hyperparathyroidism is caused by a parathyroid adenoma. Secondary hyperparathyroidism is often related to chronic kidney disease.

EXAMPLE   The patient was treated for primary hyperparathyroidism. The patient was hypercalcemic, E21.0. Note the Excludes note under E83.5. Disorders of calcium metabolism (Figure 12-10). Hypercalcemia or hypocalcemia would not be coded as an additional code with any hyperparathyroidism, E21.0-E21.3.

Hyperpituitarism

Hyperpituitarism results from increased production of pituitary hormones, particularly of human growth hormone (hGH). **Gigantism** or **acromegaly** may occur, depending on the time of life when hormonal dysfunction begins (Figure 12-11).

Gigantism occurs when hypersecretion of hGH occurs before puberty, along with proportionate overgrowth of all body tissues, especially of the long bones. Often, a pituitary adenoma results from oversecretion of hGH. Acromegaly results when hypersecretion of hGH occurs after puberty, along with overgrowth of the face, hands, feet, and soft tissues. Pituitary adenoma is often the cause.

EXAMPLE   Patient has hypersecretion of growth hormone, E22.0.

Hypopituitarism

Hypopituitarism is a condition that is caused by low levels of pituitary hormones. Hormones secreted by the pituitary gland may affect the function of other glands. Lack of

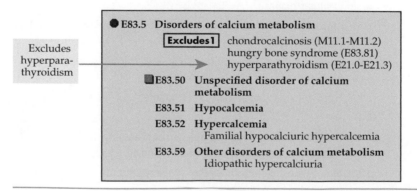

FIGURE 12-10. Disorders of calcium metabolism Excludes1 note.

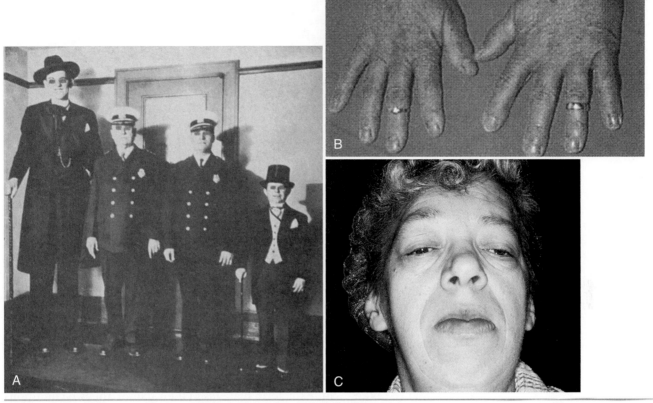

FIGURE 12-11. Effects of growth hormone. **A,** Comparison of gigantism, normal growth, and dwarfism. **B,** Hands with clinical signs of acromegaly. **C,** Face with clinical signs of acromegaly.

thyroid-stimulating hormone (TSH) affects the function of the thyroid gland. Hypopituitarism may be caused by a variety of conditions, such as the following:

- Tumor
- Head trauma
- Brain surgery
- Stroke
- Infections of brain

Occasionally, immune system or metabolic disease such as sarcoidosis, histiocytosis X, and hemochromatosis can cause hypopituitarism.

EXAMPLE   The patient has hypopituitarism due to pituitary adenoma, D35.2, E23.0.

EXAMPLE   The patient has hypopituitarism due to abscess of the brain, G06.0, E23.0.

Diabetes Insipidus

Diabetes insipidus (DI) or water diabetes is a deficiency in the release of vasopressin by the posterior pituitary gland. The patient excretes volumes of dilute urine and experiences excessive thirst, fatigue, and dehydration. The underlying cause needs to be identified and treated.

Underlying causes of DI include the following:

- Stroke
- Neoplasm
- Polycystic kidney disease
- Neurosurgery

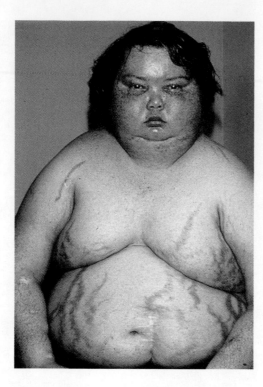

FIGURE 12-12. Cushingoid features—moon face, obesity, and cutaneous striae.

Although DI and DM both include the term diabetes in their names, the two conditions are not related.

EXAMPLE The patient suffers from diabetes insipidus, E23.2.

Cushing's Syndrome

Cushing's syndrome is a condition that results in excessive circulating cortisol levels due to chronic hypersecretion of the adrenal cortex. Common signs and symptoms include the following:

- Fatigue
- Muscle weakness
- Changes in body appearance with fat deposits in the scapular and abdominal areas
- Moon face
- Hypertension
- Edema

Other complications include hyperlipidemia, osteoporosis, diabetes, excessive hair growth, amenorrhea, impotence, and psychiatric disturbances (Figure 12-12). The skin becomes thin and bruises easily, and red or purple stretch marks develop.

Administration of glucocorticoids (steroids) to treat other diseases can result in **iatrogenic** (treatment-induced) Cushing's. The patient's appearance may be described as "cushingoid" (see Figure 12-12).

EXAMPLE Patient has Cushing's syndrome and hyperlipidemia, E24.9, E78.5.

Addison's Disease

Addison's disease is an adrenocortical insufficiency that may be caused by neoplasms, surgical removal of the adrenal gland, autoimmune processes, tuberculosis, hemorrhage, and/or infection. Addison's is characterized by the following symptoms:

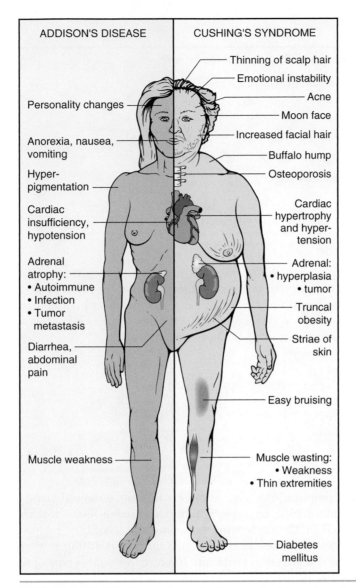

ADDISON'S DISEASE	CUSHING'S SYNDROME

Thinning of scalp hair
Emotional instability
Acne
Moon face
Increased facial hair
Buffalo hump
Osteoporosis
Cardiac hypertrophy and hypertension
Adrenal:
• hyperplasia
• tumor
Truncal obesity
Striae of skin
Easy bruising
Muscle wasting:
• Weakness
• Thin extremities
Diabetes mellitus

Personality changes
Anorexia, nausea, vomiting
Hyper-pigmentation
Cardiac insufficiency, hypotension
Adrenal atrophy:
• Autoimmune
• Infection
• Tumor metastasis
Diarrhea, abdominal pain
Muscle weakness

FIGURE 12-13. Comparison of adrenocortical hyperfunction and hypofunction.

- Hypotension
- Weight loss
- Anorexia
- Weakness
- Bronze skin coloring

Other complications include cardiovascular problems such as irregular pulse, reduced cardiac output, and orthostatic hypotension (Figure 12-13). Emotional disturbances such as depression and anxiety are common. When dehydration and electrolyte imbalances occur, medical attention is required to prevent a life-threatening situation.

EXAMPLE Patient was admitted to the hospital for treatment of dehydration and for prevention of Addison's crisis, E86.0, E27.1.

Assign codes to the following conditions.

1. Hyperparathyroidism   _____

2. Syndrome of inappropriate antidiuretic hormone secretion (SIADH)   _____

3. Vasopressin deficiency   _____

4. Multiple endocrine neoplasia, type 1   _____

5. Precocious puberty   _____

Malnutrition (E40-E46) and Other Nutritional Deficiencies (E50-E64)

Malnutrition

Malnutrition is a nutritional disorder that is caused by primary deprivation of protein energy as the result of poverty, self-imposed starvation, or in relation to deficiency diseases such as cancer. Other conditions that may cause malnutrition include Crohn's disease, short bowel syndrome, malabsorption syndrome, or severe burns or traumatic injury. Signs and symptoms of malnutrition include the following:

- Loss of energy
- Diarrhea
- Drastic weight change (loss or gain)
- Skin lesions
- Loss of hair
- Poor nails
- Edema
- Delayed healing
- Greasy stools due to loss of body fat

Other complications, such as muscle wasting, enlarged glands, and hepatomegaly, may occur as malnutrition progresses. Blood and urine tests show many abnormalities. Treatment is based on the underlying cause and the severity of malnutrition.

Kwashiorkor is a severe type of malnutrition resulting in dyspigmentation of skin and hair, edema, and growth retardation. It is rare to find this type of malnutrition in the United States. **Nutritional marasmus** is a severe form of malnutrition that is characterized by severe tissue wasting, loss of subcutaneous fat, and maybe dehydration.

EXAMPLE   The patient was found to have severe malnutrition, E43.

Vitamin Deficiencies

Vitamin deficiencies may be caused by many different factors, such as poor nutrient absorption, digestive tract disorders, lifestyle issues (e.g., alcohol, smoking, medications, over-exercising), chronic illness, age, and many other factors. Applicable codes are included in the following code categories:

E50	Vitamin A deficiency
E51-E52	Thiamine and niacin deficiency states
E53	Deficiency of B complex components
E54	Ascorbic acid deficiency
E55	Vitamin D deficiency
E63	Other nutritional deficiencies

A diagnosis can be stated as a vitamin deficiency, or a specific name may be used for that particular deficiency (Figure 12-14). Another name for vitamin C deficiency is scurvy.

EXAMPLE   Rickets due to vitamin D deficiency, E55.0.

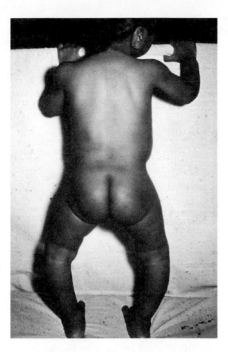

FIGURE 12-14. Rickets. The bowing of legs in a toddler due to formation of poorly mineralized bones.

EXERCISE 12-4

Assign codes to the following conditions.

1. Emaciation
   _____
2. Vitamin B_{12} deficiency
   _____
3. Night blindness due to vitamin A deficiency
   _____
4. Severe protein calorie malnutrition
   _____

Overweight, Obesity, and Other Hyperalimentation (E65-E68)

Obesity

Obesity is defined as an increase in body weight beyond the limitations of skeletal and physical requirements, as a result of excessive accumulation of fat in the body. In the United States, obesity has reached epidemic proportions, with two-thirds of American adults being overweight, and one in three considered obese. **Body mass index** (BMI) uses weight and height to estimate body fat.

According to the Centers for Disease Control and Prevention (CDC), for adults, body mass index (BMI) is defined as follows:

Below 18.5	Underweight
Between 18.5 and 24.9	Healthy weight or normal
Between 25.0 and 29.0	Overweight
30.0 and above	Obese

Z codes should be used in combination with overweight and obesity codes to indicate a patient's BMI, if documented. Assignment of codes for overweight or obesity must be based on documentation provided by the physician. According to General Coding Guidelines, it is acceptable to assign a body mass index (BMI) code based on medical record documentation from clinicians who are not the patient's provider. BMI is often documented in nurse or dietician notes. There are different BMI codes for pediatric and adult patients. The pediatric BMI codes are for use for persons 2 to 20 years of age. The adult BMI codes are for use for persons 21 years of age and older.

EXAMPLE	Adult patient is obese with a BMI of 31, E66.9, Z68.31.

Morbid obesity is the term that applies to patients who are 100 pounds overweight or over 50% above their ideal body weight. A BMI of 40 or higher defines morbid obesity. Many complications may be related to obesity, including the following:

- Diabetes
- Hypertension
- Heart disease
- Stroke
- Certain cancers such as breast and colon
- Depression
- Osteoarthritis

EXAMPLE	Adult patient is morbidly obese with a BMI of 41 and suffers from DM, E66.01, E11.9, Z68.41.

Hypervitaminosis

Hypervitaminosis is toxicity that results from an excess of any vitamin, but especially fat-soluble vitamins such as A, D, and K. If toxicity occurs because of an overdose, a poisoning code would be assigned. Poisonings are discussed in Chapter 24.

EXAMPLE	Hypervitaminosis (vitamin D), E67.3.

EXERCISE 12-5

Assign codes to the following conditions.

1. Adult patient with severe obesity with BMI of 40 _____
2. Hypoventilation syndrome in morbidly obese patient _____
3. Localized adiposity _____

Metabolic Disorders (E70-E88)

Cystic Fibrosis

Cystic fibrosis (CF) or mucoviscidosis is a genetic (inherited) condition that affects the cells that produce mucus, sweat, saliva, and digestive juices (Figure 12-15). Instead of being thin and slippery, these secretions are thick and sticky, plugging up tubes, ducts, and passageways, especially in the pancreas and lungs. No cure is available, and treatment is directed at the complications and manifestations of the disease. The most frequent complications are respiratory infections such as pneumonia, bronchitis, and bronchiectasis. Asthma may also develop. Although the organism *Pseudomonas aeruginosa* does not cause problems in a healthy person, it is a common infective organism in the patient with CF. Presence of *Pseudomonas* organism in the patient's sputum does not necessarily indicate that the patient has pneumonia due to *Pseudomonas*.

According to *Coding Clinic for ICD-9-CM* (1990:4Q:p17),[3] when a patient is admitted for a complication of CF, the complication is the principal diagnosis, and CF is a secondary diagnosis. The codes E84.0, cystic fibrosis with pulmonary manifestations, and E84.19, cystic fibrosis with intestinal manifestations, identify the two major systems that are affected by the disease. If the patient has both respiratory and intestinal manifestations, both cystic fibrosis codes are used.

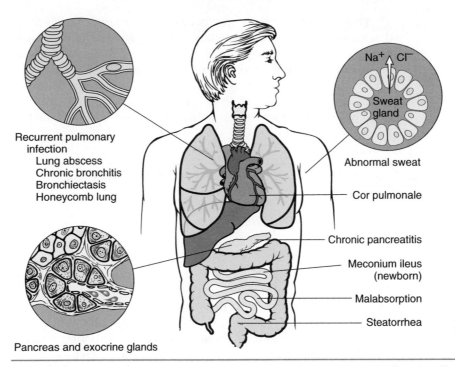

FIGURE 12-15. Abnormal chloride transport associated with cystic fibrosis affects the secretions of all exocrine glands, especially the pancreas, intestine, and bronchi.

EXAMPLE | Patient who suffers from CF is admitted because of acute bronchitis. Patient also has pancreatic insufficiency due to CF, J20.9, E84.0, E84.8, K86.8.

Disorders of Fluid, Electrolyte, and Acid-Base Balance

Fluid balance occurs when the amount of fluid taken in is equal to the amount that is lost from the body. **Euvolemia** is the state of normal body fluid volume. A patient's fluid balance provides important information about their hydration, renal and cardiovascular function. **Fluid overload** or **hypervolemia** occurs when there is too much fluid in the body. Fluid overload may be the result of too much sodium intake, due to IVs or blood transfusions, or a side effect of medication. Some conditions of the heart, kidney, and liver can affect fluid balance. The chief cause of fluid overload is heart failure. When fluid overload is due to congestive heart failure, it is not coded separately. Fluids can build up in various parts of the body causing edema. Peripheral edema is swelling that occurs in the lower extremities. Fluid can also build up in the lungs causing pulmonary edema or in the abdomen causing ascites.

EXAMPLE | Patient has volume overload due to noncompliance with dialysis for end-stage renal disease, E87.70, N18.6, Z91.15.

Hypovolemia occurs due to decreased plasma volume. **Dehydration** is when the body does not have enough water or fluids as it should. Dehydration can be caused by losing too much fluid (e.g., vomiting, diarrhea), not drinking enough water or fluids, or both. **Volume depletion** may be the result of either dehydration or hypovolemia.

EXAMPLE | Patient was seen in the Emergency Room and treated with IV fluids due to dehydration from gastroenteritis, E86.0, K52.9.

Dehydration occurs frequently as the result of other medical conditions and principal diagnosis selection and sequencing may be confusing. According to the neoplasm guidelines, if an admission occurs for the management of dehydration due to malignancy or therapy for the malignancy, or a combination of both, and only dehydration is being treated, then dehydration is designated as the principal diagnosis, followed by the code(s) for malignancy. According to *Coding Clinic for ICD-9-CM* (2002:3Q:p21-22; 2003:1Q:p22),[4-5] in admissions in which severe dehydration causes acute renal failure, acute renal failure is the principal diagnosis.

EXAMPLE Patient was admitted for dehydration and acute renal failure, N17.9, E86.0.

Tumor Lysis Syndrome

Tumor lysis syndrome (TLS) is the development of electrolyte and metabolic disturbances that can occur after treatment of cancer, usually lymphoma and leukemia, and sometimes even without treatment. Patients with preexisting kidney disease are at increased risk for developing TLS. Tumor lysis syndrome is caused by the breakdown of dying cancer cells and includes hyperkalemia, hyperphosphatemia, hyperuricemia and hyperuricosuria, and hypocalcemia. Acute renal failure and acute uric acid nephropathy can develop as a result of these electrolyte and metabolic disturbances. Although a patient may not have any symptoms in the early stages, as it progresses, symptoms include nausea and vomiting, shortness of breath, irregular heartbeat, lethargy, cloudy urine, and/or joint discomfort. Preventive measures can be taken before and during treatment that include IV hydration, and medications such as allopurinol or rasburicase, and alkalinization of urine with sodium bicarbonate. If TLS is untreated or it progresses, it can cause acute kidney failure, cardiac arrhythmias, seizures, loss of muscle control, and death.

EXAMPLE Patient was admitted to the hospital due to possible acute myeloid leukemia. After confirmation of his AML, it was decided to administer chemotherapy. His labs were followed and showed tumor lysis syndrome due to the chemo, C92.00, E88.3, T45.1x5A, 3E04305.

Dysmetabolic Syndrome X

Dysmetabolic Syndrome X is characterized by abdominal obesity, insulin resistance, dyslipidemia, and elevated blood pressure or hypertension. Patients with these conditions are considered to be at greater risk for type 2 diabetes, cardiovascular disease, and stroke. Other names for dysmetabolic syndrome X include metabolic syndrome, syndrome X, insulin resistance syndrome, obesity syndrome, and Reaven's syndrome. In the ICD-10-CM code book, there is an Instructional note to use additional codes for any associated conditions.

EXAMPLE Adult patient was seen in the clinic for dietary counseling for dysmetabolic syndrome X. Patient is obese with a BMI of 35 and has hypertriglyceridemia and hypertension, Z71.3, E88.81, E66.9, Z68.35, E78.1, I10.

EXERCISE 12-6

Assign codes to the following conditions.

1. Hypocalcemia _____

2. Hypovolemia _____

3. Alpha 1–antitrypsin deficiency _____

4. Metabolic acidosis _____

FACTORS INFLUENCING HEALTH STATUS AND CONTACT WITH HEALTH SERVICES (Z CODES)

As was discussed in Chapter 8, it is difficult to locate Z codes in the index. Coders will often say, "I did not know there was a Z code for that."

Refer to Chapter 8 for a listing of common main terms to locate Z codes. Z codes that may be used with diseases of the endocrine glands, nutritional, and metabolic diseases include the following:

Z13.1	Encounter for screening for diabetes mellitus
Z13.21	Encounter for screening for nutritional disorder
Z13.220	Encounter for screening for lipoid disorders
Z13.228	Encounter for screening for other metabolic disorders
Z13.29	Encounter for screening for other suspected endocrine disorders
Z14.1	Cystic fibrosis carrier
Z15.81	Genetic susceptibility to multiple endocrine neoplasia
Z46.51	Encounter for fitting and adjustment of gastric lap band
Z46.81	Encounter for fitting and adjustment of insulin pump
Z68.1	Body mass index (BMI) 19 or less, adult
Z68.20	Body mass index (BMI) 20.0-20.9, adult
Z68.21	Body mass index (BMI) 21.0-21.9, adult
Z68.22	Body mass index (BMI) 22.0-22.9, adult
Z68.23	Body mass index (BMI) 23.0-23.9, adult
Z68.24	Body mass index (BMI) 24.0-24.9, adult
Z68.25	Body mass index (BMI) 25.0-25.9, adult
Z68.26	Body mass index (BMI) 26.0-26.9, adult
Z68.27	Body mass index (BMI) 27.0-27.9, adult
Z68.28	Body mass index (BMI) 28.0-28.9, adult
Z68.29	Body mass index (BMI) 29.0-29.9, adult
Z68.30	Body mass index (BMI) 30.0-30.9, adult
Z68.31	Body mass index (BMI) 31.0-31.9, adult
Z68.32	Body mass index (BMI) 32.0-32.9, adult
Z68.33	Body mass index (BMI) 33.0-33.9, adult
Z68.34	Body mass index (BMI) 34.0-34.9, adult
Z68.35	Body mass index (BMI) 35.0-35.9, adult
Z68.36	Body mass index (BMI) 36.0-36.9, adult
Z68.37	Body mass index (BMI) 37.0-37.9, adult
Z68.38	Body mass index (BMI) 38.0-38.9, adult
Z68.39	Body mass index (BMI) 39.0-39.9, adult
Z68.41	Body mass index (BMI) 40.0-44.9, adult
Z68.42	Body mass index (BMI) 45.0-49.9, adult
Z68.43	Body mass index (BMI) 50.0-59.9, adult
Z68.44	Body mass index (BMI) 60.0-69.9, adult
Z68.45	Body mass index (BMI) 70 or greater, adult
Z68.51	Body mass index (BMI) pediatric, less than 5th percentile for age
Z68.52	Body mass index (BMI) pediatric, 5th percentile to less than 85th percentile for age
Z68.53	Body mass index (BMI) pediatric, 85th percentile to less than 95th percentile for age
Z68.54	Body mass index (BMI) pediatric, greater than or equal to 95th percentile for age
Z71.3	Dietary counseling and surveillance
Z79.4	Long-term (current) use of insulin

Z83.3	Family history of diabetes mellitus
Z83.41	Family history of multiple endocrine neoplasia [MEN] syndrome
Z83.49	Family history of other endocrine, nutritional, and metabolic diseases
Z86.31	Personal history of diabetic foot ulcer
Z86.32	Personal history of gestational diabetes
Z86.39	Personal history of other endocrine, nutritional, and metabolic disease
Z94.83	Pancreas transplant status
Z96.41	Presence of insulin pump (external) (internal)
Z96.49	Presence of other endocrine implants
Z98.84	Bariatric surgery status

EXAMPLE Patient has a family history of diabetes, Z83.3.

EXAMPLE Patient is a type 2 diabetic who has been treated with insulin, E11.9, Z79.4.

EXERCISE 12-7

Assign codes to the following conditions.

1. Status post pancreas transplant _____
2. Dietary counseling for patient with new diagnosis of DM _____
3. Family history of Graves' disease _____
4. History of rickets as a child _____

COMMON TREATMENTS

CONDITION	MEDICATION/TREATMENT
Goiter	Small doses of iodine if due to iodine deficiency; otherwise, radioactive iodine or surgical treatment if symptomatic
Hypothyroidism/Hashimoto's disease	Levothyroxine, Levothroid, and Synthroid, which is the most common thyroid hormone replacement medication
Hyperthyroidism/Graves' disease	Antithyroid medications such as Tapazole; radioactive iodine or surgery
Diabetes	Diet, monitoring of blood sugars, and insulins such as Regular, Lente, Humalog, NPH; oral medications such as Glyburide, Micronase, Diabeta, Glucophage, etc.
Hyperpituitarism	Decrease the amount of hormone secreted, usually with radiation or surgery
Hypopituitarism	Removal of tumor if that is the cause, or hormone replacement therapy
Diabetes insipidus	Depending on cause, vasopressin medication
Hyperparathyroidism	Treatment depends on the cause
Hypoparathyroidism	Replacement therapy with calcium and vitamin D
Cushing's syndrome	Removal of tumor if that is the cause, or medication to suppress the production of cortisol
Addison's disease	Replacement therapy with corticosteroids
Malnutrition	Treat symptoms and/or underlying cause; nutritional supplements; replace missing nutrients, possibly with TPN (total parenteral nutrition)

CONDITION	MEDICATION/TREATMENT
Vitamin deficiencies	Treat symptoms and/or underlying cause; replace missing vitamins
Hypokalemia	Replace with potassium supplement, such as K-Dur, K-Lyte, K-Tab, K-Lor, Micro-K
Hyperkalemia	Remove potassium from body with Kayexalate, diuretics, sodium bicarbonate, intravenous calcium, glucose, or insulin
Cystic fibrosis	Postural drainage and chest percussion treatments, pancreatic enzymes and vitamins, antibiotics for infection, and possibly lung transplant
Obesity	Diet, exercise, behavior modification, and bariatric surgery
Hypervitaminosis	Stop taking specific vitamin

PROCEDURES

Procedures related to the endocrine system in ICD-10-PCS can be located in the following tables:

0F1-0FY	Gastrointestinal System
0F1-0FY	Hepatobiliary System and Pancreas
0G2-0GW	Endocrine System

EXAMPLE Goiter with complete thyroidectomy, E04.9, 0GTK0ZZ.

EXAMPLE Conn's syndrome due to adenoma of right adrenal gland with diagnostic percutaneous biopsy of adrenal gland D35.01, E26.01, 0GB33ZX.

Bariatric Surgery

Bariatric surgery is surgery performed for weight loss on people who are obese, usually with a BMI (Body Mass Index) of greater than 40. To achieve weight loss the stomach must be reduced. There are several different types of surgical procedures performed to achieve this result. The four most common types being offered in the U.S. are (Figure 12-16):

- BPD-DS biliopancreatic diversion is rarely used because of troubles with malnourishment, and they now use a modification, which is known as a duodenal switch. This procedure includes three features. The first is that a large part of the stomach is removed creating a pouch. The second is that the food is rerouted away from much of the small intestine limiting the amount of food absorbed by the body, and lastly the third feature changes how bile affects the body's ability to digest and absorb food. The distal part of the small intestine is connected to the pouch bypassing the duodenum and jejunum.
- Roux-en-Y (RYGB) is a gastric bypass procedure. This procedure both restricts food intake as well as decreases how food is absorbed. The food is restricted because a small pouch is created by a stapler. A section of the small intestine is attached to the pouch, which bypasses the duodenum and part of the jejunum. Portions of the stomach are not removed in this procedure as they are in the BPD. This procedure may be performed both laparoscopically as well as open. In ICD-10-PCS when coding bypass procedures it is important to know which body part is "bypassed from" and which body part is "bypassed to." In this procedure the 4th character would represent the from (stomach) and the 7th character would represent the to (jejunum).

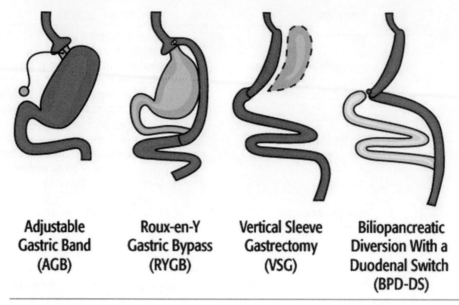

Adjustable Gastric Band (AGB)

Roux-en-Y Gastric Bypass (RYGB)

Vertical Sleeve Gastrectomy (VSG)

Biliopancreatic Diversion With a Duodenal Switch (BPD-DS)

FIGURE 12-16. Types of bariatric surgery.

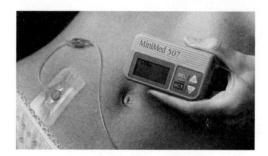

FIGURE 12-17. Insulin pump.

- Adjustable gastric banding (AGB) is a restrictive procedure. A band with an inflatable inner collar is placed around the upper stomach to restrict food intake. This makes the patient feel full earlier. Most often, this procedure is performed laparoscopically. In ICD-10-PCS the root operation is restriction.
- Vertical Sleeve Gastrectomy (VSG) both restricts food intake and decreases the amount of food used. In this procedure most of the stomach is removed. The hormone ghrelin that affects appetite appears to be decreased in this type of surgery.

EXAMPLE
Morbidly obese adult patient (BMI 42) with diabetes mellitus. A laparoscopic gastric banding with extraluminal device was performed E66.01, E11.9, Z68.41, 0DV64CZ.

Insulin Pumps

An insulin pump is a small, computerized device that is attached to the body and delivers insulin via a catheter (Figure 12-17). This pump provides a continuous drip of insulin throughout the day. The patient may also administer a bolus of insulin by pushing a button. The root operation for insulin pump implantation is insertion (putting in a nonbiological device).

EXAMPLE
Patient has brittle Type 1 diabetes and is admitted for implantation (percutaneous) of insulin pump (subcutaneous infusion device implanted in abdomen), E10.9, 0JH83VZ.

EXERCISE 12-8

Assign codes for all diagnoses and procedures.

1. Multinodular goiter which is symptomatic for dysphagia. Total   _____
   thyroidectomy was performed.

2. Pheochromocytoma with laparoscopic excision right adrenal   _____
   gland

3. Adult with morbid obesity with BMI of 40. Laparoscopic VBG   _____
   was performed.

DOCUMENTATION/REIMBURSEMENT/MS-DRGs

Often, coding difficulties are due to lack of documentation. Sometimes pathology and other test results are not available at the time of discharge, or when the physician is dictating the discharge summary or is reporting the final diagnoses.

Malnutrition may not be well documented by the physician. Nutritional consults or dietician notes should be reviewed. A physician query would be needed to confirm any diagnoses based on a dietician's assessment.

Many of the conditions and diseases related to nutritional and metabolic disorders are supported by laboratory tests. Coders should not assign a diagnosis code on the basis of abnormal laboratory findings alone. A laboratory value may be higher or lower than the normal range, but this does not necessarily indicate a disorder. If abnormal laboratory value(s) is noted and treatment is given or documentation supports monitoring, it would be appropriate to query the physician regarding the abnormal laboratory value(s). An abnormal finding must be clinically significant to be coded.

Frequently missed complications/comorbidities from this chapter include the following:

- Acidosis
- Alkalosis
- Hypernatremia
- Hyponatremia
- Malnutrition

MS-DRG With and Without MCC/CC

EXAMPLE

Patient was admitted with Addison's crisis, and sodium on admission was 115 (normal, 135-148 mEq/L).

Patient treated with hypertonic saline IVs. The physician documents in the discharge summary that the patient's sodium levels improved dramatically before discharge.

DIAGNOSES	CODES	MS-DRG	RW
Addison's crisis with hyponatremia	E27.2, E87.1	644	1.0583
Addison's crisis without hyponatremia	E27.2	645	0.7252

The presence of a complication or comorbidity can make a difference in reimbursement, depending on the principal diagnosis and the MS-DRG assigned. The code for hyponatremia is a complication/comorbidity. In this case, it would be necessary to query the physician regarding the low sodium levels and treatment with hypertonic saline IV before the hyponatremia code is assigned.

Two Diagnoses That Equally Meet the Definition for Principal Diagnosis

Dehydration may cause confusion when selecting a principal diagnosis because dehydration is often caused by other conditions. If two or more conditions are present on admission and meet the definition for principal diagnosis, either one could be selected as principal.

EXAMPLE

A patient was admitted with urinary tract infection (UTI) and moderate dehydration. The dehydration was treated aggressively with intravenous fluids, and the UTI was treated with intravenous (IV) antibiotics.

DIAGNOSES	CODES	MS-DRG	RW
Dehydration and UTI	E86.0, N39.0	641	0.6988
UTI and dehydration	N39.0, E86.0	690	0.7870

In this case, both UTI and dehydration were treated by measures that would require inpatient admission, so it would be possible to sequence either diagnosis as the principal diagnosis. If the patient had been treated with IV fluids for dehydration and oral antibiotics for the UTI, dehydration should be the principal because oral antibiotics would not typically require inpatient hospitalization.

Diabetic Manifestation versus Not Related to Diabetes

Documentation with regard to diabetes can be conflicting and/or may need clarification. Sometimes documentation is inconsistent, and diabetes has been documented as both type 1 and type 2 within the record. A patient is either type 1 or type 2, and it is necessary to query the physician to determine which type is correct. It is also important to make sure that any manifestations are documented as related to diabetes. In addition, when a principal diagnosis is selected, the diabetes codes must be sequenced before any manifestation code. This can make a significant difference in MS-DRG assignment and reimbursement.

EXAMPLE

DIAGNOSES	CODES	MS-DRG	RW
Diabetic ulcer left toe	E11.621, L97.529	639	0.5503
Ulcer left toe, diabetes	L97.529, E11.9	594	0.6981

CHAPTER REVIEW EXERCISE

Assign codes for all diagnoses and procedures.

1. Homocystinemia _____

2. Conn's syndrome _____

3. Myxedema _____

4. Idiopathic Cushing's syndrome _____

5. Testicular hypogonadism _____

6. Overproduction of growth hormone _____

7. Hypertonic dehydration _____

8. Asymptomatic hyperuricemia _____

9. Symptomatic premature menopause _____

10. Respiratory acidosis with metabolic alkalosis _____

11. Overweight adult with BMI of 26.0 _____

12. Volume depletion _____

13. Patient with cystic fibrosis admitted with exacerbation of respiratory symptoms _____

14. Hyperthyroidism with exophthalmos _____

15. Poorly controlled diabetes (type 2) with diabetic gastroparesis; _____
    patient is on insulin

16. Albinism _____

17. Amyloidosis _____

18. Proliferative retinopathy due to DM, type 2, out of control _____

19. Diabetes due to prednisone (sequela due to long term use of a _____
    prescribed drug)

20. Hyperlipidemia due to Cushing's syndrome _____

21. Thiamine deficiency due to chronic alcoholism _____

22. Phenylketonuria (PKU) _____

23. Chronic kidney disease, stage 3 due to diabetic nephropathy, _____
    juvenile-onset diabetes

24. Adult patient with severe obesity with BMI 43 and obstructive _____
    sleep apnea; patient had open Roux-en-Y gastric bypass to
    jejunum

25. Erectile dysfunction due to diabetes mellitus, type 2 _____

26. Inanition _____

27. Methylenetetrahydrofolate reductase deficiency _____

Write the correct answer(s) in the space(s) provided.

28. List a couple of conditions that qualify a person as morbidly obese.

    _____

    _____

29. What type of diabetes is the most common?

    _____

30. What organism may cause complications for a patient with cystic fibrosis?

    _____

CHAPTER GLOSSARY

Acromegaly: condition that results when hypersecretion of hGH occurs after puberty, along with overgrowth of the face, hands, feet, and soft tissues.

Addison's disease: adrenocortical insufficiency that may be caused by neoplasms, surgical removal of the adrenal gland, autoimmune processes, tuberculosis, hemorrhage, and/or infection.

Atrophy: when a gland becomes smaller.

Bariatrics: branch of medicine that is concerned with the management (prevention or control) of obesity and allied diseases.

Body mass index: uses weight and height to estimate body fat.

Cushing's syndrome: condition that results in excessive circulating cortisol levels caused by chronic hypersecretion of the adrenal cortex.

Cystic fibrosis: genetic (inherited) condition that affects the cells that produce mucus, sweat, saliva, and digestive juices. Instead of being thin and slippery, these secretions are thick and sticky, plugging up tubes, ducts, and passageways, especially in the pancreas and lungs.

Dehydration: is when the body does not have enough water or fluids as it should.

Diabetes insipidus: deficiency in the release of vasopressin by the posterior pituitary gland.

Diabetes mellitus: chronic syndrome of impaired carbohydrate, protein, and fat metabolism caused by insufficient production of insulin by the pancreas or faulty utilization of insulin by the cells.

Dysmetabolic Syndrome X: is characterized by abdominal obesity, insulin resistance, dyslipidemia, and elevated blood pressure or hypertension.

Endocrine system: body system composed of many glands that secrete hormones that regulate bodily functions; it works with the nervous system to maintain body activities and homeostasis and to respond to stress.

Euvolemia: is the state of normal body fluid volume.

Exophthalmos: bulging of the eyes.

Fluid overload: occurs when there is too much fluid in the body.

Genetic: inherited.

Gigantism: condition that occurs when hypersecretion of hGH occurs before puberty, along with proportionate overgrowth of all bodily tissues, especially the long bones.

Goiter: enlargement of the thyroid gland.

Graves' disease: the most common form of hyperthyroidism; it occurs through an autoimmune response that attacks the thyroid gland, resulting in overproduction of the thyroid hormone thyroxine.

Hashimoto's disease: inflammation of the thyroid gland that often results in hypothyroidism.

Hormones: substances secreted by glands that can regulate bodily functions, such as urinary output, cellular metabolic rate, and growth and development.

Hyperglycemia: condition that results when glucose or blood sugar becomes abnormally high. This is a relatively common event in patients with diabetes.

Hyperparathyroidism: condition that results when an overactive parathyroid gland secretes excessive parathyroid hormone, causing increased levels of circulating calcium associated with loss of calcium in the bone.

Hyperpituitarism: increased production of the pituitary hormones, particularly the human growth hormone (hGH).

Hyperplasia: enlargement of a gland.

Hyperthyroidism: abnormality of the thyroid gland in which secretion of thyroid hormone is usually increased and is no longer under the regulatory control of hypothalamic-pituitary centers.

Hypertrophy: enlargement of a gland.

Hypervitaminosis: toxicity resulting from an excess of any vitamin, especially fat-soluble vitamins such as A, D, and K.

Hypervolemia: occurs when there is too much fluid in the body.

Hypoglycemia: condition that results when glucose or blood sugar becomes abnormally low.

Hypoparathyroidism: underactive parathyroid gland that results in decreased levels of circulating calcium.

Hypopituitarism: condition caused by low levels of pituitary hormones. Hormones secreted by the pituitary gland can affect the functions of other glands.

Hypoplasia: atrophy; condition that results when a gland becomes smaller.

Hypothyroidism: condition caused by low levels of pituitary hormones. Hormones secreted by the pituitary gland can affect the functions of other glands.

Hypovolemia: occurs due to decreased plasma volume.

Iatrogenic: caused by medical treatment.

Kwashiorkor: severe type of malnutrition resulting in dyspigmentation of skin and hair, edema, and growth retardation.

Malnutrition: nutrition disorder caused by primary deprivation of protein energy caused by poverty or self-imposed starvation, or associated with deficiency diseases such as cancer.

Morbid obesity: applies to patients who are 50% to 100% or 100 pounds above their ideal body weight. A BMI of 40 or higher defines morbid obesity.

Myxedema: skin and tissue disorder that is usually due to severe prolonged hypothyroidism.

Nutritional marasmus: severe form of malnutrition that is characterized by severe tissue wasting, loss of subcutaneous fat, and maybe dehydration.

Obesity: condition defined as an increase in body weight beyond the limitation of skeletal and physical requirements, caused by excessive accumulation of fat in the body.

Secondary diabetes mellitus: form of the disease that develops as a result of another disease or condition.

Steroid-induced diabetes: diabetes that is caused by the use of steroids.

Tetany: a continuous muscle spasm.

Thyrotoxic crisis or storm: complication of hyperthyroidism associated with a sudden intensification of symptoms combined with fever, rapid pulse, and delirium.

Tumor lysis syndrome (TLS): is the development of electrolyte and metabolic disturbances that can occur after treatment of cancer, usually lymphoma and leukemia, and sometimes even without treatment.

Vitamin deficiency: condition caused by many different factors, such as poor nutrient absorption, digestive tract disorders, lifestyle issues (e.g., alcohol, smoking, medication, overexercising), chronic illness, age, and many other factors.

Volume depletion: may be the result of either dehydration or hypovolemia.

REFERENCES

1. Frazier ME, Drzymkowski JW. Essentials of Human Diseases and Conditions, 3rd ed. St. Louis: Saunders, 2004, Table 4-1, pp 150-151.
2. Chabner D. The Language of Medicine, 7th ed. St. Louis: Saunders, 2004, Table 18-13, p 745.
3. American Hospital Association. *Coding Clinic for ICD-9-CM* 1990:4Q:p17. Cystic fibrosis sequencing—Guidelines.
4. American Hospital Association. *Coding Clinic for ICD-9-CM* 2002:3Q:p21-22. ARF due to dehydration and treated with IV hydration only.
5. American Hospital Association. *Coding Clinic for ICD-9-CM* 2003:1Q:p22. Clarification—Renal failure due to dehydration with IV hydration.

13

Mental, Behavioral, and Neurodevelopmental Disorders

(ICD-10-CM Chapter 5, Codes F01-F99)

LEARNING OBJECTIVES

1. Apply and assign the correct ICD-10-CM/PCS codes in accordance with Official Guidelines for Coding and Reporting

2. Identify major differences between ICD-10-CM and ICD-9-CM related to mental disorders

3. Identify pertinent anatomy and physiology of mental, behavioral, and neurodevelopmental disorders

4. Identify various mental, behavioral, and neurodevelopmental disorders

5. Assign the correct Z codes and procedure codes related to mental, behavioral, and neurodevelopmental disorders
6. Identify common treatments and medications
7. Explain the importance of documentation in relation to MS-DRGs for reimbursement

ABBREVIATIONS/ ACRONYMS

ADD attention deficit disorder

ADHD attention deficit hyperactivity disorder

CC complication/comorbidity

DSM-IV-TR *Diagnostic and Statistical Manual of Mental Disorders, Fourth Edition, Text Revision*

DTs delirium tremens

ECT electroconvulsive therapy

ICD-9-CM *International Classification of Diseases, 9th Revision, Clinical Modification*

ICD-10-CM *International Classification of Diseases, 10th Revision, Clinical Modification*

ICD-10-PCS *International Classification of Diseases, 10th Revision, Procedure Coding System*

IQ intelligence quotient

LD learning disability/difficulty

MR mental retardation

MRCP mental retardation, cerebral palsy

MS-DRG Medicare Severity diagnosis-related group

OBS organic brain syndrome

OIG Office of the Inspector General

PKU phenylketonuria

PTSD posttraumatic stress disorder

ICD-10-CM

Official Guidelines for Coding and Reporting

Please refer to the companion Evolve website for the most current guidelines.
5. **Chapter 5: Mental, Behavioral and *Neurodevelopmental* disorders (F01-F99)**
   a. **Pain disorders related to psychological factors**
   Assign code F45.41, for pain that is exclusively **related to psychological disorders. As indicated by the Excludes 1 note under category G89, a code from category G89 should not be assigned with code F45.41**
      Code F45.42, Pain disorders with related psychological factors, should be used with a code from category G89, Pain, not elsewhere classified, if there is documentation of a psychological component for a patient with acute or chronic pain.
   See Section I.C.6. Pain

EXAMPLE Patient is receiving behavioral therapy for treatment of chronic pain syndrome with associated psychological factors, G89.4, F45.42.

---

   b. **Mental and behavioral disorders due to psychoactive substance use**
      1) **In Remission**
         Selection of codes for "in remission" for categories F10-F19, Mental and behavioral disorders due to psychoactive substance use (categories F10-F19 with -.21) requires the provider's clinical judgment. The appropriate codes for "in remission" are assigned only on the basis of provider documentation (as defined in the Official Guidelines for Coding and Reporting).

EXAMPLE Patient has a history of alcohol dependence, currently in remission, F10.21.

---

      2) **Psychoactive Substance Use, Abuse And Dependence**
         When the provider documentation refers to use, abuse and dependence of the same substance (e.g. alcohol, opioid, cannabis, etc.), only one code should be assigned to identify the pattern of use based on the following hierarchy:
         • If both use and abuse are documented, assign only the code for abuse
         • If both abuse and dependence are documented, assign only the code for dependence

> • If use, abuse and dependence are all documented, assign only the code for dependence
> • If both use and dependence are documented, assign only the code for dependence

EXAMPLE | The ER physician documents daily alcohol use. The attending documents alcohol abuse on discharge summary, F10.10.

3) Psychoactive Substance Use
As with all other diagnoses, the codes for psychoactive substance use (F10.9-, F11.9-, F12.9-, F13.9-, F14.9-, F15.9-, F16.9-) should only be assigned based on provider documentation and when they meet the definition of a reportable diagnosis (see Section III, Reporting Additional Diagnoses). The codes are to be used only when the psychoactive substance use is associated with a mental or behavioral disorder, and such a relationship is documented by the provider.

Apply General Coding Guidelines as found in Chapter 5 of this textbook and the Procedural Coding Guidelines as found in Chapters 6 and 7.

The *Diagnostic and Statistical Manual of Mental Disorders, Fourth Edition* (DSM-IV), is used by healthcare professionals to diagnose mental disorders on the basis of specific criteria. A multiaxial assessment system is used to assess clinical disorders, personality disorders and intellectual disabilities, medical conditions that may affect psychological condition, psychosocial and environmental factors (stressors such as homelessness or unemployment), and global assessment of functioning.

The DSM-IV-TR, or a text revision (TR), was published in 1996. It includes ICD-9-CM codes that should be assigned to all mental disorders and conditions. Many healthcare professionals use these ICD-9-CM codes within their documentation. These professionals may be taking the codes from the DSM-IV-TR, so it is always recommended to verify codes with the ICD-10-CM code book, to ensure accurate code assignment.

The DSM-5 is currently in development. A draft has been released for comment with an expected final publication in May 2013.

MAJOR DIFFERENCES BETWEEN ICD-10-CM AND ICD-9-CM

- ICD-10-CM does not have codes for history of drug and alcohol dependence. In ICD-10-CM, past history of drug and alcohol dependence are assigned codes for "in remission."
- There is a notation under category F10 in ICD-10-CM to use an additional code for blood alcohol level, if applicable (Y90.-).
- ICD-10-CM has expanded the nicotine abuse codes to identify the type of nicotine product (e.g., cigarettes, chewing tobacco, or other tobacco product).
- The fifth digits used to identify drug and type of alcohol usage (continuous, episodic, and unspecified) in ICD-9-CM are not applicable in ICD-10-CM.

ANATOMY AND PHYSIOLOGY

No one body system is known to cause or be affected by mental disorders because the causes of mental illness are not always known. Stress can be a contributing factor in mental disorders. Psychological issues can and do affect one's physical health.

DISEASE CONDITIONS

Mental Disorders, found in Chapter 5 in the ICD-10-CM code book, are divided into the following categories:

CATEGORY	SECTION TITLES
F01-F09	Mental disorders due to known physiological conditions
F10-F19	Mental and behavioral disorders due to psychoactive substance abuse
F20-F29	Schizophrenia, schizotypal, delusional, and other non-mood psychotic disorders
F30-F39	Mood (affective) disorders
F40-F48	Anxiety, dissociative, stress-related, somatoform, and other nonpsychotic mental disorders
F50-F59	Behavioral syndromes associated with physiological disturbances and physical factors
F60-F69	Disorders of adult personality and behavior
F70-F79	Intellectual disabilities
F80-F89	Pervasive and specific developmental disorders
F90-F98	Behavioral and emotional disorders with onset usually occurring in childhood and adolescence
F99	Unspecified mental disorder

Mental Disorders due to Known Physiological Conditions (F01-F09)

Organic psychosis occurs as the result of deterioration in the brain. It is usually progressive and irreversible, as in senile dementia and Alzheimer's disease. Organic brain damage may be produced by a variety of conditions, including arteriosclerosis, thrombi, metabolic conditions, infection, toxins, tumors, alcohol, and drugs. The onset and severity of damage depend on the cause. **Organic brain syndrome** (OBS) or disease is a general term that is used to describe the decrease in mental function caused by other physical disease(s).

Dementia

Dementia is a progressive deterioration of mental faculties that is characterized by impairment of memory and one or more cognitive impairments in areas such as language, reasoning, judgment, calculation, and problem-solving abilities. **Cognitive impairment** is a decline in mental activities associated with thinking, learning, and memory. Dementia can occur at any age but is more prevalent in the elderly. Disease processes that may be associated with dementia include the following:

- Alzheimer's disease
- Lewy body disease
- Alcoholism
- AIDS
- Parkinson's disease
- Normal pressure hydrocephalus with dementia
- Genetic or metabolic disease (e.g., thyroid)
- Toxic or traumatic injury
- Malignant disease and treatment

Although the term "senile" may be associated with those who are 65 years of age or older, it should not be assumed that because a patient is older than 65, a condition is due to senility. The physician must document within the health record the specific type of dementia. For many of the dementia codes, code assignment may depend on the presence of behavioral disturbances such as aggressiveness, combativeness, violence, or wandering off.

EXAMPLE Patient is 70 years old and has dementia with delirium, F03.90, F05.

EXAMPLE Patient is 60 years old and has senile dementia, F03.90.

EXERCISE 13-1

Assign codes to the following conditions.

1. Pre-senile dementia with depression _____
2. Organic brain syndrome _____
3. Dementia due to neurosyphilis with behavioral disturbances _____
4. Dementia due to Pick's disease _____
5. Multiple sclerosis with dementia _____
6. Postconcussion syndrome due to previous head trauma _____
7. AIDS-related dementia _____

Mental and Behavioral Disorders due to Psychoactive Substance Abuse (F10-F19)

Alcohol/Drug Dependence and Abuse and Associated Psychoses

Alcohol dependence, or alcoholism, is a chronic disease that is characterized by a strong compulsion to drink, increasing tolerance, the inability to stop drinking once the person has started, and physical dependence and withdrawal symptoms. If alcohol dependence is associated with alcoholic psychosis, drug dependence or abuse, or physical complications, all diagnoses should be coded.

Drug dependence or addiction is similar to dependence on alcohol. It includes a compulsion to take the drug, increased tolerance, an inability to stop using, and physical withdrawal if the person does not have the drug.

It may be difficult for a healthcare provider to determine whether a patient is actually dependent on alcohol or drugs, so abuse codes tend to be used more often. It is possible that a patient is dependent on one drug and is abusing another drug or alcohol. Abuse and dependence codes of different substances can be used for the same patient.

Dependence is not limited to illegal substances and can occur with prescription drugs. Because drugs have generic and brand names, and since these are used interchangeably, it may be difficult to determine which category is assigned for a particular drug dependence. A drug reference book or an Internet search can be used to determine the generic name or category of the drug.

When a patient is admitted for a medical condition, they may have a comorbidity of alcohol dependence. Along with treating the medical condition, the patient's alcohol dependence may need to be stabilized with drugs to prevent withdrawal. Because they are treating to prevent withdrawal does not mean that the patient is experiencing withdrawal and therefore withdrawal is not coded.

EXAMPLE | Alcoholic gastritis with alcohol abuse, K29.10, F10.10. Upon verification of code K29.20 in the Tabular, there are instructions to use an additional code to identify alcohol abuse and dependence.

Drug or alcohol abuse indicates a problem with the substance that occurs without craving and physical dependence. However, it is likely that substance abuse can still cause problems with work, school, and home responsibilities and can interfere with relationships.

Particularly in the emergency room setting, physicians may document that the patient is a "drug seeker" or has "drug-seeking behavior." Drug-seeking behavior is coded to F19.10, unspecified drug abuse, and Z76.5, person feigning illness.

Psychosis is an impairment in mental state by which one's perception of reality becomes distorted. It may include visual or auditory hallucinations, paranoia or delusions, personality changes, and disorganized thinking. The use of alcohol or drugs could lead to alcohol- or drug-related psychosis. Psychotic episodes vary from person to person.

> **Withdrawal state**– *see also* Dependence,
> drug by type, with withdrawal
> newborn
>   correct therapeutic substance prop-
>   erly administered P96.2
> infant of dependent mother P96.1
> therapeutic substance, neonatal P96.2

FIGURE 13-1. Cross reference for withdrawal.

Alcohol withdrawal symptoms vary in severity from mild shakiness and sweating to the worst form, **delirium tremens** (DTs). Delirium tremens may involve severe mental or neurologic changes such as delirium and/or hallucinations. This is a life-threatening condition. People who have gone through withdrawal once are more likely to have withdrawal symptoms again when they stop drinking. Seizures are also a common form of withdrawal.

When a patient is admitted for withdrawal symptoms, the withdrawal code is assigned as the principal diagnosis. In the Alphabetic Index under the term "withdrawal state," there is a cross reference to *see also* Dependence, drug by type, with withdrawal (Figure 13-1).

EXAMPLE   Seizure due to alcohol withdrawal. Patient is an alcoholic who usually drinks every day but hasn't had a drink in 2 days, F10.239, R56.9.

EXAMPLE   Patient is being treated for withdrawal due to dependence on Valium, F13.239.

Admissions to the hospital for drug psychosis are on the rise. A number of drugs can induce psychosis; cocaine and methamphetamine are the most common.

EXAMPLE   Paranoia due to methamphetamine (meth). Patient is dependent on meth, F15.259.

EXERCISE 13-2

Assign codes to the following conditions.

1. Delirium tremens due to chronic alcoholism   _____
2. Morphine-induced delirium (adverse effect)   _____
3. Addiction to heroin and OxyContin   _____
4. Cirrhosis of liver due to chronic alcoholism   _____
5. Wernicke-Korsakoff syndrome; patient is an alcoholic who has   _____
   been sober for 2 years
6. Acute alcohol intoxication with blood alcohol level of   _____
   200 mg/100 mL
7. Cocaine dependence in patient who abuses marijuana   _____

Schizophrenia, Schizotypal, Delusional, and Other Non-mood Psychotic Disorders (F20-F29)

Schizophrenia

Schizophrenia is a disorder of the brain. A person with schizophrenia may have trouble differentiating between real and unreal experiences and may not demonstrate logical thinking, normal emotional responses to others, and appropriate behavior in social situations. A genetic component is associated with the disease, in that people who have family members with the disease are more likely to exhibit the disease themselves. Schizophrenia usually has its onset during young adulthood, and it affects men and women equally. Five types of schizophrenia have been identified:

- Catatonic—withdrawn, in own world
- Paranoid—suspicious of others
- Disorganized—disorganized thought process, unable to communicate coherently
- Undifferentiated—mixed types of schizophrenia
- Residual—has milder symptoms that come and go

EXAMPLE | The patient has been in a chronic catatonic state of schizophrenia, F20.2.

Schizoaffective Disorders

Schizoaffective disorder is a condition in which a person experiences a combination of schizophrenia symptoms while exhibiting mood disorder symptoms, such as mania or depression. It can be difficult to differentiate a schizoaffective disorder from schizophrenia and from a mood disorder. Also, symptoms of schizoaffective disorder vary and may range from mild to severe.

Symptoms of schizoaffective disorder may include:

Depression
- Poor appetite
- Weight loss or gain
- Changes in sleeping patterns
- Agitation or restlessness
- Lack of energy
- Loss of interest in usual activities
- Feelings of worthlessness or hopelessness
- Guilt or self-blame
- Inability to think or concentrate
- Thoughts of death or suicide

Mania
- Increased activity (e.g., work, social, and sexual activity)
- Increased and/or rapid talking
- Rapid or racing thoughts
- Little need for sleep
- Agitation or restlessness
- Inflated self-esteem
- Distractibility
- Self-destructive or dangerous behavior (spending sprees, driving recklessly, or unsafe sex)

Schizophrenia
- Delusions
- Hallucinations
- Disorganized thinking
- Odd or unusual behavior
- Slow movements or total immobility
- Lack of emotion in facial expression and speech
- Poor motivation
- Problems with speech and communication

EXAMPLE | Patient is being treated as an outpatient for schizoaffective disorder with depression, F25.1.

Assign codes to the following conditions.

1. Paranoid schizophrenia   _____
2. Delusional disorder   _____
3. Schizo affective disorder, mixed type   _____

Mood [Affective] Disorders (F30-F39)

Mood Disorders

Mood disorders occur when a change in mood has been present for a prolonged time. The two most common mood disorders (**affective disorders**) are major depression and bipolar disorder (manic-depressive illness). Mood disorders can be triggered by a life event or by a chemical imbalance. The type of depression that is included in categories F32-F33 is different than depression, not otherwise specified (F32.9). **Bipolar disorder** is characterized by mood swings. Onset of symptoms is most likely to occur in early adulthood. A person with bipolar can have four main types of mood "episodes":

1. **Depression**—a feeling of sadness that can go on for a long period of time; lack of enjoyment of the things one would normally do
2. **Mania**—the other side of depression, in which a person feels so good, it is like a "high"; may do risky things
3. **Hypomania**—milder form of mania, but this "feel good" mood can change to depression or mania
4. **Mixed mood**—alternating between mania and depression, very quickly

Major depressive disorder is characterized by one or more major depressive episodes with a history of mania, hypomania, or mixed episodes. In major depression, more numerous symptoms of depression may be present, and usually, the symptoms are more severe. Major depression is most likely to occur in persons between the ages of 25 and 44; an episode may last from 6 to 9 months.

EXAMPLE   The patient was diagnosed with major depressive disorder of moderate severity, single episode, F32.1.

EXAMPLE   The patient is in a severe manic phase of bipolar I disorder, F31.13.

Assign codes to the following conditions.

1. Bipolar disorder, currently depressed   _____
2. Major depressive disorder, recurrent   _____
3. Bipolar disorder in full remission   _____
4. Bipolar II disorder   _____

Anxiety, Dissociative, Stress-related, Somatoform, and Other Nonpsychotic Mental Disorders (F40-F48)

Anxiety Disorders

Following is a breakdown of the different types of anxiety disorders:

- Generalized anxiety disorder
- Panic disorder

- Phobias
- Posttraumatic stress disorder

Most people experience mild anxiety and nervousness at various times during their lives, such as during a job interview, a business presentation, or social events.

Generalized anxiety disorder refers to chronic, exaggerated worry, tension, and irritability that may occur without cause or may be more intense than is warranted by the situation. Physical symptoms include restlessness, sleeping problems, headache, trembling, twitching, muscle tension, and sweating.

Panic disorder is a terrifying experience that occurs suddenly without warning. Physical symptoms include pounding heart, chest pains, dizziness, nausea, shortness of breath, trembling, choking, fear of dying, sweating, feelings of unreality, numbness, hot flashes or chills, and a feeling of going out of control or "crazy." Because panic attacks are unpredictable, many people live in fear of when the next one will occur.

Phobias are irrational anxieties or fears that can interfere with one's everyday life or daily routine. For example, if fear of heights would keep a person from visiting relatives who live on the 13th floor of an apartment building, the fear is excessive and disproportionate to the situation. A person without a phobia but with a fear of heights would still be able to go to visit the relatives. If situations are avoided because of fear, or if fear prevents one from enjoying life or preoccupies one's thinking, hindering ability to work, sleep, or do other things, then it becomes irrational.

Posttraumatic stress disorder (PTSD) is an anxiety disorder that is triggered by memories of a traumatic event. This disorder commonly affects survivors of traumatic events, such as sexual or physical assault, war, torture, a natural disaster, an automobile accident, or an airplane crash. In addition, PTSD can affect rescue workers at the site of an airplane crash or a mass shooting or someone who witnessed a tragic accident.

EXAMPLE   The patient suffers from agoraphobia, F40.00.

EXAMPLE   The patient has generalized anxiety, F41.1.

Conversion disorder is a condition in which a person has some type of sensory or motor (neurologic) symptom(s) that cannot be explained. These physical symptom(s) appear suddenly and may be the result of psychological stress or emotional conflict. Three criteria must be met to diagnose a conversion disorder:

- Neurological disease is ruled out
- Feigning illness is ruled out
- Psychological stress or emotional conflict is determined

Conversion disorder can present with many neurological symptoms. The following are some common symptoms:

- Weakness or paralysis of an extremity or the entire body (also known as hysterical paralysis)
- Vision impairment (hysterical blindness) or hearing impairment
- Alteration of sensation
- Impairment or loss of speech (hysterical aphonia)
- Psychogenic nonepileptic seizures
- Various movement disorders
- Problems with gait
- Fainting

EXAMPLE   Following numerous tests, the patient was diagnosed with conversion disorder with seizures, F44.5.

EXERCISE 13-5

Assign codes to the following conditions.

1. Obsessive-compulsive disorder   _____
2. Posttraumatic stress syndrome   _____
3. Panic attack   _____
4. Fear of thunderstorms   _____
5. Hysterical blindness   _____

Behavioral Syndromes Associated with Physiological Disturbances and Physical Factors (F50-F59)

Eating Disorders

Eating disorders refer to a group of conditions characterized by abnormal eating habits that may affect an individual's physical and psychological well-being. The most common disorders include:

■ Binge-eating disorder, characterized by eating binges without compensatory behavior.

■ Bulimia nervosa, is characterized by eating binges followed by compensatory behavior such as purging (self-induced vomiting, fasting, excessive use of laxatives/diuretics, and/or excessive exercise)

■ Anorexia nervosa, characterized by an unhealthy body weight and the fear of gaining weight. It is not about the food but is an unhealthy means of coping with emotional issues.

These disorders can have serious physical consequences and may even be life-threatening. Treatments for eating disorders usually involve psychotherapy, including family counseling, nutrition education, medications, and even hospitalization.

Sexual Problems

Sexual problems may be due to organic or medical conditions or to psychological dysfunction. Alcohol and drug use can also affect sexual function. After medical problems have been ruled out, a psychological cause can be explored.

EXAMPLE | Patient is treated for impotence due to psychogenic cause, F52.21.

EXAMPLE | Patient treated for erectile dysfunction, N52.9.

If a patient has erectile dysfunction it has to be specified as due to psychogenic causes to be coded to F52.21.

EXAMPLE | Patient is being seen for psychogenic dyspareunia, F52.6.

EXAMPLE | Female patient is being seen for dyspareunia, N94.1.

EXERCISE 13-6

Assign codes to the following conditions.

1. Anorexia nervosa with binging/purging _____

2. Adult patient was seen in the clinic because of pagophagia; _____
   tests were ordered to evaluate for iron deficiency anemia

3. Night terrors _____

4. Laxative abuse _____

Disorders of Adult Personality and Behavior (F60-F69)

Personality Disorders

A **personality disorder** is a pattern of behavior that can disrupt many aspects of a person's life. Personality disorders range from mild to severe and are often exacerbated during times of stress or external pressure. If a personality disorder is associated with neuroses, psychosis, or a physical condition, this should be coded. Personality disorders are divided into three clusters:

1. Cluster A—patients appear odd or eccentric, socially awkward
   * Paranoid—are suspicious of and do not trust others
   * Schizoid—loners who lack or do not show emotion
   * Schizotypal—seek isolation
2. Cluster B—patients appear dramatic, emotional, or erratic
   * Antisocial—disregard and tend to violate the rights of others, fail to conform to societal norms
   * Borderline—have difficulty coping with minor stress, have unstable relationships, and are self-destructive
   * Histrionic—are overly dramatic with a need to be the center of attention
   * Narcissistic—have an inflated sense of self-importance
3. Cluster C—patients appear anxious and fearful
   * Avoidant—avoid social situations because of fear of criticism, disapproval, or rejection; view themselves as inferior
   * Dependent—rely on others to make decisions for them; fear losing the support and approval of others
   * Obsessive-compulsive—are excessively preoccupied with orderliness, perfection, and mental and interpersonal control

EXAMPLE   Patient has an obsessive-compulsive personality disorder, F60.5.

EXAMPLE   Patient has a passive-aggressive personality, F60.89.

Sexual Disorder

Sexual activities that are not practiced by the majority of the population have been characterized as "deviant" or "variant" behavior. Although some may experiment with a variety of sexual behaviors, it is not until a person begins to rely on the deviant behavior as a means of sexual gratification that it becomes a more permanent trait. "Unconventional" sexual behaviors or paraphilias are coded to category 302 and include some of the following:

Transvestism—assuming the appearance, manner, or roles traditionally associated with members of the opposite sex (cross-dressing)

Exhibitionism—recurrent intense sexual urges and fantasies of exposing the genitals to an unsuspecting stranger

Fetishism—recurrent intense sexual urges and fantasies of using inanimate objects for sexual arousal or orgasm. Objects commonly used include female clothing such as shoes, earrings, or undergarments

Voyeurism—recurrent intense sexual urges and fantasies involving observing unsuspecting people who are naked, disrobing, or engaging in sexual activity

Sadism—the act or sense of gaining pleasure from inflicting physical or psychological pain on another

Masochism—the act or sense of gaining pleasure from experiencing physical or psychological pain

---

EXAMPLE   Patient is an exhibitionist, F65.2.

EXERCISE 13-7

Assign codes to the following conditions.

1. Borderline personality   _____
2. Pedophile   _____
3. Kleptomania   _____
4. Voyeurism   _____

Intellectual Disabilities (F70-F79)

Mental retardation (MR) is a disorder in which a person's overall intellectual functioning is well below average, and intelligence quotient (IQ) is around 70 or less. Mental retardation is a subtype of intellectual disability. The term intellectual disability is now preferred instead of mental retardation. Rosa's Law was passed on October 6, 2010, which required replacing the term mental retardation with intellectual disability in United States official documents. Individuals with intellectual disability also may have a significantly impaired ability to cope with common life demands and lack some of the daily living skills that are expected of people in their age group and culture. Impairment may interfere with learning, communication, self-care, independent living, social interaction, play, work, and safety. It appears in childhood, before age 18. There are a variety of causes for intellectual disability; however, often the cause is not documented. Causes of intellectual disability are discussed in the following paragraphs.

Genetic Causes

■ Defective genes, as in Fragile X syndrome, which is the most common inherited cause of intellectual disability

■ Chromosomal disorders such as Down's syndrome that are characterized by an abnormal number of chromosomes

■ Congenital hypothyroidism, which can result in intellectual disability and stunted growth if the patient is not treated with thyroid replacement

■ Inborn errors of metabolism may result in intellectual disability. More than 300 gene disorders involve inborn errors of metabolism. These include the following:
   • Phenylketonuria (PKU)
   • Tay-Sachs disease
   • Galactosemia
   • Homocystinuria
   • Maple syrup urine disease
   • Biotinidase deficiency

External Causes

■ During pregnancy, the following factors can result in intellectual disability:
   • Malnutrition
   • Mother's use of alcohol and drugs

- Environmental toxins such as lead and mercury
- Viral infections such as rubella and cytomegalovirus
- Untreated diabetes mellitus
◼ During birth, the following conditions can result in intellectual disability:
- Low birth weight
- Premature birth
- Deprivation of oxygen
◼ After birth, the following conditions can result in intellectual disability:
- Complications from infectious diseases such as measles, chickenpox, and whooping cough
- Exposure to lead and mercury
- Accidental injury to the brain
- Severe child abuse
- Poverty

At the beginning of this section, instructions state an additional code(s) should be assigned to identify any associated psychiatric or physical condition(s). A number of congenital syndromes may have some form of associated intellectual disability. The most common severity level is mild mental retardation; 85% of those affected have the mild type.

ICD-10-CM codes for intellectual disability are classified by IQ, as follows:

IQ 50-55 to 70	Mild intellectual disability
IQ 35-40 to 50-55	Moderate intellectual disability
IQ 20-25 to 35-40	Severe intellectual disability
IQ below 20-25	Profound intellectual disability

Documentation of intellectual disability in the health record may not include the IQ, but the condition often is described by severity.

EXAMPLE	Fragile X syndrome with mild intellectual disability, Q99.2, F70.

EXAMPLE	MRCP with IQ of 45, G80.9, F71.

EXERCISE 13-8

Assign codes to the following conditions.

1. Shaken baby syndrome with profound intellectual disability; injury happened 2 years ago   _____

2. Trisomy 21 with moderate intellectual disability   _____

3. Severe intellectual disability due to Angelman's syndrome   _____

4. Mild intellectual disability due to Lesch-Nyhan syndrome   _____

5. Cerebral palsy with intellectual disability   _____

Pervasive and Specific Developmental Disorders and Behavioral (F80-F89) and Emotional Disorders With Onset Usually Occurring in Childhood and Adolescence (F90-F98)

Learning Disorders

Learning disabilities or differences (LDs) affect a person's ability to understand or use spoken or written language (**dyslexia**), to do mathematical calculations (**dyscalculia**), to coordinate movements such as writing (**dysgraphia**), or to direct attention. Although LDs may occur in very young children, these disorders usually are not recognized until the child reaches school age.

EXAMPLE Patient's test results show a developmental mathematics disorder, F81.2.

Attention Deficit Disorder

Attention deficit disorder (ADD) and **attention deficit hyperactivity disorder** (ADHD) are common childhood disorders. ADHD and ADD are not learning disabilities, but they are characterized by inattention, hyperactivity, and impulsivity. Three subtypes of ADHD have been identified:

1. Hyperactive/impulsive type—patient does not show significant inattention
2. Inattentive type—patient does not show significant hyperactive-impulsive behavior; sometimes called ADD
3. Combined type—patient displays both inattentive and hyperactive-impulsive symptoms

Other disorders that sometimes accompany ADHD include Tourette's syndrome, oppositional defiant disorder, conduct disorder, anxiety and depression, and bipolar disorder. Attention deficit hyperactivity disorder continues into adulthood in about 50% of persons with childhood ADHD.

EXAMPLE Patient takes medication for ADHD, combined type, F90.2.

Oppositional Defiant Disorder

Oppositional defiant disorder is defined as a pattern of uncooperative, defiant, and hostile behavior toward authority figures that does not involve major antisocial violations, is not normal for the patient's developmental stage, and results in significant functional impairment. A certain level of oppositional behavior is common in children and adolescents. It should be considered a disorder only when behaviors are more frequent and intense than in unaffected peers, and when they cause dysfunction in social, academic, or work-related arenas.

EXERCISE 13-9

Assign codes to the following conditions.

1. Attention deficit disorder with overactivity _____
2. Dyslexia, developmental _____
3. Asperger's syndrome _____
4. Conduct disorder _____

FACTORS INFLUENCING HEALTH STATUS AND CONTACT WITH HEALTH SERVICES (Z CODES)

As discussed in Chapter 8, it may be difficult for the coder to locate Z codes in the index. Coders often say, "I did not know there was a Z code for that." Refer to Chapter 8 for a listing of common main terms used to locate Z codes.

A review of the Tabular reveals that some Z codes pertain to mental and behavioral disorders.

Z02.83	Encounter for blood-alcohol and blood-drug test
Z04.6	Encounter for general psychiatric examination, requested by authority
Z13.4	Encounter for screening for certain developmental disorders in childhood

Z55.0	Illiteracy and low-level literacy
Z55.1	Schooling unavailable and unattainable
Z55.2	Failed school examinations
Z55.3	Underachievement in school
Z55.4	Educational maladjustment and discord with teachers and classmates
Z55.8	Other problems related to education and literacy
Z55.9	Problems related to education and literacy, unspecified
Z56.0	Unemployment, unspecified
Z56.1	Change of job
Z56.2	Threat of job loss
Z56.3	Stressful work schedule
Z56.4	Discord with boss and workmates
Z56.5	Uncongenial work environment
Z56.6	Other physical and mental strain related to work
Z56.81	Sexual harassment on the job
Z56.82	Military deployment status
Z56.89	Other problems related to employment
Z56.9	Unspecified problems related to employment
Z59.0	Homelessness
Z59.1	Inadequate housing
Z59.2	Discord with neighbors, lodgers, and landlord
Z59.3	Problems related to living in residential institution
Z59.4	Lack of adequate food and safe drinking water
Z59.5	Extreme poverty
Z59.6	Low income
Z59.7	Insufficient social insurance and welfare support
Z59.8	Other problems related to housing and economic circumstances
Z59.9	Problem related to housing and economic circumstances, unspecified
Z60.0	Problems of adjustment to life-cycle transitions
Z60.2	Problems related to living alone
Z60.3	Acculturation difficulty
Z60.4	Social exclusion and rejection
Z60.5	Target of (perceived) adverse discrimination and persecution
Z60.8	Other problems related to social environment
Z60.9	Problem related to social environment, unspecified
Z62.0	Inadequate parental supervision and control
Z62.1	Parental overprotection
Z62.21	Child in welfare custody
Z62.22	Institutional upbringing
Z62.29	Other upbringing away from parents
Z62.3	Hostility towards and scapegoating of child
Z62.6	Inappropriate (excessive) parental pressure
Z62.810	Personal history of physical and sexual abuse in childhood
Z62.811	Personal history of psychological abuse in childhood
Z62.812	Personal history of neglect in childhood
Z62.819	Personal history of unspecified abuse in childhood
Z62.820	Parent-biological child conflict
Z62.821	Parent-adopted child conflict
Z62.822	Parent-foster child conflict
Z62.890	Parent-child estrangement NEC
Z62.891	Sibling rivalry
Z62.898	Other specified problems related to upbringing

Z62.9	Problem related to upbringing, unspecified
Z63.0	Problems in relationship with spouse or partner
Z63.1	Problems in relationship with in-laws
Z63.31	Absence of family member due to military deployment
Z63.32	Other absence of family member
Z63.4	Disappearance and death of family member
Z63.5	Disruption of family by separation and divorce
Z63.6	Dependent relative needing care at home
Z63.71	Stress on family due to return of family member from military deployment
Z63.72	Alcoholism and drug addiction in family
Z63.79	Other stressful life events affecting family and household
Z63.8	Other specified problems related to primary support group
Z63.9	Problem related to primary support group, unspecified
Z64.0	Problems related to unwanted pregnancy
Z64.1	Problems related to multiparity
Z64.4	Discord with counselors
Z65.0	Conviction in civil and criminal proceedings without imprisonment
Z65.1	Imprisonment and other incarceration
Z65.2	Problems related to release from prison
Z65.3	Problems related to other legal circumstances
Z65.4	Victim of crime and terrorism
Z65.5	Exposure to disaster, war, and other hostilities
Z65.8	Other specified problems related to psychosocial circumstances
Z65.9	Problem related to unspecified psychosocial circumstances
Z69.010	Encounter for mental health services for victim of parental child abuse
Z69.011	Encounter for mental health services for perpetrator of parental child abuse
Z69.020	Encounter for mental health services for victim of nonparental child abuse
Z69.021	Encounter for mental health services for perpetrator of nonparental child abuse
Z69.11	Encounter for mental health services for victim of spousal or partner abuse
Z69.12	Encounter for mental health services for perpetrator of spousal or partner abuse
Z69.81	Encounter for mental health services for victim of other abuse
Z69.82	Encounter for mental health services for perpetrator of other abuse
Z70.0	Counseling related to sexual attitude
Z70.1	Counseling related to patient's sexual behavior and orientation
Z70.2	Counseling related to sexual behavior and orientation of third party
Z70.3	Counseling related to combined concerns regarding sexual attitude, behavior, and orientation
Z70.8	Other sex counseling
Z70.9	Sex counseling, unspecified
Z71.41	Alcohol abuse counseling and surveillance of alcoholic
Z71.42	Counseling for family member of alcoholic
Z71.51	Drug abuse counseling and surveillance of drug abuser
Z71.52	Counseling for family member of drug abuser
Z71.6	Tobacco abuse counseling
Z71.81	Spiritual or religious counseling
Z71.89	Other specified counseling
Z71.9	Counseling, unspecified
Z72.0	Tobacco use
Z72.3	Lack of physical exercise
Z72.4	Inappropriate diet and eating habits
Z72.51	High-risk heterosexual behavior
Z72.52	High-risk homosexual behavior

Z72.53	High-risk bisexual behavior
Z72.6	Gambling and betting
Z72.810	Child and adolescent antisocial behavior
Z72.811	Adult antisocial behavior
Z72.820	Sleep deprivation
Z72.821	Inadequate sleep hygiene
Z72.89	Other problems related to lifestyle
Z72.9	Problem related to lifestyle, unspecified
Z73.0	Burn-out
Z73.1	Type A behavior pattern
Z73.2	Lack of relaxation and leisure
Z73.3	Stress, not elsewhere classified
Z73.4	Inadequate social skills, not elsewhere classified
Z73.5	Social role conflict, not elsewhere classified
Z73.6	Limitation of activities due to disability
Z73.810	Behavioral insomnia of childhood, sleep-onset association type
Z73.811	Behavioral insomnia of childhood, limit-setting type
Z73.812	Behavioral insomnia of childhood, combined type
Z73.819	Behavioral insomnia of childhood, unspecified type
Z73.82	Dual sensory impairment
Z73.89	Other problems related to life management difficulty
Z73.9	Problem related to life management difficulty, unspecified
Z76.5	Malingerer [conscious simulation]
Z81.0	Family history of intellectual disability
Z81.1	Family history of alcohol abuse and dependence
Z81.2	Family history of tobacco abuse and dependence
Z81.3	Family history of other psychoactive substance abuse and dependence
Z81.4	Family history of other substance abuse and dependence
Z81.8	Family history of other mental and behavioral disorders
Z87.890	Personal history of sex reassignment
Z87.891	Personal history of nicotine dependence
Z91.410	Personal history of adult physical and sexual abuse
Z91.411	Personal history of adult psychological abuse
Z91.412	Personal history of adult neglect
Z91.419	Personal history of unspecified adult abuse
Z91.49	Other personal history of psychological trauma, not elsewhere classified
Z91.5	Personal history of self-harm

EXAMPLE Adjustment disorder with depressed mood due to unemployment, F43.21, Z56.0.

EXAMPLE Counseling regarding marital problems, Z71.89.

EXERCISE 13-10

Assign codes to the following conditions.

1. Screening for depression _____
2. Malingerer _____
3. Examination for blood alcohol test _____

4. Counseling for mother and son due to son's ADHD   _____

5. Laboratory testing (liver function tests) on patient who takes   _____
   Cognex for Alzheimer's disease with dementia

COMMON TREATMENTS

Many of the mental disorders can be treated with psychotherapy. Often, a combination of psychotherapy and medication is necessary for effective treatment.

CONDITION	MEDICATIONS
Dementia	Depends on type of dementia
Alcohol withdrawal	Benzodiazepam, such as diazepam (Valium) or chlordiazepoxide (Librium or Libritabs), may be used to reduce anxiety
	Multivitamin; thiamine and folate
	Beta blockers such as propranolol (Inderal) or atenolol (Tenormin) reduce heart rate and tremors
	Phenytoin (Dilantin), carbamazepine (Tegretol), and divalproex sodium (Depakote) are antiseizure medications that can be used to treat or prevent seizures
Drug withdrawal	Treatment would depend on the drug
Schizophrenia	Often requires a combination of antipsychotic, antidepressant, and antianxiety medications such as haloperidol (Haldol), chlorpromazine (Thorazine), thioridazine (Mellaril), fluphenazine (Prolixin), Serentil, Seroquel, Clozaril, and Zyprexa
Depression	Antidepressants such as fluoxetine (Prozac), paroxetine (Paxil), sertraline hydrochloride (Zoloft), citalopram hydrobromide (Celexa), nefazodone (Serzone), mirtazapine (Remeron), venlafaxine (Effexor), and bupropion hydrochloride (Wellbutrin)
Bipolar disorder	Medications include lithium; anticonvulsants such as carbamazepine (Tegretol), divalproex sodium (Depakote), gabapentin (Neurontin), and lamotrigine (Lamictal); antidepressants such as bupropion hydrochloride (Wellbutrin) or sertraline hydrochloride (Zoloft); neuroleptics (e.g., Haldol); and benzodiazepines (e.g., lorazepam)
Anxiety	Diazepam (Valium), lorazepam (Ativan), clorazepate (Tranxene), alprazolam (Xanax), paroxetine (Paxil), buspirone (Buspar)
Panic disorder	Alprazolam (Xanax), paroxetine (Paxil)
Phobias	Amitriptyline (Elavil), desipramine (Norpramin), imipramine (Tofranil), nortriptyline (Pamelor), phenelzine (Nardil)
PTSD	Medications to reduce anxiety, depression, and insomnia associated with PTSD
ADD/ADHD	Methylphenidate (Ritalin, Concerta), amphetamine dextroamphetamine (Adderall), pemoline (Cylert), atomoxetine (Strattera)

PROCEDURES

Procedures related to mental disorders in ICD-10-PCS can be located in the following tables:

GZ1-GZJ	Mental Health
HZ2-HZ9	Substance Abuse

Some procedures would be appropriate for mental disorders such as detoxification and/or rehabilitation for alcohol and drug abuse. Sometimes, a patient's medical condition is stabilized in a hospital setting, and then the patient is transferred to a facility that is better equipped to offer specialized mental health care. Facility policy may determine which procedures are coded or provided by the facility.

Electroconvulsive Therapy

Electroconvulsive therapy (ECT) is a treatment in which electricity is used to induce seizures. The procedure root type is electroconvulsive therapy. ECT is usually only considered when patients have not responded well to drug therapies. It is primarily used to treat severe depression and other disorders such as schizophrenia, mania, or catatonia. A course of treatments usually consists of 6-12 treatments, but may be more or may be less.

Detoxification and Rehabilitation

Detoxification is the active management of withdrawal symptoms in a patient who is physically dependent on alcohol or drugs. The procedure root type for detoxification is detoxification services. It consists of evaluation, observation, and monitoring, along with administration of thiamine, multivitamins, and other medications as needed. Detoxification for alcohol may require a 4- to 5-day period; depending on the drug, it may go on for days or months.

Rehabilitation is a structured program with the goal to stop and recover from the use of alcohol and/or drugs. The procedure root type for rehabilitation is counseling and/or psychotherapy. Many different types of programs are available in a variety of settings; these include inpatient, outpatient, day treatment, residential treatment, half-way houses, and so forth.

Facility policy will determine the coding of these procedures. In the hospital setting, a patient may be treated to prevent alcohol and drug withdrawal, or to alleviate symptoms of withdrawal, but this may not constitute true detoxification.

EXERCISE 13-11

Assign codes for all diagnoses and procedures.

1. Electroconvulsive therapy for schizophrenia   _____

2. Detoxification and rehabilitation (12-step group counseling)   _____
   for chronic alcoholism, continuous

3. Detoxification for heroin dependence, daily use   _____

DOCUMENTATION/REIMBURSEMENT/MS-DRGs

Often, coding difficulties are due to lack of documentation. Sometimes test results are not available at the time of discharge or when the physician is dictating the discharge summary or is reporting the final diagnoses.

In the inpatient setting, mental health disorders are often secondary to a more acute medical condition. Many physicians are vague in their descriptions of mental disorders. They may not say that a patient is dependent on drugs or alcohol and may document the condition as drug and/or alcohol abuse. A number of patients are being treated for depression and are on medications. The F32.9 depression code is often used because of insufficient documentation regarding whether this is an adjustment disorder, a single episode, recurrent, and/or a mood disorder. If they are available, the coder should review consultation reports from the psychologist or the psychiatrist for more specific diagnoses. The coder may need to query the physician to get needed documentation and assign the most appropriate diagnosis code. The presence of an MCC (major complication/comorbidity) or CC (complication/comorbidity) can make a difference in reimbursement, depending on the principal diagnosis and the MS-DRG assigned.

Frequently missed complications/comorbidities from this chapter include the following:

- Alcohol withdrawal
- Drug withdrawal
- Major depressive disorder
- Autism

Detoxification and Rehabilitation

EXAMPLE

The patient is admitted for detoxification and rehabilitation (Group 12-step) of heroin and alcohol dependence. The patient uses $30 of heroin per day and drinks 1 quart of wine every day. No IV drug use.

DIAGNOSES	CODES	MS-DRG	RW
Heroin and alcohol dependence Detox/Rehab	F11.20 F10.20 HZ2ZZZZ, HZ43ZZ	895	1.0952
Heroin and alcohol dependence Detox only	F11.20 F10.20 HZ2ZZZZ	897	0.6687

It is important to code the appropriate procedure code to include both the detoxification and rehabilitation if performed, as it may affect MS-DRG assignment.

CHAPTER REVIEW EXERCISE

Assign codes for all diagnoses and procedures.

1. Dysthymic disorder _____
2. Panic disorder with agoraphobia _____
3. Fragile X syndrome with IQ of 25; family history of intellectual disability _____
4. Inhalant abuse _____
5. Tourette's syndrome _____
6. Malnutrition due to anorexia nervosa _____
7. History of alcoholism with 1 year of sobriety _____
8. Intellectual disability due to chickenpox 2 years ago _____
9. Alcoholic cardiomyopathy _____
10. Holiday heart syndrome with atrial fibrillation; patient had a drinking binge over Labor Day weekend, history of alcohol abuse _____
11. Depression with anxiety _____
12. Social phobia _____
13. Dementia with wandering _____
14. Adjustment disorder with conduct disturbance due to parents' divorce _____
15. Hypochondria _____
16. Gambling addiction _____
17. Psychogenic asthma _____
18. Pica in an adult patient _____
19. Enuresis, psychogenic _____
20. Fear of flying _____
21. Adult patient with history of emotional abuse _____

22. Parkinson's disease with dementia and related behavioral disturbances   _____

23. Suicidal ideation   _____

24. Unable to tolerate CT scan due to claustrophobia   _____

Write the correct answer(s) in the space(s) provided.

25. Which procedure code groups into the higher paying MS-DRG in the Detoxification and Rehabilitation example?

_____

26. List four types of Cluster B personality disorders.

_____

_____

_____

_____

27. When are learning disabilities usually recognized?

_____

28. List four causes of intellectual disability.

_____

_____

_____

_____

CHAPTER GLOSSARY

Affective disorders: a category of mental health problems that include major depressive disorders and bipolar disorders.

Attention deficit disorder: a common childhood disorder characterized by inattention and impulsivity.

Attention deficit hyperactivity disorder: a common childhood disorder characterized by inattention, hyperactivity, and impulsivity.

Bipolar disorder: brain disorder that causes unusual shifts in a person's mood, energy, and ability to function; different from the normal ups and downs that everyone goes through; symptoms of bipolar disorder can be severe.

Cognitive impairment: a decline in mental activities associated with thinking, learning, and memory.

Conversion disorder: condition in which a person has some type of sensory or motor (neurologic) symptom(s) that cannot be explained.

Delirium tremens: life-threatening condition that may involve severe mental or neurologic changes such as delirium and/or hallucinations.

Dementia: progressive deterioration of mental faculties characterized by impairment of memory and one or more cognitive impairments such as language, reasoning and judgment, and calculation and problem-solving abilities.

Depression: affective disorder that is characterized by sadness, lack of interest in everyday activities and events, and a sense of worthlessness.

Detoxification: active management of withdrawal symptoms in a patient who is physically dependent on alcohol or drugs.

Dyscalculia: learning disability that affects a child's ability to do mathematical calculations.

Dysgraphia: learning disability that affects a child's ability to coordinate movements such as writing.

Dyslexia: learning disability that affects a child's ability to understand or use spoken or written language.

Eating disorders: a group of conditions characterized by abnormal eating habits that may affect an individual's physical and psychological well-being. The most common eating disorders are binge-eating disorder, bulimia nervosa, and anorexia nervosa.

Electroconvulsive therapy: psychiatric treatment in which electricity is used to induce seizures.

Exhibitionism: recurrent intense sexual urges and fantasies of exposing the genitals to an unsuspecting stranger.

Fetishism: recurrent intense sexual urges and fantasies of using inanimate objects for sexual arousal or orgasm. Objects commonly used include female clothing such as shoes, earrings, or undergarments.

Generalized anxiety disorder: chronic, exaggerated worry, tension, and irritability that may be without cause or may be more intense than the situation warrants.

Hypomania: milder form of mania, but this "feel good" mood can change to depression or mania.

Intellectual disabilities: disorder in which a person's overall intellectual functioning is well below average, with an intelligence quotient (IQ) around 70 or less.

Major depressive disorder: characterized by one or more major depressive episodes with a history of mania, hypomania, or mixed episodes.

Mania: the other side of depression, in which a person feels so good, it is like a "high"; may do risky things.

Masochism: the act or sense of gaining pleasure from experiencing physical or psychological pain.

Mental retardation: a disorder in which a person's overall intellectual functioning is well below average, and intelligence quotient (IQ) is around 70 or less.

Mixed mood: alternating between mania and depression, very quickly.

Mood disorder: condition that occurs with a change in mood over a prolonged period.

Oppositional defiant disorder: pattern of uncooperative, defiant, and hostile behavior toward authority figures that does not involve major antisocial violations, is not accounted for by the child's developmental stage, and results in significant functional impairment.

Organic brain syndrome: general term used to describe a decrease in mental function due to other physical disease(s).

Panic disorder: terrifying experience that occurs suddenly without warning. Physical symptoms include pounding heart, chest pains, dizziness, nausea, shortness of breath, trembling, choking, fear of dying, sweating, feelings of unreality, numbness, hot flashes or chills, and a feeling of going out of control or "crazy."

Personality disorder: a pattern of behavior that can disrupt many aspects of a person's life.

Phobia: irrational anxiety or fear that can interfere with one's everyday life or daily routine.

Posttraumatic stress disorder: anxiety disorder that is triggered by memories of a traumatic event.

Psychosis: impairment in mental state in which perception of reality has become distorted.

Rehabilitation: structured program with the goal of stopping and recovering from the use of alcohol and/or drugs.

Sadism: the act or sense of gaining pleasure from inflicting physical or psychological pain on another.

Schizoaffective disorder: condition in which a person experiences a combination of schizophrenia symptoms while exhibiting mood disorder symptoms, such as mania or depression.

Schizophrenia: disorder of the brain characterized by trouble differentiating between real and unreal experiences, along with problems with logical thinking, normal emotional responses to others, and appropriate behavior in social situations.

Transvestism: assuming the appearance, manner, or roles traditionally associated with members of the opposite sex (cross-dressing).

Voyeurism: recurrent intense sexual urges and fantasies involving observing unsuspecting people who are naked, disrobing, or engaging in sexual activity.

14

Diseases of the Nervous System, Diseases of the Eye and Adnexa, and Diseases of the Ear and Mastoid Process

(ICD-10-CM Chapter 6, Codes G00-G99, Chapter 7, Codes H00-H59, and Chapter 8, Codes H60-H95)

Vagal Nerve Stimulation
Photodynamic Therapy
Cataract Extraction

Documentation/Reimbursement/MS-DRGs
Causative Organism
Shunt Revision

Chapter Review Exercise
Chapter Glossary

LEARNING OBJECTIVES

1. Apply and assign the correct ICD-10-CM/PCS codes in accordance with Official Guidelines for Coding and Reporting

2. Identify major differences between ICD-10-CM and ICD-9-CM related to the nervous system and sense organs

3. Identify pertinent anatomy and physiology of the nervous system and sense organs

4. Identify diseases of the nervous system and sense organs

5. Assign the correct Z codes and procedure codes related to the nervous system and sense organs

6. Identify common treatments, medications, laboratory values, and diagnostic tests

7. Explain the importance of documentation in relation to MS-DRGs for reimbursement

ABBREVIATIONS/ ACRONYMS

CNS central nervous system

CPAP continuous positive airway pressure

CSF cerebrospinal fluid

CVA cerebrovascular accident

DBS deep brain stimulation

EEG electroencephalogram

EMG electromyelogram

ICD-9-CM *International Classification of Diseases, 9th Revision, Clinical Modification*

ICD-10-CM *International Classification of Diseases, 10th Revision, Clinical Modification*

ICD-10-PCS *International Classification of Diseases, 10th Revision, Procedure Coding System*

IOL intraocular lens

IOP intraocular pressure

IV intravenous

LP lumbar puncture

MCI mild cognitive impairment

MRI magnetic resonance imaging

MS-DRG Medicare Severity diagnosis-related group

NPH normal pressure hydrocephalus

OM otitis media

OSA obstructive sleep apnea

PDT photodynamic therapy

SIRS systemic inflammatory response syndrome

SOM serous otitis media

SZ seizure

TIA transient ischemic attack

VPS ventriculoperitoneal shunt

VNS vagal nerve stimulator

ICD-10-CM

Official Guidelines for Coding and Reporting

Please refer to the companion Evolve website for the most current guidelines.

6. Chapter 6: Diseases of Nervous System and Sense Organs (G00-G99)

a. Dominant/nondominant side

Codes from category G81, Hemiplegia and hemiparesis, and subcategories, G83.1, Monoplegia of lower limb, G83.2, Monoplegia of upper limb, and G83.3, Monoplegia, unspecified, identify whether the dominant or nondominant side is affected. Should the affected side be documented, but not specified as dominant or nondominant, and the classification system does not indicate a default, code selection is as follows:

- For ambidextrous patients, the default should be dominant.
- If the left side is affected, the default is non-dominant.
- If the right side is affected, the default is dominant.

EXAMPLE   Patient is seen at physician's office following discharge from the hospital following a CVA. Patient has hemiparesis of the right side, G81.91.

b. Pain—Category G89

1) General coding information

Codes in category G89, Pain, not elsewhere classified, may be used in conjunction with codes from other categories and chapters to provide more detail about acute or chronic pain and neoplasm-related pain, unless otherwise indicated below.

If the pain is not specified as acute or chronic, post-thoracotomy, postprocedural, or neoplasm-related, do not assign codes from category G89.

A code from category G89 should not be assigned if the underlying (definitive) diagnosis is known, unless the reason for the encounter is pain control/ management and not management of the underlying condition.

When an admission or encounter is for a procedure aimed at treating the underlying condition (e.g., spinal fusion, kyphoplasty), a code for the underlying condition (e.g., vertebral fracture, spinal stenosis) should be assigned as the principal diagnosis. No code from category G89 should be assigned.

EXAMPLE

The patient is admitted with acute chest pain due to pneumonia, J18.9. Only the code for pneumonia would be assigned.

EXAMPLE

The patient is admitted for acute pain control after failing off a ladder and suffering two broken ribs on the right side. The patient was admitted for pain control, G89.11, S22.41xA, W11.xxxA.

EXAMPLE

Patient with acute back pain secondary to an acute vertebral fracture of the C3 vertebra is admitted for a kyphoplasty. Patient fell while walking the dog, S12.201A, W18.39xA, 0PU33JZ, Y93.k1.

(a) Category G89 Codes as Principal or First-Listed Diagnosis

Category G89 codes are acceptable as principal diagnosis or the first-listed code:

- When pain control or pain management is the reason for the admission/ encounter (e.g., a patient with displaced intervertebral disc, nerve impingement and severe back pain presents for injection of steroid into the spinal canal). The underlying cause of the pain should be reported as an additional diagnosis, if known.

EXAMPLE

Patient is admitted to the hospital with acute testicular pain. The patient had a vasectomy yesterday and the physician documents postprocedural pain, G89.18, N50.8

- When a patient is admitted for the insertion of a neurostimulator for pain control, assign the appropriate pain code as the principal or first-listed diagnosis. When an admission or encounter is for a procedure aimed at treating the underlying condition and a neurostimulator is inserted for pain control during the same admission/encounter, a code for the underlying condition should be assigned as the principal diagnosis and the appropriate pain code should be assigned as a secondary diagnosis.

EXAMPLE

Patient has acute pain secondary to lumbar spinal stenosis. She is admitted for insertion of a neurostimulator for pain control. The generator is inserted into the chest pocket and the leads are inserted into the spinal canal via open approach, M54.5, M48.06, 0JH60MZ, 00HU0MZ.

(b) Use of Category G89 Codes in Conjunction with Site Specific Pain Codes

(i) Assigning Category G89 and Site-Specific Pain Codes

Codes from category G89 may be used in conjunction with codes that identify the site of pain (including codes from chapter 18) if the category G89 code provides additional information. For example, if the code describes the site of the pain, but does not fully describe whether the pain is acute or chronic, then both codes should be assigned.

EXAMPLE   Patient is admitted with acute back pain after being rear-ended by a vehicle while driving her children to school, M54.9, G89.11, V43.52xA.

(ii) Sequencing of Category G89 Codes with Site-Specific Pain Codes

The sequencing of category G89 codes with site-specific pain codes (including chapter 18 codes), is dependent on the circumstances of the encounter/ admission as follows:

- If the encounter is for pain control or pain management, assign the code from category G89 followed by the code identifying the specific site of pain (e.g., encounter for pain management for acute neck pain from trauma is assigned code G89.11, Acute pain due to trauma, followed by code M54.2, Cervicalgia, to identify the site of pain).
- If the encounter is for any other reason except pain control or pain management, and a related definitive diagnosis has not been established (confirmed) by the provider, assign the code for the specific site of pain first, followed by the appropriate code from category G89.

EXAMPLE   Patient presents to the ER with acute chest pain secondary to being kicked in the chest by a horse, R07.9, G89.11, W55.12xA.

2) Pain due to devices, implants and grafts

See Section I.C.19. Pain due to medical devices

3) Postoperative Pain

The provider's documentation should be used to guide the coding of postoperative pain, as well as *Section III. Reporting Additional Diagnoses* and *Section IV. Diagnostic Coding and Reporting in the Outpatient Setting.*

The default for post-thoracotomy and other postoperative pain not specified as acute or chronic is the code for the acute form.

Routine or expected postoperative pain immediately after surgery should not be coded.

EXAMPLE   Patient is seen in physician's office after having a lesion removed from the lung. Patient presents complaining of chest pain. The physician's diagnosis is post-thoracotomy pain, G89.12, R07.9.

(a) Postoperative pain not associated with specific postoperative complication

Postoperative pain not associated with a specific postoperative complication is assigned to the appropriate postoperative pain code in category G89.

(b) Postoperative pain associated with specific postoperative complication

Postoperative pain associated with a specific postoperative complication (such as painful wire sutures) is assigned to the appropriate code(s) found in Chapter 19, Injury, poisoning, and certain other consequences of external causes. If appropriate, use additional code(s) from category G89 to identify acute or chronic pain (G89.18 or G89.28).

EXAMPLE
> Patient is 1 month status post TURP. Patient presents to physician's office with acute abdominal pain. After examination and assessment the physician documents acute post–TURP pain, G89.18, R10.9.

4) Chronic pain
Chronic pain is classified to subcategory G89.2. There is no time frame defining when pain becomes chronic pain. The provider's documentation should be used to guide use of these codes.

EXAMPLE
> Patient is 2 years status post lumbar laminectomy and is being seen again for chronic low back pain, G89.28, M54.5.

5) Neoplasm Related Pain
Code G89.3 is assigned to pain documented as being related, associated or due to cancer, primary or secondary malignancy, or tumor. This code is assigned regardless of whether the pain is acute or chronic.

This code may be assigned as the principal or first-listed code when the stated reason for the admission/encounter is documented as pain control/pain management. The underlying neoplasm should be reported as an additional diagnosis.

When the reason for the admission/encounter is management of the neoplasm and the pain associated with the neoplasm is also documented, code G89.3 may be assigned as an additional diagnosis. It is not necessary to assign an additional code for the site of the pain.

See Section I.C.2 for instructions on the sequencing of neoplasms for all other stated reasons for the admission/encounter (except for pain control/pain management).

EXAMPLE
> Patient is admitted for pain control due to metastatic bone cancer. Patient has a past history of breast cancer treated with surgical removal, G89.3, C79.51, Z85.3.

EXAMPLE
> Patient was admitted for back pain due to vertebral metastasis. An MRI indicates that the disease has progressed. Patient has a history of prostate cancer with surgical removal, C79.51, G89.3, Z85.46. Patient's bone mets treated with external beam radiation via the linear accelerator using electrons, DP0C3ZZ.

6) Chronic pain syndrome
Central pain syndrome (G89.0) and chronic pain syndrome (G89.4) are different than the term "chronic pain," and therefore codes should only be used when the provider has specifically documented this condition.
See Section I.C.5. Pain disorders related to psychological factors
7. Chapter 7: Diseases of the Eye and Adnexa (H00-H59)
   a. Glaucoma
     1) Assigning Glaucoma Codes
     Assign as many codes from category H40, Glaucoma, as needed to identify the type of glaucoma, the affected eye, and the glaucoma stage.
     2) Bilateral glaucoma with same type and stage
     When a patient has bilateral glaucoma and both eyes are documented as being the same type and stage, and there is a code for bilateral glaucoma, report only the code for the type of glaucoma, bilateral, with the seventh character for the stage.

When a patient has bilateral glaucoma and both eyes are documented as being the same type and stage, and the classification does not provide a code for bilateral glaucoma (i.e. subcategories H40.10, H40.11 and H40.20) report only one code for the type of glaucoma with the appropriate seventh character for the stage.

3) Bilateral glaucoma stage with different types or stages

When a patient has bilateral glaucoma and each eye is documented as having a different type or stage, and the classification distinguishes laterality, assign the appropriate code for each eye rather than the code for bilateral glaucoma.

When a patient has bilateral glaucoma and each eye is documented as having a different type, and the classification does not distinguish laterality (i.e. subcategories H40.10, H40.11 and H40.20), assign one code for each type of glaucoma with the appropriate seventh character for the stage.

When a patient has bilateral glaucoma and each eye is documented as having the same type, but different stage, and the classification does not distinguish laterality (i.e. subcategories H40.10, H40.11 and H40.20), assign a code for the type of glaucoma for each eye with the seventh character for the specific glaucoma stage documented for each eye.

4) Patient admitted with glaucoma and stage evolves during the admission

If a patient is admitted with glaucoma and the stage progresses during the admission, assign the code for highest stage documented.

5) Indeterminate stage glaucoma

Assignment of the seventh character "4" for "indeterminate stage" should be based on the clinical documentation. The seventh character "4" is used for glaucomas whose stage cannot be clinically determined. This seventh character should not be confused with the seventh character "0", unspecified, which should be assigned when there is no documentation regarding the stage of the glaucoma.

EXAMPLE   Patient presents to ophthalmologist's office and is diagnosed with bilateral chronic angle closure glaucoma. Both eyes are mild stage, H40.2231.

EXAMPLE   Patient presets to ophthalmologist's office with bilateral acute angle closure glaucoma, right eye with moderate stage and left eye with severe, H40.2112, H40.2123.

EXAMPLE   Glaucoma suspect in both eyes, H40.003.

---

8. **Chapter 8: Diseases of Ear and Mastoid Process (H60-H95)**
   Reserved for future guideline expansion

Apply General Coding Guidelines as found in Chapter 5 and the Procedural Coding Guidelines as found in Chapters 6 and 7.

MAJOR DIFFERENCES BETWEEN ICD-10-CM AND ICD-9-CM

- Codes for TIA are now included in the nervous system chapter in ICD-10-CM.
- Codes for migraine have been expanded to fifth and sixth characters to indicate whether the migraine is intractable and to reflect additional specificity.
- Codes for secondary parkinsonism have been expanded at the fourth or fifth characters for more specificity.
- Codes for hemiplegia and monoplegia identify whether the dominant or nondominant side is affected. If the information is not available, the default is dominant. The default for ambidextrous people is also dominant.

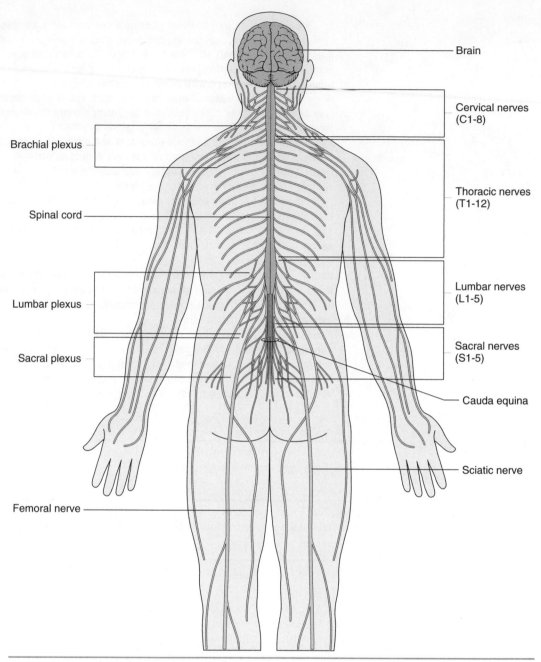

FIGURE 14-1. The brain and the spinal cord, spinal nerves, and spinal plexuses.

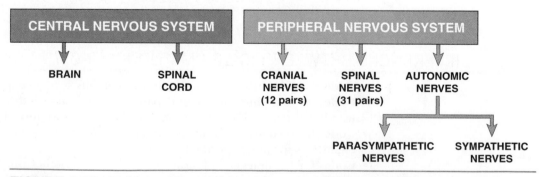

FIGURE 14-2. Divisions of the central nervous system (CNS) and peripheral nervous system (PNS). The autonomic nervous system is a part of the peripheral nervous system.

ANATOMY AND PHYSIOLOGY

The nervous system is composed of specialized tissue that controls the actions and reactions of the body and the way it adjusts to changes that occur inside and outside the body. The nervous system is divided into two main systems: the central nervous system and the peripheral nervous system (Figures 14-1 and 14-2). The central nervous system and the peripheral nervous system are each further divided into two parts. The central nervous system is made up of the brain and the spinal cord, and the peripheral nervous system is made up of the somatic nervous system and the autonomic nervous system.

Central Nervous System

Different areas of the brain are in control of different functions of the body (Figure 14-3). For example, the cerebral cortex controls thought, language, and reasoning; the brain stem is in control of breathing and blood pressure; and the hippocampus is in control of memory and learning. The spinal cord serves as a pathway for information passing from the brain to the peripheral nervous system. Both the brain and the spinal cord are covered by bone— the brain by the skull, and the spinal cord by the vertebral column; both are covered by membranes called the meninges. The meninges (Figure 14-4) are made up of three layers: dura, arachnoid, and pia. In the spinal column, the dura is not attached to the vertebrae but is separated from them by the epidural space. The purpose of these membranes is to protect the brain and the spinal cord.

The spinal cord, which is located in the vertebral foramen, consists of 31 segments, each of which has a pair of spinal nerves that exit from the segment. The purpose of the spinal cord is to conduct nerve impulses and spinal reflexes.

Peripheral Nervous System

The peripheral nervous system connects the central nervous system to other parts of the body. It may be broken down into two parts: the somatic nervous system and the autonomic

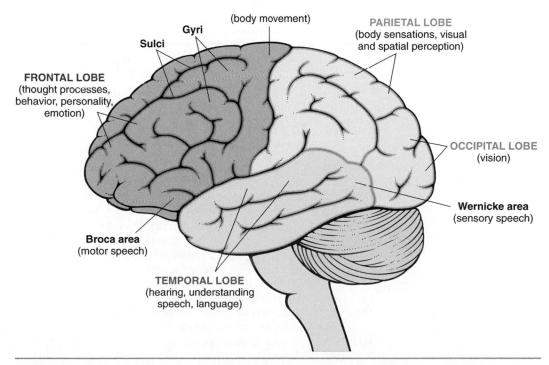

FIGURE 14-3. Left cerebral hemisphere (lateral view). Gyri (convolutions) and sulci (fissures) are indicated. Note the lobes of the cerebrum and the functional centers that control speech, vision, movement, hearing, thinking, and other processes.

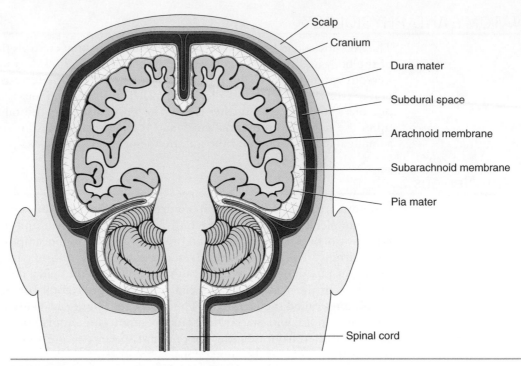

FIGURE 14-4. Meninges, frontal view.

nervous system. The **somatic nervous system** sends sensory information (taste, hearing, smell, and vision) to the central nervous system (CNS) and motor nerve impulses to the skeletal muscles.

The **autonomic nervous system** has both sensory and motor functions that involve the CNS and the internal organs. Actions produced by this system, such as beating of the heart muscle, are for the most part involuntary.

DISEASE CONDITIONS

Diseases of the Nervous System (G00-G99), Chapter 6 in the ICD-10-CM code book, Diseases of the Eye and Adnexa (H00-H59), Chapter 7 in the ICD-10-CM code book, and Diseases of the Ear and Mastoid Process (H60-95), Chapter 8 in the ICD-10-CM code book, are divided into the following categories:

CATEGORY	SECTION TITLE
G00-G009	Inflammatory diseases of the central nervous system
G10-G13	Systemic atrophies primarily affecting the central nervous system
G20-G26	Extrapyramidal and movement disorders
G30-G32	Other degenerative diseases of the nervous system
G35-G37	Demyelinating diseases of the central nervous system
G40-G47	Episodic and paroxysmal disorders
G50-G59	Nerve, nerve root, and plexus disorders
G60-G64	Polyneuropathies and other disorders of the peripheral nervous system
G70-G73	Diseases of myoneural junction and muscle
G80-G83	Cerebral palsy and other paralytic syndromes
G89-G99	Other disorders of the nervous system
H00-H05	Disorders of eyelid, lacrimal system, and orbit
H10-H11	Disorders of the conjunctiva
H15-H21	Disorders of sclera, cornea, iris, and ciliary body
H25-H28	Disorders of the lens
H30-H36	Disorders of the choroid and retina
H40-H42	Glaucoma
H43-H44	Disorders of the vitreous body and globe

CATEGORY	SECTION TITLE
H46-H47	Disorders of the optic nerve and visual pathways
H49-H52	Disorders of ocular muscles, binocular movement, accommodation, and refraction
H53-H54	Visual disturbances and blindness
H55-H57	Other disorders of eye and adnexa
H59	Intraoperative and postprocedural complications and disorders of eye and adnexa, not elsewhere classified
H60-H62	Diseases of external ear
H65-H75	Diseases of middle ear and mastoid
H80-H83	Diseases of the inner ear
H90-H94	Other disorders of ear
H95	Intraoperative and postprocedural complications and disorders of ear and mastoid process, not elsewhere classified

Inflammatory Diseases of the Central Nervous System (G00-G09)

Meningitis is an infection or inflammation of the meninges. Meningitis is caused by a viral or bacterial organism and may be treated with antibiotics. Vaccines are available to prevent meningitis that is due to *Streptococcus pneumoniae*. It should be noted that often, coding of meningitis requires two codes, and in most cases, the Tabular List instructs to code the underlying condition first. For more information on coding guidelines for underlying conditions, refer to Chapter 5 in this text, General Coding Guidelines.

EXAMPLE   The patient was treated for meningitis due to Lyme disease, A69.21.

The signs and symptoms of meningitis include high fever, headache, and stiff neck. Other symptoms that may be present are nausea, vomiting, sleepiness, and sensitivity to bright lights. To diagnose meningitis, physicians perform a lumbar puncture (Figure 14-5) to obtain spinal fluid and to look for organisms that may be present. Bacterial meningitis is treated with antibiotics, and the treatment for viral meningitis (aseptic) is usually limited to treating the symptoms.

EXAMPLE   Patient is admitted for meningitis due to chickenpox, B01.0.

EXAMPLE   Patient is being treated for *Pseudomonas* meningitis, G00.8, B96.5.

Additional disease conditions found in the section on Inflammatory Diseases of the Central Nervous System often require the use of two codes and include the instruction to code first the underlying condition. It is also important to follow the Excludes notes for further instruction (Figure 14-6).

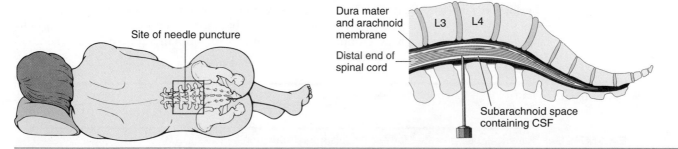

FIGURE 14-5. Lumbar (spinal) puncture. The patient lies laterally, with the knees drawn up to the abdomen and the chin brought down to the chest. This position increases the spaces between the vertebrae. The lumbar puncture needle is inserted between the third and fourth (or fourth and fifth) lumbar vertebrae, and it enters the subarachnoid space.

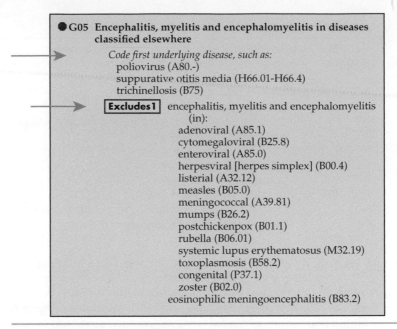

● **G05 Encephalitis, myelitis and encephalomyelitis in diseases
classified elsewhere**

   Code first underlying disease, such as:
      poliovirus (A80.-)
      suppurative otitis media (H66.01-H66.4)
      trichinellosis (B75)

   Excludes1   encephalitis, myelitis and encephalomyelitis
         (in):
            adenoviral (A85.1)
            cytomegaloviral (B25.8)
            enteroviral (A85.0)
            herpesviral [herpes simplex] (B00.4)
            listerial (A32.12)
            measles (B05.0)
            meningococcal (A39.81)
            mumps (B26.2)
            postchickenpox (B01.1)
            rubella (B06.01)
            systemic lupus erythematosus (M32.19)
            toxoplasmosis (B58.2)
            congenital (P37.1)
            zoster (B02.0)
      eosinophilic meningoencephalitis (B83.2)

FIGURE 14-6. Refer to the Excludes notes for further instruction if an underlying disease is causing encephalitis, myelitis, and encephalomyelitis.

EXAMPLE   Patient is being treated for encephalitis due to infectious mononucleosis, B27.92.

EXAMPLE   The patient was admitted with herpes encephalitis, B00.4.

EXERCISE 14-1

Assign codes to the following conditions.

1. Meningitis due to *Salmonella*   _____
2. *Klebsiella pneumoniae* meningitis   _____
3. Gram-negative meningitis   _____
4. Spinal meningitis   _____
5. Encephalitis following chickenpox   _____

Extrapyramidal and Movement Disorders (G20-G26)

Parkinson's disease (Figure 14-7) is a progressive and chronic motor system disorder. Symptoms may include tremor, rigidity, and impaired balance or coordination. It is usually treated with drugs such as L-dopa and sometimes with implantation of an intracranial neurostimulator.

EXAMPLE   Patient with Parkinson's disease, G20.

EXAMPLE   Patient is being treated for parkinsonism in Huntington's disease, G10.

EXAMPLE   Patient has parkinsonism due to Risperdal, G21.11, T43.595A.

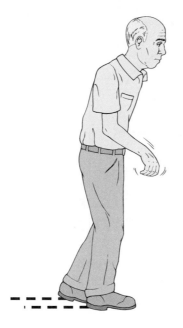

FIGURE 14-7. Typical shuffling gait and posture of patients with Parkinson's disease.

Other Degenerative Diseases of the Nervous System (G30-G32)

Alzheimer's disease (Figure 14-8) is a disorder of the brain that causes a progressive decline in mental and physical function. This disease is the most common cause of mental deterioration, and medications are available now and others are in development to assist in the treatment of this disease. When a physician documents the condition as Alzheimer's dementia, it is necessary to use two codes, with Alzheimer's disease sequenced first. For many of the dementia codes, code assignment may depend on the presence of behavioral disturbances such as aggressiveness, combativeness, violence, or wandering off.

EXAMPLE   Patient has Alzheimer's dementia without behavioral disturbance, G30.9, F02.80.

Cognitive impairment is characterized by problems with memory or thinking beyond that explained by normal aging. There is a higher risk for developing Azheimer's for those diagnosed with mild cognitive impairment. The symptoms of MCI include forgetting recent events or conversations, difficulty performing more than one task at a time, difficulty solving problems, and taking a longer time to perform difficult mental activities.

Episodic and Paroxysmal Disorders (G40-G47)

Epilepsy is a disorder of the brain that is characterized by abnormal electrical discharges from the brain cells. Recurrent seizures are the main symptom of epilepsy. Two major types of seizures can occur: generalized and partial. Seizures may present in a variety of forms; patients may lose consciousness, their arms and legs may jerk, they may become incontinent, or they may stare blankly, unaware of their surroundings.

Epilepsy has many causes; however, in approximately half of the cases, the cause is unknown. Epilepsy may be inherited, or it may be caused by injury to the brain, metabolic disturbances, alcohol and drug abuse, brain tumor, infection, stroke, fever, or it may occur in pregnancy. Epilepsy is generally treated with anticonvulsants such as Dilantin or Depakote, although in severe uncontrolled cases, surgery may be performed on the brain to remove the area of the brain where seizures originate. The most common diagnostic test for epilepsy is an electroencephalogram (EEG).

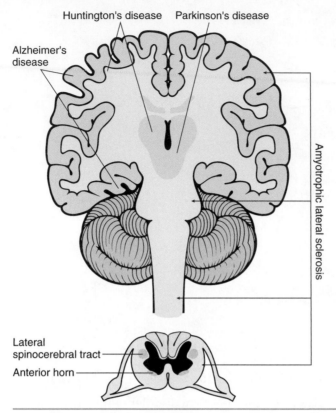

FIGURE 14-8. Degenerative diseases of the brain preferentially involve various parts of the brain. Alzheimer's disease causes atrophy of the frontal and occipital cortical gyri. Huntington's disease affects the frontal cortex and basal ganglia. Parkinson's disease is marked by changes in the substantia nigra. Amyotrophic lateral sclerosis affects the motor neurons in the anterior horn of the spinal cord, brain stem, and frontal cortex of the brain.

Different Types of Seizures

- Localization-related (begin in a specific part of the brain)
  - Simple partial—a seizure that presents with abnormal sensations (jerking, smells, abnormal motor movements) where the patient does not lose consciousness
  - Complex partial—a seizure that presents with alteration in consciousness causing confusion
- Generalized seizures (affect both hemispheres of the brain)
  - Absence—a seizure that presents with a short lapse of consciousness, most often seen in children
  - Atonic, myoclonic, and tonic-clonic—loss of muscle control resulting in collapse or jerking movements

Epilepsy may be defined as intractable or not intractable. Intractable epilepsy is defined as epilepsy that is not controlled by medication. Some of the other terms that are synonymous with intractable are pharmacoresistant, treatment resistant, refractory, and poorly controlled. In ICD-10-CM the sixth digit defines whether the patient has status epilepticus. Status epilepticus occurs when the brain is in a continous state of seizure. Status epilepticus is a medical emergency.

EXAMPLE | Patient was admitted for intractable epilepsy, G40.919.

EXAMPLE | Patient is being treated for progressive myoclonic epilepsy, G40.309.

Transient Ischemic Attack

A **transient ischemic attack** (TIA) is a stroke that lasts for only a few minutes. Patients who present with a TIA usually have the same symptoms as occur with a stroke. Most symptoms of a TIA are gone within an hour, but they may last up to 24 hours.

Sleep Disorders

Some typical sleep problems include **insomnia**, (difficulty falling asleep, staying asleep, wakefulness, and early morning awakening) and **hypersomnia** (excessive sleep). These problems are classified in this section when they are caused by a physiological condition.

EXAMPLE The patient is being treated for insomnia, G47.00.

Sleep apnea is a disorder that is characterized by breathing interruption during sleep. These patients awaken many times during the night to regain their breathing. This disorder results in sleep deprivation and can be life threatening. Sleep apnea can result in a drop in the oxygen saturation of blood and is a cause of daytime **somnolence** (sleepiness). A person is more likely to have obstructive sleep apnea (OSA) if they are overweight, snore loudly, are hypertensive, or have a family history of sleep apnea. This obstruction occurs when there is a blockage in the airway. Obstructive sleep apnea is diagnosed by a sleep study or polysomnogram. Patients may be treated with a CPAP (continuous positive airway pressure) mask. This mask helps push air into the breathing pathway. There are also surgical procedures to correct the obstruction.

Central sleep apnea occurs when the brain does not signal the muscles to breathe. This might occur in a stroke victim that has nervous system dysfunction or in patients that have neurodegenerative illnesses such as Lou Gehrig's disease.

EXAMPLE Patient has obstructive sleep apnea, G47.33.

Polyneuropathy and Other Disorders of the Peripheral Nervous System (G60-G65)

Critical illness polyneuropathy and myopathy are diseases of the nerves and muscles that occur as a complication of severe trauma or infection. These conditions are often diagnosed when there is an unexplained difficulty in weaning the patient from mechanical ventilation. These conditions are often associated with sepsis and are thought to be a manifestation of the systemic inflammatory response syndrome (SIRS).

EXAMPLE Patient is diagnosed with critical illness polyneuropathy, G62.81.

EXAMPLE Patient has polyneuropathy in type 2 diabetes, E11.42.

Diseases of the Myoneural Junction and Muscle (G70-G73)

Myasthenia gravis is a chronic **autoimmune disorder** that manifests as muscle weakness of varying degrees. The most frequently affected muscles are those that control the eye, eyelid, face, and swallowing. Myasthenia gravis may be treated with medication, thymectomy, and/or plasmapheresis. Patients who present in crisis may have difficulty breathing and require a ventilator to assist with breathing. These crises may be brought on by many different events, such as infection, stress, or fever.

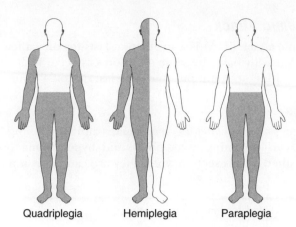

Quadriplegia Hemiplegia Paraplegia

FIGURE 14-9. Types of paralysis.

EXAMPLE | Patient was admitted for an acute exacerbation of myasthenia gravis, G70.01.

Muscular dystrophy is a type of myopathy. **Myopathies** are general disorders that affect muscles and usually result in muscle weakening or atrophy. Many disease processes involve myopathies.

EXAMPLE | Patient has Graves' myopathy, E05.00, G73.7.

Cerebral Palsy and Other Paralytic Syndromes (G80-G83)

Hemiplegia and hemiparesis (Figure 14-9) describe paralysis of the body that could have a number of causes. One of the most common causes of hemiplegia is a cerebrovascular accident (CVA) (Figure 14-10). When a patient is admitted with an acute CVA and has hemiplegia, it is appropriate to code this condition.

EXAMPLE | Patient has right-sided dominant spastic hemiparesis, G81.11.

Codes in category G81 and G83.1-G83.3 hemiplegia, heimparesis, and monoplegia have a fifth digit that identifies whether the dominant or non-dominant side is affected. If dominance is not documented in the record but the affected side is documented and there is no default indicated in the classification system, then the default would be as follows:
If the left side is affected, the default is non-dominant.
If the right side is affected, the default is dominant.
Hemiplegia is total paralysis of one side of the body, either of the leg or arm. Hemiparesis is incomplete paralysis of one side of the body or a generalized weakness. Flaccid hemiplegia results in muscle loss, whereas spastic hemiplegia will be defined by uncontrollable muscle spasms.
Sometime hemiplegia/hemiparesis may be a sequela of a stroke. This is not always the case, and sometimes it is just transient in that it rapidly clears. If it were a sequela (late effect) of a stroke, codes would be assigned from category I69. This will be described in more detail in Chapter 15, the circulatory chapter of this book.

Other Disorders of the Nervous System (G89-G99)

To use codes from category G89 the pain should be specified as:
- Pain due to trauma
- Postthoracotomy
- Postprocedural
- Neoplasm-related
- Central pain syndrome or chronic pain syndrome

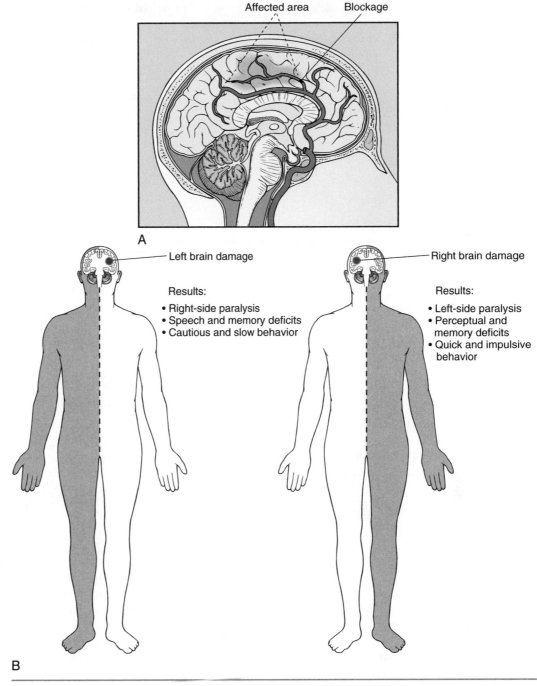

FIGURE 14-10. A, Cerebrovascular accident (CVA). **B,** Areas of the body affected by CVA.

These codes may be used with other codes to provide more detail about acute or chronic pain. If the cause of the pain (i.e, the underlying condition) is known, then a code from G89 is not used unless the purpose of the encounter is strictly for pain control or management and not for management of the underlying condition.

EXAMPLE   Patient is seen in the ER for acute tooth pain. He is given pain meds and told to see his dentist as soon as possible, K08.8.

Use category G89 codes as the principal or first-listed diagnosis when:

- The patient is admitted for pain management or control that is posttraumatic, postprocedural, postthoracotomy, or neoplasm-related (assign the specific site of the pain secondarily)
- The patient is admitted for the insertion of a neurostimulator for pain control

EXAMPLE

> The patient has chronic lumbar pain secondary to an old automobile accident and is now admitted for pain control, G89.21, M54.5, V89.2xxS.

Sequencing of Pain With Site-Specific Pain Codes

If assigning a site of pain code and there is no description in the code of acute or chronic, then the G89 code may be assigned as an additional code.

EXAMPLE

> Patient is seen in the physician's office with acute right shoulder pain following a fall, M25.511, G89.11, W19.xxxA.

If postoperative pain is not specified as acute or chronic, then the default is acute. It is important to note that routine postoperative pain following surgery is not assigned a G89 code.

EXAMPLE

> Patient is admitted from the ER with acute chest pain due to pneumonia, J18.9.
> The cause of the acute chest pain is known; therefore no pain code is necessary.

EXAMPLE

> Patient presents to the ER in acute pain after falling off a horse at riding camp. Patient is admitted for acute pain control because of two broken ribs, G89.11, S22.49xA, V80.018A, Y93.52, Y92.39.
> Even though there is a definitive diagnosis for the pain, the reason for admission is for pain control, not treatment of the broken ribs.

Hydrocephalus is excessive water (cerebrospinal fluid) on the brain. Cerebrospinal fluid (CSF) surrounds the brain and the spinal cord, and when this fluid accumulates on the brain, it causes pressure on brain tissue. Hydrocephalus may be acquired or congenital and communicating or obstructive. In communicating hydrocephalus, CSF can flow between ventricles of the brain, but it is blocked upon exit of the ventricle as opposed to obstructive hydrocephalus, in which the flow between ventricles is blocked. In addition, a condition known as normal pressure hydrocephalus (NPH) occurs in the elderly population and often occurs with dementia. Hydrocephalus is most often treated with a ventricular shunt (Figure 14-11). Hydrocephalus that is left untreated is a fatal condition.

EXAMPLE

> The patient has a shunt for noncommunicating hydrocephalus, G91.1, Z98.2.

Metabolic encephalopathy is temporary or permanent damage to the brain due to lack of glucose, oxygen, metabolic agents, or organ dysfunction. Another term used by physicians to describe this disorder may be acute confusional state. A patient with this condition usually presents with a change in mental status that could denote delirium and may be confused or agitated. Metabolic encephalopathy is a medical emergency. The causes of metabolic encephalopathy include brain tumors, cerebral infarcts, nutritional deficiency, poisoning, alcohol withdrawal, and systemic infection, to name a few. The treatment depends on the underlying cause.

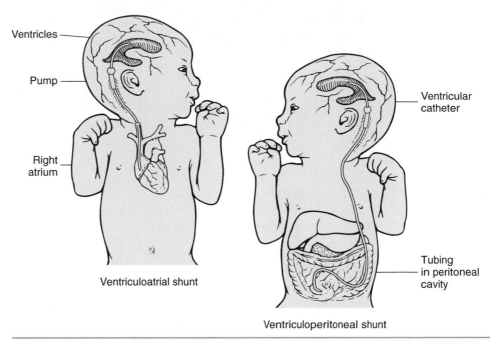

FIGURE 14-11. Shunting procedures for hydrocephalus. Ventriculoperitoneal shunt is the preferred procedure.

Cerebral edema is an accumulation of water on the brain either intracellular or extracellular. Vasogenic cerebral edema may be caused by malignant hypertension, brain cancer, altitude sickness, or hypertensive encephalopathy. There are other forms of cerebral edema that may be caused by SIADH (syndrome of inappropriate antidiuretic hormone), acidosis, hydrocephalus, and pseudotumor cerebri, and stroke, to name a few. Cerebral edema is not always clinically significant. If a patient has undergone brain surgery, some amount of cerebral edema may be expected and therefore no code would be assigned. Likewise, in a stroke patient, some amount of cerebral edema is usually present as a reaction to the infarction. If the cerebral edema is being treated with drainage, steroids, or other type of medications to decrease the pressure, then this condition should probably be assigned a code. If there is any doubt as to the significance of this condition, it is best to query the health care provider.

EXAMPLE | Patient is admitted to the hospital with acute mental status changes. The physician documents that the patient has metabolic encephalopathy secondary to hypernatremia, E87.0, G93.41.

EXAMPLE | Patient has a known glioblastoma multiforme. They are being seen in the ER for severe headache and neck pain. The patient is admitted with cerebral edema, G93.6, C71.9.

EXERCISE 14-2

Assign codes to the following conditions.

1. Parkinson's dementia   _____
2. Normal pressure hydrocephalus   _____
3. Seizure disorder   _____

4. Epilepsy, visual type   _____

5. Uncontrolled grand mal epilepsy   _____

6. Status epilepticus   _____

7. Organic hypersomnia   _____

8. Febrile seizures   _____

9. Patient has hemiplegia, which is a late effect of a CVA   _____

10. Patient is left handed and has hemiparesis affecting the nondominant side   _____

11. Patient is admitted for pain control with acute abdominal pain related to pancreatic cancer   _____

12. Patient is admitted with back pain for intravenous (IV) pain management after a fall down the stairs   _____

13. Patient is admitted for acute neck pain after an automobile accident. Attending plans magnetic resonance imaging (MRI) of the neck to rule out fracture   _____

14. Patient is readmitted for postoperative pain control after emergency appendectomy   _____

15. Patient is admitted for narcotics to treat chronic pain syndrome   _____

DISEASES OF THE EYE AND ADNEXA (H00-H59)

Many eye disorders are treated in the outpatient setting. Some of the conditions commonly found in inpatient records involve injuries to the eye (Figure 14-12), glaucoma, cataracts, macular degeneration, and visual impairment such as blindness. Injuries to the eye are covered in Chapter 19.

Disorders of the Lens (H25-H28)

Cataract (Figure 14-13) is a clouding of the lens of the eye that can cause obstructed vision. Most cataracts are related to the aging process; however, do not use the code for senile

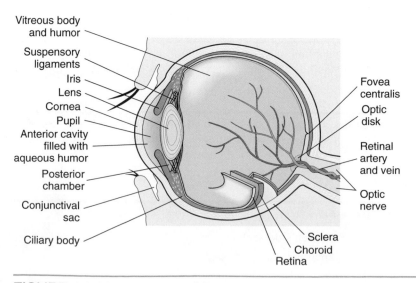

FIGURE 14-12. Normal eye anatomy.

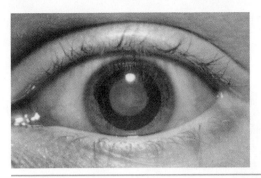

FIGURE 14-13. Cataract. The lens appears cloudy.

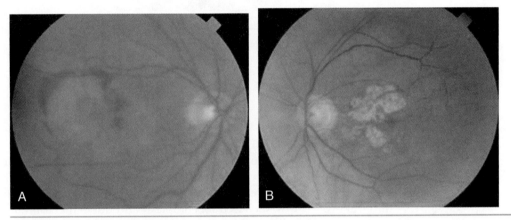

FIGURE 14-14. Macular degeneration. **A,** Wet, atrophic, age-related macular degeneration. **B,** Dry, atrophic, age-related macular degeneration.

cataract just because of a patient's age. The physician must document the type of cataract the patient has. Other risk factors for development of cataracts include smoking, diabetes, and prolonged exposure to sunlight. Cataracts are most often treated by surgery. Possible complications of cataract surgery include retinal detachment, anterior capsule contracture, and aftercataract.

EXAMPLE   Patient has a mature senile cataract, H25.89.

Disorders of the Choroid and the Retina (H30-H36)

Macular degeneration (Figure 14-14) is the leading cause of vision loss in the United States. Persons affected by this disease tend to be elderly; vision is lost in the central portion of the eye, leaving the patient with peripheral vision or low vision. Two common types of this disease have been identified: dry and wet. The dry form is more common and is less aggressive than the wet type.

EXAMPLE   Patient has exudative macular degeneration, H35.32.

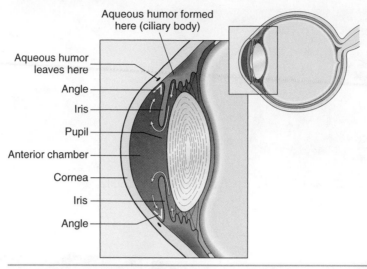

FIGURE 14-15. Glaucoma and circulation of aqueous humor. Circulation is impaired in glaucoma, so that aqueous fluid builds up in the anterior chamber.

Glaucoma (H40-H42)

Glaucoma (Figure 14-15) is a disorder of the optic nerve that may result in vision loss. The most common form is primary open angle glaucoma, in which the drainage canals of the eye become clogged over time and cause intraocular pressure (IOP) to rise; this damages the optic nerve. Glaucoma is most often treated with medicines in the form of eye drops. Surgical procedures, such as trabeculoplasty and trabeculectomy, may assist in the treatment of glaucoma. It is important to note that there is a specific code for borderline glaucoma or glaucoma suspect.

EXAMPLE | Patient is treated for open angle glaucoma, mild stage, left eye, H40.10x1.

Visual Disturbances and Blindness (H53-H54)

Category H54, Blindness and low vision has a note which instructs the coder to list first any associated underlying cause of blindness. This category also refers the coder to the visual impairment category table (Figure 14-16). The most severely affected eye is first in the code title, and the least affected eye is listed secondarily in the code title.

EXAMPLE | Blind in the right eye and normal vision in the left eye, H54.41.

EXAMPLE | Low vision, both eyes, H54.2.

DISEASES OF THE EAR AND THE MASTOID PROCESS (H60-H95)

Diseases of the Middle Ear and Mastoid (H65-H75)

As with eye conditions, many disorders of the ear (Figure 14-17) are treated in the outpatient setting. At times, inpatient coders see patients with the diagnoses of otitis media, mastoiditis, vertigo, and cholesteatoma, and of course, patients with hearing loss.

Category of visual impairment	Visual acuity with best possible correction	
	Maximum less than:	*Maximum equal to or better than:*
1	6/18 3/10 (0.3) 20/70	6/60 1/10 (0.1) 20/200
2	6/60 1/10 (0.1) 20/200	3/60 1/20 (0.05) 20/400
3	3/60 1/20 (0.05) 20/400	1/60 (finger counting of 1 meter) 1/50 (0.02) 5/300 (20/1200)
4	1/60 (finger counting of meter) 1/50 (0.02) 5/300	Light perception
5	No light perception	
9	Undetermined or unspecfied	

FIGURE 14-16. Visual impairment category table.

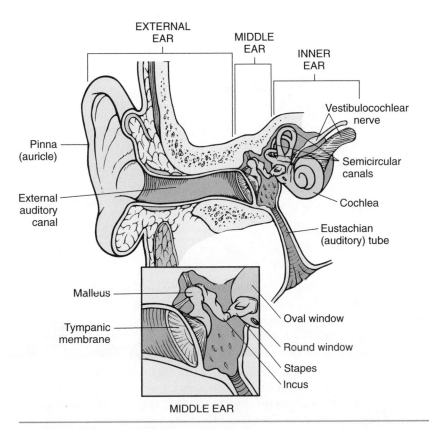

FIGURE 14-17. Normal ear anatomy.

Otitis media (OM) is a middle ear infection. It is the most common illness among children and babies. OM often occurs after another illness such as a cold. If the physician describes OM as suppurative, it is purulent or is expressing pus.

EXAMPLE | Patient has acute allergic serous otitis media, right ear, H65.111.

Mastoiditis is an infection of the mastoid bone of the skull. It is often the consequence of untreated OM and may be difficult to treat. Treatment usually consists of antibiotics and, as a last resort, a mastoidectomy to drain and remove the mastoid.

EXAMPLE | Patient is being treated for chronic recurrent mastoiditis in left ear, H70.12.

A **cholesteatoma** is a growth in the middle ear that usually results from repeated ear infections. Cholesteatomas may cause hearing loss or dizziness and may require surgery.

EXAMPLE | Patient was diagnosed with a right attic cholesteatoma, H71.01.

EXERCISE 14-3

Answer the following questions and assign codes to the following conditions as appropriate.

1. What is the leading cause of vision loss in the United States?   _____
2. SOM (serous otitis media)   _____
3. Acute and chronic mastoiditis   _____
4. Glaucoma suspect   _____
5. Cataract due to diabetes   _____
6. Meniere's disease, bilateral   _____
7. Papilledema   _____
8. Acquired aphakia, bilateral   _____
9. Acute uveitis   _____
10. Unstable keratoconus of the left eye   _____

FACTORS INFLUENCING HEALTH STATUS AND CONTACT WITH HEALTH SERVICES (Z CODES)

As was discussed in Chapter 8, it is difficult to locate Z codes in the Index. Coders will often say, "I did not know there was a Z code for that." Refer to Chapter 8 for a listing of common main terms used to locate Z codes. A review of the Tabular reveals that some Z codes pertain to diseases of the nervous system.

Z01.00	Encounter for examination of eyes and vision without abnormal findings
Z01.01	Encounter for examination of eyes and vision with abnormal findings
Z01.10	Encounter for examination of eyes and vision without abnormal findings

Z01.110	Encounter for hearing examination following failed hearing screening
Z01.118	Encounter for examination of ears and hearing with other abnormal findings
Z01.12	Encounter for hearing conservation and treatment
Z13.5	Encounter for screening for eye and ear disorders
Z13.858	Encounter for screening for other nervous system disorders
Z44.20	Encounter for fitting and adjustment of artificial eye, unspecified
Z44.21	Encounter for fitting and adjustment of artificial right eye
Z44.22	Encounter for fitting and adjustment of artificial left eye
Z45.320	Encounter for adjustment and management of bone conduction device
Z45.321	Encounter for adjustment and management of cochlear device
Z45.328	Encounter for adjustment and management of other implanted hearing device
Z45.41	Encounter for adjustment and management of cerebrospinal fluid drainage device
Z45.42	Encounter for adjustment and management of neuropacemaker (brain) (peripheral nerve) (spinal cord)
Z45.49	Encounter for adjustment and management of other implanted nervous system device
Z45.82	Encounter for adjustment or removal of myringotomy device (stent) (tube)
Z46.0	Encounter for fitting and adjustment of spectacle and contact lenses
Z46.1	Encounter for fitting and adjustment of hearing aid
Z46.2	Encounter for fitting and adjustment of other devices related to nervous system and special senses
Z52.5	Cornea donor
Z57.0	Occupational exposure to noise
Z79.891	Long-term (current) use of opiate analgesic
Z82.0	Family history of epilepsy and other diseases of the nervous system
Z82.1	Family history of blindness and visual loss
Z82.2	Family history of blindness and hearing loss
Z82.3	Family history of stroke
Z83.511	Family history of glaucoma
Z83.518	Family history of other specified eye disorders
Z83.52	Family history of ear disorders
Z86.61	Personal history of infections of the central nervous system
Z86.69	Personal history of other diseases of the nervous system and sense organs
Z90.01	Acquired absence of eyes
Z94.7	Corneal transplant status
Z96.1	Presence of intraocular lens
Z96.20	Presence of otological and audiological implant, unspecified
Z96.21	Cochlear implant status
Z96.22	Myringotomy tube(s) status
Z96.29	Presence of other otological and audiological implants
Z97.0	Presence of artificial eye
Z97.3	Presence of spectacles and contact lenses
Z97.4	Presence of external hearing aid
Z98.2	Presence of cerebrospinal fluid drainage device
Z98.41	Cataract extraction status, right eye
Z98.42	Cataract extraction status, left eye
Z98.49	Cataract extraction status, unspecified eye
Z98.83	Filtering (vitreous) bleb after glaucoma surgery status

EXAMPLE Patient with previous cornea transplant, Z94.7.

EXERCISE 14-4

Assign codes to the following conditions.

1. Encounter for fitting of glasses _____
2. Patient is status cataract removal and has a history of cornea _____
   transplant
3. Patient previously had enucleation of right eye _____
4. Patient was screened for glaucoma _____

COMMON TREATMENTS

CONDITION	MEDICATION/TREATMENT
Alzheimer's	Tacrine (Cognex), donepezil hydrochloride (Aricept), rivastigmine tartrate (Exelon), galantamine (Reminyl), memantine HCl (Namenda)
Parkinson's	Entacapone (Comtan), pramipexole dihydrochloride (Mirapex), ropinirole hydrochloride (Requip), Carbidopa-Levodopa (Sinemet)
Epilepsy	Carbamazepine (Tegretol), clonazepam (Klonopin), phenytoin (Dilantin), sodium valproate and valproic acid (Depakote), levetiracetam (Keppra), topiramate (Topamax)
Myasthenia gravis	Neostigmine bromide—oral (Prostigmin), Pyridostigmine (Regonol), (Mestinon)
Muscular dystrophy	Phenytoin (Dilantin), phenytoin (Phenytek), Deltasone
Macular degeneration	Vitamins/Photodynamic surgery
Glaucoma	Eye drops such as Xalatan (prostaglandins), Iopidine (adrenergics), Carbachol (miotic), Timoptic (beta blocker), and Diamox (carbonic anhydrase inhibitors)

PROCEDURES

Procedures related to the nervous system and sense organs in ICD-10-PCS may be found in the following tables:

Central Nervous System	001-00X
Peripheral Nervous System	012-01X
Eye	080-08Y
Ear, Nose, Sinus	090-09W

Lumbar Puncture

Lumbar puncture (LP), also known as spinal tap or spinal puncture, is used both diagnostically and therapeutically. The root operation in ICD-10-PCS for a lumbar puncture is drainage. When LP is performed for diagnosis, the cerebrospinal fluid (CSF) is analyzed for infection, inflammatory diseases such as multiple sclerosis, subarachnoid hemorrhage, and certain types of carcinoma. When LP is done therapeutically, it may be done to decrease spinal fluid pressure in conditions such as normal pressure hydrocephalus, benign intracranial hypertension, or pseudotumor cerebri. When LP is done therapeutically, the coder will find this code listed in the index under "Drainage, canal, spinal."

EXAMPLE | Patient presents to the ER with high fever and neck pain. The physician performs a lumbar puncture to rule out meningitis, R50.9, M54.2, 009U3ZX.

Deep Brain Stimulation

A brain stimulator, also known as an intracranial neurostimulator, a **deep brain stimulator** (DBS) or a thalamic stimulator, is used to control tremors in patients with Parkinson's and in those who have the condition of essential tremor. The root operation in ICD-10-PCS for insertion of a neurostimulator is insertion. An electrode is implanted, usually into the thalamus, and then is connected by a wire under the skin to a pulse generator implanted in the chest. Electrical impulses are sent to the thalamus, which in turn, controls tremors.

Ventricular Shunting

Shunting treatment of hydrocephalus is done to drain fluid from the brain to relieve pressure. The most common type of shunting (ventriculoperitoneal shunt) occurs between the ventricles of the brain and the abdominal cavity. The root operation in ICD-10-PCS for insertion of a ventricular shunt is bypass of the ventricle, cerebral. In this case, the excess fluid is drained from the ventricles into the peritoneal cavity, where it is reabsorbed. Sometimes, complications can occur in either the ventricular or the peritoneal part of the shunt. It may be necessary to perform surgery only at the site with the complication. This is a shunt revision. The code will be determined by the site that is revised. It is important to review the operative record to determine which site (peritoneal or ventricular) is being revised.

When coding these cases, it is important to look in the index under "Complication, ventricular, shunt" for the appropriate diagnosis code.

EXAMPLE   Patient admitted for insertion of ventriculoperitoneal shunt for communicating hydrocephalus, G91.0, 00160J6.

Electromyelogram

An **electromyelogram** (EMG) is a diagnostic test that measures electrical activity in muscles and nerves. The root operation in ICD-10-PCS for an EMG is measurement of musculoskeletal contractility. It is used to determine whether a patient has a disease that is damaging muscles, such as myasthenia gravis, or nerves, such as amyotrophic lateral sclerosis.

Hemispherectomy

Surgery for epilepsy currently consists of four basic types: amygdalohippocampectomy, lobectomy (temporal), hemispherectomy, and corpus callosotomy. The root operation in ICD-10-PCS for a hemispherectomy is resection of cerebral hemisphere. Surgery is not the norm for treatment of epilepsy, but it is used in the most severe cases when medications have failed to control seizures. Many tests must be performed before a person is considered a candidate for surgery and prior to the surgery itself.

Lobectomy, usually in the temporal region, is performed for partial seizures; during this surgery, the seizure focus is removed. During hemispherectomy, approximately half of the brain is removed. This procedure is usually performed on children.

EXAMPLE   A patient with intractable epilepsy is admitted for a temporal lobectomy, G40.919, 00B70ZZ.

Vagal Nerve Stimulation

A **vagal nerve stimulator** is a device that is used to treat intractable epilepsy. The root operation in ICD-10-PCS for a vagal nerve stimulator is insertion of a stimulator and insertion of

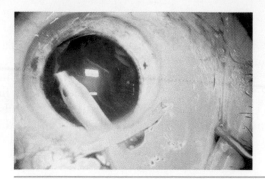

FIGURE 14-18. Phacoemulsification of a cataractous lens through a small, self-sealing, scleral tunnel incision.

an electrode. This device, which is similar to a heart pacemaker, is inserted into the upper chest and sends electrical current to the vagus nerve in the neck, which in turn travels to the brain and reduces or controls seizures.

EXAMPLE A patient with intractable epilepsy presents for implantation of a single array neurostimulator pulse generator with leads. The generator was placed in the chest via open procedure and the leads were placed in the neck via open procedure attached to the vagus nerve, G40.919, 00HE3MZ, 0JH60BZ.

Photodynamic Therapy

Photodynamic therapy (PDT) is used in treatment of the wet form of macular degeneration. The root operation in ICD-10-PCS for PDT for macular degeneration is destruction of the retina.

This procedure is usually performed in a doctor's office. The patient is injected with the drug and the drug travels to the vessels in the back of the eye where it is activated by shining a laser into the patient's eye.

Cataract Extraction

Cataract extraction is usually performed by **phacoemulsification** (Figure 14-18), wherein an incision is made on the side of the cornea and the lens material is softened, broken, and suctioned out. Usually after the lens is removed, an artificial lens is inserted (intraocular lens [IOL]). The root operation in ICD-10-PCS for cataract removal is extraction, and the root operation for lens insertion is replacement.

EXAMPLE Patient is admitted for a mature senile cataract in the right eye to be removed by phacoemulsification with IOL replacement, H25.89, 08RJ3JZ, 08DJ3ZZ.

It is important to remember that when bilateral procedures are coded, the procedure code should be coded twice, unless a code is classified as bilateral. This follows the coding guideline from Chapter 6.

EXERCISE 14-5

Answer the following questions, and code all diagnoses and procedures as appropriate.

1. What is the name of the test used to measure electrical activity in muscles? _____

2. Name one reason a surgeon may perform a hemispherectomy. _____

3. What is PDT used to treat? _____

4. Patient with pseudotumor cerebri is treated with a therapeutic spinal tap. _____

5. Patient presents with malfunctioning ventriculoperitoneal shunt, and revision of the shunt is performed at the peritoneal site. _____

6. Patient with Parkinson's disease is admitted for insertion of a thalamic stimulator. Single array generator inserted in the chest. _____

7. Patient admitted with nuclear senile cataract in the left eye and an extracapsular cataract extraction with Yag laser with lens implant was performed. _____

8. A patient who had a cornea transplant on his right eye now has glaucoma in his left eye. He is admitted for a trabeculectomy ab externo. _____

DOCUMENTATION/REIMBURSEMENT/MS-DRGs

Often, coding difficulties are due to lack of documentation. Sometimes pathology and other test results are not available at the time of discharge or when the physician is dictating the discharge summary or is reporting the final diagnoses.

When coding meningitis, the causative organism may affect MS-DRG assignment.

Frequently missed complications/comorbidities from this chapter include the following:

- Seizure, petit mal, with intractable epilepsy
- Communicating hydrocephalus
- Secondary parkinsonism
- Reflex sympathetic dystrophy
- Cauda equina syndrome
- Leukodystrophy
- Progressive muscular dystrophy
- Idiopathic transverse myelitis
- Quadraplegia

Causative Organism

EXAMPLE	DIAGNOSES	CODE	MS-DRG	RW
	Viral meningitis	A87.9	076	0.8751
	Salmonella meningitis	A02.21	096	1.9069

Shunt Revision

	DIAGNOSES/PROCEDURES	CODE	MS-DRG	RW
EXAMPLE	Hydrocephalus	G91.9	033	1.4085
	Revision ventriculoperitoneal shunt (revision of ventricular site)	00W000Z		
	Hydrocephalus	G91.9	042	1.7442
	Revision ventriculoperitoneal shunt (revision peritoneal site)	0DWW00Z		

CHAPTER REVIEW EXERCISE

Answer the following questions and where applicable, assign codes for diagnoses, procedures, Z codes, and external cause codes.

1. Candidal meningitis _____

2. Meningitis with a headache due to herpes zoster virus _____

3. Meningitis due to whooping cough _____

4. Normal pressure hydrocephalus treated with a ventriculocisternal shunt _____

5. Congenital hydrocephalus with lumbosacral spina bifida _____

6. Parkinsonism in Shy-Drager syndrome _____

7. Benign essential tremor _____

8. Lou Gehrig's disease _____

9. Hemiplegia of the right side _____

10. Recurrent seizures _____

11. History of seizures _____

12. Jacksonian seizure _____

13. Intractable epileptic convulsions _____

14. Addison's disease with myopathy _____

15. Intensive care unit myopathy _____

16. Glaucoma suspect _____

17. Aftercataract obscuring vision _____

18. One eye blind, the other with near normal vision _____

19. Lumbar puncture performed on a patient with probable diagnosis of multiple sclerosis. The patient is currently inpatient _____

Write the correct answer(s) in the space(s) provided.

20. What procedure would a surgeon use to treat tremors in Parkinson's disease?

_____

21. Patient with macular degeneration has the drug Visudyne injected, and then a laser is used. What is this procedure known as?

_____

22. What is the most common diagnostic test for epilepsy?

_____

23. If a surgeon performed a trabeculectomy, what would he or she be treating?

_____

CHAPTER GLOSSARY

Alzheimer's disease: disorder of the brain that causes a progressive decline in mental and physical function.

Autoimmune disorder: disorder that occurs when the immune system attacks itself inappropriately.

Autonomic nervous system: consists of both sensory and motor functions that involve the central nervous system and internal organs.

Cataract: clouding of the lens of the eye causing obstructed vision.

Cerebral edema: an accumulation of water on the brain either intracellular or extracellular.

Cholesteatoma: growth in the middle ear that usually results from repeated ear infections.

Cognitive impairment: decline in mental activities associated with thinking, learning, and memory.

Deep brain stimulator: a device implanted to control tremors.

Electromyelogram: test that measures electrical activity in muscles and nerves.

Epilepsy: disorder of the brain that is characterized by abnormal electrical discharges from the brain cells.

Glaucoma: disorder of the optic nerve that may result in vision loss.

Hemiplegia: paralysis of half of the body.

Hydrocephalus: cerebrospinal fluid collection in the skull.

Hypersomnia: excessive sleep.

Insomnia: difficulty falling asleep, wakefulness, and early morning awakening.

Intractable: not manageable.

Legal blindness: severe or profound impairment in both eyes.

Macular degeneration: vision loss in the central portion of the eye, leaving the patient with peripheral vision or low vision.

Mastoiditis: infection of the mastoid bone of the skull.

Meningitis: infection or inflammation of the meninges.

Metabolic encephalopathy: temporary or permanent damage to the brain due to lack of glucose, oxygen, metabolic agents, or organ dysfunction.

Muscular dystrophy: type of myopathy.

Myasthenia gravis: chronic autoimmune disorder that manifests as muscle weakness of varying degrees.

Myopathy: disorder that affects muscles, usually resulting in weakness or atrophy.

Otitis media: middle ear infection.

Parkinson's disease: progressive and chronic motor system disorder.

Phacoemulsification: incision is made on the side of the cornea and the lens material is softened, broken, and suctioned out.

Shunting: procedure to drain fluid from the brain to relieve pressure.

Sleep apnea: disorder characterized by breathing interruption during sleep.

Somatic nervous system: sends sensory (taste, hearing, smell) information to the central nervous system.

Somnolence: sleepiness.

Transient ischemic attack: a stroke that lasts only for a few minutes.

Vagal nerve stimulator: a device to control seizures.

15

Diseases of the Circulatory System

(ICD-10-CM Chapter 9, Codes I00-I99)

CHAPTER OUTLINE

ICD-10-CM Official Guidelines for Coding and Reporting

Major Differences Between ICD-10-CM and ICD-9-CM

Anatomy and Physiology
- The Heart
- Blood Vessels
- Lymphatic System

Disease Conditions
- Acute Rheumatic Fever (I00-I02) and Chronic Rheumatic Heart Disease (I05-I09)
- Hypertensive Diseases (I10-I15)
- Ischemic Heart Disease (I20-I25)
- Pulmonary Heart Disease and Diseases of Pulmonary Circulation (I26-I28)
- Other Forms of Heart Disease (I30-I52)
- Cerebrovascular Diseases (I60-I69)
- Diseases of the Arteries, Arterioles, and Capillaries (I70-I79)
- Diseases of Veins, Lymphatic Vessels, and Lymph Nodes, Not Elsewhere Classified (I80-I89)

Factors Influencing Health Status and Contact With Health Services (Z Codes)

Common Treatments

Procedures
- Diagnostic Cardiac Catheterization
- Angioplasty
- Coronary Artery Bypass Graft
- Electrophysiologic Studies/Procedures
- Pacemaker/Defibrillators (AICD)
- Aneurysm Repair
- Central Lines/Catheters

Documentation/Reimbursement/MS-DRGs
- MS-DRG With and Without MCC/CC
- Pacemakers/ICDs/Cardioverter/Defibrillators

Chapter Review Exercise

Chapter Glossary

Reference

LEARNING OBJECTIVES

1. Apply and assign the correct ICD-10-CM/PCS codes in accordance with Official Guidelines for Coding and Reporting
2. Identify major differences between ICD-10-CM and ICD-9-CM related to diseases of the circulatory system
3. Identify pertinent anatomy and physiology of the circulatory system

4. Identify diseases of the circulatory system
5. Assign the correct Z codes and procedure codes related to the circulatory system
6. Identify common treatments, medications, laboratory values, and diagnostic tests
7. Explain the importance of documentation in relation to MS-DRGs for reimbursement

ABBREVIATIONS/ ACRONYMS

ACS acute coronary syndrome

AF atrial fibrillation

AICD automatic implantable cardioverter-defibrillator

AIDS acquired immunodeficiency syndrome

AMI acute myocardial infarction

AV atrioventricular

AVM arteriovenous malformation

AVR aortic valve replacement

BNP brain natriuretic peptide

BP blood pressure

CAB coronary artery bypass

CABG coronary artery bypass graft

CAD coronary artery disease

CAT computerized axial tomography

CCU coronary care unit

CHB complete heart block

CHF congestive heart failure

CKD chronic kidney disease

COPD chronic obstructive pulmonary disease

CPK creatine phosphokinase

CPK-MB creatine phosphokinase, isoenzyme MB

CRT cardiac resynchronization therapy

CRT-D cardiac resynchronization treatment defibrillator

CRT-P cardiac resynchronization treatment pacemaker

CT computerized tomography

CVA cerebrovascular accident

CVL central venous line

CXR chest x-ray

DES drug-eluting stent

DOE dyspnea on exertion

DM diabetes mellitus

DVT deep vein thrombosis

EKG/ECG electrocardiogram

EP electrophysiologic

ER Emergency Room

HCVD hypertensive cardiovascular disease

HTN hypertension

ICD internal cardiac defibrillator

ICD-9-CM *International Classification of Diseases, 9th Revision, Clinical Modification*

ICD-10-CM *International Classification of Diseases, 10th Revision, Clinical Modification*

ICD-10-PCS *International Classification of Diseases, 10th Revision, Procedure Coding System*

ICV implantable cardioverter

IV intravenous

IVDU intravenous drug user

LAD left anterior descending

LCA left coronary artery

MI myocardial infarction

MRI magnetic resonance imaging

MS-DRG Medicare Severity diagnosis-related group

MUGA multiple-gated acquisition

MVR mitral valve replacement

NQMI non–Q wave myocardial infarction

NSTEMI non–ST elevation myocardial infarction

OM obtuse marginal

OSA obstructive sleep apnea

PCI percutaneous coronary intervention

PDA posterior descending artery

PHT pulmonary hypertension

PICC peripherally inserted central catheter

PPH primary pulmonary hypertension

PTCA percutaneous transluminal coronary angioplasty

RA right atrium

RBBB right bundle branch block

RCA right coronary artery

RFA radiofrequency ablation

RHD rheumatic heart disease

RW relative weight

SOB shortness of breath

SSS sick sinus syndrome

STEMI ST elevation myocardial infarction

SVT supraventricular tachycardia

TIA transient ischemic attack

TPA tissue plasminogen activator

TPN total parenteral nutrition

USA unstable angina

ICD-10-CM

Official Guidelines for Coding and Reporting

Please refer to the companion Evolve website for the most current guidelines.

9. Chapter 9: Diseases of Circulatory System (I00-I99)

a. Hypertension

1) Hypertension with Heart Disease

Heart conditions classified to I50.- or I51.4-I51.9, are assigned to a code from category I11, Hypertensive heart disease, when a causal relationship is stated (due to hypertension) or implied (hypertensive). Use an additional code from category I50, Heart failure, to identify the type of heart failure in those patients with heart failure.

The same heart conditions (I50.-, I51.4-I51.9) with hypertension, but without a stated causal relationship, are coded separately. Sequence according to the circumstances of the admission/encounter.

EXAMPLE Congestive heart failure due to hypertensive heart disease, I11.0, I50.9.

EXAMPLE Congestive heart failure in a patient with hypertension, I50.9, I10.

2) Hypertensive Chronic Kidney Disease

Assign codes from category I12, Hypertensive chronic kidney disease, when both hypertension and a condition classifiable to category N18, Chronic kidney disease (CKD), are present. Unlike hypertension with heart disease, ICD-10-CM presumes a cause-and-effect relationship and classifies chronic kidney disease with hypertension as hypertensive chronic kidney disease.

The appropriate code from category N18 should be used as a secondary code with a code from category I12 to identify the stage of chronic kidney disease.

See Section I.C.14. Chronic kidney disease.

If a patient has hypertensive chronic kidney disease and acute renal failure, an additional code for the acute renal failure is required.

EXAMPLE The patient was admitted with acute renal failure. The patient was given secondary diagnoses of benign hypertension and chronic kidney disease, stage III, N17.9, I12.9, N18.3.

3) Hypertensive Heart and Chronic Kidney Disease

Assign codes from combination category I13, Hypertensive heart and chronic kidney disease, when both hypertensive kidney disease and hypertensive heart disease are stated in the diagnosis. Assume a relationship between the hypertension and the chronic kidney disease, whether or not the condition is so designated. If heart failure is present, assign an additional code from category I50 to identify the type of heart failure.

The appropriate code from category N18, Chronic kidney disease, should be used as a secondary code with a code from category I13 to identify the stage of chronic kidney disease.

See Section I.C.14. Chronic kidney disease.

The codes in category I13, Hypertensive heart and chronic kidney disease, are combination codes that include hypertension, heart disease and chronic kidney disease. The Includes note at I13 specifies that the conditions included at I11 and I12 are included together in I13. If a patient has hypertension, heart disease and chronic kidney disease then a code from I13 should be used, not individual codes for hypertension, heart disease and chronic kidney disease, or codes from I11 or I12.

For patients with both acute renal failure and chronic kidney disease an additional code for acute renal failure is required.

EXAMPLE Patient has stage III chronic kidney disease. They are admitted with acute on chronic diastolic congestive heart failure which is hypertensive in nature, I13.0, I50.33, N18.3.

4) Hypertensive Cerebrovascular Disease

For hypertensive cerebrovascular disease, first assign the appropriate code from categories I60-I69, followed by the appropriate hypertension code.

EXAMPLE Cerebrovascular accident in a patient with malignant hypertension, I63.9, I10.

5) Hypertensive Retinopathy

Subcategory H35.0, Background retinopathy and retinal vascular changes, should be used with a code **from category** I10 – **I15, Hypertensive** disease to include the systemic hypertension. The sequencing is based on the reason for the encounter.

EXAMPLE The patient is being treated for bilateral retinopathy due to labile hypertension, H35.033, I10.

6) Hypertension, Secondary

Secondary hypertension is due to an underlying condition. Two codes are required: one to identify the underlying etiology and one from category I15 to identify the hypertension. Sequencing of codes is determined by the reason for admission/ encounter.

EXAMPLE Hypertension due to periarteritis nodosa, M30.0, I15.8.

7) Hypertension, Transient

Assign code R03.0, Elevated blood pressure reading without diagnosis of hypertension, unless patient has an established diagnosis of hypertension. Assign code O13.-, Gestational [pregnancy-induced] hypertension without significant proteinuria, or O14.-, Pre-eclampsia, for transient hypertension of pregnancy.

EXAMPLE The patient has an elevated blood pressure caused by the stress of being in an MVA, R03.0.

8) Hypertension, Controlled

This diagnostic statement usually refers to an existing state of hypertension under control by therapy. Assign the appropriate code from categories I10-I15, Hypertensive diseases.

9) Hypertension, Uncontrolled

Uncontrolled hypertension may refer to untreated hypertension or hypertension not responding to current therapeutic regimen. In either case, assign the appropriate code from categories I10-I15, Hypertensive diseases.

EXAMPLE The patient's benign hypertension has been well controlled since the patient lost 20 pounds and started a regular exercise program, I10.

EXAMPLE The patient's hypertension has been uncontrolled for the past 2 months in spite of changes in medication, I10.

b. Atherosclerotic Coronary Artery Disease and Angina

ICD-10-CM has combination codes for atherosclerotic heart disease with angina pectoris. The subcategories for these codes are I25.11, Atherosclerotic heart disease of native coronary artery with angina pectoris and I25.7, Atherosclerosis of coronary artery bypass graft(s) and coronary artery of transplanted heart with angina pectoris.

When using one of these combination codes it is not necessary to use an additional code for angina pectoris. A causal relationship can be assumed in a patient with both atherosclerosis and angina pectoris, unless the documentation indicates the angina is due to something other than the atherosclerosis.

If a patient with coronary artery disease is admitted due to an acute myocardial infarction (AMI), the AMI should be sequenced before the coronary artery disease. *See Section I.C.9. Acute myocardial infarction (AMI)*

EXAMPLE Patient with a previous coronary artery bypass is admitted with unstable angina. It is determined that the patient's angina is due to a blockage in the bypass grafts, I25.700.

c. Intraoperative and Postprocedural Cerebrovascular Accident

Medical record documentation should clearly specify the cause- and-effect relationship between the medical intervention and the cerebrovascular accident in order to assign a code for intraoperative or postprocedural cerebrovascular accident.

Proper code assignment depends on whether it was an infarction or hemorrhage and whether it occurred intraoperatively or postoperatively. If it was a cerebral hemorrhage, code assignment depends on the type of procedure performed.

EXAMPLE The patient had a postoperative cerebrovascular accident, which was embolic in nature. The patient had initially been admitted for treatment of coronary artery arteriosclerosis with CABG (left internal mammary artery and two open saphenous vein grafts from the left greater saphenous vein were used). Cardiopulmonary bypass was used during the surgery. I25.10, I97.820, I63.40, 021109W, 02100A9, 5A1221Z, 06BQ0ZZ.

d. Sequelae of Cerebrovascular Disease

1) Category I69, Sequelae of Cerebrovascular disease

Category I69 is used to indicate conditions classifiable to categories I60-I67 as the causes of **sequela** (neurologic deficits), themselves classified elsewhere. These "late effects" include neurologic deficits that persist after initial onset of conditions classifiable to categories I60-I67. The neurologic deficits caused by cerebrovascular disease may be present from the onset or may arise at any time after the onset of the condition classifiable to categories I60-I67.

2) Codes from category I69 with codes from I60-I67

Codes from category I69 may be assigned on a health care record with codes from I60-I67, if the patient has a current cerebrovascular disease and deficits from an old cerebrovascular disease.

3) Code Z86.73

Assign code Z86.73, Personal history of transient ischemic attack (TIA), and cerebral infarction without residual deficits (and not a code from category I69) as an additional code for history of cerebrovascular disease when no neurologic deficits are present.

EXAMPLE Aphasia due to cerebrovascular accident 3 months ago, I69.320.

EXAMPLE The patient was admitted with left-sided hemiparesis due to a cerebrovascular accident. The patient has a history of previous CVA with residual facial droop, I63.9, G81.94, I69.392.

EXAMPLE The patient had a CVA in 2002 with no residuals, Z86.73.

e. **Acute myocardial infarction (AMI)**

1) **ST elevation myocardial infarction (STEMI) and non ST elevation myocardial infarction (NSTEMI)**

The ICD-10-CM codes for acute myocardial infarction (AMI) identify the site, such as anterolateral wall or true posterior wall. Subcategories I21.0-I21.2 and code I21.4 are used for ST elevation myocardial infarction (STEMI). Code I21.4, Non-ST elevation (NSTEMI) myocardial infarction, is used for non ST elevation myocardial infarction (NSTEMI) and nontransmural MIs.

If NSTEMI evolves to STEMI, assign the STEMI code. If STEMI converts to NSTEMI due to thrombolytic therapy, it is still coded as STEMI.

For encounters occurring while the myocardial infarction is equal to, or less than, four weeks old, including transfers to another acute setting or a postacute setting, and the patient requires continued care for the myocardial infarction, codes from category I21 may continue to be reported. For encounters after the 4 week time frame and the patient **is still receiving** care related to the myocardial infarction, the appropriate aftercare code should be assigned, rather than a code from category I21. **For old or healed myocardial infarctions not requiring further care,** code I25.2, Old myocardial infarction, may be assigned.

EXAMPLE The patient was admitted with NSTEMI, I21.4.

EXAMPLE The patient was admitted with anterolateral wall STEMI, I21.09.

2) **Acute myocardial infarction, unspecified**

Code I21.3, ST elevation (STEMI) myocardial infarction of unspecified site, is the default for the unspecified term acute myocardial infarction. If only STEMI or transmural MI without the site is documented, query the provider as to the site, or assign code I21.3.

3) **AMI documented as nontransmural or subendocardial but site provided**

If an AMI is documented as nontransmural or subendocardial, but the site is provided, it is still coded as a subendocardial AMI. If NSTEMI evolves to STEMI, assign the STEMI code. If STEMI converts to NSTEMI due to thrombolytic therapy, it is still coded as STEMI.

See Section I.C.21.3 for information on coding status post administration of tPA in a different facility within the last 24 hours.

EXAMPLE Patient is admitted with an NSTEMI of the anterolateral wall, I21.4.

4) **Subsequent acute myocardial infarction**

A code from category I22, Subsequent ST elevation (STEMI) and non ST elevation (NSTEMI) myocardial infarction, is to be used when a patient who has suffered an AMI has a new AMI within the 4 week time frame of the initial AMI. A code from category I22 must be used in conjunction with a code from category I21. The sequencing of the I22 and I21 codes depends on the circumstances of the encounter.

EXAMPLE Patient is admitted with an STEMI of the anterolateral wall. During initial recovery in the hospital, the patient experiences a subsequent NSTEMI, I21.09, I22.2.

EXAMPLE Patient was discharged 3 weeks ago following an inferolateral STEMI. She presents today with unstable angina determined to be a posterolateral MI, I22.8, I21.19.

Apply the General Coding Guidelines as found in Chapter 5 and the Procedural Coding Guidelines as found in Chapters 6 and 7.

MAJOR DIFFERENCES BETWEEN ICD-10-CM AND ICD-9-CM

- The code for gangrene has been moved from the symptom chapter in ICD-9-CM to Diseases of the Circulatory System in ICD-10-CM.
- The section Late Effects of Cerebrovascular Disease has been expanded to include more specificity and laterality.
- The time limit for assigning the acute MI code is 28 days in ICD-10-CM, whereas in ICD-9-CM, it was 8 weeks.
- A new category has been added for coding a subsequent acute MI, which is an MI that occurs within 28 days of a previous acute MI.
- A new category for complications within 28 days of acute MI has been added.
- Transient ischemic attack has been reclassified to the nervous system chapter.
- Stages of chronic kidney disease are no longer found as fifth digits but are assigned a separate code.
- Subsequent acute MI is new to I10. This is a new MI that occurs in a patient who suffered a previous new MI within the last 4 weeks.
- There is no Hypertension Table in ICD-10-CM.
- There are no fourth digits to classify hypertension as benign, malignant, or unspecified; all are included in the code for hypertension.
- A causal relationship can be assumed when a patient has both atherosclerosis and angina, and an additional code for the angina is not assigned, the combination code is used.

ANATOMY AND PHYSIOLOGY

The circulatory system is composed of the heart and blood vessels (Figure 15-1). Its function is to supply tissue in the body with oxygen and nutrients. This function is accomplished when the arteries carry blood (oxygen) to the cells. The largest artery, the aorta, branches off the heart and divides into many smaller arteries. The veins carry deoxygenated blood to the lungs to acquire oxygen and then to the heart, whose job it is to pump oxygenated blood back to the arteries.

The Heart

The function of the heart is to pump oxygen-rich blood to the cells of the body. The heart itself receives oxygenated blood from the coronary arteries; the two major coronary arteries branch off the aorta.

The heart is enclosed laterally by the lungs, posteriorly by the backbone, and anteriorly by the sternum. The wall of the heart is composed of three layers: epicardium, myocardium, and endocardium (Figure 15-2). The epicardium is the outer protective layer, the myocardium is the middle layer and is composed of cardiac muscle, and the endocardium is the inner layer that lines all the heart chambers and covers the heart valves.

The heart consists of four chambers: right atrium, left atrium, right ventricle, and left ventricle. The atrium and the ventricle on the right side are separated from the left by a septum. The top two chambers, the atria, receive blood via the veins from the body or the lungs. The right ventricle pumps blood to the lungs to pick up oxygen, and the left ventricle pumps blood to the rest of the body. Within the heart are four valves (Figure 15-3), and their job is to direct blood flow. The tricuspid valve is located between the right atrium and the right ventricle. The valve between the left atrium and the left ventricle is the mitral or bicuspid valve. The aortic valve is located in the aorta at the point at which the left ventricle empties into the aorta. The pulmonary valve is located in the pulmonary artery at the point of exit from the right ventricle.

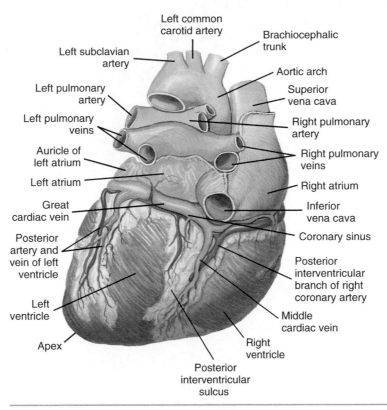

FIGURE 15-1. The heart and great vessels, posterior view.

Blood Vessels

Blood vessels are the tubes that transport blood from the heart to the cells and back to the heart. Most arteries carry oxygenated blood away from the heart. They continue to get smaller the farther away they are from the heart (arterioles). At this point, arterioles lead to **capillaries**, and exchange is made between blood and body cells; venules and veins return blood back to the heart. The circulation of blood that moves throughout the body is referred to as systemic circulation. Blood pressure measured at the arm indicates systemic pressures.

Lymphatic System

The lymphatic system is closely related to the circulatory system. The lymphatic drainage system returns back to the bloodstream products that have leaked out from the capillaries. The lymph system is also made up of lymph nodes, as well as spleen, thymus, tonsils, and adenoids. The lymph system fights infection by filtering out viruses and bacteria by attacking them with lymphocytes.

DISEASE CONDITIONS

Diseases of the Circulatory System (I00-I99), Chapter 9 in the ICD-10-CM code book, is divided into the following categories:

CATEGORY	SECTION TITLES
I00-I02	Acute rheumatic fever
I05-I09	Chronic rheumatic heart disease
I10-I15	Hypertensive diseases

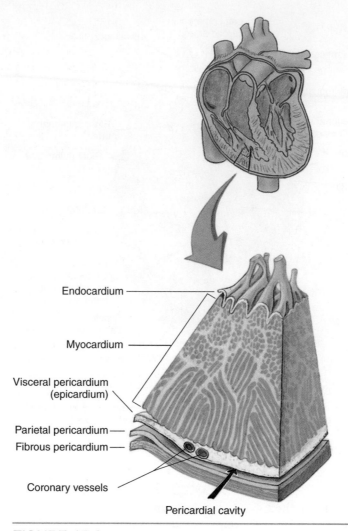

Endocardium

Myocardium

Visceral pericardium
(epicardium)

Parietal pericardium

Fibrous pericardium

Coronary vessels

Pericardial cavity

FIGURE 15-2. Layers of the heart wall.

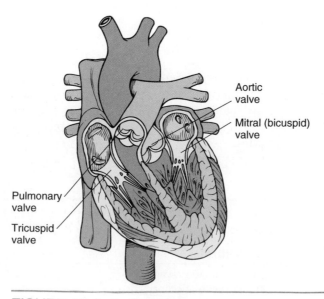

Aortic
valve

Mitral (bicuspid)
valve

Pulmonary
valve

Tricuspid
valve

FIGURE 15-3. Cardiac valves.

CATEGORY	SECTION TITLES
I20-I25	Ischemic heart diseases
I26-I28	Pulmonary heart disease and diseases of pulmonary circulation
I30-I52	Other forms of heart disease
I60-I69	Cerebrovascular diseases
I70-I79	Diseases of arteries, arterioles, and capillaries
I80-I89	Diseases of veins, lymphatic vessels, and lymph nodes, not elsewhere classified
I95-I99	Other and unspecified disorders of the circulatory system

Acute Rheumatic Fever (I00-I02) and Chronic Rheumatic Heart Disease (I05-I09)

Acute rheumatic fever is an inflammatory disease usually found in children that may affect the heart, joints, skin, or brain following an infection with streptococcal bacteria such as strep throat or scarlet fever.

EXAMPLE   Patient was admitted with acute rheumatic fever with endocarditis, I01.1.

EXAMPLE   Patient has rheumatic chorea without heart involvement, I02.9.

Chronic rheumatic heart disease is a chronic condition that is usually a late effect of attacks of acute rheumatic fever and most often involves the heart valves. When mitral and aortic valves are involved, ICD-10-CM assumes a causal relationship to rheumatic heart disease unless specified as nonrheumatic. Tricuspid valve disorders are assumed rheumatic unless specified as nonrheumatic in origin (Figure 15-4).

Mitral stenosis with insufficiency, incompetence or regurgitation, and mitral valve failure are presumed by ICD-10-CM to be rheumatic in origin.

EXAMPLE   Stenosis, mitral, I05.0.

Hypertensive Diseases (I10-I15)

Hypertension is classified as primary (essential) or secondary. Primary hypertension, or high **blood pressure** (BP), is a condition that is defined as abnormally high blood pressure in the arterial system. The American Heart Association defines hypertension as pressures exceeding 140/90. A diagnosis of hypertension can be made only by a physician and should

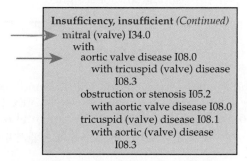

FIGURE 15-4. Mitral insufficiency with aortic valve disease.

not be assigned on the basis of BP readings alone. Essential hypertension has no known origin, and its symptoms are insidious.

Secondary hypertension is a consequence of other diseases such as kidney diseases, brain tumor, or polycythemia. When secondary hypertension is documented, two codes are required. The additional code required for secondary hypertension is the underlying condition code. The sequencing of these two codes depends on the circumstances of the admission.

EXAMPLE   Patient is admitted with hypercalcemia due to hyperparathyroidism. The patient also has hypertension due to the hyperparathyroidism, E21.3, I15.2.

EXAMPLE   Patient has hypertension due to Cushing's disease, E24.9, I15.2.

Medications often used for treating hypertension include Accupril, Aldomet, captopril, Cardizem, diltiazem, Cozaar, losartan, Coreg, dyazide, Hytrin, Inderal, Lopressor, Norvasc, Procardia, Tenormin, atenolol, Vasotec, Toprol, Calan, verapamil, Zestril, and lisinopril.

EXAMPLE   Patient has a past history of hypertension, currently taking verapamil, I10.

For a variety of reasons, patients may have elevated blood pressure readings. Unless a patient has an established diagnosis of hypertension, the code R03.0 elevated blood pressure, should be assigned.

EXAMPLE   The patient has high blood pressure; will recheck at next clinic visit. No medications were given, R03.0.

Hypertensive Heart, Renal, and Heart and Renal Disease

ICD-10-CM assumes a cause-and-effect relationship and classifies chronic kidney disease with hypertension as hypertensive renal disease. This indicates to the coder that any time hypertension and chronic kidney disease (codes from category N18) occur in a patient, category (I12) should be assigned. The only time the (I12) category code would not be selected is when the physician documents CKD not due to hypertension. On occasion, a patient will have CKD due to diabetes and also have hypertension; diabetic kidney disease and hypertensive kidney disease would both be assigned in these cases.

Hypertensive heart disease, in contrast to hypertensive renal disease, does not assume a cause-and-effect relationship. A causal relationship must be stated by the physician. For a code from this category to be assigned, the physician must document hypertensive heart disease or must say that heart disease is due to hypertension. It is important to note that if a patient has hypertensive congestive heart failure, at least two codes—I11.0 and I50.-—are required; if known, the codes for systolic (I50.2-), diastolic (I50.3-), or a combination systolic and diastolic (I50.4-) should also be assigned.

EXAMPLE   Patient is admitted with both diastolic and systolic congestive heart failure due to long history of hypertension, I11.0, I50.40.

Hypertensive heart and renal disease requires that the condition be classified to I13.–. It is important to become familiar with the Includes as well as Excludes notes in all of the above categories. It is also important to note that if a patient also has acute renal failure with any of the above conditions, an additional code for the acute renal failure is also assigned.

EXAMPLE | Patient is admitted with hypertensive renal disease. The patient also has hypertensive cardiomyopathy, I13.10, N18.9.

EXERCISE 15-1

Assign codes to the following conditions.

1. Patient is admitted with a diagnosis of hypertensive urgency _____
2. Aortic stenosis with mitral insufficiency _____
3. Malignant hypertension _____
4. Labile hypertension _____
5. Portal hypertension _____
6. Congestive heart failure due to hypertensive heart disease _____
7. Cardiomegaly with hypertension _____
8. Hypertension secondary to coarctation of aorta _____
9. Ocular hypertension, right eye _____
10. Essential hypertension _____
11. HCVD (hypertensive cardiovascular disease) with chronic renal failure _____
12. High blood pressure reading _____

Ischemic Heart Disease (I20-I25)

Acute Myocardial Infarction

Acute **myocardial infarction** (AMI, or MI) in layman's terms is known as a heart attack. An MI occurs when complete blockage of blood flow occurs in a coronary artery. When this occurs, blood is prevented from reaching the heart muscle (Figure 15-5). Blockage may be caused by fatty deposits (also known as plaque or atherosclerosis) or blood clots. When the blood cannot reach the heart, the heart muscle may become damaged. Signs of a heart attack include chest pain, shortness of breath, nausea, and pain in the arms and chest.

To determine whether a patient is having a heart attack, several tests, including various types of blood tests, may be performed. One of these tests is called CPK (creatine phosphokinase, or creatine kinase). CPK is an isoenzyme that occurs in high concentration in the heart and skeletal muscle. The level of CPK-MB (creatine phosphokinase, MB isoenzyme) in the blood rises 3 to 6 hours after an MI and returns to normal 12 to 48 hours after the infarct. Usually, CPK is measured every 8 to 12 hours, and patterns are determined. The normal value for males is 25 to 90; for females, it is 10 to 70. Another type of blood test that is often performed is the measurement of cardiac muscle proteins called troponins. Testing for troponin levels and CPK levels is performed serially. Troponin levels are usually very low, and elevated levels can indicate damage to the heart. Healthcare providers also perform electrocardiograms (EKGs) to determine whether an MI has occurred.

Types of MI may be classified as to the area of heart that suffers damage or the extent of damage, as evidenced by an EKG (Figure 15-6). The most common areas are the following:

- Anterior
- Inferior
- Lateral
- Posterior
- Right ventricular

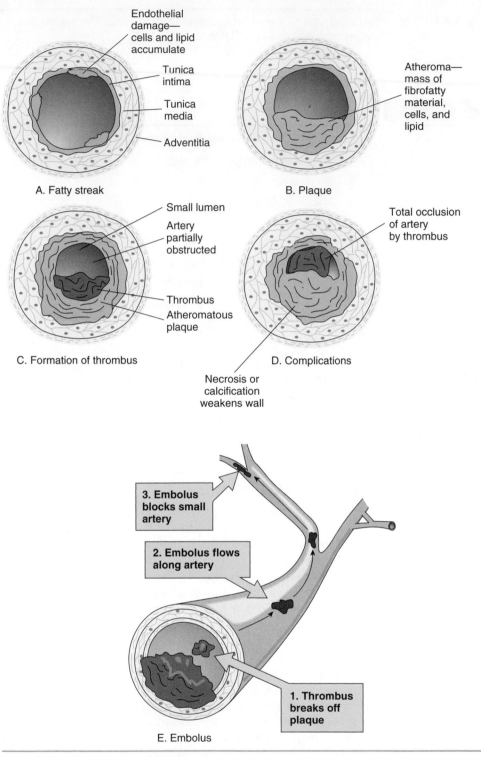

Endothelial damage—cells and lipid accumulate

Tunica intima

Tunica media

Adventitia

A. Fatty streak

Atheroma—mass of fibrofatty material, cells, and lipid

B. Plaque

Small lumen

Artery partially obstructed

Thrombus

Atheromatous plaque

C. Formation of thrombus

Total occlusion of artery by thrombus

Necrosis or calcification weakens wall

D. Complications

3. Embolus blocks small artery

2. Embolus flows along artery

1. Thrombus breaks off plaque

E. Embolus

FIGURE 15-5. Development of an atheroma, leading to arterial occlusion.

STEMI (ST elevation MI) occurs when complete obstruction of the coronary artery causes damage involving the full thickness of the heart muscle. This type of MI is also known as an ST elevation MI or a Q wave MI. **NSTEMI** (non–ST elevation) occurs when a coronary artery is partially obstructed and damage does not involve the full thickness of the heart muscle. This type of MI is often referred to as non–Q wave MI. Old terminology for transmural or nontransmural MI has been replaced by Q or non–Q MI.

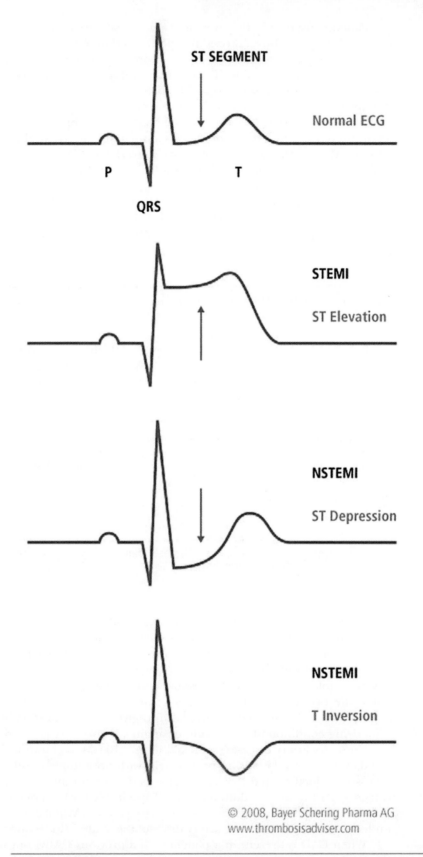

FIGURE 15-6. Illustration of normal ECG as well as STEMI and NSTEMI.

Patients suspected of having an MI are usually treated with a combination of medications and/or procedures. Procedures performed to treat the causes of MI include coronary angioplasty (percutaneous transluminal coronary angioplasty [PTCA]), stenting (percutaneous coronary intervention [PCI]), and possibly coronary artery bypass surgery (CABG or CAB). Often, upon presentation of the patient to the Emergency Room (ER), thrombolytic therapy is initiated. Thrombolytics (tissue plasminogen activator [TPA], streptokinase) are used to dissolve blood clots that may be blocking a coronary artery. Thrombolytics must be administered within 6 hours of the onset of chest pain to avoid heart damage. A potential adverse effect of the use of these drugs is severe bleeding; for this reason, they are contraindicated in many patients. All of these procedures are discussed in greater detail in the procedure section of this chapter.

When assigning a code for an acute MI in ICD-10-CM, it is important to find documentation of the site of the MI for a STEMI. It is also important to note that a code from I21 is assigned for an MI that has occurred within 28 days of the current admission. If the MI is older than 28 days, then code I25.2 is assigned.

EXAMPLE | Patient was admitted with NSTEMI, I21.4.

ICD-10-CM also has codes for subsequent MIs that occur within 28 days of the previous MI. The code category assigned for these subsequent MIs is I22. Category I22 can never be assigned without a code from I21 for the original. The sequencing of these codes is dependent upon the conditions of the admission to the hospital.

EXAMPLE | Patient is admitted to the hospital with chest pain. After testing, it is determined that the patient has suffered a NSTEMI. Patient is discharged home. Two weeks later, patient returns to the hospital with severe chest pain. It is now determined that the patient has suffered a STEMI of the inferolateral wall, I22.0, I21.4.

EXAMPLE | Patient is admitted to the hospital with chest pain. Five weeks ago, the patient had been admitted for a NSTEMI, R07.9, I25.2.

Prior to having an MI, a patient may have had symptoms such as unstable angina (USA), which is often described in today's vernacular as acute coronary syndrome, or ACS. A patient with this condition requires immediate medical treatment, but a patient with chronic angina may be treated with medications on a long-term basis as necessary. Patients with ACS may have unstable angina or could possibly have a non–Q MI. It may at times be necessary to query the provider for more specificity when ACS has been documented. Patients with angina may be prescribed sublingual nitroglycerin to relieve pain symptoms. Often, the underlying condition of chest pain, or angina, is coronary artery disease.

Coronary artery disease is indexed in ICD-10-CM as shown in Figure 15-7. ICD-10-CM assumes a causal relationship in a patient with both angina and coronary atherosclerosis unless it is documented that the angina is due to another cause. There is a note under category I25.1 to use an additional code if applicable for lipid rich plaque. Lipid rich plaque is the accumulation of lipids within coronary plaques. When coding an acute MI where the underlying cause is coronary artery disease, the acute MI is sequenced first.

When CAD is present in a patient with a previous CABG but it is not known whether the CAD is of a graft or a native artery, the code I25.10 should be used. Also assign code Z95.1 to show that the patient had coronary artery bypass surgery. When there is no documentation that the patient had a CABG procedure in the past, then the code for CAD should be assigned to native arteries I25.10.

> **Disease, diseased** (*Continued*)
>   heart (*Continued*)
>   hyperthyroid (*see also* Hyperthyroidism) E05.90 [I43]
>   with thyroid storm E05.91 [I43]
>   ischemic (chronic or with a stated duration of over 4 weeks) I25.9
> → atherosclerotic (of) I25.10
>   with angina pectoris - *see* Arteriosclerosis, coronary (artery)
>   coronary artery bypass graft - *see* Arteriosclerosis, coronary (artery),
>   cardiomyopathy I25.5
>   diagnosed on ECG or other special investigation, but currently presenting no symptoms I25.6
>   silent I25.6
>   specified form NEC I25.89

FIGURE 15-7. Coronary artery disease in ICD-10-CM Alphabetic Index.

Cardiologists may select a particular type of stent based on the presence of lipid rich plaque. Identification of plaque as being lipid rich or non–lipid rich is important diagnostic information for the interventional cardiologist. This diagnostic information can assist the cardiologist in determining the most appropriate type of stent (i.e., drug-eluting vs. bare metal) to use based on the present location and amount of lipid-rich plaque. The code for coronary atherosclerosis is sequenced before the code for lipid-rich plaque.

EXERCISE 15-2

Assign codes to the following conditions.

1. Patient had an MI 1 year prior to this admission _____

2. Patient had a nontransmural MI 6 weeks ago and now presents with chest pain _____

3. Patient has CAD and a history of CABG. Recent coronary catheterization shows coronary artery disease of the native arteries _____

4. Patient has CAD and a previous MI and coronary artery bypass _____

5. Patient with an anterolateral MI is transferred to this hospital for further evaluation and treatment _____

Pulmonary Heart Disease and Diseases of Pulmonary Circulation (I26-I28)

Pulmonary Embolism

A **pulmonary embolism** is a blood clot(s) in the pulmonary artery that causes blockage in the artery. Most often, clots originate in the legs and then travel to the lung. A blood clot that forms and remains in a vein is a **thrombus**. A clot that travels to another part of the body is an **embolus**. Common symptoms of pulmonary embolism include shortness of breath, chest pain, and cough.

A pulmonary embolism may be diagnosed via lung scan or computed tomography (CT) scan. A pulmonary embolism can be life threatening, and once you have had one, the risk for recurrence is increased.

An acute pulmonary embolism may be treated with anticoagulant therapy (heparin or Coumadin) for 3 to 6 months and generally does not cause chronic disease. Once the embolism dissolves, therapy is discontinued. When a patient has a chronic pulmonary embolism, treatment may be longstanding, and sometimes surgery is performed to remove the clot.

EXAMPLE | Patient is admitted to the hospital with chest pain. Two weeks prior to this admit, the patient had been treated for an acute pulmonary embolism for which he is receiving Coumadin. The discharge summary documents the reason for admission to be chest pain due to GERD, K21.9, I26.99.

Pulmonary Hypertension

Pulmonary hypertension (PHT) is high blood pressure in the arteries that supply blood to the lungs. Normal pulmonary systolic pressure is 18 to 25 mm Hg. Two types of pulmonary hypertension—primary and secondary—have been identified. Primary pulmonary hypertension (PPH) is a rare condition of unknown origin that is both progressive and ultimately fatal. In recent years, this condition has been linked with the use of anti-obesity drugs such as Fen/Phen. Secondary pulmonary hypertension is caused by other conditions such as chronic obstructive pulmonary disease (COPD), emphysema, pulmonary embolism, or obstructive sleep apnea (OSA). Patients who have prolonged untreated pulmonary hypertension often develop right ventricular failure. Doppler echocardiography is the most useful test for determining the diagnosis of pulmonary hypertension.

Symptoms of pulmonary hypertension may include dyspnea on exertion (DOE), syncope, fatigue, and chest pain. Treatment for this disease may involve correcting the underlying cause, if possible. Medical treatments may include vasodilators, diuretics, anticoagulants, oxygen, and digoxin. In some cases, lung transplantation may be considered.

EXAMPLE | Patient has pulmonary hypertension due to COPD, I27.2, J44.9.

Other Forms of Heart Disease (I30-I52)

Pericarditis

Pericarditis is inflammation of the covering of the heart. It is often a complication of viral infection and systemic disease such as acquired immunodeficiency syndrome (AIDS). Sometimes, pericarditis follows an MI; it may also arise from bacterial infection. The disease presents with symptoms such as chest pain, breathing difficulties, fever, and cough. The heart sound heard through the stethoscope by the physician in cases of pericarditis is called a pericardial rub. Pericarditis is diagnosed through the use of chest x-ray (CXR), echocardiography, and magnetic resonance imaging (MRI). Usually, these patients also have abnormal EKG results.

EXAMPLE | Acute pericardial effusion, I30.9.

EXAMPLE | Uremic pericarditis, N18.9, I32.

EXAMPLE | Acute viral pericarditis, I30.1, B97.89.

Endocarditis

Endocarditis is inflammation of the lining of the heart chambers and valves. Most often, bacterial infection is the cause of endocarditis. Patients with intravenous drug use (IVDU), central venous lines, and valve replacements (aortic valve replacement [AVR], mitral valve replacement [MVR]) are at greater risk for developing endocarditis. Patients with endocarditis might present with fever, shortness of breath (SOB), fatigue, night sweats, and muscle aches. In determining this diagnosis, physicians order blood cultures and perform echocardiograms. Treatment always consists of intravenous (IV) antibiotics; therefore, the patient may be hospitalized. IV antibiotic treatment may take up to 6 weeks.

EXAMPLE   Patient admitted for antibiotics for subacute endocarditis, I33.9.

EXAMPLE   Patient admitted for endocarditis caused by typhoid, A01.02.

Non–rheumatic Valve Disorders

Non–rheumatic valve disorders of incompetence, insufficiency, and regurgitation may be classified to categories I35-I39. A leaking valve is another name for regurgitation, incompetence, or insufficiency. When this occurs, blood flows backward within the valve. If a valve's opening is blocked or flow of blood is diminished, this is called stenosis. Coding of valve disorders requires the user to pay close attention to the Alphabetic Index and all Instruction notes. When coding a combination of mitral, aortic, or tricuspid valve disorders together, ICD-10-CM assumes a causal relationship and defaults to rheumatic.

EXAMPLE   Non-rheumatic tricuspid stenosis, I36.0.

EXAMPLE   Mitral insufficiency, I34.0.

EXAMPLE   Mitral valve prolapse, I34.1.

Cardiomyopathy

Cardiomyopathy is a disorder of the muscle of the heart chambers that impedes the functioning of the heart. Another term for congestive cardiomyopathy is dilated cardiomyopathy. Cardiomyopathy can be caused by disorders such as CAD, infection, diabetes, or alcohol abuse. Two codes may be required to code cardiomyopathy—one for the underlying condition and one for cardiomyopathy. Cardiomyopathy is diagnosed by echocardiography and is treated with antibiotics if due to an infection or treatment may be targeted to the underlying cause. Congestive cardiomyopathy may be associated with congestive heart failure. When they occur together, congestive heart failure would be the principal diagnosis, because it is often the focus of treatment. The cardiomyopathy would be assigned as an additional code.

EXAMPLE   Obstructive hypertrophic cardiomyopathy, I42.1.

EXAMPLE   Alcoholic cardiomyopathy, I42.6, F10.20.

Cardiomyopathy due to amyloidosis, E85.4, I43.

Conduction Disorders

A **conduction disorder** is a problem that occurs in the electrical impulses that regulate heartbeat. A heartbeat begins when an electrical impulse is sent through the upper chambers of the heart. A human heart usually beats from 60 to 100 times per minute. **Tachycardia** (fast heart rate) means the heartbeat is greater than 100 beats per minute; **bradycardia** (slow heart rate) is a heartbeat of fewer than 60 beats per minute.

Electrophysiologic studies are often performed after a device is implanted to test if the device is working. If an arrhythmia is induced to test a device, the arrhythmia is not coded. If however, the arrhythmia or condition is discovered during testing, then this diagnosis would be coded.

Heart blocks occur when impulses originating in the upper chambers are unable to pass to the lower chambers at the correct rate. Three types of blocks have been observed:
- First degree: Conduction of beats from upper to lower is slower than normal.
- Second degree: Not all beats pass from upper to lower.
- Third degree: Impulses cannot pass from upper to lower.

EXAMPLE ECG shows left bundle branch block, anterior fascicular block with posterior fascicular block, I44.7, I44.4, I44.5.

EXAMPLE The patient has a bifascicular block, I45.2.

Cardiac arrhythmias (Table 15-1) occur when the normal sequence of electrical impulses changes, or the rhythm of the heartbeat is disturbed. (Normal sequence = RA [right atrium] through atrioventricular [AV] node through His bundle to ventricles.)

EXAMPLE Atrial fibrillation (AF), I48.91.

EXAMPLE Sick sinus syndrome (SSS), I49.5.

EXAMPLE Supraventricular tachycardia (SVT), I47.1.

Cardiac arrest, the sudden loss of heart function, is assigned code I46.9. This may be coded as the principal diagnosis in only two instances:
1. When the patient presents to the ER in cardiac arrest and dies before the underlying cause of the arrest has been established
2. When the patient presents to the hospital in cardiac arrest, is resuscitated, admitted as an inpatient, and subsequently dies before the underlying cause of the arrest has been established

Cardiac arrest may be coded as a secondary diagnosis when a patient has a cardiac arrest and is resuscitated on arrival or during the inpatient stay. The arrest is not coded when a physician documents cardiac arrest as the cause of death.

Heart failure is impaired function of the heart's pumping ability. The heart is unable to pump with enough force or to fill with enough blood. This damage to the heart muscle

TABLE 15-1 ARRYTHMIAS[1]

Types	Symptoms and Signs	Etiology	Diagnosis	Treatment
Normal sinus rhythm	Rate of 60-100 bpm, regular, P wave uniform	Impulse originates in SA node, conduction normal	Normal	None indicated
Sinus tachycardia	Rate >100 bpm, regular, P wave uniform	Rapid impulse originates in SA node, conduction normal	Rapid rate	Beta blockers, calcium channel blockers
Sinus brachycardia	Rate <60 bpm, regular, P wave uniform	Slow impulse originates in SA node, conduction normal	Slow rate	Atropine
Premature atrial contraction	Rate depends on underlying rhythm, usually normal P wave, morphology different from other P waves	Irritable atrium, single ectopic beat that arises prematurely, conduction through ventricle normal	Irregular heartbeat, diagnosis by ECG	Treatment usually unnecessary; if needed, antiarrhythmic drugs
Atrial tachycardia	Rate of 150-250 bpm, rhythm normal, sudden onset	Irritable atrium, firing at rapid rates, normal conduction	Rapid rate with atrial and ventricular rates identical, diagnosis by ECG	Reflex vagal stimulation, calcium channel–blocking drugs (verapamil), cardioversion
Atrial fibrillation	Atrial rate >350 bpm, ventricular rate <100 bpm (controlled) or ≥100 bpm (rapid ventricular response)	Atrial ectopic foci discharging at too rapid and chaotic a rate for muscles to respond and contract, resulting in quivering of atrium; AV node blocks some impulses, and ventricle responds irregularly	ECG show no P waves, grossly irregular ventricular rate	IV verapamil; if unsuccessful, procainamide; if unsuccessful, cardioversion
First-degree heart block	Rate depends on rate of underlying rhythm, PR interval >0.20 second	Delay at AV node, impulse eventually conducted	ECG shows PR interval >0.20 second	Atropine; if unsuccessful, artificial pacemaker insertion
Second-degree heart block, Wenckebach block	Intermittent block with progressively longer delay in conduction until one beat is blocked; atrial rate normal, ventricular rate slower than normal, rhythm irregular	SA node initiates impulse, conduction through AV node is blocked intermittently	ECG shows normal P waves, some P waves not followed by QRS complex; PR interval progressively longer, followed by block of impulse	Mild forms, no treatment; severe, insertion of artificial pacemaker
Classic second-degree heart block	Ventricular rate slow (½, ⅓, or ¼ of atrial rate); rhythm, regular; P waves normal, QRS complex dropped every 2nd, 3rd, or 4th beat	SA node initiates impulse, conduction through AV node is blocked	ECG shows P waves present, QRS complex blocked every 2nd, 3rd, or 4th impulse	Artificial pacemaker is inserted
Third-degree heart block	Atrial rate normal, ventricular rate 20-40 or 40-60 bpm; no relationship between P wave and QRS complex	SA node initiates impulse, which is completely blocked from conduction, causing atria and ventricles to beat independently	ECG shows P waves and QRS complexes with no relationship to each other; rhythms are regular but independent of each other	Insertion of artificial pacemaker is needed

AV, Atrioventricular; *bpm*, beats per minute; *ECG*, electrocardiogram; *IV*, intravenous; *PR*, pulse rate; *PVC*, premature ventricular contraction; *SA*, sinoatrial.

Continued

TABLE 15-1 ARRYTHMIAS[1]—cont'd

Types	Symptoms and Signs	Etiology	Diagnosis	Treatment
Premature ventricular contraction (single focus)	Single ectopic beat, arising from ventricle, followed by compensatory pause	Ectopic beat originates in irritable ventricle	ECG shows a wide, bizarre QRS complex >0.12 second, usually followed by a compensatory pause	Usually, no treatment if <6 per minute and single focus
Multifocal arrhythmia Coupling, 2 in a row Bigeminy, every other beat Trigeminy, every 3rd beat Quadrigeminy, every 4th beat	Rate dependent on underlying rhythm; rhythm regular or irregular; P wave absent before ectopic beat	Same as single focus	Same as single focus	Same as single focus
Ventricular tachycardia	Rate of 150-250 bpm, rhythm usually regular; focus of pacemaker normally single; patient experiences palpitations, dyspnea, and anxiety followed by chest pain	Four or more consecutive PVCs at a rapid rate due to advanced irritability of myocardium, indicating ventricular command of heart rate	ECG show runs of four or more PVCs; P was buried in QRS complex	Often forerunner of ventricular fibrillation; immediate intervention necessary; IV lidocaine; if unsuccessful, follow by cardioversion; procainamide or bretylium may be used
Ventricular fibrillation (lethal arrhythmia)	Patient loses consciousness immediately after onset; no peripheral pulses palpable, no heart sounds, no blood pressure	Ventricular fibers twitch rather than contract; reason unknown	Pulseless, unconscious patient; ECG shows rapid, repetitive, chaotic waves originating in ventricle	Recognize and terminate rhythm; precordial shock (defibrillation)

AV, Atrioventricular; *bpm*, beats per minute; *ECG*, electrocardiogram; *IV*, intravenous; *PR*, pulse rate; *PVC*, premature ventricular contraction; *SA*, sinoatrial.

may be caused by a variety of heart conditions such as CAD, MI, cardiomyopathy, hypertension (HTN), valve disease, diabetes mellitus (DM), and chronic kidney disease (CKD). This impaired pumping function in turn results in insufficient blood reaching the kidneys, which causes the body to retain fluid (Figure 15-8). Symptoms of heart failure include congested lungs, edema, fatigue, and irregular heartbeat.

Two types of heart failure may occur: systolic and diastolic. Systolic heart dysfunction, also known as systolic heart failure, occurs when the heart muscles are not contracting with enough force, and therefore, not enough blood is being pumped to the body. Diastolic cardiac dysfunction, also known as diastolic heart failure, occurs when the contraction is normal but the ventricle does not allow enough blood to enter the heart. Physicians can measure the percentage of blood that is pumped out of a filled ventricle with each heartbeat (known as ejection fraction) to determine how the heart is functioning. A normal ejection fraction measures 55% to 70%. Ejection fraction can be determined in several ways: echocardiography, MRI, multiple-gated acquisition (MUGA scan), or computerized tomography (CT) scan. Another test used to determine whether a patient is in heart failure is the brain natriuretic peptide (BNP) test. **BNP** is a hormone that is produced by the heart; a BNP test measures the amount of BNP that is found in the blood. Normally, levels of BNP are low, but in heart failure, these levels become elevated. A normal value of BNP would be 0 to 99 pg/mL. If this level is greater than 100, heart failure is indicated. Sometimes a provider

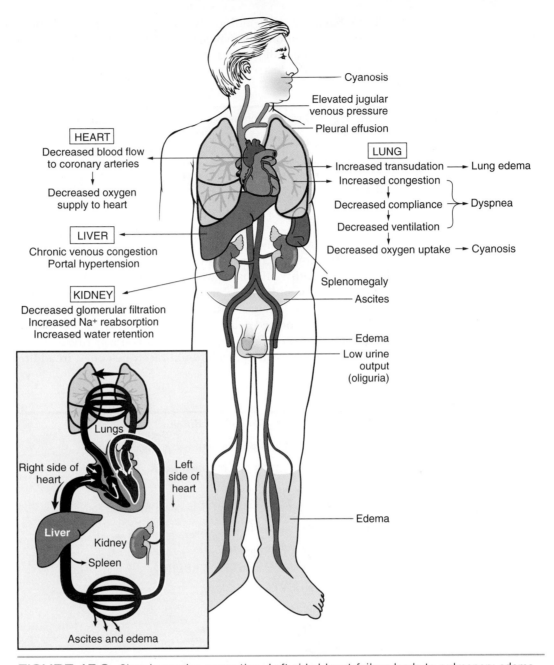

FIGURE 15-8. Chronic passive congestion. Left-sided heart failure leads to pulmonary edema. Right ventricular failure causes peripheral edema that is most prominent in the lower extremities.

will document the stage of heart failure. This may be described by a classification of the New York Heart Association (NYHA):

- NYHA Class I   Asymptomatic
- NYHA Class II   Symptoms with moderate exertion
- NYHA Class III   Symptoms with minimal exertion
- NYHA Class IV   Symptoms at rest

When coding heart failure, if the clinician documents systolic or diastolic heart failure along with congestive heart failure, only one code for the diastolic and/or systolic is assigned. The congestive heart failure is included in the codes of diastolic, systolic, or a combination. It is also important to look for documentation of acute, chronic, or acute on chronic. It is important to recognize that the terms "exacerbated" and "decompensated" indicate that a chronic condition is now in an acute phase. Patients may be treated for CHF as a chronic condition and may never be hospitalized. To assign a code for rheumatic congestive heart failure, the heart failure must be classified as rheumatic, or the physician must document that the heart failure is rheumatic in nature.

EXAMPLE | Patient admitted with decompensated diastolic congestive heart failure, I50.30.

EXAMPLE | Patient admitted with congestive heart failure, acute on chronic combined systolic and diastolic, I50.43.

In many cases, physicians will refer to heart failure as pulmonary edema or volume overload. Pulmonary edema has other causes, but one of its main causes is heart failure. Also, patients with CHF may have pleural effusions. A pleural effusion is commonly seen with CHF with or without pulmonary edema. In cases in which the patient has CHF, pulmonary edema, and pleural effusions, CHF would always be the principal diagnosis. Pleural effusion may be reported as an additional diagnosis if it was specifically evaluated or treated. Evaluation may consist of special x-rays to confirm presence, treatment, or a diagnostic thoracentesis. Pulmonary edema would rarely be coded in addition to CHF.

EXERCISE 15-3

Assign codes to the following conditions.

1. Pulmonary hypertension with cor pulmonale _____
2. Acute pericarditis due to tuberculosis _____
3. Acute bacterial endocarditis _____
4. Chronic hypertension and pulmonary hypertension _____
5. Aortic regurgitation _____
6. Dilated cardiomyopathy _____
7. Right bundle branch block (RBBB) _____
8. Wenckebach heart block _____
9. Atrial flutter _____
10. Persistent sinus bradycardia _____
11. Thyrotoxic cardiomyopathy _____
12. Hypertensive cardiomyopathy _____
13. Another name for inflammation of the lining of the heart chambers _____

Cerebrovascular Diseases (I60-I69)

A patient who is admitted with a diagnosis of **stroke** (brain infarction or cerebrovascular accident [CVA]) is similar to a patient who is admitted with a diagnosis of heart attack or MI. The blood supply to a part of the brain is blocked by a broken blood vessel, ischemia, or blood clots (Figure 15-9). When the blood supply is cut off, brain cells die. Several types of stroke or brain infarcts may occur (Figure 15-10). Ischemic stroke, which accounts for 80% of all strokes, happens when blockage to the brain, usually by a blood clot, occurs. A clot that develops in another part of the body and then becomes wedged in a brain artery is a free-roaming clot or an embolus (Figure 15-11).

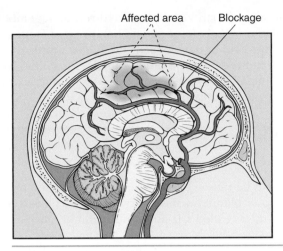

FIGURE 15-9. Cerebrovascular accident (CVA).

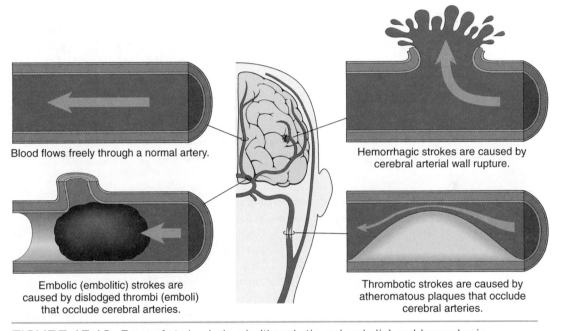

Blood flows freely through a normal artery.

Embolic (embolitic) strokes are caused by dislodged thrombi (emboli) that occlude cerebral arteries.

Hemorrhagic strokes are caused by cerebral arterial wall rupture.

Thrombotic strokes are caused by atheromatous plaques that occlude cerebral arteries.

FIGURE 15-10. Types of stroke: ischemic (thrombotic and embolic) and hemorrhagic.

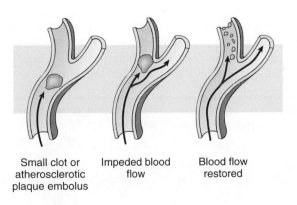

Small clot or atherosclerotic plaque embolus

Impeded blood flow

Blood flow restored

FIGURE 15-11. Embolus.

The most common type of stroke is ischemic (thrombotic/embolic). An ischemic stroke occurs when a blood clot or a piece of plaque breaks loose from an artery and lodges in a blood vessel of the brain, which then cuts off the blood supply to that area of the brain. A blood clot that forms and remains in a vein is called a thrombus, whereas a clot that travels to another part of the body is an **embolus**. Sometimes plaque is dislodged and becomes an embolus. The other type of stroke is hemorrhagic.

EXAMPLE   Embolic right middle cerebral infarction, I63.411.

Ischemic stroke may be caused by narrowing of the arteries, or **stenosis**. Stenosis is often caused by the buildup of plaque in the artery. This may be referred to as small- or large-vessel disease. Often, this is called a lacunar infarction.

EXAMPLE   Ischemic stroke, I63.9.

Hemorrhagic stroke occurs when an artery in the brain bursts and blood seeps into the surrounding tissue, causing the tissue to malfunction. When bleeding from the artery goes into the brain itself, this is called an intracerebral hemorrhage. When bleeding seeps into the meninges or outer membranes, this is called a subarachnoid hemorrhage. Hemorrhagic stroke may be caused by aneurysms, arteriovenous malformations (AVMs), and, possibly, plaque-encrusted walls that rupture. Hypertension can increase the risk of rupture of the artery wall.

EXAMPLE   Nontraumatic subarachnoid hemorrhage, I60.7.

Symptoms of a stroke often appear suddenly. These may occur as weakness or numbness of one side of the body, arm, leg, or face; confusion; difficulty talking or speaking; trouble walking or seeing; dizziness; and headache. A CT scan is often used to determine whether a patient has had a hemorrhagic stroke; MRI is another useful tool in the diagnosis of stroke. The benefit of MRI is that it can rapidly detect small infarcts.

Medication is the most common treatment for stroke patients. Patients with ischemic stroke may be treated with thrombolytic agents such as TPA. Similar to heart attack victims, stroke patients need to be treated with TPA soon after onset of symptoms. There is a code (Z92.82) for a patient who was administered TPA at a different facility. Most patients are treated with anticoagulants or with antiplatelet agents.

Sometimes a patient will present to the hospital with symptoms of a stroke, such as difficulty speaking or weakness on one side. TPA may be administered with considerable improvement in the patient's symptoms. If the TPA aborts the patient's cerebral infarction code I63.9 is assigned. Often, a patient is admitted with a stroke with deficits. These deficits are often gone by the time the patient is discharged. Any deficits that a patient exhibits from the stroke, whether present at discharge or not, should be assigned codes.

EXAMPLE   Patient suffered an embolic stroke in the middle cerebral artery. She presented with hemiparesis of the right side and aphasia both of which were not present at discharge, I63.419, I69.351, I69.320.

EXAMPLE   Subdural hemorrhage, with dysphagia at time of discharge, I62.00, I69.291, R13.10.

EXAMPLE   Stenosis of the carotid artery with cerebral infarction, I63.239.

Carotid artery stenosis is indexed in ICD-10-CM under occlusion, artery, carotid (Figures 15-12 and 15-13). It is important to take note of laterality if a patient has an infarct as a result of this stenosis and a known history of bilateral carotid stenosis—two codes are required.

EXAMPLE Patient with a history of bilateral carotid stenosis is admitted to the hospital with symptoms of a stroke. A workup is initiated, and it is determined that the patient had a ischemic stroke due to a thrombosis of the right carotid artery. The left carotid was recorded as a 65% blockage, I63.031, I65.22.

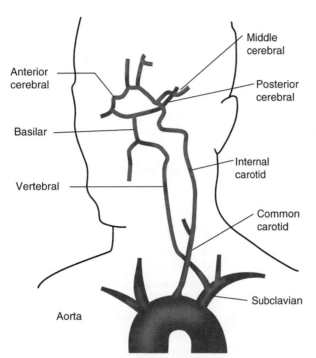

FIGURE 15-12. Cerebral and precerebral arteries.

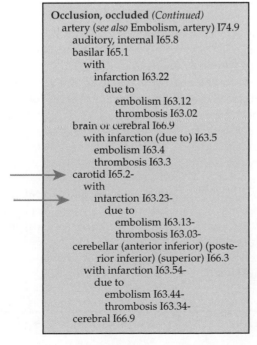

Occlusion, occluded *(Continued)*
 artery *(see also* Embolism, artery) I74.9
  auditory, internal I65.8
  basilar I65.1
   with
    infarction I63.22
     due to
      embolism I63.12
      thrombosis I63.02
  brain or cerebral I66.9
   with infarction (due to) I63.5
    embolism I63.4
    thrombosis I63.3
  carotid I65.2-
   with
    infarction I63.23-
     due to
      embolism I63.13-
      thrombosis I63.03-
  cerebellar (anterior inferior) (posterior inferior) (superior) I66.3
   with infarction I63.54-
    due to
     embolism I63.44-
     thrombosis I63.34-
  cerebral I66.9

FIGURE 15-13. Carotid artery stenosis with infarction.

Sequelae of Cerebrovascular Disease

Stroke is one of the leading causes of disability in the United States. Types of disability that may result from stroke consist of paralysis, particularly on one side of the body (hemiplegia), or weakness on one side (hemiparesis). Other disabilities include **cognitive deficits**, **aphasia** (impairment of language comprehension and production), emotional problems, and pain. When an inpatient has had a stroke, has current deficits, and also has late effects from a previous stroke, all codes should be assigned. Late effect codes may be listed as principal diagnoses when the purpose of the admission is to treat the late effect. The code for a history of CVA with no residuals is Z86.73.

EXAMPLE | Patient presents with carotid artery stenosis with infarct and current hemiparesis. Patient has residual aphasia from a previous stroke, I63.239, I69.359, I69.320.

EXERCISE 15-4

Assign codes to the following conditions.

1. Cerebral hemorrhage   _____

2. Patient was admitted with CVA and aphasia; the aphasia cleared before discharge   _____

3. Cerebral thrombosis without infarction   _____

4. Ruptured berry aneurysm   _____

5. Patient with a history of cerebrovascular accident, no residuals   _____

6. Quadriplegia resulting from a stroke last year   _____

7. Patient is being treated for cognitive deficits following a stroke   _____

Diseases of the Arteries, Arterioles, and Capillaries (I70-I79)

Atherosclerosis or arteriosclerosis is a stricture or hardening of the artery that is caused by deposits of plaque. These deposits restrict blood flow through the artery; plaques can rupture and travel to other parts of the body or can form blood clots that block a blood vessel. If a blood vessel to the heart is blocked, this causes a heart attack; if a vessel to the brain is blocked, this causes a stroke; and if vessels to the extremities are blocked, this can cause claudication, ulcers, and eventually, gangrene. Codes found in subcategory I70.2 are hierarchical. For example, if a patient has atherosclerosis of a native artery of the right leg with ulceration of the heel, rest pain, and claudication of the right leg, then only the code from I70.234 would be assigned, for the ulceration.

Atherosclerosis may continue to progress and in that case code only the most severe form:

- I70.21- atherosclerosis of the extremity with intermittent claudication
- I70.22- atherosclerosis of the extremity with intermittent claudication and rest pain
- I70.23-, I70.24-, I70.25- atherosclerosis of the extremity with intermittent claudication, rest pain, and ulceration
- I70.26- atherosclerosis of the extremity with intermittent claudication, rest pain, ulceration, and gangrene

---

EXAMPLE | Stenosis of renal artery, I70.1.

EXAMPLE Atherosclerosis of left leg autologous bypass graft with intermittent claudication, I70.412.

An **aneurysm** is a bulging or ballooning out of a vessel. Aneurysms are often caused by atherosclerosis and tend to have no symptoms, unless dissection occurs. Dissection is typically accompanied by severe pain in the area of dissection. Aneurysms tend to form in areas where vessels branch out. Aortic aneurysms (Figure 15-14) can occur anywhere along the aorta, which is the largest artery in the body; it runs from the heart through the chest into the abdominal area and then divides into vessels that supply blood to the legs. The most common aneurysms occur in the abdominal area. Rupture of an aneurysm is a life-threatening event. The risk of rupture increases as the aneurysm becomes larger. Sometimes, an aneurysm becomes **dissecting**, which means a tear begins in the wall of the vessel that causes layers to separate. Physicians use the terms type I, type II, and type III to describe dissecting aneurysms.

EXAMPLE   Patient presents to hospital with Type I thoracoabdominal aneurysm, I71.03.

Aneurysms are usually not treated until they reach a certain size or begin to enlarge quickly. Treatment for an aneurysm consists of open or endovascular surgery, which is discussed in the Procedure section of this chapter.

EXAMPLE   Abdominal aortic aneurysm, I71.4.

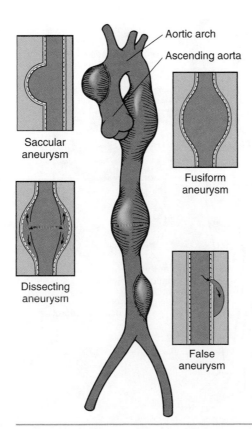

Saccular aneurysm

Aortic arch

Ascending aorta

Fusiform aneurysm

Dissecting aneurysm

False aneurysm

FIGURE 15-14. Types of aortic aneurysm.

| EXAMPLE | Ruptured thoracic aneurysm, I71.1. |

| EXAMPLE | Femoral aneurysm, I72.4. |

An arteriovenous **fistula** is an abnormal passage between an artery and a vein. Blood typically flows from arteries into capillaries and then to veins; however, when blood bypasses the capillaries and goes directly to the vein, an arteriovenous fistula results.

| EXAMPLE | Patient has an arteriovenous fistula, acquired, I77.0. |

Diseases of Veins, Lymphatic Vessels, and Lymph Nodes, Not Elsewhere Classified (I80-I89)

Phlebitis, Thrombophlebitis, and Deep Vein Thrombosis

Phlebitis is inflammation of a vein; thrombophlebitis occurs when a clot forms in the vein and then causes inflammation or phlebitis. **Deep vein thrombosis** (DVT) is a blood clot that forms in a deep vein, usually in the leg or hip (Figures 15-15 and 15-16). A DVT is indexed

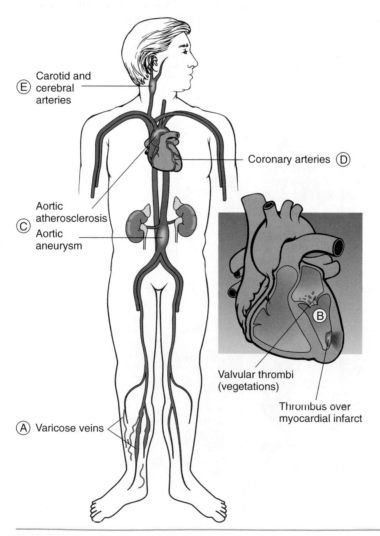

FIGURE 15-15. Common sites of thrombus formation.

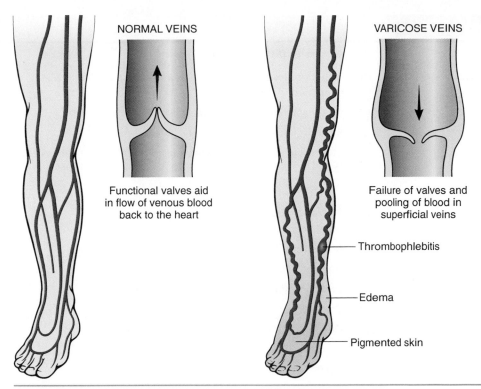

NORMAL VEINS

Functional valves aid
in flow of venous blood
back to the heart

VARICOSE VEINS

Failure of valves and
pooling of blood in
superficial veins

—— Thrombophlebitis

—— Edema

—— Pigmented skin

FIGURE 15-16. Normal and varicose veins. Slow flow in the veins makes an individual susceptible to clot formation. Thrombotic occlusion of varicose veins is known as thrombophlebitis. If a thrombus becomes loosened from its place in a vein, it can travel to the lungs (pulmonary embolism) and block a blood vessel there. Then blood pools in the lower part of the leg and fluid leaks from distended small capillaries, causing edema.

in ICD-10-CM under Embolism, vein, lower extremity. DVTs are treated with anticoagulants such as heparin or warfarin. In some cases a filter may need to be inserted in the vena cava to prevent clots from traveling to the lungs or the heart.

EXAMPLE | Patient admitted with an acute femoral DVT of the right leg with inflammation, I82.411.

Varicose veins are enlarged, twisted veins that usually occur in the legs. Varicose veins can be found in other areas of the body such as the esophagus. Varicose veins often develop complications that require surgical treatment. Stasis dermatitis with varicose veins of the leg is assigned code I83.10.

Stasis dermatitis is a skin condition caused by poor circulation (venous insufficiency) that is characterized by swelling, skin discoloration, weeping, itching, and scaly skin. The legs and particularly the ankles are the areas most often affected. This condition is often seen in the elderly, and risk for developing this condition increases when any of the following conditions is present: obesity, high blood pressure, varicose veins and heart, and/or kidney failure. A common complication of stasis dermatitis is cellulitis.

EXAMPLE | Patient with stasis dermatitis of the left leg with a Stage 1 calf ulcer, I83.222, L97.221.

EXAMPLE | Patient with alcoholic cirrhosis of the liver with esophageal varices with bleeding, K70.30, I85.11, F10.20.

Assign codes to the following conditions.

1. Atherosclerosis of the extremities with rest pain and gangrene _____

2. Arteriosclerotic cardiovascular disease _____

3. Arteriosclerosis of a left carotid artery _____

4. Atherosclerosis of a nonautologous bypass graft of the left leg _____

5. Dissection of the thoracic aorta _____

6. Type II dissection of the aorta _____

7. Iliac artery aneurysm _____

8. Acquired arteriovenous aneurysm of the brain _____

9. Buerger's disease _____

10. Embolic infarction of the abdominal aorta _____

11. Thrombosis of the subclavian artery _____

12. Deep vein thrombosis of the right lower extremity _____

13. Peroneal DVT of the left leg _____

14. Scrotal varices _____

15. Bilateral varicose veins, asymptomatic _____

FACTORS INFLUENCING HEALTH STATUS AND CONTACT WITH HEALTH SERVICES (Z CODES)

As was discussed in Chapter 8, it may be difficult to locate Z codes in the index. Coders often say, "I did not know there was a Z code for that."

Refer to Chapter 8 for a listing of common main terms used to locate Z codes. A review of the Tabular reveals that some Z codes pertain to diseases of the circulatory system:

Z01.30	Encounter for examination of blood pressure without abnormal findings
Z01.31	Encounter for examination of blood pressure with abnormal findings
Z13.6	Encounter for screening for cardiovascular disorders
Z45.010	Encounter for checking and testing of cardiac pacemaker pulse generator [battery]
Z45.018	Encounter for adjustment and management of other part of cardiac pacemaker
Z45.02	Encounter for adjustment and management of automatic implantable cardiac defibrillator
Z45.09	Encounter for adjustment and management of other cardiac device
Z45.1	Encounter for adjustment and management of infusion pump
Z45.2	Encounter for adjustment and management of vascular access device
Z82.41	Family history of sudden cardiac death
Z82.49	Family history of ischemic heart disease and other diseases of the circulatory system
Z86.711	Personal history of pulmonary embolism
Z86.718	Personal history of other venous thrombosis and embolism
Z86.72	Personal history of thrombophlebitis
Z86.73	Personal history of transient ischemic attack (TIA) and cerebral infarction without residual deficits
Z86.74	Personal history of sudden cardiac arrest
Z86.79	Personal history of other diseases of the circulatory system

Z92.82	Status post administration of tPA (rtPA) in a different facility within the last 24 hours prior to admission to current facility
Z94.1	Heart transplant status
Z94.3	Heart and lungs transplant status
Z95.0	Presence of cardiac pacemaker
Z95.1	Presence of aortocoronary bypass graft
Z95.2	Presence of prosthetic heart valve
Z95.3	Presence of xenogenic heart valve
Z95.4	Presence of other heart-valve replacement
Z95.5	Presence of coronary angioplasty implant and graft
Z95.810	Presence of automatic (implantable) cardiac defibrillator
Z95.811	Presence of heart-assist device
Z95.812	Presence of fully implantable artificial heart
Z95.818	Presence of other cardiac implants and grafts
Z95.820	Presence vascular angioplasty status with implants and grafts
Z95.828	Presence of other vascular implants and grafts
Z95.9	Presence of cardiac and vascular implant and graft, unspecified
Z98.61	Coronary angioplasty status
Z98.62	Peripheral vascular angioplasty status

EXAMPLE Patient admitted with chest pain. Has a history of PTCA, R07.9, Z98.61.

EXAMPLE Patient admitted for DVT right lower extremity. On Coumadin for previous stroke, I82.401, Z79.01, Z86.73.

EXAMPLE Patient admitted to Hospital A with a CVA and tPA was administered percutaneously via a peripheral vein. The patient was stabilized and 8 hours later transferred to Hospital B for treatment of CVA.
　　Hospital A: I63.50; 3E03317.
　　Hospital B: I63.50, Z92.82, 3E03317.

EXERCISE 15-6

Assign codes to the following conditions.

1. Patient is admitted to the hospital with chest pain; the only　＿＿＿＿＿＿＿
   risk factor he has is a family history of CAD

2. Patient is admitted with acute pulmonary edema, history of　＿＿＿＿＿＿＿
   CHF, patient currently on lasix, and history of a heart valve
   replaced by a prosthesis

3. Patient is admitted to the hospital with an acute MI and　＿＿＿＿＿＿＿
   history of a five-vessel CABG

4. Patient is admitted to the hospital with ACS and has a　＿＿＿＿＿＿＿
   history of angioplasty

5. Patient is admitted to the hospital with syncope and has　＿＿＿＿＿＿＿
   previously had a pacemaker inserted

6. Patient is awaiting a heart transplant and is on a heart assist　＿＿＿＿＿＿＿
   device

COMMON TREATMENTS

CONDITION	MEDICATION/TREATMENT
Angina	Nitroglycerin, beta blockers, and calcium channel blockers Coreg, Lopressor, Norvasc, Verapamil, Procardia
Atrial fibrillation	Blood thinners (Coumadin, Plavix, Ticlid) Rate control: calcium channel blockers: Cardizem, verapamil Beta blockers: atenolol, Lopressor, Inderal, Digoxin, Lanoxin, Amiodarone
Congestive heart failure	Diuretics such as Lasix, Bumex, Zaroxolyn, Furosemide Beta blockers: Dyazide, Lanoxin, HCTZ
Hypertension	Diuretics, Aldactone Beta blockers: atenolol, Vasotec, Cozaar, Calan, Cardizem, Aldomet (for additional antihypertensive drugs)
Stroke/CVA (nonhemorrhagic)	Blood thinners (Coumadin, Plavix, Ticlid) and clot busting agents such as tPA and streptokinase

PROCEDURES

Procedures related to the cardiovascular system in ICD-10-PCS may be found in the following tables:

Heart and Great Vessels	021-02Y
Upper Arteries	031-03W
Lower Arteries	041-04W
Upper Veins	051-05W
Lower Veins	061-06W

Diagnostic Cardiac Catheterization

Diagnostic cardiac catheterization (Figure 15-17) is a procedure that may be performed on a patient with chest pain, angina, or an acute MI to determine if coronary artery disease is present. This procedure allows the physician to view the heart chambers, valves, and arteries. A hollow needle or catheter is inserted into the vein for a right heart catheterization

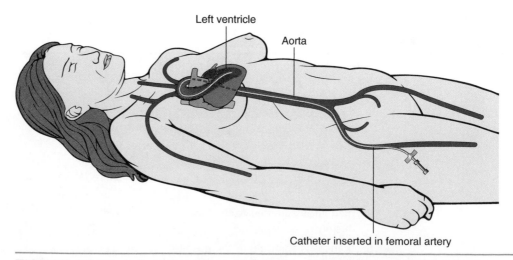

FIGURE 15-17. Left-sided cardiac catheterization. The catheter is passed retrograde (backward) from the femoral artery into the aorta and then into the left ventricle. For right-sided cardiac catheterization, the cardiologist inserts a catheter through the femoral vein and advances it to the right atrium and right ventricle and into the pulmonary artery.

and into an artery in the arm or groin for a left heart catheterization. Usually, this catheter is inserted into the groin in the femoral artery and winds its way up into the coronary artery. Pictures of the arteries are then taken. These pictures are called coronary arteriograms or angiograms. When a cardiac catheterization is coded, the procedure codes listed in Table 15-2 may be assigned. In ICD-10-PCS, cardiac caths are found in the measurement and monitoring section, with the root operation being measurement (determining the level of a physiologic function at a point in time).

Once the cardiologist has determined the extent of the patient's problem, he or she decides on medical therapy, refers the patient for bypass, or performs a therapeutic procedure right then and there, while the catheter is in place. The cardiologist may go on to perform the procedures as described below.

Angioplasty

Angioplasty is a procedure for widening a diseased vessel, which is usually either obstructed or narrowed. The device is inserted, the balloon inflated, and the plaque is compressed against the wall of the artery (Figure 15-18). Angioplasty can be performed on both coronary and noncoronary vessels. In ICD-10-PCS the vessels are determined to be upper if they are above the diaphragm or lower if they are below the diaphragm. When angioplasty is performed on the coronary arteries it is often abbreviated PTCA (percutaneous transluminal coronary angioplasty). The root operation for an angioplasty procedure in ICD-10-PCS is dilation (expanding an orifice or lumen). In ICD-10-PCS it is important to know that coronary arteries are classified as a single body part. Attention must be paid to the number of sites treated and not by name or number of arteries. In ICD-10-PCS, character 6 identifies whether the stent being inserted is drug eluting, non–drug eluting, radioactive, or no device. If different types of stents are inserted into different arteries two codes would be required to identify the stent.

EXAMPLE Patient has a PTCA of the LAD and LCD with a drug-eluting stent placed in the LCD, 02703ZZ, 027034Z.

EXAMPLE Patient with CAD presents for PTCA of left anterior descending and left circumflex, I25.10, 02713ZZ.

TABLE 15-2 COMMON PROCEDURE CODES FOR CARDIAC CATHETERIZATION

Test	Procedure	Comment
Left heart cath	4A023N7	Most commonly done alone when used to diagnose coronary artery disease (CAD)
Right heart cath	4A023N6	This is used most commonly for assessment of ventricular function, especially for patients who also have congestive heart failure (CHF)
Combined right and left heart catherization	4A023N8	
Right angiogram	B204YZZ	All of these angiograms are also called ventriculograms
Left angiogram	B205YZZ	
Combined right and left angiogram	B206YZZ	
Coronary arteriography	B200YZZ	Also known as Sones technique; uses single cath
Coronary arteriography	B200YZZ	Also known as Judkins technique; uses two catheters
Coronary arteriography	B200YZZ	Other and unspecified coronary arteriography

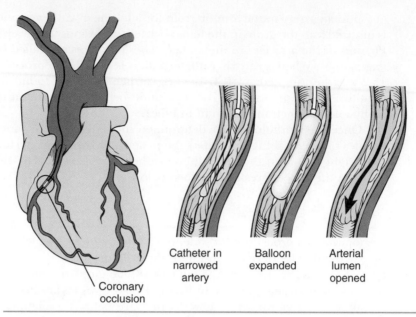

FIGURE 15-18. Angioplasty.

One of the most common complications of angioplasty is restenosis, which occurs in about one-third of cases. To try to avoid restenosis, physicians may use a stent. Sometimes, they also treat a restenosed patient with intravascular radiation therapy. Most often, an angioplasty is performed prior to insertion of a stent.

Atherectomy is the removal of plaque from a vessel. This may be done with the use of a catheter with a shaver or rotablator on the end. A laser is also used to perform atherectomy.

Stent insertion into the coronary artery is a procedure that may be performed after completion of an angioplasty (Figure 15-19). The stent helps to keep the artery open. Inserted stents may be drug-eluting (DES) or non–drug-eluting.

Three types of drug-eluting stents that are currently used in the United States are a paclitaxel-eluting stent, a sirolimus-eluting stent, and an everolimos. These drug-eluting stents are not to be confused with a stent that may be coated with antiplatelet drug.

EXAMPLE The patient had a percutaneous coronary intervention (PCI), which included inserting a drug-eluting stent into the LAD for coronary atherosclerosis, I25.10, 027034Z.

Coronary Artery Bypass Graft

Coronary artery bypass graft (CABG or CAB) is surgery that is performed to bypass blood around the clogged arteries to the heart (Figure 15-20). The procedure is done by taking a healthy blood vessel from another part of the body, usually the internal mammary artery or the saphenous vein. Surgeons should document in their operative notes the number of arteries bypassed and the types of blood vessels used. The root operation for a CABG in ICD-10-PCS is bypass (altering a root of passage of a tubular body part).

When reading a bypass operative report, it is helpful to know the coronary arteries that may be bypassed (Figure 15-22). Two main coronary arteries are located on the left (LCA) and on the right (RCA). The LCA divides into two arteries: the LAD and the circumflex. The RCA divides into the posterior descending artery (PDA) and the marginal branch. Smaller branches consist of the acute marginal, the obtuse marginal (OM), and the diagonals.

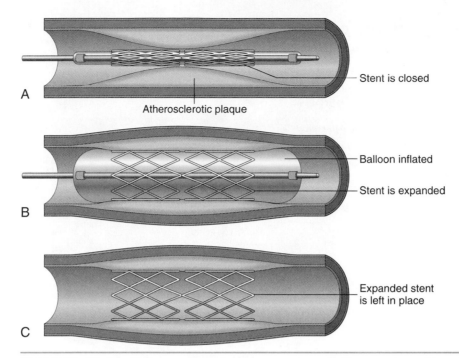

FIGURE 15-19. Placement of an intracoronary stent. **A,** The stent is positioned at the site of the lesion. **B,** The balloon is inflated, thereby expanding the stent. **C,** The balloon is then deflated and removed, and the implanted stent is left in place. Coronary stents are stainless steel scaffolding devices that help hold open arteries such as the coronary, renal, and carotid arteries.

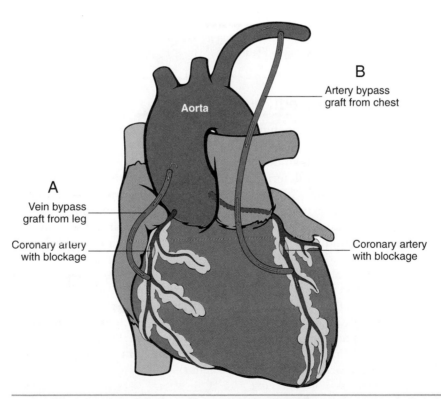

FIGURE 15-20. Coronary artery bypass graft (CABG) surgery with anastomosis of vein and arterial grafts. **A,** Section of a vein is removed from the leg and is anastomosed (upside down because of its directional valves) to a coronary artery to bypass the area of arteriosclerotic blockage. **B,** An internal mammary artery is grafted to a coronary artery to bypass a blockage.

SECTION: 0 MEDICAL AND SURGICAL
BODY SYSTEM: 2 HEART AND GREAT VESSELS
OPERATION: 1 BYPASS: *(on multiple pages)*

Altering the route of passage of the contents of a tubular body part

Body Part	Approach	Device	Qualifier
0 Coronary Artery, One Site 1 Coronary Artery, Two Sites 2 Coronary Artery, Three Sites 3 Coronary Artery, Four or More Sites	0 Open	9 Autologous Venous Tissue A Autologous Arterial Tissue J Synthetic Substitute K Nonautologous Tissue Substitute	3 Coronary Artery 8 Internal Mammary, Right 9 Internal Mammary, Left C Thoracic Artery F Abdominal Artery W Aorta
0 Coronary Artery, One Site 1 Coronary Artery, Two Sites 2 Coronary Artery, Three Sites 3 Coronary Artery, Four or More Sites	0 Open	Z No Device	3 Coronary Artery 8 Internal Mammary, Right 9 Internal Mammary, Left C Thoracic Artery F Abdominal Artery

FIGURE 15-21. Coronary artery bypass table.

To code coronary artery bypasses in ICD-10-CM, the coder must review the operative report for the number of sites bypassed. A separate procedure is coded for each coronary artery site that uses a different device (i.e., saphenous vein, internal mammary). The qualifier identifies the origin of the bypass or the vessel bypassed from. A separate code is assigned for the harvesting of the bypass graft.

EXAMPLE	Patient has CABG of three coronary arteries, using a greater saphenous vein from the left leg, 021209W, 06BQ4ZZ (Figure 15-21).

Electrophysiologic Studies/Procedures

Electrophysiologic studies (EPS) are used to analyze the electrical conduction system of the heart. The root operation for eletrophysiologic studies is found in the medical- and surgical-related sections under measurement and monitoring (with a root operation of measurement, which is determining the level of a physiological or physical function at a point in time). Patients with symptoms such as light-headedness, palpitations, or syncope may have EP tests done to determine the cause of these symptoms. Other patients with known heart rhythm disturbances may have EP studies so that the severity of the heart disturbance can be determined. During these studies, catheters are inserted into a vein in the leg and are threaded to the heart. They measure electrical signals and conduction of these signals and look for abnormal heart rhythms. The **electrophysiologist** (physician trained in electrical disorders of the heart) may administer electrical stimuli to check the heart's response.

Ablation is correction of abnormal heart rhythm by destroying of abnormal heart tissue through radiofrequency or other methods such as laser, microwave, or freezing. Radiofrequency ablation (RFA) can be performed with the use of an EP catheter. The root operation for ablation in ICD-10-PCS is destruction (eradicating all or a portion of a body part by energy, force, or a destructive agent).

EXAMPLE	Patient is admitted through the ER with atrial fibrillation and a history of COPD. She is taken to the EPS lab for EPS testing, mapping, and a minimaze ablation of the left atrium, I48.91, J44.9, 02574ZZ, 02K83ZZ, 4A023FZ.

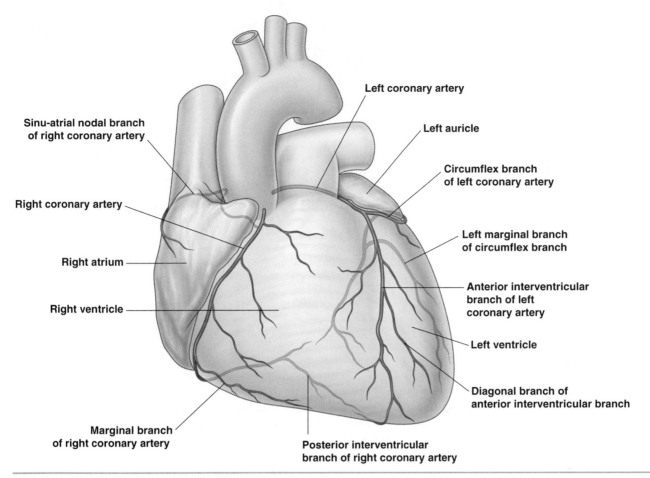

FIGURE 15-22. Anterior view of coronary arterial system.

Pacemaker/Defibrillators (AICD)

A pacemaker is a device that is used to correct abnormally slow heartbeats, complete heart blocks (CHB), and other abnormalities of heart conduction. The root operation for pacemaker generator insertion is insertion of device into subcutaneous tissue of the chest. The root operation for insertion of leads (electrodes) is insertion of intraluminal device into the atrium (putting in a non–biologic device that monitors, assists, performs, or prevents a physiological function but does not take the place of a body part). Using the Index to locate the pacemaker insertion, the coder would look in the Alphabetic Index under insertion, subcutaneous, chest, pacemaker. Under the root operation, insertion, in the Alphabetic Index, not only are there Index listings for body system, but there are also subterms for the device being inserted. Patients who present with syncope and studies determined that they have a heart block often require a pacemaker. A pacemaker has two functions: sensing and pacing. Pacing is the sending of electrical signals to the heart from the pacemaker via the lead. If the rhythm of the heart is too slow, the pacemaker paces the heart to a faster rhythm. Sensing involves monitoring the heart's electrical activity; when the heart is functioning normally, no pacing is required.

The pacemaker system consists of the pulse generator (device, battery) and the leads (electrodes) (Figure 15-23). Leads are placed into the heart chambers and are then attached to the generator. These can be temporary or permanent. A temporary pacemaker is used for emergencies or intraoperatively. Code assignment for a temporary pacemaker does not require codes for the leads or codes for removal.

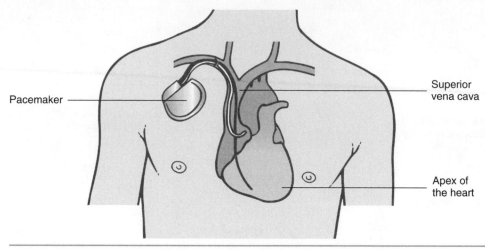

FIGURE 15-23. Cardiac leads in the atrium and in the ventricle enable a dual-chamber pacemaker to sense and pace in both heart chambers.

A permanent pacemaker is usually implanted through an incision near the collarbone. Wires are inserted into a vein and are advanced into the heart; they are then connected to a generator, which is implanted under the skin. Coding of initial insertion of permanent pacemakers requires two codes: one for the insertion of the generator/device, and one for insertion of the leads or electrodes. Leads can be placed inside the heart or outside the heart (epicardially). Pacemaker pockets for epicardial leads are usually placed in the abdominal wall; this is typically done for children who are still growing.

Insertion/replacement/revision requires that the coder must know the type of device that is being inserted. Codes for initial insertion and replacement require knowledge as to whether this is a single-chamber or a dual-chamber device and whether the device is rate responsive. A rate-responsive device has a sensor that detects changes in movement of the body and reacts accordingly.

EXAMPLE Initial open insertion of a single-chamber device into the chest with percutaneous insertion of a single lead into the right atrium, 0JH604Z, 02H63JZ.

EXAMPLE Initial open insertion of a dual-chamber pacemaker into the subcutaneous tissue of the chest with percutaneous insertion of leads into the right atrium and right ventricle, 0JH606Z, 02H63JZ, 02HK3JZ.

Separate codes are used for replacement of devices and leads and removal of devices and leads. When a patient is admitted for removal, replacement, or reprogramming the codes Z45.010 (Encounter for checking and testing of cardiac pacemaker pulse generator) or Z45.018 (Encounter for adjustment and management of other part of cardiac pacemaker) are assigned. Often, surgeons document that a patient is being admitted for end of life of the battery or pacemaker. In ICD-10-PCS the removal of a pacemaker and leads is found under the root operation removal (taking out a device). It is important to remember that if a device is removed and then a new device reinserted, both removal and insertion are assigned codes in ICD-10-PCS.

EXAMPLE Admission for removal of a pacemaker and leads. Leads removed percutaneously and device via open approach, Z45.010, Z45.018, 02PA3MZ, 0JPT0PZ.

EXAMPLE | Replacement of a single-chamber pacemaker with a dual-chamber device, 0JPT0PZ, 02HK0JZ, 02HK0JZ; with retention of the atrial lead and open removal of the single chamber device with transvenous right ventricle lead insertion.

An automatic implantable cardioverter-defibrillator (AICD) is a device that is used for treating patients with tachyarrhythmias. Similar to a pacemaker, it has a pulse generator and electrodes that both sense and defibrillate. The root operation for insertion of an AICD is insertion for both the leads and the generator (putting in a nonbiologic device). Defibrillators give shocks that attempt to convert the heart rhythm. Implantation of this system is usually done via thoracotomy or sternotomy.

EXAMPLE | Patient is admitted with ventricular tachycardia and has an AICD placed in the chest in the subcutaneous tissue, via open approach with leads inserted percutaneously in the right atrium and right ventricle, I47.2, 0JH608Z, 02H63KZ, 02HK3KZ.

Biventricular pacing is also known as cardiac resynchronization therapy (CRT). Biventricular pacemakers come as a stand-alone device or with a built-in implantable cardioverter (ICV). They are used primarily to treat heart failure. Similar to a pacemaker, a generator and leads are included. The biventricular pacemaker uses a third lead. This third lead, which is attached to the wall of the left ventricle in the vein of the coronary sinus, causes both ventricles to contract at the same time or in sync. In contrast to regular pacemakers, biventricular pacemakers do not increase heart rate. Some biventricular pacers include internal cardiac defibrillators (ICDs) for patients with fast irregular rhythms. These systems have biventricular pacing, anti-tachycardia pacing, and internal defibrillators. There are codes for implantation and replacement of both systems, with the ICD and without. The root operation for insertion of a biventricular pacemaker and leads is insertion (putting in a nonbiologic device). The root operation for insertion of a cardiac resynchronization defibrillator pulse generator and the insertion of leads is insertion.

EXAMPLE | Percutaneous implantation of a cardiac resynchronization pacemaker pulse generator into the chest with percutaneous insertion of left ventricular lead, 0JH637Z, 02HL3JZ.

EXAMPLE | Percutaneous implantation of cardiac resynchronization treatment defibrillator (CRT-D), total system CRT-D into chest, or biventricular pacing and ICD total system with percutaneous insertion of leads into right ventricle, left ventricle, and coronary vein, 0JH639Z, 02HK3KZ, 02H43KZ, 02HL3KZ.

Aneurysm Repair

Aneurysms can be repaired either by resection using an open transperitoneal approach, with either an anastomosis or graft repair or endovascular repair where an endograft is introduced through the femoral artery via a catheter, which avoids the major abdominal incision. The root operations for an abdominal aortic aneurysm repair depend on the type of procedure performed. If the aneurysm is repaired openly by replacement with a graft, the root operation is replacement (putting in a device that replaces some or all of a body part). Taking out the body part is included in replacement. If the aneurysm is repaired openly by an anastomosis, the root operation is excision of an abdominal aorta (cutting out or off without replacement). Lastly, if the repair is performed endovascularly, the root operation is restriction of the abdominal aorta (partially closing off an orifice of a tubular body), if done with stent insertion or if done by synthetic or biologic graft, the root operation is supplement.

EXAMPLE Patient presents for repair of an abdominal aortic aneurysm. The repair is performed endovascularly with restriction by an intraluminal device, I71.4, 04U04JZ.

Central Lines/Catheters

Central venous lines are used for several purposes. They may be used to administer chemotherapy, total parenteral nutrition (TPN), antibiotics, and for dialysis. Hickman, Groshong, triple lumen, and double lumen are all types of central lines. Usually, central venous catheters are inserted into the subclavian or jugular vein and are then advanced into the vena cava. The root operation for insertion of a central line is insertion (putting in a non–biological device). A central line has a catheter that is NOT totally implanted under the skin. A peripherally inserted central catheter (PICC) (Figure 15-24) is assigned the same code as a central line. It is inserted in a slightly different manner. Sometimes a provider will document a diagnosis of poor IV access when a line is being inserted. There is no diagnosis code for poor IV access, and in these cases the underlying condition should be coded.

EXAMPLE Patient is admitted to the hospital for bacterial endocarditis. A central line is inserted into the right subclavian vein for administration of antibiotics to treat the endocarditis, I33.0, 05H533Z.

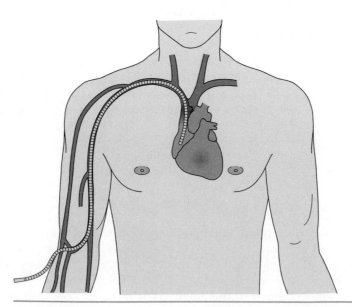

FIGURE 15-24. A peripherally inserted central catheter is threaded through the vein until the end is near the heart.

EXERCISE 15-7

Assign codes to the following conditions.

1. Patient is admitted for a diagnostic left cardiac
    catheterization with a diagnosis of chest pain   _____

2. Patient is admitted with a diagnosis of CAD for a PTCA with   _____
    CYPHER stent insertion into the LAD

3. Patient is admitted 3 days status post angioplasty with   _____
    restenosis of a stent; a non–drug-eluting stent is inserted
    into the RCA

4. Patient with CAD is admitted, and a bypass of four coronary   _____
    arteries is performed; bypass grafts were performed with use
    of the left internal mammary to the LAD, and saphenous
    vein grafts were used to bypass PDA, circumflex, and obtuse
    marginal

5. Patient is admitted with ventricular fibrillation, and   _____
    percutaneous RF ablation is performed

6. Patient is admitted with bradycardia, and a complete   _____
    dual-chamber pacemaker system is inserted. The generator
    is inserted into a chest pocket and one lead is inserted in
    the right atrium, and the other lead is inserted into the right
    ventricle via a percutaneous approach

7. Patient is admitted for a pacemaker battery change for the   _____
    end of life of the battery. The generator is inserted into a
    subcutaneous chest pocket

8. Patient with CHF is admitted for total biventricular pacing   _____
    with internal cardiac defibrillation

9. Patient is admitted with cerebral aneurysm, and a clipping   _____
    is performed

10. Patient with a tachyarrhythmia has a total AICD placed. The   _____
    generator is placed in a chest pocket, and leads are placed
    percutaneously in the right atrium and right ventricle

DOCUMENTATION/REIMBURSEMENT/MS-DRGs

Often, documentation difficulties are due to lack of documentation. Sometimes pathology
and other test results are not available at the time of discharge, or when the physician is
dictating the discharge summary or is reporting the final diagnoses.

Frequently missed complications/comorbidities from this chapter include:

- Prinzmetal angina
- Cardiac arrest
- Cardiomyopathy
- Cor pulmonale
- Hypertensive heart and kidney disease
- Ventricular fibrillation
- Atrial flutter
- Myocardial infarction
- Coronary ischemia, acute
- Phlebitis
- Paroxysmal supraventicular tachycardia
- Cardiogenic shock
- Gangrene

MS-DRG With and Without MCC/CC

EXAMPLE   Patient was admitted with subendocardial MI; patient also was treated for acidosis, I21.4, E87.2.

DIAGNOSES	CODES	MS-DRG	RW
Acute subendocardial MI	I21.4	282	0.7856
Acute subendocardial MI with acidosis	I21.4	281	1.1478
	E87.2		

Pacemakers/ICDs/Cardioverter/Defibrillators

Insertion of pacemakers, as mentioned earlier in the chapter, more often than not will require two codes. One code will be assigned for insertion of the generator, and the other for insertion of the leads. As illustrated below, if the leads are not coded, the payment would be significantly lower.

EXAMPLE

DIAGNOSES/PROCEDURES	CODES	MS-DRG	RW
Sick sinus syndrome (SSS) with open insertion of dual chamber pacemaker (coded only the device, not the leads) into chest	I49.5 0JH60PQ	310	0.5608
SSS with insertion of dual chamber pacemaker (both leads and device) generator inserted openly into chest subcutaneous via percutaneous insertion of leads in right atrium and right ventricle	I49.5 0JH60P2, 02H63MA, 02HK3MA	244	2.0538

EXAMPLE

DIAGNOSES/PROCEDURES	CODES	MS-DRG	RW
SSS with open insertion of total biventricular pacemaker CRT-P generator inserted into chest subcutaneous, percutaneous insertion of leads in right atrium and right ventricle	I49.5 0JH60P3, 02HK3MA, 02H63MA	244	2.0538
SSS with open insertion of total biventricular defibrillator CRT-D generator inserted into chest subcutaneous 3 leads inserted, one in right atrium, one in left ventricle, and one in coronary sinus via percutaneous approach	I49.5 0JH60P5 02HL3ME 02H43ME	227	5.1500

CHAPTER REVIEW EXERCISE   *Assign codes for all diagnoses and procedures including all applicable Z codes and external cause codes.*

1. Patient has atrial fibrillation with rapid ventricular response   _____

2. Patient had a previous CVA and now has left hemiparesis   _____

3. Patient has orthostatic hypotension   _____

4. Patient has mitral and tricuspid insufficiency   _____

5. Patient has congestive heart failure, rheumatic   _____

6. Patient has both acute and chronic renal failure and a history of   _____
   hypertension; patient is currently taking verapamil

7. Patient has congestive heart failure with pleural effusion and hypertension _____

8. Patient has chest pain and elevated troponins _____

9. Patient presents with a non–Q wave myocardial infarction (NQMI), is taken to the cath lab for a left heart cath, and has a drug-eluting stent inserted in RCA for coronary artery disease _____

10. Patient with a previous CABG presents to the hospital with USA _____

11. Patient with ACS presents to the hospital; patient is taken to the cath lab and following a left cardiac cath and diagnosis of CAD, the patient was immediately taken to surgery, where a 2-vessel CABG is performed LIMA to LAD and an autologous saphenous vein graft to RCA. Procedure performed under bypass and the right lesser saphenous vein was harvested via an open approach _____

12. Patient has a left anterior fascicular block _____

13. Patient is admitted through the ER with chest pain that is determined to be coronary artery disease following a left heart cath. Following the cath procedure, the patient dies of cardiac arrest _____

14. Patient has congestive systolic and diastolic heart failure _____

15. Patient presents to the hospital with pulmonary edema and a history of hypertensive congestive heart failure for which the patient currently takes Lasix and verapamil _____

16. Patient is admitted for a stroke with left side weakness and dysphagia. Upon discharge the weakness has resolved. _____

17. Patient has a history of stroke and is currently admitted with atrial fibrillation and dysphagia due to the old stroke _____

18. Patient has arteriosclerosis of the extremities and is admitted with a stage 1 ulcer and gangrene of the right foot _____

19. Patient is admitted to the hospital with deep vein thrombosis of the left calf and a pulmonary embolism _____

20. History of heart valve replaced with porcine valve _____

21. Patient had a left heart catheterization, a left ventriculography fluoroscopy with low osmolar contrast, and a single-catheter coronary arteriography with low osmolar contrast to determine the cause of chest pain _____

22. Patient had an angioplasty with atherectomy of the right coronary artery for CAD _____

23. Patient with CAD had a coronary bypass times two using one saphenous vein LAD and left internal mammary RCA; the cardiac bypass pump was used and vein was taken from left greater saphenous _____

24. Patient had a dual chamber pacemaker inserted for syncope, which was attributed to bradycardia. Generator inserted into the chest and leads into the right atrium and right ventricle _____

25. Patient had congestive heart failure and was treated with a cardiac resynchronization pacemaker with leads inserted into both ventricles and the right atrium _____

26. Patient had an abdominal aortic aneurysm (AAA) and was treated with endovascular repair _____

27. Patient was admitted with endocarditis and had a Hickman catheter inserted into the left subclavian percutaneously for antibiotic administration _____

CHAPTER GLOSSARY

Ablation: correction of abnormal heart rhythm by burning of abnormal heart tissue through radiofrequency or other methods such as laser, microwave, or freezing.

Aneurysm: bulging or ballooning out of a vessel.

Angioplasty: a procedure performed to treat coronary artery disease. An inflated balloon compresses plaque against artery walls.

Aphasia: impairment of speech expression and/or word understanding.

Atherosclerosis: type of arteriosclerosis wherein fatty substances such as plaque block or clog the arteries.

Blood pressure: the force that blood puts on the arterial walls when the heart beats.

BNP: (brain natriuretic peptide) a hormone that is produced by the heart; a BNP test measures the amount of BNP that is found in the heart.

Bradycardia: slow heart rate, generally fewer than 60 beats per minute.

Capillaries: smallest blood vessel through which material passes to and from the bloodstream.

Cardiac arrest: sudden loss of heart function.

Cardiomyopathy: a disorder of the muscles of the heart chambers that impedes heart function.

Cognitive deficit: disorder in thinking, learning, awareness, or judgment.

Conduction disorder: abnormalities of cardiac impulses.

Coronary artery bypass graft: surgery performed to bypass an occluded coronary artery.

Deep vein thrombosis: a blood clot that forms in a deep vein.

Dissection: a tear in wall of a vessel.

Electrophysiologist: physician trained in electrical disorders of the heart.

Embolus: clot that travels to another part of the body.

Endocarditis: inflammation of the lining of the heart chambers and valves.

Fistula: an abnormal passage between an artery and a vein.

Heart failure: impaired function of the heart's pumping ability.

Malignant hypertension: rapidly rising blood pressure, usually in excess of 140 mm Hg diastolic with findings of visual impairment and symptoms or signs of progressive cardiac failure.

Myocardial infarction: heart attack.

NSTEMI: non–ST elevation myocardial infarction.

Pericarditis: inflammation of the covering of the heart.

Phlebitis: inflammation of a vein.

Pulmonary embolism: a blood clot(s) in the pulmonary artery that causes blockage in the artery.

Pulmonary hypertension: high blood pressure in the arteries that supply blood to the lungs.

Stasis dermatitis: skin condition due to poor circulation (venous insufficiency) that is characterized by swelling, skin discoloration, weeping, itching, and scaly skin.

STEMI: ST elevation myocardial infarction.

Stenosis: abnormal narrowing.

Stroke: cerebrovascular accident or brain infarction.

Tachycardia: fast heart rate, generally greater than 100 beats per minute.

Thoracentesis: puncture of the chest wall to remove fluid (pleural effusion) from the space between the lining of the outside of the lungs (pleura) and the wall of the chest.

Thrombus: a blood clot that forms and remains in a vein.

Varicose veins: enlarged, twisted veins that usually occur in the legs.

REFERENCE

1. From Frazier ME, Drzymkowski JW. *Essentials of Human Diseases and Conditions,* 3rd ed. St. Louis: Saunders, 2004, Table 10-1, pp 457-459.

16

Diseases of the Respiratory System

(ICD-10-CM Chapter 10, Codes J00-J99)

CHAPTER OUTLINE

ICD-10-CM Official Guidelines for Coding and Reporting

Major Differences Between ICD-10-CM and ICD-9-CM Guidelines

Anatomy and Physiology

Disease Conditions

Acute Upper Respiratory Infections (J00-J06) and Other Diseases of Upper Respiratory Tract (J30-J39)

Influenza and Pneumonia (J09-J18)

Other Acute Lower Respiratory Infections (J20-J22)

Chronic Lower Respiratory Diseases (J40-J47)

Lung Diseases Due to External Agents (J60-J70)

Other Respiratory Diseases Principally Affecting the Interstitium (J80-J84)

Suppurative and Necrotic Conditions of the Lower Respiratory Tract (J85-J86) and Other Diseases of the Pleura (J90-J94)

Other Diseases of the Respiratory System (J96-J99)

Factors Influencing Health Status and Contact With Health Services (Z Codes)

Common Treatments

Procedures

Mechanical Ventilation

Noninvasive Ventilation

Bronchoscopy

Thoracentesis

Thoracostomy

Tracheostomy

Pulmonary Resection

Documentation/Reimbursement/MS-DRGs

Pneumonia and Causative Organism

Two Diagnoses That Equally Meet the Definition for Principal Diagnosis

MS-DRG With and Without MCC/CC

Respiratory Failure versus Another Acute Condition

Chapter Review Exercise

Chapter Glossary

References

LEARNING OBJECTIVES

1. Apply and assign the correct ICD-10-CM/PCS codes in accordance with Official Guidelines for Coding and Reporting
2. Identify major differences between ICD-10-CM and ICD-9-CM related to the respiratory system
3. Identify pertinent anatomy and physiology of the respiratory system
4. Identify diseases of the respiratory system

5. Assign the correct Z codes and procedure codes related to the respiratory system
6. Identify common treatments, medications, laboratory values, and diagnostic tests
7. Explain the importance of documentation in relation to MS-DRGs for reimbursement

---

ABBREVIATIONS/ ACRONYMS

ABG arterial blood gas

AIDS acquired immunodeficiency syndrome

AMI acute myocardial infarction

BIPAP bilevel positive airway pressure

CAP community-acquired pneumonia

CC complication/comorbidity

CHF congestive heart failure

COPD chronic obstructive pulmonary disease

CPAP continuous positive airway pressure

CVA cerebrovascular accident

E. coli Escherichia coli

ER Emergency Room

GERD gastroesophageal reflux disease

H. flu Haemophilus influenzae

HIV human immunodeficiency virus

ICD-9-CM *International Classification of Diseases, 9th Revision, Clinical Modification*

ICD-10-CM *International Classification of Diseases, 10th Revision, Clinical Modification*

ICD-10-PCS *International Classification of Diseases, 10th Revision, Procedure Coding System*

IPPV intermittent positive pressure ventilation

IV intravenous

LLL left lower lobe

MS-DRG Medicare Severity diagnosis-related group

NEC not elsewhere classifiable

NOS not otherwise specified

NPPV noninvasive positive pressure ventilation

O₂ oxygen

OIG Office of the Inspector General

OR Operating Room

Paco₂ partial pressure of carbon dioxide in arterial blood

Pao₂ partial pressure of oxygen in arterial blood

PCP *Pneumocystis carinii* pneumonia

RAD reactive airway disease

RSV respiratory syncytial virus

RUL right upper lobe

RW relative weight

STAPH aureus Staphylococcus aureus

TRALI transfusion-related acute lung injury

VATS video-assisted thoracic surgery

ICD-10-CM	Please refer to the companion Evolve website for the most current guidelines.

Official Guidelines for Coding and Reporting	**10. Chapter 10: Diseases of Respiratory System (J00-J99)**
	  a. Chronic Obstructive Pulmonary Disease [COPD] and Asthma
	    1) Acute exacerbation of chronic obstructive bronchitis and asthma
	    The codes in categories J44 and J45 distinguish between uncomplicated cases and those in acute exacerbation. An acute exacerbation is a worsening or a decompensation of a chronic condition. An acute exacerbation is not equivalent to an infection superimposed on a chronic condition, though an exacerbation may be triggered by an infection.

EXAMPLE	Patient is seen by the pulmonologist for management of exacerbation of COPD. The exacerbation was triggered by the patient's pneumonia, J18.9, J44.1 or J44.1, J18.9.

EXAMPLE	Patient has asthma and is being treated for pneumonia, J18.9, J45.909.

b. **Acute Respiratory Failure**
1) **Acute respiratory failure as principal diagnosis**
   A code from subcategory J96.0, Acute respiratory failure, or **subcategory** J96.2, Acute and chronic respiratory failure, may be assigned as a principal diagnosis when it is the condition established after study to be chiefly responsible for occasioning the admission to the hospital, and the selection is supported by the Alphabetic Index and Tabular List. However, chapter-specific coding guidelines (such as obstetrics, poisoning, HIV, newborn) that provide sequencing direction take precedence.

EXAMPLE   The patient presented to the ER in acute respiratory failure and was intubated and admitted to ICU. Following admission, the patient was started on antibiotics for pneumonia. The patient was on mechanical ventilation for 24 hours, J96.00, J18.9, 5A1945Z, 0BH17EZ.
   (Per guidelines, if respiratory failure and another acute condition are equally responsible for occasioning the admission, the guidelines regarding two or more diagnoses that equally meet the definition for principal diagnoses may be applied.)

2) **Acute respiratory failure as secondary diagnosis**
   Respiratory failure may be listed as a secondary diagnosis if it occurs after admission, or if it is present on admission, but does not meet the definition of principal diagnosis.

EXAMPLE   The patient was admitted from the clinic for IV antibiotics for pneumonia. A couple of hours after admission, the patient's condition deteriorated and acute respiratory failure developed, J18.9, J96.00.

3) **Sequencing of acute respiratory failure and another acute condition**
   When a patient is admitted with respiratory failure and another acute condition, (e.g., myocardial infarction, cerebrovascular accident, aspiration pneumonia), the principal diagnosis will not be the same in every situation. This applies whether the other acute condition is a respiratory or nonrespiratory condition. Selection of the principal diagnosis will be dependent on the circumstances of admission. If both the respiratory failure and the other acute condition are equally responsible for occasioning the admission to the hospital, and there are no chapter-specific sequencing rules, the guideline regarding two or more diagnoses that equally meet the definition for principal diagnosis *(Section II, C.)* may be applied in these situations.
   If the documentation is not clear as to whether acute respiratory failure and another condition are equally responsible for occasioning the admission, query the provider for clarification.

EXAMPLE   Patient was admitted to the hospital in acute respiratory failure due to congestive heart failure. The patient was intubated and placed on mechanical ventilation for 2 days. The patient responded well to IV diuretics, J96.00, I50.9, 5A1945Z, 0BH17EZ.

c. Influenza due to certain identified influenza viruses

Code only confirmed cases of influenza **due to certain identified influenza viruses (category J09)**. This is an exception to the hospital inpatient guideline Section II, H. (Uncertain Diagnosis).

In this context, "confirmation" does not require documentation of positive laboratory testing specific for avian or **other** novel influenza **A**. However, coding should be based on the provider's diagnostic statement that the patient has avian influenza, **or other novel influenza A**.

If the provider records "suspected" or "possible" or "probable" avian influenza," the appropriate influenza code from category J11, Influenza due to **unidentified** influenza virus, should be assigned. A code from category J09, Influenza due to certain identified influenza viruses, should not be assigned.

EXAMPLE | Patient was admitted with a confirmed case of avian influenza, J09.X2.

EXAMPLE | Patient was admitted with possible H1N1 influenza, J11.1.

d. Ventilator associated Pneumonia

1) Documentation of Ventilator associated Pneumonia

As with all procedural or postprocedural complications, code assignment is based on the provider's documentation of the relationship between the condition and the procedure.

Code J95.851, Ventilator associated pneumonia, should be assigned only when the provider has documented ventilator associated pneumonia (VAP). An additional code to identify the organism (e.g., Pseudomonas aeruginosa, code B96.5) should also be assigned. Do not assign an additional code from categories J12-J18 to identify the type of pneumonia.

Code J95.851 should not be assigned for cases where the patient has pneumonia and is on a mechanical ventilator **and** the provider has not specifically stated that the pneumonia is ventilator-associated pneumonia. If the documentation is unclear as to whether the patient has a pneumonia that is a complication attributable to the mechanical ventilator, query the provider.

2) Ventilator associated Pneumonia Develops after Admission

A patient may be admitted with one type of pneumonia (e.g., code J13, Pneumonia due to Streptococcus pneumonia) and subsequently develop VAP. In this instance, the principal diagnosis would be the appropriate code from categories J12-J18 for the pneumonia diagnosed at the time of admission. Code J95.851, Ventilator associated pneumonia, would be assigned as an additional diagnosis when the provider has also documented the presence of ventilator associated pneumonia.

Apply the General Coding Guidelines as found in Chapter 5 and the Procedural Coding Guidelines as found in Chapters 6 and 7.

MAJOR DIFFERENCES BETWEEN ICD-10-CM AND ICD-9-CM GUIDELINES

- ICD-10-CM uses codes that identify acute recurrent sinusitis to the individual sinuses.
- In ICD-9-CM, asthma is coded by specific type (e.g., extrinsic, intrinsic, chronic obstructive, or unspecified) and by whether the condition is exacerbated or status asthmaticus is present. ICD-10-CM divides asthma into the following subcategories:

- Mild intermittent asthma
- Mild persistent asthma
- Moderate persistent asthma
- Severe persistent asthma
- Other and unspecified asthma

■ Under code category J44, Other chronic obstructive pulmonary disease, there is an instructional notation to code also the type of asthma if applicable (J45.-). In ICD-9-CM, asthma associated with COPD is only one combination code. In ICD-10-CM, both conditions are assigned codes if the specific type of asthma is documented.

■ In ICD-10-CM, an instructional note at the beginning of the chapter states that if a respiratory condition occurs in more than one site, and it is not specifically indexed, it should be classified to the lower anatomic site, such as tracheobronchitis would be classified to bronchitis.

■ Procedural complications affecting the respiratory system are included in Chapter 10, Diseases of the Respiratory System, of ICD-10-CM. Some of the complications include:
  - Tracheostomy complication
  - Acute pulmonary insufficiency following thoracic surgery
  - Acute pulmonary insufficiency following nonthoracic surgery
  - Postprocedural pneumothorax
  - Postprocedural respiratory failure
  - Intraoperative hemorrhage, hematoma, or accidental laceration
  - Transfusion-related acute lung injury (TRALI)
  - Mechanical complication of respiratory (ventilator)

ANATOMY AND PHYSIOLOGY

The primary function of the **respiratory system** (Figure 16-1) is to supply the body with oxygen (O_2). Respiration occurs through the nose and mouth, bringing oxygen through the larynx and trachea and into the lungs, where oxygen is delivered and carbon dioxide is exhaled. Dome-shaped muscles at the bottom of the lungs, or the **diaphragm**, assist in the process of breathing and in the exchange of oxygen/carbon dioxide. The lungs are the major organ of the respiratory system. The right lung is made up of three lobes; the left lung is smaller and contains two lobes. The **bronchi** are the two air tubes that branch off the trachea and deliver air to both lungs. The **trachea**, or windpipe, is responsible for filtering the air that we breathe.

DISEASE CONDITIONS

Diseases of the Respiratory System, Chapter 10 in the ICD-10-CM code book, are divided into the following categories:

CATEGORY	SECTION TITLES
J00-J06	Acute upper respiratory infections
J09-J18	Influenza and pneumonia
J20-J22	Other acute lower respiratory infections
J30-J39	Other diseases of upper respiratory tract
J40-J47	Chronic lower respiratory diseases
J60-J70	Lung diseases due to external agents
J80-J84	Other respiratory diseases principally affecting the interstitium
J85-J86	Suppurative and necrotic conditions of the lower respiratory tract
J90-J94	Other diseases of the pleura
J95	Intraoperative and postprocedural complications and disorders of respiratory system, not elsewhere classified
J96-J99	Other diseases of the respiratory system

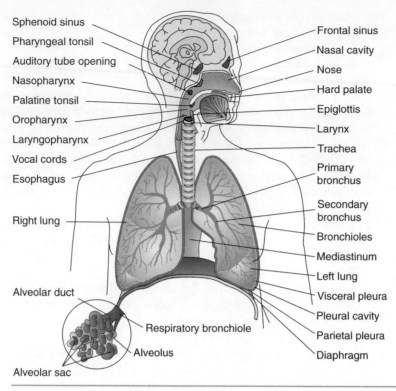

FIGURE 16-1. Anatomy of the respiratory system.

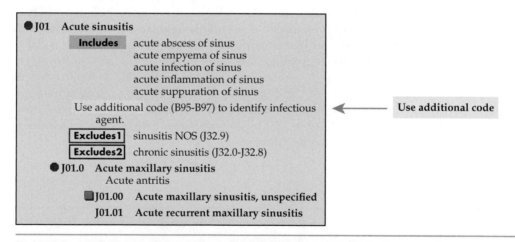

FIGURE 16-2. Instruction to use additional code to identify infectious agent.

In the Respiratory chapter, some codes are provided that do include the organisms. When the organism is included, it is not necessary to assign an additional code for the organism. There will be an Instructional note if it is necessary to use an additional code to identify the infectious agent (Figure 16-2).

EXAMPLE Pneumonia due to respiratory syncytial virus, J12.1.

This is a combination code that includes the disease process, pneumonia, and the causative organism, respiratory syncytial virus (RSV). No additional code is necessary to identify the organism.

EXAMPLE
> Acute laryngitis due to *Haemophilus influenzae,* J04.0, B96.3.

In this case, laryngitis is due to *Haemophilus influenzae* bacteria *(H flu).* The code for acute laryngitis, J04.0, makes no mention of the causative bacteria; therefore, code B96.3 is assigned as an additional code to identify the bacteria.

Infection is invasion of the body by organisms that have the potential to cause disease. In the respiratory chapter there are infections and/or inflammations of the upper and lower respiratory tract. It is possible that an acute infection may be superimposed upon a chronic infection or inflammation. Following general guidelines, "If the same condition is described as both acute (subacute) and chronic, and separate subentries exist in the Alphabetic Index at the same indentation level, code both and sequence the acute (subacute) code first" (Figure 16-3).

ICD-10-CM also has some codes to identify an infection that is acute and recurrent. An infection would be classified as recurrent if a patient has had multiple episodes within a year. Recurrent does not necessarily mean the condition is chronic. In a patient with recurrent acute infection a different approach in treating the infection may be necessary. For example, a patient with acute recurrent tonsillitis may require a tonsillectomy. A patient with acute tonsillitis may be treated with antibiotics.

EXAMPLE
> Acute and chronic bronchitis, J20.9, J42.

Acute Upper Respiratory Infections (J00-J06) and Other Diseases of Upper Respiratory Tract (J30-J39)

Acute **sinusitis** occurs when the linings of one or more sinuses become infected, usually because of viruses or bacteria. Sinuses may swell, causing an obstruction and interfering with the normal drainage of mucus. This may occur as the result of a cold. Sinusitis can cause considerable discomfort and may lead to more serious infection.

EXAMPLE
> Acute maxillary sinusitis, J01.00.

Chronic sinusitis occurs when the sinuses become inflamed and swollen. Chronic sinusitis may be caused by an infection but could also be due to conditions such as nasal polyps or a deviated nasal septum. It can be difficult to treat and may last 12 weeks or longer.

EXAMPLE
> Chronic maxillary sinusitis, J32.0.

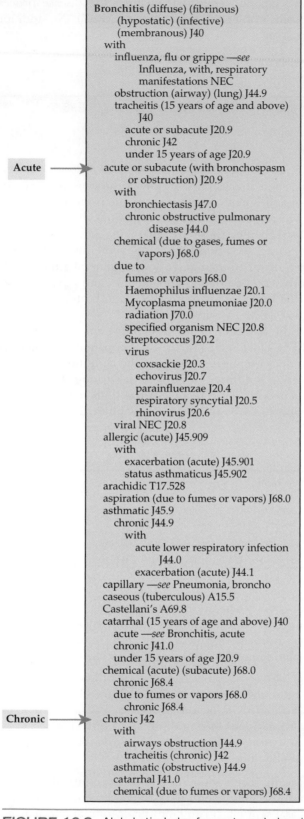

FIGURE 16-3. Alphabetic Index for acute and chronic bronchitis.

EXERCISE 16-1

Assign codes to the following conditions.

1. Headache due to acute pansinusitis   _____
2. Laryngotracheitis   _____
3. Acute streptococcal pharyngitis   _____
4. Nasal polyp   _____
5. Upper respiratory infection   _____
6. Acute and chronic maxillary sinusitis   _____
7. Deviated nasal septum   _____
8. Paralysis, vocal cords, bilateral   _____
9. Allergic rhinitis   _____
10. Spasm larynx   _____

Influenza and Pneumonia (J09-J18)

Influenza is a contagious viral infection of the respiratory tract that causes coughing, difficulty breathing, headache, muscle aches, and weakness. Possible complications include pneumonia, encephalitis, bronchitis, and sinus and ear infections. Three types of influenza virus have been identified: Types A, B, and C. Types A and B cause flu epidemics each winter and are the types that may be prevented with a flu shot. Type A is the most common and the most serious type. Influenza C is a very mild respiratory illness that is not thought to be responsible for epidemics.

H1N1 influenza is an influenza virus that is a subtype of influenza A. Because it is a new virus, people may not have any immunity to it. H1N1 influenza poses a greater risk to certain groups of people such as:

- Pregnant women
- Persons who are 6 months to 24 years of age
- Persons who are 25 to 64 years who have health conditions that put them at risk for medical complications due to influenza

Bacterial pneumonia is the most common complication of influenza.

EXAMPLE   Influenza with *Klebsiella* pneumonia, J11.08, J15.0.

Pneumonia is an infection of the lungs that can be caused by a variety of organisms, including viruses, bacteria, and parasites. Pneumonia frequently follows an upper respiratory infection, and symptoms depend on age and cause of the pneumonia. More than 50 different types of pneumonia have been identified. High-risk individuals include the elderly, the very young, and those with underlying health problems such as chronic obstructive pulmonary disease (COPD), diabetes mellitus, congestive heart failure, asthma, and sickle cell anemia. Those with impaired immune systems as the result of human immunodeficiency virus (HIV) or acquired immunodeficiency syndrome (AIDS), cancer therapy, steroid therapy, or anti-rejection medications are also at risk for developing pneumonia.

Some common symptoms of pneumonia include the following:

- Fever/chills
- Cough
- Chest pain
- Shortness of breath
- Rapid breathing and heart rate

Community-acquired pneumonia (CAP) is a broad term that is used to refer to pneumonias that are contracted outside of the hospital or nursing home setting. The most common cause of CAP is *Streptococcus pneumoniae*. **Nosocomial pneumonia** refers to a pneumonia that is acquired while the patient is hospitalized. Hospital patients are most susceptible to Gram-negative bacteria and staphylococcal pneumonia. **Nursing home–acquired pneumonia** refers to a pneumonia that is acquired in a nursing home or extended care facility. More than one organism may be responsible for pneumonia. In this case, pneumonia codes would be assigned to identify both types of pneumonia. If this was the reason for the hospital stay, either could be sequenced as the principal diagnosis. See Table 16-1 for other pathogens responsible for pneumonia. Complications of pneumonia include the formation of abscesses, respiratory failure, bacteremia, pleural effusion, empyema, and pneumothorax.

A diagnostic workup may be performed to determine the infectious agent that is responsible for the patient's condition. This could include various cultures, x-rays, other minimally invasive tests, such as bronchoscopy, or a lung biopsy, if necessary. A sputum culture from a healthy person would generally have no growth. A mixture of microorganisms, normally found in or on a patient's body, may be identified in a culture. This does not necessarily mean that this organism is responsible for a particular infection. A physician may document that a particular organism is a **contaminant**. This means that the physician does not believe that this organism is responsible for causing the infection. No code would be assigned for an organism that was described as a contaminant. Coders should not assume a causal organism on the basis of laboratory findings alone. All code assignments should be based on the physician's documentation. A physician query may be necessary to confirm whether the culture findings identify the causative agent or identify a contaminant.

Sometimes, pneumonia may be described as to the lobe that it is located in; for example, right upper lobe (RUL) pneumonia or left lower lobe (LLL) pneumonia. Both of these diagnostic statements are coded to J18.9, pneumonia, unspecified. The location of the pneumonia should not be misinterpreted to mean lobar pneumonia.

Often, **empiric** treatment (initiation of treatment prior to making a definite diagnosis) with antibiotic will be administered before the organism has been identified or the type of pneumonia determined. For example, patients with HIV may be treated empirically with antibiotics that treat both *Pneumocystis carinii* pneumonia (PCP) and CAP. Once PCP has been ruled out, the treatment and the type of antibiotic used may be modified. Because *Pneumocystis carinii* pneumonia was ruled out, it cannot be coded, even though the condition was treated as such until test results were complete.

TABLE 16-1 COMMON CAUSES OF PNEUMONIA[1]

Causative Agents	Percentage of All Diagnosed Cases
Bacteria	50
Streptococcus pneumoniae	10
Haemophilus influenzae	5
Staphylococcus aureus	5
Mycobacterium tuberculosis	10
Viruses	
Influenza virus	–
Fungi*	
Aspergillus fumigatus	–
Candida albicans	–
Pneumocystis jiroveci	–
Bacterium-like organisms	
Mycoplasma pneumoniae	10

*Opportunistic infection: rare except in immunosuppressed, debilitated, or terminally ill patients.

| EXAMPLE | Pneumonia due to Gram-negative bacteria, J15.6. |

| EXAMPLE | Bronchopneumonia, J18.0. |

EXERCISE 16-2

Assign codes to the following conditions.

1. Influenza with *Staph aureus* pneumonia   _____
2. Viral pneumonia   _____
3. *Mycoplasma* pneumonia   _____
4. Possible Avian influenza   _____
5. Pneumonia due to *E. coli*   _____
6. Cough and fever due to pneumonitis   _____
7. Community-acquired pneumonia; empiric treatment was   _____
   started for *Pneumocystis carinii* pneumonia. PCP was ruled
   out. Patient has AIDS.
8. Headache and weakness due to influenza A   _____

Other Acute Lower Respiratory Infections (J20-J22)

Acute **bronchitis** is a lower respiratory tract or bronchial tree infection that may be characterized by cough, sputum production, and wheezing. Most cases of acute bronchitis are caused by viruses such as RSV, influenza, and parainfluenza. Bacterial infection with *Mycoplasma pneumoniae*, *Chlamydia pneumoniae*, and *Bordetella pertussis* (whooping cough), particularly in young adults, can lead to acute bronchitis. Bronchitis may progress to pneumonia or may aggravate respiratory symptoms in those who have chronic respiratory conditions.

| EXAMPLE | Subacute bronchitis with bronchospasm, J20.9. |

EXERCISE 16-3

Assign codes to the following conditions.

1. Acute bronchiolitis due to RSV   _____
2. Acute bronchitis due to *Hemophilus influenzae*   _____
3. Acute on chronic bronchitis   _____

Chronic Lower Respiratory Diseases (J40-J47)

COPD, or **chronic obstructive pulmonary disease**, is a general term that is used to describe a lung disease in which the airways become obstructed, making it difficult for air to get into and out of the lungs. Although cigarette smoking is the most common culprit, other irritants such as pollution, chemicals, or dust can also play a role. Various diseases can be classified as COPD; these include chronic asthmatic bronchitis, chronic obstructive bronchitis, and emphysema. All three affect the bronchial tree and result in wheezing, coughing, and shortness of breath. It may be clinically difficult to distinguish among these disorders.

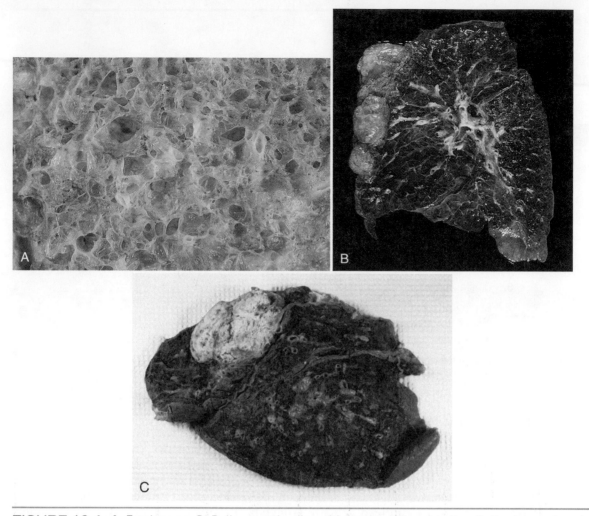

FIGURE 16-4. A, Emphysema. **B,** Bullous emphysema with large subpleural bullae. **C,** Emphysematous lung with tumor.

Chronic bronchitis is characterized by a mucus-producing cough most days of the month, 3 months out of a year, for 2 successive years, with no other underlying disease that explains the cough. Smoking cigarettes is the most common cause of chronic bronchitis. Chronic bronchitis often remains untreated because it is thought to be just a "smoker's cough."

Emphysema is a chronic lung disease of gradual onset that can be attributed to chronic infection and inflammation or irritation from cigarette smoke (Figure 16-4).

EXAMPLE Patient was admitted with exacerbation of chronic obstructive bronchitis, J44.1.

Asthma is a disease that affects the airways that carry air into and out of the lungs. Asthma can be controlled to minimize serious symptoms or attacks. Physicians use the terms "asthma" and "reactive airway disease" (RAD) interchangeably.

Asthma can be classified into four severity stages based on the frequency of symptoms, the frequency of nocturnal symptoms, and the results of spirometry testing. Those stages are:

- Mild intermittent asthma
- Mild persistent asthma
- Moderate persistent asthma
- Severe persistent asthma

Status asthmaticus can be described with the following terms:

- Intractable asthmatic attack
- Refractory asthma
- Severe, prolonged asthmatic attack
- Airway obstruction (mucous plug) not relieved by bronchodilators
- Severe, intractable wheezing

The presence of status asthmaticus should be queried if it is not documented by the physician.

If respiratory failure occurs, it should also be coded, and sequencing would depend on whether respiratory failure was present on admission and meets the criteria for principal diagnosis.

Asthmatic bronchitis refers to an underlying asthmatic problem in patients in whom asthma has become so persistent that clinically significant chronic airflow obstruction is present, despite antiasthmatic therapy. Symptoms of chronic bronchitis are generally also present.

EXAMPLE

Patient was admitted in acute hypoxemic respiratory failure caused by severe persistent asthma with status asthmatics, J96.01, J45.52.

(Per guidelines, if both the respiratory failure and another acute condition are equally responsible for occasioning the admission, the guidelines regarding two or more diagnoses that equally meet the definition for principal diagnosis may be applied.)

EXAMPLE

Patient was admitted with acute exacerbation of chronic asthmatic bronchitis. The patient went into acute respiratory failure 6 hours after admission, J44.1, J96.00.

EXERCISE 16-4

Assign codes to the following conditions.

1. Mild persistent asthma _____
2. Bronchiectasis _____
3. Asthma exacerbation with pneumonia _____
4. Emphysema with chronic bronchitis _____
5. Asthma with allergic rhinitis _____
6. Acute bronchitis with COPD _____
7. Decompensated COPD _____
8. Moderate persistent asthma with exacerbation of COPD _____

Lung Diseases Due to External Agents (J60-J70)

Pneumoconioses are lung diseases that are caused by chronic inhalation of inorganic (mineral) dust and are often due to occupational exposure. Examples include **siderosis**, which results from inhalation of iron oxide; **baritosis**, caused by inhalation of barium; **stannosis**, resulting from inhalation of tin particles; **black lung or coal workers' pneumoconiosis**

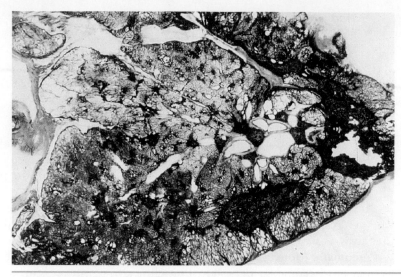

FIGURE 16-5. Coal workers' lung shows deposits of carbon particles *(black areas)*.

(Figure 16-5), caused by inhalation of coal dust; and **asbestosis**, which is caused by inhalation of asbestos.

> **EXAMPLE** Patient has silicosis, caused by working as a sandblaster for many years, J62.8.

Category J67.–, Extrinsic allergic alveolitis, includes conditions that are due to inhalation of organic materials such as grain dust, cotton dust, or animal dander.

> **EXAMPLE** Patient was diagnosed with farmers' lung, J67.0.

Aspiration pneumonia is an inflammation of the lungs and bronchial tubes that is due to the aspiration of foreign material (e.g., food, saliva, vomit) into the lung. Disorders that affect normal swallowing include disorders of the esophagus, decreased or absent gag reflex, old age, dental problems, use of sedative drugs, anesthesia, coma, and excessive alcohol consumption. These disorders may cause aspiration.

If both aspiration pneumonia and bacterial pneumonia are present, it is acceptable to assign codes for both.

> **EXAMPLE** Aspiration pneumonia with superimposed pneumonia due to *Staphylococcus aureus*, J69.0, J15.211.
> If both were present on admission, either could be sequenced as the principal diagnosis.

Several respiratory conditions can be induced by chemical fumes and vapors. These range from acute conditions such as bronchitis and pneumonitis to chronic respiratory conditions such as emphysema and pulmonary fibrosis.

> **EXAMPLE** Acute pulmonary edema due to smoke inhalation from grass fire, T59.811A, J70.5, X01.1xxA.

Assign codes to the following conditions.

1. Aspiration pneumonia; patient has dysphagia due to old CVA   _____
2. Fibrosis lung due to radiation treatments (isotope)   _____
3. Black lung disease   _____
4. Pleural effusion due to asbestosis   _____
5. Ventilation pneumonitis   _____
6. Mushroom worker's lung   _____

Other Respiratory Diseases Principally Affecting the Interstitium (J80-J84)

Pulmonary Edema

Pulmonary edema is a condition whereby fluid accumulates in the lungs. In most cases, heart problems are the cause. Pulmonary edema that is associated with heart failure is included in the heart failure codes and should not be assigned as an additional code.

EXAMPLE   Patient admitted with exacerbation of left ventricular heart failure with pulmonary edema confirmed by chest x-ray, I50.1.

Acute Pulmonary Edema of Noncardiac Origin

Pulmonary edema is not always related to a cardiac condition. The "noncardiogenic" type of acute pulmonary edema may also be caused by lung disease or related to patient trauma, and occurs in a variety of conditions. Some of these conditions include the following:

- Postoperative pulmonary edema that is not caused by left ventricular failure or CHF, both of which are cardiac in nature.
- Postoperative pulmonary edema specifically caused by fluid overload is reported with J81.0 and E87.7.
- Acute pulmonary edema caused by bacterial pneumonia, or viral pneumonia, is reported with J81.0 unless caused by left ventricular failure or congestive heart failure, because the latter conditions are cardiac in nature.
- Acute pulmonary edema is reported with an additional code when in conjunction with endotoxic shock, uremia, or septicemia.

Assign codes to the following conditions.

1. Patient with hypertensive heart disease with CHF and   _____
   pulmonary edema
2. Acute pulmonary edema due to pneumonia   _____
3. Acute pulmonary edema in patient with no history of CHF   _____
4. Acute pulmonary edema following surgery   _____

Suppurative and Necrotic Conditions of the Lower Respiratory Tract (J85-J86) and Other Diseases of the Pleura (J90-J94)

Empyema and Lung Abscess

A **lung abscess** is an infection that forms in the lung parenchyma. It occurs more often in the right lung and often develops following an aspiration event. An **empyema** forms when pus collects in the pleural space. An empyema can be a complication of pneumonia. Many patients with pneumonia will develop a parapneumonic effusion in the pleural space. If this fluid becomes infected and turns to pus, it is called an empyema. Both of these conditions are more common in children and the elderly.

Pleural Effusion

Pleural effusion is accumulation of fluid in the pleural space caused by trauma or disease. If blood is present in the accumulating fluid, the condition is called **hemothorax**; if pus is present, it is called **empyema**; if chyle (milky fluid consisting of lymph and fat) is present, it is called **chylothorax**. The most common causes of pleural effusion include the following:

- Cardiac: congestive heart failure
- Liver: liver failure
- Kidney: nephrotic syndrome, peritoneal dialysis, uremia
- Lung: infection, pulmonary embolism, pulmonary infarction, cancer (primary lung and metastatic), asbestosis
- Vascular: collagen vascular disease (systemic lupus erythematosus, rheumatoid arthritis)
- Trauma: hemothorax, chylothorax, rupture of the esophagus
- Miscellaneous: pancreatitis, post abdominal or coronary artery bypass graft surgery, and drug reactions

According to *Coding Clinic for ICD-9-CM* (1991:3Q:p19-20),[2] pleural effusion is not usually reported if it appears in conjunction with congestive heart failure because the condition is not separately treated. When the only documentation is a diagnostic x-ray, the coder should not report the condition. However, in certain cases, "special x-rays such as decubitus views are required to confirm the presence of pleural effusion or diagnostic thoracentesis may be performed to identify its etiology. In other cases, it may be necessary to address the effusion by therapeutic thoracentesis or chest tube drainage. In any of these situations, it is acceptable to report pleural effusion as an additional diagnosis since the condition was specifically evaluated or treated, but reporting is not required."

EXAMPLE Hemothorax due to pulmonary embolism, I26.99, J94.2.

Pneumothorax

When air enters the pleural space, this is called **pneumothorax**. A pneumothorax may be classified as spontaneous (not caused by trauma), traumatic, or iatrogenic. **Spontaneous pneumothorax** may occur in individuals who have no history of lung disease and often is the result of a ruptured subpleural bleb. **Iatrogenic** pneumothorax is the result of a complication of a diagnostic or therapeutic intervention or procedure. Traumatic pneumothorax occurs as the result of an injury and is assigned an injury code.

EXAMPLE Spontaneous pneumothorax, no specific cause found, J93.83.

EXERCISE 16-7

Assign codes to the following conditions.

1. Empyema due to *streptococcus pneumoniae*   _____

2. Pleural plaque with asbestos   _____

3. Hemopneumothorax   _____

4. Lung abscess due to *pseudomonas aeruginosa*   _____

Other Diseases of the Respiratory System (J96-J99)

Respiratory Failure

Respiratory failure is a general term that describes ineffective gas exchange across the lungs by the respiratory system. An arterial blood gas (ABG) measurement may be used to detect the presence of respiratory failure. A partial pressure of oxygen in arterial blood (Pao$_2$) of less than 60 torr and a partial pressure of carbon dioxide in arterial blood (Paco$_2$) greater than 50 torr indicate respiratory failure.

Some of the most common causes of respiratory failure include the following:

- Obstruction of the airways (chronic bronchitis, emphysema, cystic fibrosis, etc.)
- Weak breathing due to drugs and alcohol, extreme obesity, or sleep apnea
- Muscle weakness from muscular dystrophy, polio, stroke, spinal cord injury, or Lou Gehrig's disease
- Abnormality of lung tissue such as pneumonia, fluid in lungs, lung cancer, pulmonary fibrosis, sarcoidosis, and radiation
- Abnormal chest wall from scoliosis or severe injury to chest wall

Respiratory failure is classified on the basis of acuity. Acute respiratory failure is the result of a sudden, catastrophic event. Chronic respiratory failure is the result of a gradual worsening of respiratory function. Acute on chronic respiratory failure occurs when a patient has chronic respiratory failure that has decompensated or deteriorated.

EXAMPLE   Patient presents to the emergency room (ER) in acute respiratory failure and is admitted. Following admission, the patient was started on antibiotics for pneumonia, J96.00, J18.9.
   (Per guidelines, if both the respiratory failure and another acute condition are equally responsible for occasioning the admission, the guidelines regarding two or more diagnoses that equally meet the definition for principal diagnosis may be applied in these situations.)

EXAMPLE   Patient is admitted from the clinic for intravenous (IV) antibiotics for pneumonia. A couple of hours after admission, the patient deteriorated and developed acute respiratory failure, J18.9, J96.00.

EXAMPLE   Patient is admitted to the hospital in acute respiratory failure and is found to have suffered a myocardial infarction, I21.3, J96.00 or J96.00, I21.3.
   (Per guidelines, if both the respiratory failure and another acute condition are equally responsible for occasioning the admission, the guidelines regarding two or more diagnoses that equally meet the definition for principal diagnosis may be applied in these situations.)

Respiratory Disorders in Diseases Classified Elsewhere

Code J99 identifies respiratory disorders in diseases that are classified elsewhere. There is a *code first* Instructional note that states the underlying disease should be coded first (Figure 16-6). There may be some combination codes such as systemic lupus erythematosus that involve the lung that are coded elsewhere. The Excludes1 note shows some of the more common conditions that are coded elsewhere (see Figure 16-6).

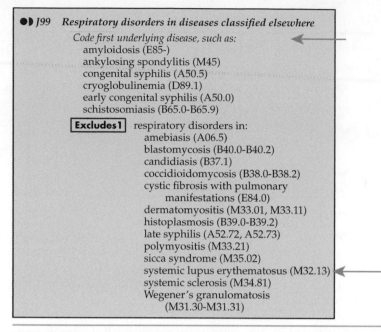

FIGURE 16-6. Code-first Instructional note and Excludes1 note.

EXAMPLE   Systemic lupus erythematosus that has affected the patient's lungs, M32.13.

EXERCISE 16-8

Assign codes to the following conditions.

1. Sickle cell disease with vaso-occlusive crisis with acute chest syndrome   _____

2. Acute respiratory failure due to pneumonia; patient was intubated and was placed on mechanical ventilation for 48 hours; the respiratory failure developed after admission   _____

3. Acute respiratory failure due to Lou Gehrig's disease   _____

4. Acute pulmonary insufficiency following thoracic surgery   _____

5. Acute on chronic respiratory failure in patient with severe emphysema; patient is oxygen dependent   _____

6. Respiratory failure due to exacerbation of COPD   _____

FACTORS INFLUENCING HEALTH STATUS AND CONTACT WITH HEALTH SERVICES (Z CODES)

As was discussed in Chapter 8, it is difficult to locate Z codes in the Index. Coders will often say, "I did not know there was a Z code for that." Refer to Chapter 8 for a listing of common main terms to locate Z codes.

Z codes that may be used with diseases of the respiratory system include the following:

EXAMPLE   Exposure to asbestos, Z77.090.

Z01.811	Encounter for preprocedural respiratory examination
Z13.83	Encounter for screening for respiratory disorder NEC
Z43.0	Encounter for attention to tracheostomy
Z48.24	Encounter for aftercare following lung transplant
Z48.813	Encounter for surgical aftercare following surgery on the respiratory system
Z57.2	Occupational exposure to dust
Z57.31	Occupational exposure to environmental tobacco smoke
Z57.39	Occupational exposure to other air contaminants
Z71.6	Tobacco abuse counseling
Z77.090	Contact with and (suspected) exposure to asbestos
Z77.110	Contact with and (suspected) exposure to air pollution
Z77.22	Contact with and (suspected) exposure to environmental tobacco smoke (acute) (chronic)
Z82.5	Family history of asthma and other chronic lower respiratory diseases
Z83.6	Family history of other diseases of the respiratory system
Z87.01	Personal history of pneumonia (recurrent)
Z87.09	Personal history of other diseases of the respiratory system
Z90.02	Acquired absence of larynx
Z90.2	Acquired absence of lung [part of]
Z92.81	Personal history of extracorporeal membrane oxygenation (ECMO)
Z93.0	Tracheostomy status
Z94.2	Lung transplant status
Z94.3	Heart and lungs transplant status
Z96.3	Presence of artificial larynx
Z98.3	Post therapeutic collapse of lung status
Z99.0	Dependence on aspirator
Z99.11	Dependence on respirator [ventilator] status
Z99.12	Encounter for respirator [ventilator] dependence during power failure
Z99.81	Dependence on supplemental oxygen

EXERCISE 16-9

Assign codes to the following conditions.

1. Status post lung transplant _____

2. Preoperative examination to assess COPD status prior to elective surgery for cholelithiasis _____

3. Patient has a tracheostomy and is dependent on a respirator _____

4. Personal history of lung cancer with previous surgery to remove lung; no recurrence _____

5. Family history of asthma _____

COMMON TREATMENTS

Smoking cessation may be beneficial in the prevention of exacerbations and progression of many respiratory conditions. Annual vaccinations against influenza and a once-only vaccination against bacterial pneumococcal pneumonia may help prevent the pulmonary complications of infection.

CONDITION	MEDICATION/TREATMENT
Sinusitis	Decongestant to help sinuses drain; antibiotics
Bronchitis	If viral—rest, fluids, cough medicine If bacterial—an antibiotic may be prescribed
Asthmatic bronchitis	Bronchodilators, steroids, and antibiotics for acute infection
Chronic bronchitis	Bronchodilators, steroids, and antibiotics for acute infection
Emphysema	Bronchodilators, steroids, oxygen therapy, and antibiotics for acute infection
Asthma	Corticosteroids, albuterol (Proventil, Ventolin), theophylline (TheoDur, Slo-Bid, Uniphyl), Serevent, Xopenex, Azmocort, Advair, Singulair, and Symbicort
COPD	Prednisone, albuterol (Proventil, Ventolin), Combivent, Serevent, Alupent, and Atrovent
Pneumonia	Sputum culture and antibiotics, if suspected to be bacterial
Influenza	Influenza vaccination, nasal swab, amantadine, zanamivir, and treatment of symptoms
Respiratory failure	Oxygen, mechanical ventilation, treatment of underlying cause
Pleural effusion	Treatment of underlying cause
Pulmonary edema	Treatment of underlying cause

PROCEDURES

Procedures related to the respiratory system in ICD-10-PCS can be located in the following tables:

0B1-0BY	Respiratory System
0C0-0CX	Mouth and Throat
5A0-5A2	Extracorporeal Assistance and Performance

Mechanical Ventilation

Mechanical ventilation is the use of a machine to induce alternating inflation and deflation of the lungs for the purpose of regulating the exchange rate of gases in the blood. The root operation for mechanical ventilation is performance (completely taking over a physiological function by extracorporeal means). The most common type of ventilator (or respirator) delivers inspiratory gases directly into the person's airway. Mechanical ventilation codes are time-based as follows:

- Less than 24 consecutive hours
- 24 to 96 consecutive hours
- Greater than 96 consecutive hours

To calculate the number of hours (duration) of continuous mechanical ventilation during a hospitalization, begin the count from the start of the (endotracheal) intubation. The duration ends with (endotracheal) extubation. If a patient is intubated prior to admission, begin counting the duration from time of admission. If a patient is transferred (discharged) while intubated, the duration would end at the time of transfer (discharge).

For patients who have been (endotracheal) intubated and subsequently undergo a tracheostomy, duration begins with the (endotracheal) intubation and ends when the mechanical ventilation is turned off (after the weaning period).

In a patient with a tracheostomy, to calculate the number of hours of continuous mechanical ventilation during hospitalization, begin counting the duration when mechanical ventilation is started. Duration ends when the mechanical ventilator is turned off (after the weaning period). If a patient has received a tracheostomy prior to admission and is on mechanical ventilation at the time of admission, begin counting the duration from the time of admission. If a patient is transferred (discharged) while still on mechanical ventilation via tracheostomy, duration would end at the time of transfer (discharge).

For certain procedures or for particular patients, mechanical ventilation may be used during surgery and in the immediate postoperative period. Mechanical ventilation during surgery does not require a code assignment, unless the ventilation is required for "an extended period (several days)" during the post surgical period. *Coding Clinic for ICD-9-CM* (2004:3Q:p11)[3] states "the term 'several' is defined as more than two. Therefore, unless the physician has clearly documented an unexpected extended period of mechanical ventilation (several days), do not assign a code for the mechanical ventilation."

If ventilation is required for a longer period than normal, a medical reason for continuing ventilation should be documented. If this is not well documented, the coder may have to query the physician. To calculate the hours, begin counting from the time of intubation.

If a patient has been extubated and is no longer on mechanical ventilation, but his or her condition deteriorates, requiring reintubation and mechanical ventilation, this would begin a new ventilation period, and a second code based on hours of ventilation would be assigned.

EXAMPLE Patient was intubated and placed on mechanical ventilation for respiratory failure due to myasthenia gravis in crisis. Patient was ventilated for 3 days, J96.90, G70.01, 5A1945Z, 0BH17EZ.

Noninvasive Ventilation

Noninvasive ventilation is a form of ventilation without an invasive artificial airway (endotracheal tube or tracheostomy). The root operation for noninvasive ventilation is assistance (taking over a portion of a physiological function by extracorporeal means). The use of noninvasive ventilation preserves the speech, swallowing, and cough functions of the patient. Noninvasive ventilation is divided into two categories:

- Negative-pressure ventilation
- Noninvasive positive-pressure ventilation (NPPV)

Negative-pressure ventilators provide ventilatory support by reducing the pressure surrounding the chest wall during inspiration and reversing the pressure during expiration. Machines such as iron lungs and body ventilators are used.

Noninvasive positive-pressure ventilation is being used more often in the hospital setting. NPPV is delivered by a nasal or face mask and may be administered with the following devices:

- Intermittent positive-pressure ventilation (IPPV)
- Bilevel positive airway pressure (BIPAP)
- Continuous positive airway pressure (CPAP)

NPPV is more comfortable for the patient and complications that are associated with invasive ventilation such as pneumothorax, airway injury, and ventilator-associated pneumonia can be minimized.

Bronchoscopy

Bronchoscopy is a diagnostic endoscopic procedure in which a tube with a tiny camera on the end is inserted through the nose or mouth into the lungs (Figure 16-7). The root operation for a diagnostic bronchoscopy is inspection (visual/manual exploration). This procedure provides a view of the airways of the lung and allows doctors to collect lung secretions or tissue specimens (biopsy).

EXAMPLE Transbronchial biopsy of the right lung, which confirmed carcinoma of the lung, C34.91, 0BBK8ZX.

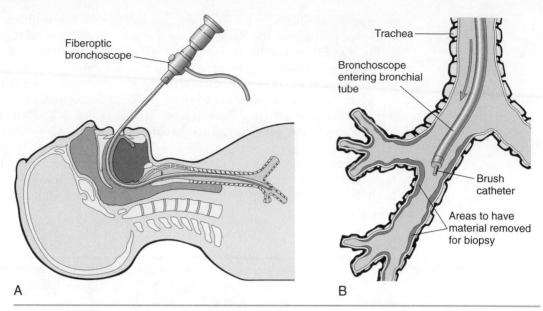

FIGURE 16-7. A, Fiberoptic bronchoscopy—a bronchoscope is passed through the nose, throat, larynx, and trachea into the bronchus. **B,** A bronchoscope with a brush catheter, ready for biopsy of bronchial tissue.

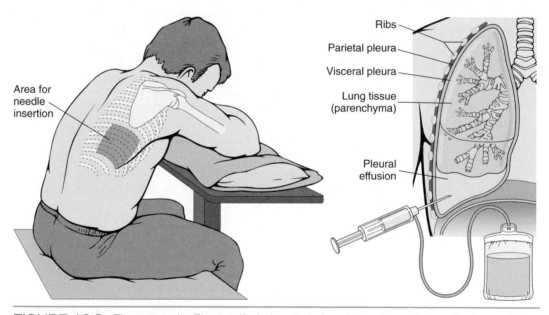

FIGURE 16-8. Thoracentesis. The needle is inserted close to the base of the effusion so that gravity will help with drainage.

Thoracentesis

Thoracentesis is puncture of the chest wall to remove fluid (pleural effusion) from the space (cavity) between the lining of the outside of the lungs (pleura) and the wall of the chest (pleural cavity) (Figure 16-8). The root operation for thoracentesis is drainage (taking or letting out fluids or gases). Physicians may perform a diagnostic thoracentesis or a therapeutic thoracentesis. The fluid collected is sent to the laboratory for analysis. This may also relieve any shortness of breath caused by compression on the lung by the fluid.

Thoracostomy

Tube thoracostomy is the term used for insertion of chest tube(s) to drain blood, fluid, or air and to allow full expansion of the lungs. The root operation for tube thoracostomy is drainage (taking or letting out fluids or gases). A tube is placed between the ribs and into the space between the inner lining and the outer lining of the lung (pleural space); fluid is allowed to drain. A suction machine may be used to facilitate drainage. Reasons why chest tubes may be used include pneumothorax, hemothorax, abscess, empyema, and cancer; they also may be used after surgery.

EXAMPLE   Insertion of chest tube on the right side for continuous drainage of empyema, J86.9, 0W9930Z.

Tracheostomy

Tracheostomy is a procedure in which an artificial opening is made in the front of the windpipe (trachea) through the skin of the neck (Figure 16-9). The root operation for tracheostomy is bypass (altering the route of passage of the contents of a tubular body part). A tube is inserted, through which breathing may continue until the normal airway can be restored. A tracheostomy may be performed during an emergency at the patient's bedside. In some cases, a tracheostomy is planned and is performed in the Operating Room (OR).

EXAMPLE   Temporary open tracheostomy was performed in the OR because of the patient's recurrent aspiration pneumonitis, J69.0, 0B110F4.

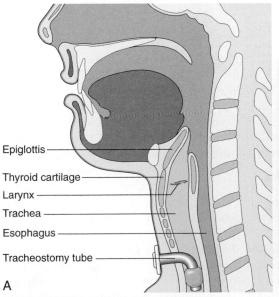

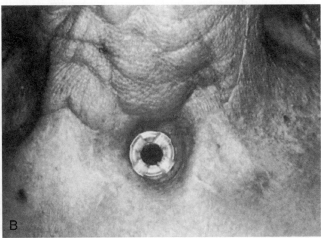

Epiglottis

Thyroid cartilage

Larynx

Trachea

Esophagus

Tracheostomy tube

A

B

FIGURE 16-9. A, Tracheostomy with tube in place. **B,** Healed tracheostomy incision.

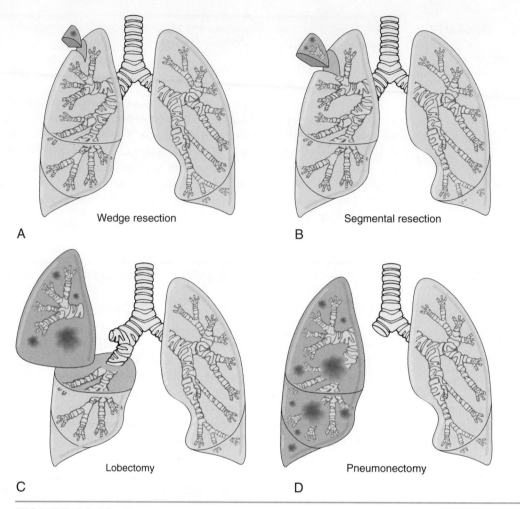

A Wedge resection

B Segmental resection

C Lobectomy

D Pneumonectomy

FIGURE 16-10. Pulmonary resections. **A,** Wedge resection. **B,** Segmental resection. **C,** Lobectomy. **D,** Pneumonectomy.

Pulmonary Resection

The type of pulmonary resection undertaken may depend on the condition that is being diagnosed and/or treated. Wedge resection (Figure 16-10, *A*) is the removal of a small, localized area of diseased tissue near the surface of the lung. Segmental resection (Figure 16-10, *B*) involves the removal of a bronchiole and its alveoli in one or more lung segments. Removal of an entire lobe of the lung is a lobectomy (Figure 16-10, *C*), and the removal of an entire lung is known as pneumonectomy (Figure 16-10, *D*). The root operation for resection of any part of the lung will depend on the portion of the lung that is resected. Resection is the root operation when all of a body part is cut out or off without replacement. "All of a body part" includes any anatomical subdivision that has its own body part value (Figure 16-11). Although a lobectomy is not the removal of the entire lung, it is the removal of a body part that has its own value, therefore it is a resection. For partial resections the root operation is excision (cutting out/off without replacement some of a body part).

A surgical technique known as video-assisted thoracic surgery (VATS) has allowed surgeons to perform thoracic surgery in a minimally invasive manner. Depending on the type of procedure performed, a hospital stay may last only 1 to 3 days, intensive care may not be needed, and recovery may be quicker. Patients may return to their normal activities much sooner than when an "open" procedure is performed.

SECTION: 0 MEDICAL AND SURGICAL
BODY SYSTEM: B RESPIRATORY SYSTEM
OPERATION: T RESECTION: Cutting out or off, without replacement, all of a body part

Body Part	Approach	Device	Qualifier
1 Trachea	0 Open	Z No Device	Z No Qualifier
2 Carina	4 Percutaneous Endoscopic		
3 Main Bronchus, Right			
4 Upper Lobe Bronchus, Right			
5 Middle Lobe Bronchus, Right			
6 Lower Lobe Bronchus, Right			
7 Main Bronchus, Left			
8 Upper Lobe Bronchus, Left			
9 Lingula Bronchus			
B Lower Lobe Bronchus, Left	Anatomical subdivisions of the lung		
C Upper Lung Lobe, Right			
D Middle Lung Lobe, Right			
F Lower Lung Lobe, Right			
G Upper Lung Lobe, Left			
H Lung Lingula			
J Lower Lung Lobe, Left			
K Lung, Right			
L Lung, Left			
M Lungs, Bilateral			
R Diaphragm, Right			
S Diaphragm, Left			

FIGURE 16-11. PCS table showing anatomical subdivisions of the lung.

EXERCISE 16-10

Assign codes for all diagnosis and procedures.

1. Thoracoscopy with excision of primary lung cancer from the left lower lobe (not a lobectomy) _____

2. Thorascopic pleurodesis with administration of talc for recurrent spontaneous pneumothorax on the right _____

3. Diagnostic thoracentesis for large right-sided pleural effusion _____

4. Bronchoalveolar lavage of right lung to assess type of pneumonia _____

5. Temporary percutaneous tracheostomy in patient with laryngeal cancer who will be having surgery in a couple of weeks _____

6. Endotracheal intubation with mechanical ventilation for 3 days because of acute respiratory failure due to exacerbation of congestive heart failure _____

7. Lobectomy for squamous cell carcinoma, right lung, upper lobe _____

8. Transbronchial biopsy of the left lung and mainstem bronchus; histologic exam confirms pulmonary tuberculosis _____

DOCUMENTATION/REIMBURSEMENT/MS-DRGs

Often, coding difficulties are due to lack of documentation. Sometimes pathology and other test results are not available at the time of discharge or when the physician is dictating the discharge summary or is reporting the final diagnoses.

Assigning the correct code to identify the COPD can be difficult because of conflicting documentation. Physicians frequently use the general term COPD rather than more specific terminology.

Documentation of pneumonia and the causative organism or sputum culture results may not be directly linked, making it necessary to query the physician. Physicians often document exacerbation of COPD but fail to document any condition that may be responsible for the exacerbation such as pneumonia.

It may be difficult to calculate mechanical ventilation time with the use of physician documentation, and it may be necessary to use respiratory therapy notes to determine the exact length of time. It is also possible that a patient could have more than one continuous episode of ventilation.

Procedures that can be performed at bedside such as tracheostomy, thoracentesis, and insertion of a chest tube may not be well documented by the physician or may be documented only within a progress note and therefore are easy to miss.

An abnormal laboratory test may not necessarily be clinically significant. If abnormal laboratory tests are noted and treatment is given, it would be appropriate to query the physician regarding the abnormal laboratory test(s). An abnormal laboratory test must be clinically significant to be coded.

Frequently missed complications/comorbidities from the respiratory chapter include the following:

- Atelectasis
- Bronchiectasis with acute exacerbation
- Bronchitis, chronic obstructive, with exacerbation
- COPD exacerbation
- Effusion, pleural
- Failure, respiratory
- Pneumonia
- Pneumothorax

Pneumonia and Causative Organism

EXAMPLE Patient has a long history of chronic obstructive pulmonary disease and was admitted for the treatment of pneumonia. Sputum cultures grew *Klebsiella*. The physician should be queried to determine whether the pneumonia is due to *Klebsiella*. The patient's COPD was treated due to flare up.

DIAGNOSES	CODES	MS-DRG	RW
Pneumonia in patient with COPD	J18.9, J44.1	194	1.0026
Klebsiella pneumonia with COPD	J15.0, J44.1	178	1.4653

The causative organism of pneumonia can make a significant difference in the MS-DRG assignment. Also, the presence of a complication/comorbidity such as an exacerbation of COPD can make a difference in reimbursement, depending on the principal diagnosis and the MS-DRG assigned.

Two Diagnoses That Equally Meet the Definition for Principal Diagnosis

EXAMPLE Patient was admitted with aspiration pneumonia and *pneumococcal* pneumonia. Patient had severe gastroesophageal reflux disease (GERD). The patient was admitted with both types of pneumonia, and both diagnoses fit the definition of principal diagnosis.

DIAGNOSES	CODES	MS-DRG	RW
Aspiration pneumonia with *pneumococcal* pneumonia	J69.0, J13, K21.9	179	1.0025
Pneumococcal pneumonia with aspiration pneumonia	J13, J69.0, K21.9	195	0.7037

Note that the aspiration pneumonia groups to an MS-DRG with a higher weight. If both pneumonias meet the definition of a principal diagnosis, it is perfectly acceptable to sequence aspiration pneumonia as the principal. If a patient was admitted with *pneumococcal* pneumonia, and a couple of days after admission aspirated and developed aspiration pneumonia, *pneumococcal* pneumonia is the principal diagnosis and aspiration pneumonia is a secondary diagnosis.

MS-DRG With and Without MCC/CC

In other MS-DRGs, either of the pneumonia diagnoses would qualify as complications/comorbidities, but with pneumonia as the principal and pneumonia as a secondary diagnosis, these case scenarios are grouped into MS-DRGs without complications/comorbidities. Further optimization could be accomplished by reviewing the chart for additional diagnoses, as in the following example:

EXAMPLE Patient was admitted with aspiration pneumonia and *pneumococcal* pneumonia. Patient has severe GERD. The patient was admitted with both types of pneumonia, and both diagnoses fit the definition of principal diagnosis. It is noted on the history and physical that the patient has a chronic kidney disease, stage IV.

DIAGNOSES	CODES	MS-DRG	RW
Aspiration pneumonia with *pneumococcal* pneumonia CKD, stage IV	J69.0, J13, K21.9, N18.4	178	1.4653
Pneumococcal pneumonia with aspiration pneumonia, CKD, stage IV	J13, J69.0, K21.9, N18.4	194	1.0026

Both MS-DRGs are optimized by the addition of N18.4 stage IV CKD, which is a complication/comorbidity in these cases. The difference in relative weight when aspiration pneumonia is sequenced as the principal diagnosis should also be noted.

Respiratory Failure versus Another Acute Condition

EXAMPLE Patient was admitted with acute respiratory failure due to pneumonia.
(Per guidelines, if both the respiratory failure and another acute condition are equally responsible for occasioning the admission, the guidelines regarding two or more diagnoses that equally meet the definition for principal diagnosis may be applied in these situations.)

DIAGNOSES	CODES	MS-DRG	RW
Respiratory failure due to pneumonia	J96.00, J18.9	189	1.2694
Pneumonia with respiratory failure	J18.9, J96.00	193	1.4948

In this case, either the respiratory failure or the pneumonia could be selected as the principal diagnosis; the reimbursement is higher if the respiratory failure is the principal diagnosis. In MS-DRG 193, the respiratory failure is an MCC.

Assign codes for all diagnoses and procedures.

1. Cough due to *Streptococcus pneumoniae* pneumonia _____

2. Patient with severe emphysema who is dependent on oxygen; quit _____
smoking 5 years ago. NPPV (48 hours) was initiated for the
patient's chronic respiratory failure

3. Patient is high risk for lung disease due to on-the-job exposure to _____
asbestos; patient has a 20–pack-year history of smoking
cigarettes, currently active

4. Croup _____

5. Left tonsillar abscess; abscess was drained _____

6. Patient with whooping cough has pneumonia _____

7. *Haemophilus influenzae* pneumonia in a patient who is being _____
treated for influenza

8. Edema larynx _____

9. Status asthmaticus in patient with severe persistent asthma _____

10. Acute bronchitis with acute exacerbation of COPD _____

11. Acute on chronic respiratory failure due to sarcoidosis involving the _____
lungs; mechanical ventilation for 3 days; patient was intubated at
transferring facility and was transferred for evaluation of sarcoidosis

12. Reactive airway disease _____

13. Patient tested positive for H1N1 influenza _____

14. Bronchiolitis obliterans organizing pneumonia _____

15. Acute and chronic sinusitis _____

16. Chronic tonsillitis and adenoiditis; tonsillectomy with _____
adenoidectomy performed

17. Nasal cavity polyps with endoscopic polypectomy _____

18. Solitary pulmonary nodule _____

19. Empyema with insertion of left chest tube; empyema was due to _____
Staphylococcus aureus

20. Double lung transplant for diffuse idiopathic pulmonary fibrosis; _____
cardiopulmonary bypass was performed in this transplant from a
cadaver

21. Congestive heart failure with left pleural effusion that was treated _____
with thoracentesis at bedside

22. Granuloma lung _____

23. Tension pneumothorax _____

24. Acute bronchitis with chronic obstructive bronchitis _____

25. Pulmonary edema _____

Write the correct answer(s) in the space(s) provided.

26. Define contamination of a culture.

_____

27. Define empiric treatment.

_____

28. Define iatrogenic.

_____

29. List two problems/conditions that could cause a patient to aspirate.

_____

_____

30. List two terms that describe status asthmaticus.

_____

_____

CHAPTER GLOSSARY

Asbestosis: lung disease due to inhalation of asbestos.

Aspiration pneumonia: inflammation of the lungs and bronchial tubes due to aspiration of foreign material into the lung.

Asthma: chronic disease that affects the airways that carry air into and out of the lungs.

Asthmatic bronchitis: underlying asthmatic problem in patients in whom asthma has become so persistent that clinically significant chronic airflow obstruction is present despite antiasthmatic therapy.

Baritosis: lung disease due to inhalation of barium.

Black lung: lung disease due to inhalation of coal dust.

Bronchi: the two air tubes that branch off the trachea and deliver air to both lungs.

Bronchitis: lower respiratory tract or bronchial tree infection characterized by cough, sputum production, and wheezing.

Bronchoscopy: diagnostic endoscopic procedure in which a tube with a tiny camera on the end is inserted through the nose or mouth into the lungs.

Chronic bronchitis: condition defined by a mucus-producing cough most days of the month, 3 months out of a year for 2 successive years, with no other underlying disease to explain the cough.

Chronic obstructive pulmonary disease: general term used to describe a lung disease in which the airways become obstructed, making it difficult for air to get into and out of the lungs.

Chronic sinusitis: occurs when the sinuses become inflamed and swollen.

Chylothorax: milky fluid consisting of lymph and fat (chyle) that accumulates in the pleural space.

Coal workers' pneumoconiosis: lung disease due to inhalation of coal dust.

Community-acquired pneumonia: broad term used to define pneumonias that are contracted outside of the hospital or nursing home setting.

Contaminant: a cultured organism that a physician does not believe is responsible for causing a particular infection.

Diaphragm: dome-shaped muscles at the bottom of the lungs that assist in the process of breathing and in the exchange of oxygen/carbon dioxide.

Emphysema: chronic lung disease of gradual onset that can be attributed to chronic infection and inflammation or irritation from cigarette smoke.

Empiric: initiation of treatment prior to making a definite diagnosis.

Empyema: pus that accumulates in the pleural space.

Hemothorax: blood that accumulates in the pleural space.

Iatrogenic: caused by medical treatment.

Infection: invasion of the body by organisms that have the potential to cause disease.

Influenza: contagious viral infection of the respiratory tract that causes coughing, difficulty breathing, headache, muscle aches, and weakness.

Lung abscess: infection that forms in the lung parenchyma.

Mechanical ventilation: use of a machine to induce alternating inflation and deflation of the lungs and to regulate the exchange rate of gases in the blood.

Noninvasive ventilation: ventilation without an invasion artificial airway (endotracheal tube or tracheostomy).

Nosocomial pneumonia: pneumonia that is acquired while the patient is residing in a hospital-type setting.

Nursing home–acquired pneumonia: pneumonia that is acquired in a nursing home or extended care facility.

Pleural effusion: fluid that accumulates in the pleural space because of trauma or disease.

Pneumoconioses: lung diseases due to chronic inhalation of inorganic (mineral) dust that are often due to occupational exposure.

Pneumonia: infection of the lungs that may be caused by a variety of organisms, including viruses, bacteria, and parasites.

Pneumothorax: air in space around the lung.

Pulmonary edema: condition in which fluid accumulates in the lungs.

Respiratory failure: general term that describes ineffective gas exchange across the lungs by the respiratory system.

Respiratory system: system that supplies the body with oxygen (O_2).

Siderosis: lung disease due to inhalation of iron oxide.

Sinusitis: a condition in which the linings of one or more sinuses become infected, usually because of viruses or bacteria.

Spontaneous pneumothorax: pneumothorax that is not caused by trauma.

Stannosis: lung disease due to inhalation of tin particles.

Thoracentesis: puncture of the chest wall to remove fluid (pleural effusion) from the space between the lining of the outside of the lungs (pleura) and the wall of the chest.

Trachea (windpipe): body part that is responsible for filtering the air that we breathe.

Tracheostomy: procedure in which an artificial opening is made in the front of the windpipe (trachea) through the skin of the neck.

Tube thoracostomy: insertion of chest tube(s) to drain blood, fluid, or air and allow full expansion of the lungs.

REFERENCES

1. Damjanov I. *Pathology for the Health Professions,* 3rd ed. St. Louis: Saunders, 2006, Table 8-1, p 177.
2. American Hospital Association. *Coding Clinic for ICD-9-CM* 1991:3Q:p19-20. Pleural effusion with congestive heart failure.
3. American Hospital Association. *Coding Clinic for ICD-9-CM* 2004:3Q:p11. Clarification—Postoperative mechanical ventilation.

Diseases of the Digestive System

(ICD-10-CM Chapter 11, Codes K00-K95)

LEARNING OBJECTIVES

1. Apply and assign the correct ICD-10-CM/PCS codes in accordance with Official Guidelines for Coding and Reporting
2. Identify major differences between ICD-10-CM and ICD-9-CM related to diseases of the digestive system
3. Identify pertinent anatomy and physiology of the digestive system

4. Identify diseases of the digestive system
5. Assign the correct Z codes and procedure codes related to the digestive system
6. Identify common treatments, medications, laboratory values, and diagnostic tests
7. Explain the importance of documentation in relation to MS-DRGs for reimbursement

ABBREVIATIONS/ ACRONYMS

AVM arteriovenous malformation

EGD esophagogastroduodenoscopy

ERCP endoscopic retrograde cholangiopancreatography

ESWL extracorporeal shock wave lithotripsy

GERD gastroesophageal reflux disease

GI gastrointestinal

ICD-9-CM *International Classification of Diseases, 9th Revision, Clinical Modification*

ICD-10-CM *International Classification of Diseases, 10th Revision, Clinical Modification*

ICD-10-PCS *International Classification of Diseases, 10th Revision, Procedure Coding System*

IV intravenous

LGIB lower gastrointestinal bleed

MS-DRG Medicare Severity diagnosis-related group

NSAID nonsteroidal antiinflammatory drug

PEG percutaneous endoscopic gastrostomy

PUD peptic ulcer disease

TIPS transjugular intrahepatic portosystemic shunt

UGIB upper gastrointestinal bleed

ICD-10-CM OFFICIAL GUIDELINES FOR CODING AND REPORTING

There are currently no official guidelines for diseases of the digestive system. Apply the General Coding Guidelines as found in Chapter 5 of this text and the Procedural Coding Guidelines as found in Chapters 6 and 7.

MAJOR DIFFERENCES BETWEEN ICD-10-CM AND ICD-9-CM

- ICD-10-CM has expanded Crohn's disease to fourth, fifth, and sixth characters. These characters specify site, whether there was a complication present, and what the specific complication was.
- ICD-9-CM classified GI ulcers by the presence or absence of an obstruction. ICD-10-CM eliminates the reference to obstruction.
- ICD-10-CM expands on the hernia categories with characters for laterality and recurrence.
- ICD-10-CM expands the section on cholelithiasis to incorporate cholangitis.

ANATOMY AND PHYSIOLOGY

The digestive system (Figure 17-1) consists of the mouth, pharynx, esophagus, stomach, small intestine and large intestine (the **alimentary canal**), and accessory organs, which include the salivary glands, liver, gallbladder, and pancreas. The purpose of the digestive system is to process food so that it may be absorbed by cells.

The mouth is where digestion begins. The tongue, which is composed of muscle, the teeth, and saliva, facilitates **mastication** and assists in moving food to the pharynx, where

ACCESSORY ORGANS   MAIN ORGANS

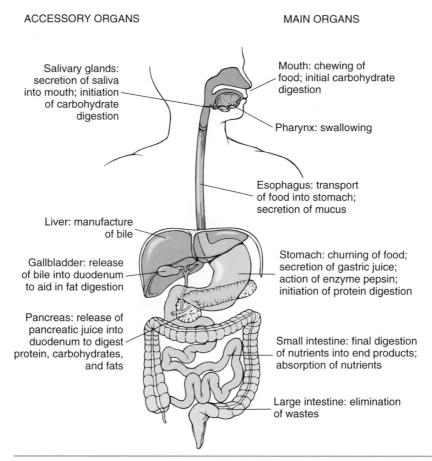

FIGURE 17-1. Main and accessory organs of the digestive system.

swallowing occurs and food moves to the esophagus. **Peristalsis**, or the squeezing movement of food toward the stomach, occurs in the esophagus. Once the food arrives in the stomach, it is churned with gastric juices and begins the movement toward the small intestine.

The pancreas, the liver, and the gallbladder all aid in the digestive process. The purpose of the pancreas is to excrete juices that aid in the digestive process. The pancreatic duct connects with the duodenum in the same area in which the bile duct from the liver and the gallbladder intersect the duodenum. The liver secretes bile to aid in the digestive process, and the gallbladder stores bile and releases it as needed. The gallbladder is attached to the liver by the cystic duct, which joins the hepatic duct. Together, they form the common bile duct, which enters into the duodenum.

The function of the liver, in addition to aiding the digestive process, is to remove poisons from the blood, produce immune agents to control infection, and remove germs and bacteria from the blood. The liver serves as a filter for the body; a person cannot live without a functioning liver.

The small intestine contains three areas: the duodenum, the jejunum, and the ileum. The small intestine completes the digestion begun in the stomach, absorbs products of digestion, and transports residue to the large intestine. The small intestine is suspended and is attached to the abdomen by a fold of peritoneum known as the mesentery. The small intestine joins the large intestine at the ileocecal valve.

The large intestine (Figure 17-2) is composed of the cecum, colon, rectum, and anal canal. The appendix is an appendage off the cecum. The purpose of the large intestine is to absorb electrolytes and store feces until the time of elimination.

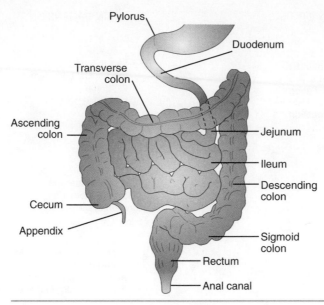

FIGURE 17-2. Small and large intestines.

DISEASE CONDITIONS

Diseases of the Digestive System (K00-K95), Chapter 11 in the ICD-10-CM code book, are divided into the following categories:

CATEGORY	SECTION TITLES
K00-K14	Diseases of oral cavity and salivary glands
K20-K31	Diseases of esophagus, stomach, and duodenum
K35-K38	Diseases of appendix
K40-K46	Hernia
K50-K52	Noninfective enteritis and colitis
K55-K63	Other diseases of intestines
K65-K68	Diseases of peritoneum and retroperitoneum
K70-K77	Diseases of liver
K80-K87	Disorders of gallbladder, biliary tract, and pancreas
K90-K95	Other diseases of the digestive system

Diseases of the Oral Cavity and Salivary Glands (K00-K14)

Many of the conditions in these categories concern the teeth and their structures which are often treated in the outpatient setting. Some of these conditions, however, may be treated when a patient is admitted for another condition. In the exam section of the record a healthcare provider might document whether the patient has dentures due to **edentulism**, which is the complete loss of teeth. The loss of teeth might affect the patient's ability to eat and therefore their nutritional state.

EXAMPLE

Patient is admitted to the hospital with severe malnutrition and dehydration. During the exam it is identified that the patient has Class I complete edentulism, E43, E86.0, K08.101.

Sialolithiasis is caused by stones in the salivary glands. Patients usually present with swollen, painful glands around the neck. When the stones are obstructing the gland, an infection, which is known as sialoadenitis, can result. Surgery may be required to remove the stone.

EXAMPLE | Patient with known sialolithiasis is admitted thru the ER with very painful glands in the neck and fever. After CT scan to determine the location of the stones and administration of antibiotics, the patient is taken to the OR for open removal, K11.5, 0CCJ0ZZ.

Mucositis is an inflammation/ulceration of the digestive tract commonly occurring in the oral cavity. It can be found in up to 40% of patients being treated with chemotherapy. The condition can range from mild to severe. In the severest cases the patient may be unable to eat due to the pain caused by ulcerations in the mouth. It can be treated with viscous lidocaine.

EXAMPLE | Patient admitted for chemotherapy for pancreatic cancer and develops ulcerative mucositis due to gemcitabine, Z51.11, K12.31, T45.1x5A, C25.9, 3E04305.

EXERCISE 17-1

Assign codes to the following conditions.

1. Canker sore   _____
2. Ulcerative stomatitis   _____
3. Hypertrophy of the salivary gland   _____
4. Impacted teeth   _____

Diseases of the Esophagus, Stomach, and Duodenum (K20-K31)

Esophageal Conditions

Esophageal varices (Figure 17-3), one of the most common causes of esophageal hemorrhage, are excluded from the code for gastrointestinal hemorrhage. The codes for esophageal hemorrhage due to esophageal varices are found in the Circulatory System chapter.

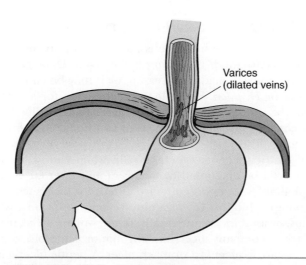

Varices
(dilated veins)

FIGURE 17-3. Esophageal varices.

> **K22.1 Ulcer of esophagus**
>   **Code first**
>   poisoning due to drug or toxin, if applicable (T36-T65 with fifth or sixth character 1–4 or 6)
>   **Use additional** code for adverse effect if applicable to identify drug (T36-T50 with fifth or sixth character 5)
>   **Excludes1:** Barrett's esophagus (K22.87-)

FIGURE 17-4. If an esophageal ulcer is drug or chemical induced, use an additional code to identify the drug.

EXAMPLE   Patient has esophageal varices due to cirrhosis of the liver, K74.60, I85.10.

Mallory-Weiss is the name for bleeding laceration of the esophagogastric junction that usually occurs after severe vomiting. If the bleeding is severe, an EGD may be performed to control bleeding. One of the most common conditions is esophageal reflux, which is also known as gastroesophageal reflux disease (GERD). It is treated with proton pump inhibitors such as Prilosec or, in more severe cases, by Nissen fundoplication surgery.

Ulcers of the esophagus are often caused by drugs or medications (Figure 17-4).

Barrett's esophagus is a precancerous condition that usually occurs in people with chronic GERD. The normal cells lining the esophagus change type. Symptoms may include heartburn, indigestion, difficulty swallowing solid foods, and nocturnal regurgitation.

EXAMPLE   Patient with chronic GERD who is having difficulty swallowing is found to have Barrett's esophagus, K22.70, K21.9, R13.10.

EXERCISE 17-2

Assign codes to the following conditions.

1. Esophageal ulcer due to ingestion of aspirin   _____
2. Inflammation of the esophagus due to reflux   _____
3. Mallory-Weiss tear   _____
4. GERD   _____

Ulcers of the Stomach and Small Intestine

An ulcer of the stomach or the intestine is an open sore in the lining of the stomach or intestine. An ulcer occurs when the lining is damaged. Damage to the lining may occur when production of stomach acid is increased, or it may be caused by a bacterium known as *Helicobacter pylori*, or *H. pylori*. When locating the code for a bacterium, the main term "Infection" should be referenced in the Alphabetic Index. Ulcers may be drug induced. The Tabular List contains instructions to use an additional code for adverse effect, if applicable to identify drug (T36-T50).

Symptoms of gastric ulcer may include pain when eating, vomiting, and tarry bowel movements. Ulcers can be diagnosed by means of an upper GI x-ray, blood tests that look for *H. pylori*, stool samples, or endoscopy. Treatment for ulcers may include antacids, drugs such as proton pump inhibitors or histamine receptor blockers, which stop the stomach from making acids, or antibiotics, and finally, in the worst case scenario, gastrectomy. Some conditions that may accompany ulcers are chronic or acute blood loss anemia and gastric outlet syndrome. A gastric ulcer is a stomach ulcer. A peptic ulcer can occur in the esophagus, stomach, duodenum, jejunum, and/or ileum.

EXAMPLE | Patient has a peptic ulcer of the esophagus, secondary to aspirin use, K22.10, T39.015A.

EXAMPLE | Patient is admitted for a bleeding gastric ulcer with obstruction and perforation, K25.6.

Gastrointestinal Hemorrhage

Gastrointestinal (GI) hemorrhage is a common reason for a patient to seek medical attention. The healthcare provider must determine whether the bleed is lower or upper GI in origin, so appropriate treatment can be provided. To make this determination, the provider must evaluate how the patient presents.

- In lower GI bleeds (LGIB), the patient may present with the following:
  Hematochezia—bright red blood in stool
- In upper GI bleeds (UGIB), the patient may present with the following:
  Hematemesis—vomiting of blood

If a patient presents with **melena** (dark blood in stool) or **occult blood** in the stool (this can be found only by laboratory inspection), it is unknown without further workup whether this is an upper or a lower GI bleed. Often, when a patient presents with acute anemia without a causative condition, the healthcare provider may suspect a GI bleed.

EXAMPLE | Blood in feces, occult, lab finding, R19.5.

GI hemorrhage has many causes; the most common causes consist of gastric or intestinal ulcers, hemorrhoids, diverticulitis, and angiodysplasia of the intestine.

EXAMPLE | Patient admitted with GI bleed caused by angiodysplasia of the stomach, K31.811.

EXAMPLE | Patient is being treated for diverticulitis of the sigmoid colon with hemorrhage, K57.33.

When a patient presents with a GI bleed and then undergoes diagnostic testing such as esophagogastroduodenoscopy (EGD) to determine the site of the bleed, unless the physician specifies a causal relationship between the findings on this test and the bleed, the code K92.2 should be assigned. Codes for any other findings such as gastritis should be coded as without hemorrhage.

EXERCISE 17-3

Assign codes to the following conditions.

1. Angiodysplasia with hemorrhage of the duodenum and chronic blood loss anemia   _____
2. Acute penetrating peptic ulcer of the duodenum   _____
3. GI bleed due to peptic ulcer   _____
4. Dyspepsia, gastrointestinal   _____
5. Blood in stool   _____

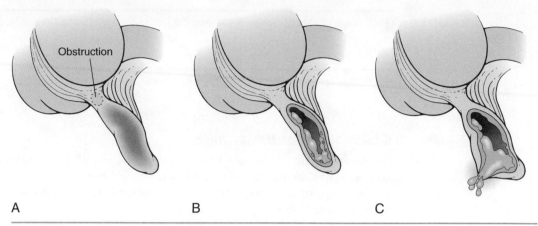

A   B   C

FIGURE 17-5. Stages of appendicitis. **A,** Obstruction that causes inflammation. **B,** Pus and bacteria invade the wall of the appendix. **C,** Pus perforates the wall of the appendix, leading to peritonitis.

Diseases of the Appendix (K35-K38)

Appendicitis is inflammation of the appendix that is usually caused by obstruction, which, in turn, results in infection (Figure 17-5). A patient who presents with appendicitis may have some or all of the following signs and symptoms: abdominal pain (right lower quadrant, also known as **McBurney's point**), vomiting, **anorexia** (loss of appetite), fever, constipation, and elevated white blood cell count.

If the appendix ruptures, peritonitis develops. Patients with appendicitis are usually treated with antibiotics and surgery (appendectomy). It is important to review the pathology report for documentation of abscess or perforation of appendix.

On occasion, all signs and symptoms lead the surgeon to believe that a patient has appendicitis, but the pathology report does not confirm this diagnosis. When the pathology report indicates a normal appendix, the symptom the patient presented with should be the principal diagnosis.

EXAMPLE | Patient admitted with acute appendicitis with peritoneal abscess, K35.3.

EXAMPLE | Patient has a ruptured appendicitis, K35.2.

Hernia (K40-K46)

A **hernia** (Figure 17-6) is a protrusion of an organ or tissue through an abnormal opening in the body. Hernias can be present at birth or may develop over time. Most commonly, a hernia is a protrusion of the intestine through a weakness in the abdominal cavity. Hernias are classified by type or site. Once the site of the hernia is known, then it must be determined whether it is obstructed or gangrenous. An obstructed abdominal hernia is one in which the bowel is trapped and obstructed but viable (still working); when it becomes nonviable, it can become gangrenous (deficient blood supply to trapped bowel, making it **necrotic**). There is a note in ICD-10-CM that if a hernia is both obstructed and gangrenous, it should be classified to a hernia with gangrene. Some codes require documentation as to whether the hernia is unilateral or bilateral. Hernia repairs require more information and are discussed in the procedure section of this chapter.

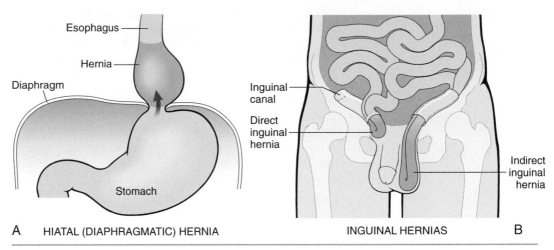

FIGURE 17-6. **A,** Hiatal hernia. **B,** Inguinal hernia. Direct inguinal hernia passes through the abdominal wall. Indirect hernia passes through the inguinal canal.

Some types of hernias:
- Inguinal—common in men, intestines protrude in the inguinal canal
- Femoral—more common in women, intestine protrudes through the femoral canal at the top of the thigh
- Umbilical—most common in children, abdominal wall is weakened at the point of the umbilical cord
- Ventral—this is when scar tissue in the abdominal wall weakens following surgery or trauma. May also be known as an incisional hernia
- Diaphragmatic—abnormal opening in the diaphragm that allows parts of organs from the abdominal cavity (i.e., intestines, stomach) to move into the chest cavity. Also known as a hiatal hernia

EXAMPLE | Patient was seen in consultation for an inguinal hernia, unilateral, recurrent, with obstruction, K40.31.

Noninfectious Enteritis and Colitis (K50-K52)

Crohn's Disease

Crohn's disease is characterized by inflammation of the GI tract, especially the small and large intestine. It is an inflammatory bowel disease that appears to run in families. It is typically diagnosed first at the age of 20 to 30. Often there is difficulty determining Crohn's versus ulcerative colitis. Crohn's may also be known as ileitis or enteritis. People presenting with Crohn's may exhibit symptoms of abdominal pain and diarrhea. Depending on the severity and location of the disease, patients may be treated with drugs to control inflammation, steroids, immunosuppressive agents, biologic response modifiers, antibiotics, and medications to control diarrhea, along with fluid replacement. Almost 75% of the patients with Crohn's require surgery at some point in their lives to remove the diseased intestine, and they often require an ostomy.

Ulcerative Colitis

Ulcerative colitis, like Crohn's disease, is an inflammatory bowel disease. Ulcerative colitis is a disease that produces ulcers in the lining of the rectum and colon, whereas Crohn's disease causes inflammation deep within the intestinal wall and can occur in other parts of the digestive system, including the small intestine, mouth, esophagus, and stomach.

EXAMPLE | Patient is admitted to the hospital with abdominal pain and dehydration. After testing is completed, a diagnosis of ulcerative enterocolitis is confirmed, K51.80, E86.0.

Gastroenteritis is an inflammation of the stomach and intestines. Two of the main causes of this condition are viruses and bacteria. Viral gastroenteritis usually runs its course in 1 to 2 days, whereas bacterial gastroenteritis can last for up to a week or more. The most common causes of viral gastroenteritis, which often spreads via poor handwashing habits in schools and daycare centers, are adenoviruses, rotaviruses, and norovirus. The noroviruses are the leading cause of acute gastroenteritis. The most common bacterial causes are *E. coli*, salmonella, campylobacter, and shigella. Gastroenteritis due to particular viruses or bacteria may be indexed under "Gastroenteritis" with a subterm for the bacterium/virus. If the bacterium/virus is not listed, the Index has an instruction to *see also* enteritis. Codes for gastroenteritis caused by viruses or bacteria may be located in the infectious and parasitic diseases chapter. Gastroenteritis may also be caused by chemical toxins such as those found in medications or foods. These types of gastroenteritis are not infectious.

The symptoms of gastroenteritis can include vomiting, diarrhea, low-grade fever, and abdominal pain. Treatment in a hospital usually consists of IV fluids for rehydration, and if the patient is suffering from bacterial gastroenteritis, antibiotics may be used. If vomiting is severe, antiemetics and antidiarrheal agents may also be used.

EXAMPLE | Patient is seen in physician's office with severe vomiting and diarrhea. After testing is performed it is determined that she is suffering from a bout of gastroenteritis, K52.9.

Other Diseases of Intestines and Peritoneum (K55-K63)

Intestinal Obstruction

This condition occurs when the content of the intestines cannot move forward. The intestines can be completely blocked or partially blocked. Obstruction may be mechanical or functional. Mechanical obstruction can be caused by a variety of conditions, such as neoplasm, **impaction**, stricture, adhesion, **intussusception**, **volvulus**, and herniation (Figure 17-7). When the obstruction is functional, it is called an **ileus.**

EXAMPLE | Patient with intestinal obstruction due to fecal impaction, K56.41.

EXAMPLE | Patient with obstruction due to ileus, K56.69.

EXAMPLE | Patient has intussusception of the intestine, K56.1.

Diverticulitis and Diverticulosis

Diverticula (Figure 17-8), also known as tics, are small pouches in the lining of the mucous membranes of an organ. When a patient has diverticula, the condition is referred to as diverticulosis. If these pouches become inflamed or infected, the condition becomes diverticulitis. Diverticulitis can result in peritonitis, perforation, fistula, bowel obstruction, or abscess. If a patient has diverticulitis, diverticula are assumed to be present and only the code for diverticulitis is assigned.

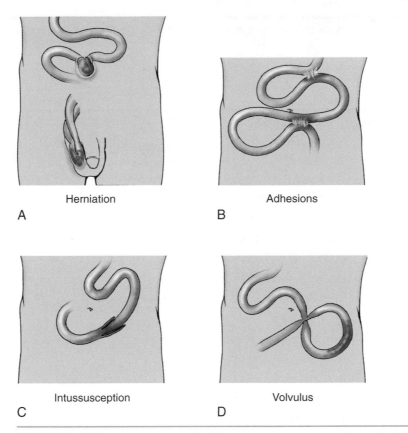

FIGURE 17-7. A, Herniation. **B,** Adhesions. **C,** Intussusception. **D,** Volvulus.

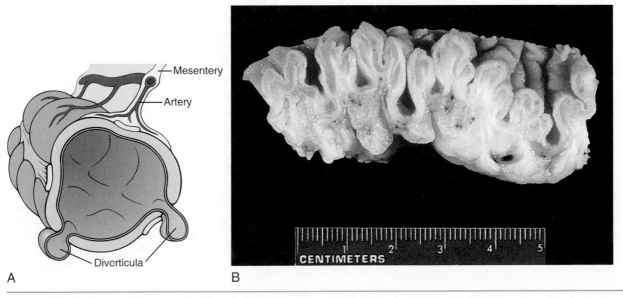

FIGURE 17-8. A, Diverticula. **B,** Diverticulosis.

EXAMPLE | Patient has diverticulosis of the duodenum with diverticulitis and hemorrhage, K57.13.

EXERCISE 17-4

Assign codes to the following conditions.

1. Patient with acute abdominal pain is taken to the Operating Room (OR) for appendectomy with suspected appendicitis. Pathology report reveals normal appendix _____
2. Incisional hernia _____
3. Gangrenous ventral hernia _____
4. Congenital diaphragmatic hernia _____
5. Obstructed unilateral femoral hernia _____
6. Meckel's diverticulitis _____
7. Hemorrhagic diverticulitis of the large intestine _____
8. Diverticulosis _____
9. Volvulus causing intestinal obstruction _____
10. Adhesions causing intestinal obstruction _____
11. Regional enteritis of the colon _____
12. Gastroenteritis due to *E. coli* _____
13. Allergic gastroenteritis due to milk allergy _____
14. Gastroenteritis due to radiation _____
15. Pseudopolyposis of the colon _____

Diseases of Peritoneum and Retroperitoneum (K65-K68)

Peritonitis is an inflammation of the peritoneum (membrane covering the organs of the abdominal cavity), usually an infection caused either by bacteria or fungus. The symptoms of peritonitis can include fever, abdominal pain or distention, and nausea and vomiting. The most common causes of peritonitis include peritoneal dialysis, cirrhosis of the liver, ascites, and peritonitis caused by conditions that allow bacteria to get into the peritoneum such as ruptured appendix, stomach ulcer, perforated colon, pancreatitis, and diverticulitis. Peritonitis can be life threatening and is generally treated with IV antibiotics and possibly surgery. In ICD-10-CM there is a note to use an additional code from B95-B97 to identify the organism responsible for the peritonitis.

EXAMPLE | Patient with known alcoholic cirrhosis of the liver is admitted with ascites and acute bacterial peritonitis due to staph aureus. Patient is a recovering alcoholic who has been in remission for 2 years, K65.0, K70.31, F10.21, B95.61.

Diseases of the Liver (K70-K77)

Cirrhosis of the Liver

Cirrhosis of the liver is degeneration of liver tissue that causes blockage of blood through the organ and inhibits the function of this organ. Cirrhosis may be caused by a variety of factors; alcoholism and hepatitis are the most common.

EXAMPLE   Alcoholic cirrhosis of liver. Patient is a recovering alcoholic and no longer drinking, K70.30, F10.21.

Hepatitis

Hepatitis, which is an inflammation of the liver, can last for a short time, or it may be chronic and last a lifetime. Most commonly, hepatitis is caused by a virus. When it is caused by a virus, hepatitis is coded from the infectious disease chapter of ICD-10-CM. However, other less common types of hepatitis are coded to the chapter on Digestive Diseases. Because the liver metabolizes both alcohol and drugs, a patient may develop alcoholic hepatitis or drug-induced hepatitis. When coding drug-induced hepatitis, it is important to also assign a code from T36-T65 to identify the responsible drug.

EXAMPLE   Patient has chronic hepatitis C, B18.2.

EXAMPLE   Patient has chronic hepatitis, K73.9.

Toxic hepatitis occurs when the liver is damaged by chemicals or drugs. Toxic hepatitis may come on very quickly or may take months of exposure to the drug or chemical. Likewise when the chemical or drug exposure stops the toxic hepatitis may clear, but sometimes permanent liver damage may have already occurred. Idiosyncratic toxins are those that cause damage in some people but not in others. Some common over the counter drugs can be toxic to the liver. These would include drugs such as Advil, Motrin, Aleve, and Tylenol. Some prescription drugs such as Isoniazid, methotrexate, and statins can potentially cause liver damage.

Disorders of the Gallbladder, Billiary Tract, and Pancreas (K80-K87)

Cholelithiasis and Cholecystitis

Cholelithiasis is an abnormal condition of stones in the gallbladder (gallstones). The condition is generally asymptomatic until gallstones block the cystic duct or the common bile duct, which does not allow the gallbladder to drain stored bile; the patient then develops acute cholecystitis (Figure 17-9). If the cystic duct is blocked, a patient generally has right upper quadrant crampy abdominal pain. This pain is often made worse by ingestion of fatty or greasy foods. When the common bile duct is blocked, a patient may develop cholangitis; when the stone is blocking the lower end of the common bile duct, secretion from the pancreas may be blocked, and pancreatitis may occur. **Choledocholithiasis** is the term used for a stone lodged in the bile duct. Endoscopic retrograde cholangiopancreatography (ERCP) may be used to detect the presence of gallstones.

In ICD-10-CM it is important to look for documentation of where the gallstones are located, i.e., in the gallbladder, the bile duct, or both; if cholecystitis is present and if it is acute or chronic; if the stone(s) are obstructing; and if there is cholangitis present.

EXAMPLE   Patient has acute cholecystitis with cholelithiasis and choledocholithiasis, K80.62.

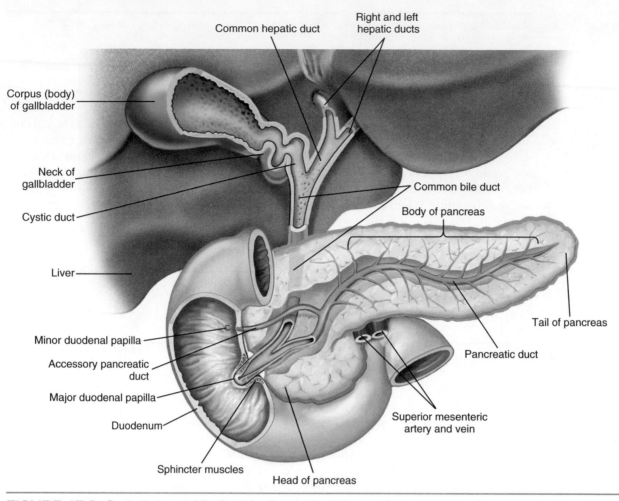

FIGURE 17-9. Ducts that carry bile from the liver and gallbladder. Obstruction of either the common hepatic duct or the common bile duct by a stone or spasm prevents bile from being ejected into the duodenum. (From Patton KT. *Anatomy and Physiology, 7th edition.* St. Louis: Mosby, 2010.)

Pancreatitis is an inflammation of the pancreas often caused by gallstones or chronic heavy alcohol use. Pancreatitis can be acute or chronic. Acute pancreatitis often presents with upper abdominal pain that extends through the back and is often severe. When a patient is experiencing acute pancreatitis, their bloodwork usually has elevated amylase and lipase, which are digestive enzymes found in the pancreas. Acute pancreatitis is treated with IV fluids, antibiotics, and pain meds. If the cause of the pancreatitis is not clear, an ERCP (endoscopic retrograde cholangiogram) may be peformed. During an ERCP a physician may perform one or more of the following procedures:

- Sphincterotomy—opens the pancreatic or bile duct
- Gallstone removal
- Stent placement—keeps the duct open
- Balloon dilation—opens or stretches the duct

Chronic pancreatitis is an inflammation that does not get better and most often gets worse and can lead to permanent damage. The most common cause of chronic pancreatitis is chronic heavy alcohol use. In chronic pancreatitis the pancreas may no longer be making the digestive enzymes and then other complications may occur such as malabsorption or diabetes.

EXERCISE 17-5

Assign codes to the following conditions.

1. Alcoholic hepatitis   _____

2. Type A viral hepatitis with coma   _____

3. Hepatitis due to cytomegalovirus   _____

4. Fatty liver   _____

5. Portal hypertension due to cirrhosis   _____

6. Patient admitted to hospital with chronic cholecystitis for a   _____
   laparoscopic cholecystectomy; during the surgery, the surgeon
   decides to convert to open

7. Patient is admitted with gallstone pancreatitis; this is treated   _____
   and the patient is sent home

FACTORS INFLUENCING HEALTH STATUS AND CONTACT WITH HEALTH SERVICES (Z CODES)

As was discussed in Chapter 8, it is difficult to locate Z codes in the Index. Coders will often say, "I did not know there was Z code for that." Refer to Chapter 8 for a listing of common main terms used to locate Z codes.

Z codes that may be used with digestive system conditions include the following:

Z01.20	Encounter for dental examination and cleaning without abnormal findings
Z01.21	Encounter for dental examination and cleaning with abnormal findings
Z13.810	Encounter for screening for upper gastrointestinal disorder
Z13.811	Encounter for screening for lower gastrointestinal disorder
Z13.818	Encounter for screening for other digestive system disorders
Z43.1	Encounter for attention to gastrostomy
Z43.2	Encounter for attention to ileostomy
Z43.3	Encounter for attention to colostomy
Z43.4	Encounter for attention to other artificial openings of digestive tract
Z46.2	Encounter for fitting and adjustment of dental prosthetic device
Z46.4	Encounter for fitting and adjustment of orthodontic device
Z46.51	Encounter for fitting and adjustment of gastric lap band
A46.59	Encounter for fitting and adjustment of other gastrointestinal appliance and device
Z52.6	Liver donor
Z83.71	Family history of colonic polyps
Z83.79	Family history of other diseases of the digestive system
Z87.11	Personal history of peptic ulcer disease
Z87.19	Personal history of other diseases of the digestive system
Z90.3	Acquired absence of stomach [part of]
Z90.4	Acquired absence of other parts of digestive tract
Z93.1	Gastrostomy status
Z93.2	Ileostomy status
Z93.3	Colostomy status
Z93.4	Other artificial openings of gastrointestinal tract status
Z94.4	Liver transplant status

Z94.82	Intestine transplant status
Z94.83	Pancreas transplant status
Z96.5	Presence of tooth-root and mandibular implants
Z97.2	Presence of dental prosthetic device (complete) (partial)
Z98.0	Intestinal bypass and anastomosis status
Z98.810	Dental sealant status
Z98.811	Dental restoration status
Z98.818	Other dental procedure status
Z98.84	Bariatric surgery status

EXAMPLE Patient is admitted to donate a liver. An open right liver lobectomy is performed, Z52.6, OFT10ZZ.

EXERCISE 17-6

Assign codes to the following conditions.

1. Patient is admitted for takedown of a colostomy   _____
2. Patient had gastric bypass 1 year ago   _____
3. Physician notes that the patient has a history of having the   _____
   pancreas replaced by a transplant
4. Patient has a remote history of PUD   _____

COMMON TREATMENTS

Many digestive disorders are treated with surgery.

CONDITION	MEDICATION
GERD	Propulsid, Reglan, Prilosec, Prevacid, Zantac, Tagamet
Crohn's disease	Azulfidine, Remicade, corticosteroids, Rowasa
Diverticulitis	Metronidazole, Ciprofloxacin
Gastric ulcer	Pepcid, Axid, Prilosec, Nexium
Gastroenteritis	Antiemetics such as Promethazine (Phenergan), prochlorperazine (Compazine), ondansetron (Zofran)
	Antidiarrheals, such as diphenoxylate atropine (Lomotil, Lofene, Lonox) or loperamide hydrochloride (Imodium)
	IV fluids
Pancreatitis	Antibiotics such as gentamicin, clindamycin

PROCEDURES

Procedures related to the digestive system in ICD-10-PCS may be found in the following tables:

Mouth and Throat	0C0-0CX
Gastrointestinal System	0D1-0DY
Hepatobiliary System and Pancreas	0F1-0FY

Procedures of the Stomach

Nissen **fundoplication** (Figure 17-10) is a surgical treatment for GERD. The root operation in ICD-10-PCS for a Nissen fundoplication is restriction (meaning partially closing an orifice or lumen) of the esophagogastric junction. This procedure takes the fundus (the upper

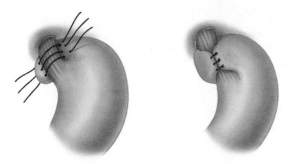

FIGURE 17-10. Nissen fundoplication.

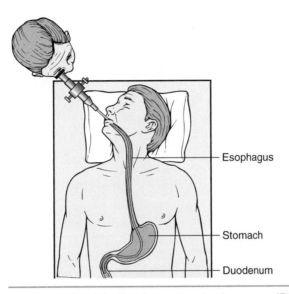

FIGURE 17-11. Esophagogastroduodenoscopy (EGD).

portion) of the stomach and wraps it around the lower portion of the esophagus to prevent the reflux of stomach contents back into the esophagus.

Percutaneous endoscopic gastrostomy (PEG) is the placement of a tube through the abdominal wall into the stomach with the use of a scope. The root operation for a PEG in ICD-10-PCS is insertion (putting in a nonbiological appliance that monitors, assists, performs, or prevents a physiological function but does not physically take the place of a body part) of a feeding device into the stomach. PEGs are used as feeding tubes for patients who are having difficulty eating (e.g., malnourished patients, patients who aspirate food). If a patient is admitted for insertion of a PEG tube because of carcinoma of the soft palate, and he or she now has dysphagia and dehydration, the principal diagnosis would be C05.1, carcinoma, and additional codes R13.10 for dysphagia and E86.0 for dehydration would be assigned.

If a patient presents to the hospital with a chief complaint of a PEG tube falling out, the principal diagnosis would be Z43.1, or attention to gastrostomy, because no complications resulted from the gastrostomy itself.

Procedures of the Intestine

Esophagogastroduodenoscopy (EGD) (Figure 17-11) is a diagnostic procedure that is used to identify disease conditions in the esophagus, stomach, and duodenum. The root

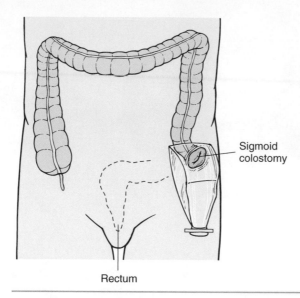

Sigmoid colostomy

Rectum

FIGURE 17-12. Colostomy. The opening of the colon is brought to the surface of the skin to divert feces into an external pouch worn by the patient.

operation for an EGD in ICD-10-PCS is inspection (visual or manual exploration of a body part). Many times additional procedures are performed, such as biopsy, lesion removal, ablation, hemorrhage control, and dilations.

EXAMPLE Patient with bleeding gastric ulcer taken to OR for EGD to control bleed; bleeding in the stomach controlled by electrocautery, K25.4, 0D568ZZ.

Colostomy (Figure 17-12) is a procedure that uses the colon to create an artificial opening (**stoma**) to the exterior of the abdomen. The root operation for a colostomy in ICD-10-PCS is bypass (altering route of passage of the contents of a tubular body part). This artificial opening serves as a substitute anus through which the intestines excrete waste until the colon heals or other corrective surgery is performed. The location of the stoma depends on which part of the colon is involved in the surgery. Most colostomies are temporary. A sigmoid colostomy is the most commonly performed type.

When a patient is admitted for a colostomy closure (takedown), the principal diagnosis should be Z43.3. Most often, when closing a colostomy, the surgeon must perform minor trimming of the colon to complete the anastomosis, but sometimes, it is necessary to actually excise portions of the colon; in that case, it would be appropriate to code the intestinal resection as an additional code.

An **ileostomy** is very similar to a colostomy, except that the end of the small intestine is brought out through the abdominal wall.

Bowel resection can be performed for many reasons (i.e., neoplasms, severe diverticulitis, bowel perforation, and bowel obstruction). Surgeons remove a portion of the bowel and then connect the bowel back together (anastomosis). In bowel resection in which an end-to-end anastomosis is performed, an additional code for the anastomosis is not assigned. This includes small intestine anastomosed to large intestine. Figure 17-13 illustrates various types of anastomoses.

EXAMPLE Patient with malignant neoplasm of the descending colon is admitted for an open left hemicolectomy, and temporary colostomy, C18.6, 0DTG0ZZ, 0DIM0Z4.

ANASTOMOSES

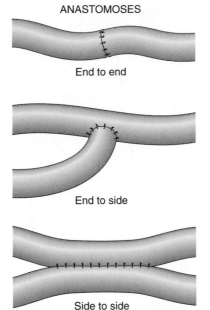

End to end

End to side

Side to side

FIGURE 17-13. Types of anastomoses.

Appendectomy is removal of the appendix. The root operation for an appendectomy in ICD-10-PCS is resection (cutting out or off without replacement all of a body part). Codes assigned will be different depending on the approach, i.e., open or laparoscopic. Often, when a surgeon is performing an abdominal operation, an incidental appendectomy may be performed. An **incidental appendectomy** is one that is performed at the time of another procedure with no known disease process in the appendix.

EXAMPLE   Patient with acute appendicitis is admitted for a laparoscopic appendectomy, K35.80, 0DTJ4ZZ.

Procedures of the Gallbladder and Biliary System

Cholecystectomy, or removal of the gallbladder, can be performed by incision or by laparoscope (Figure 17-14). The root operation for a cholecystectomy in ICD-10-PCS is resection (cutting out or off without replacement, all of a body part). Cholecystotomy may also be performed to remove stones from the gallbladder. This can be performed by open incision as well as by scope.

EXAMPLE   Patient with acute cholecystitis with cholelithiasis has a laparoscopic cholecystectomy, K80.00, 0FT44ZZ.

Common bile duct stones can be removed in three different ways (i.e., by incision, endoscopy, or percutaneously). Occasionally a cholecystectomy is performed along with removal of common duct stones. Codes should be assigned for both the cholecystectomy and the common bile duct stone removal. Fragmentation of stones of the gallbladder by extracorporeal shock wave lithotripsy, or ESWL, is the breaking apart of stones by shock waves.

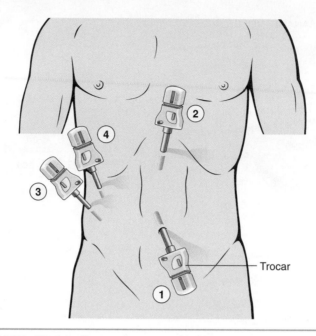

FIGURE 17-14. Trocar placement for laparoscopic cholecystectomy.

EXAMPLE | Patient with common bile duct stones presents for stone removal by ERCP, K80.50, 0FC98ZZ.

An endoscopic retrograde cholangiopancreatography (ERCP) is often done for diagnosis, but it may be done for stent insertion, or may be done in combination with a sphincterotomy or for removal of stones. In all of these cases, both the ERCP and the additional codes are assigned. The root operation in ICD-10-PCS for a diagnostic ERCP is fluoroscopy of biliary and pancreatic ducts. If the ERCP is done for stent insertion, the root operation is dilation (expanding an orifice or lumen of a tubular body part). If the ERCP is done for stone removal, the root operation is extirpation (taking or cutting out solid matter from a body part).

EXAMPLE | Patient with abdominal pain that is suspected to be due to a pancreatic malignancy presents for a diagnostic ERCP with low osmolar contrast. The ERCP reveals no malignancy, R10.9, BF111ZZ.

Lysis of Adhesions

Lysis of adhesions is a procedure that is performed to destroy adhesions. The root operation in ICD-10-PCS for lysis of adhesions is release (freeing a body part from an abnormal physical constraint). **Adhesions,** which are very often found in the peritoneal area, are fibrous bands of tissue that adhere abdominal organs to one another or to the abdominal wall. Adhesions are often synonymous with scar tissue and can develop after surgery, often causing abdominal pain. Significant adhesions and the lysis thereof are to be assigned codes only if the significance is documented by the surgeon. The surgeon may document extensive adhesions, extensive lysis, or lysis requiring significant time. If there is any question as to the significance of the adhesions, the surgeon should be queried.

EXAMPLE | Patient with chronic cholecystitis admitted for laparoscopic cholecystectomy. The surgeon performed manual lysis of adhesions of the gallbladder, prior to laparoscopic cholecystectomy, K81.1, 0FT44ZZ. No code for lysis of adhesions required.

EXAMPLE   Patient with abdominal pain is admitted. The surgeon performed laparoscopic lysis of adhesions of the peritoneum, K66.0, 0DNW4ZZ.

Hernia Repair

Herniorrhaphy is repair of a hernia. The root operation in ICD-10-PCS for hernia repair is repair (restoring a body part to its normal structure and function). When the hernia is repaired with mesh, the root operation becomes supplement (putting in or on biological or synthetic material that physically reinforces and/or augments the function of a portion of a body part.) Coding hernia repairs requires attention to location, laterality, and whether performed with a prosthesis or a graft.

EXAMPLE   Patient had a bilateral inguinal hernia repair direct and indirect with prosthesis, K40.20, 0YUA0JZ.

Whipple Procedure

Whipple procedure is also known as a pancreaticoduodenectomy. This procedure generally involves removal of the gallbladder, common bile duct, part of the duodenum, and the head of the pancreas. The root operation in ICD-10-PCS for a Whipple procedure includes both resection and bypass. This procedure may be performed for chronic pancreatitis, pancreatic pseudocysts, or pancreatic malignancies.

EXAMPLE   Patient with pancreatic cancer in the head of the pancreas presents for Whipple procedure. The head of the pancreas, a portion of the bile duct, the gallbladder, and part of the duodenum were removed during this procedure, C25.0, 0FT40ZZ, 0FBG0ZZ, 0FB90ZZ, 0D160ZA, 0DB90ZZ, 0F190Z3, 0F1G0ZC.

Transjugular Intrahepatic Portosystemic Shunt (TIPS)

TIPS (transjugular intrahepatic portosystemic shunt): This procedure is often performed by interventional radiologists for patients with severe complications of liver disease. The root operation in ICD-10-PCS for a TIPS procedure is bypass (altering the route of passage of a tubular body part). The interventionalist percutaneously makes a tunnel through the liver with a needle and connects the portal vein to one of the hepatic veins. A stent is inserted into this tunnel to keep the tract open. This procedure does not improve the functioning of the liver but helps in treatment of the complications.

EXAMPLE   A patient with portal hypertension is admitted for a TIPS procedure, K76.6, 06183DY.

EXERCISE 17-7

Assign codes to the following conditions.

1. Insertion of percutaneous endoscopic gastrostomy for dysphagia _____

2. Incidental appendectomy during cholecystectomy for gallstones in the gallbladder _____

3. Open repair of ventral hernia _____

4. ERCP with endoscopic pancreatic sphincterotomy and stone removal from pancreatic duct, fluoroscopy performed with low osmolar contrast _____

5. Patient with GERD admitted for Nissen fundoplication _____

DOCUMENTATION/REIMBURSEMENT/MS-DRGs

Often, coding difficulties are due to lack of documentation. Sometimes pathology and other test results are not available at the time of discharge or when the physician is dictating the discharge summary or is reporting the final diagnoses.

Frequently missed complications/comorbidities from this chapter include the following:

- Cholangitis
- Hematemesis
- GI hemorrhage
- Ileus
- Melena
- Pancreatitis
- Peritonitis

Types of Appendicitis

It is important to check pathology reports when appendectomies are performed and to review the record for documentation of appendiceal rupture, abscess, or generalized peritonitis. Different MS-DRGs are assigned for appendicitis with a complicated principal diagnosis.

EXAMPLE

DIAGNOSES/PROCEDURES	CODES	MS-DRG	RW
Acute appendicitis with	K35.9	343	0.9587
Appendectomy, laparoscopic	0DTJ8ZZ		
Ruptured appendicitis with	K35.0	340	1.2308
Appendectomy, laparoscopic	0DTJ8ZZ		

Two or More Interrelated Conditions, Each Potentially Meeting the Definition of Principal Diagnosis

EXAMPLE

DIAGNOSES	CODES	MS-DRG	RW
Dehydration	E86.0	641	0.6988
Gastroenteritis	K52.9		
Gastroenteritis	K52.9	392	0.7241
Dehydration	E86.0		

If the patient had dehydration caused by gastroenteritis and was admitted for IV fluids, then the principal diagnosis would be the dehydration. However, if the patient had gastroenteritis and dehydration and the patient was admitted for treatment of both of these diagnoses, then either diagnosis could be sequenced as the principal.

Lysis of Adhesions

It is always important to review the operative report for lysis of adhesions. Coding the lysis of the adhesions may be required if they are significant and require considerable time. If in doubt the surgeon should be queried.

EXAMPLE

DIAGNOSES/PROCEDURES	CODES	MS-DRG	RW
Acute appendicitis	K35.9	343	0.9587
Adhesions	K66.0		
Appendectomy	0DTJ8ZZ		
Acute appendicitis	K35.9	337	1.4956
Adhesions	K66.0		
Appendectomy	0DTJ8ZZ		
Lysis of adhesions	0DNW4ZZ		

When minor adhesions exist and are easily lysed as part of the principal procedure, coding a diagnosis of adhesions and the procedure would be inappropriate.

Blood Loss Anemia With GI Bleeds

In cases of GI bleed, it would be prudent to check laboratory values with regard to falling hematocrit or hemoglobin, as well as orders for transfusions. Many GI bleeds have as a common comorbidity acute or chronic blood loss anemia. This is often not well documented by physicians, and a query may be required.

EXAMPLE

DIAGNOSES	CODES	MS-DRG	RW
GI bleed	K92.2	379	0.7067
GI bleed with acute blood loss anemia	K92.2	378	1.0238
	D62		

Types of Cholecystectomies and Additional Procedures Performed

Cholecystectomies have a separate set of MS-DRGs for those done with common bile duct exploration. Common bile duct exploration is a procedure that allows the clinician to see whether a stone is blocking the flow of bile from the liver and gallbladder to the intestine. Close attention must be paid to the method by which the cholecystectomy is performed as there is a separate MS-DRG for cholecystectomies performed by laparoscopy.

EXAMPLE

DIAGNOSES/PROCEDURES	CODES	MS-DRG	RW
Calculus of bile duct with acute cholecystitis and cholecystectomy	K80.62 0FT40ZZ	416	1.3588

EXAMPLE

DIAGNOSES/PROCEDURES	CODES	MS-DRG	RW
Calculus of bile duct with acute cholecystitis and cholecystectomy with exploration of the common bile duct	K80.62 0FT40ZZ 0FJ90ZZ	413	1.7409

EXAMPLE

DIAGNOSES/PROCEDURES	CODES	MS-DRG	RW
Calculus of bile duct with acute cholecystitis and laparoscopic cholecystectomy	K80.62 0FB44ZZ	419	1.1814

CHAPTER REVIEW EXERCISE

Where applicable, assign codes for diagnoses, procedures, Z codes, and external cause codes.

1. What makes up the alimentary canal?

   _____

2. What are the three areas of the small intestines?

   1. _____

   2. _____

   3. _____

3. What three organs assist the digestive process?

   1. _____

   2. _____

   3. _____

4. A patient is admitted to the hospital with severe indigestion. An EGD is performed, and it is discovered that the patient has acute gastritis due to *H. pylori.*   _____

5. A patient presents to the Emergency Room (ER) with hematochezia. The patient is admitted, and it is determined that acute blood loss anemia is caused by diverticulosis.   _____

6. A patient has a bleeding gastric ulcer caused by *Helicobacter pylori.*   _____

7. A patient is admitted to the hospital with what the surgeon believes to be acute appendicitis. The surgeon takes the patient to the Operating Room (OR) and removes the appendix; the pathology report reveals a ruptured appendix.   _____

8. A patient is admitted to the hospital with an incisional hernia. The patient is taken to the OR, and open herniorrhaphy is performed with a graft.   _____

9. A patient is admitted to the hospital with a bilateral indirect inguinal hernia that is repaired with a graft.   _____

10. A patient with diverticulitis and diverticulosis is taken to the OR for an endoscopic diverticulectomy of the large intestine.   _____

11. A patient with cholecystitis presents to the ER. ERCP reveals cholelithiasis. The surgeon performs a laparoscopic partial cholecystectomy.   _____

12. A patient with severe Crohn's disease is taken to the OR for a Hartmann procedure on the left with an end-to-end anastomosis and a temporary colostomy.   _____

13. A patient with cholelithaisis has an ESWL.   _____

14. A patient with severe chronic pancreatitis is admitted to the hospital, where a surgeon performs a Whipple procedure.   _____

15. A patient with ascites due to alcoholic cirrhosis is admitted to the hospital for a TIPS procedure. Procedure was performed via a laproscopic approach.   _____

16. A patient with a bleeding duodenal ulcer is admitted to the hospital, where the gastroenterologist provides endoscopic control of the hemorrhage by ablation.   _____

17. A patient with severe malnutrition is admitted to the hospital for endoscopic placement of a gastrostomy tube.   _____

18. Acute hemorrhagic gastric ulcer caused by NSAID   _____

19. Gallstone of common bile duct, status post cholecystectomy, 1   _____
    year PTA

20. GI bleed due to acute vascular insufficiency   _____

CHAPTER GLOSSARY

Adhesion: scar tissue that forms an abnormal connection between body parts.

Alimentary canal: comprises the mouth, pharynx, esophagus, stomach, small intestine, and large intestine.

Angiodysplasia: type of AVM characterized by dilated or fragile blood vessels.

Anorexia: loss of appetite.

Appendectomy: removal of the appendix.

Appendicitis: inflammation of the appendix.

Arteriovenous malformation: defect that arises during fetal development.

Barrett's esophagus: precancerous condition that usually occurs in people with chronic GERD.

Bowel resection: removal of a portion of the bowel.

Choledocholithiasis: stone lodged in the bile duct.

Cholelithiasis: an abnormal condition of stones in the gallbladder.

Cirrhosis: liver disease wherein scar tissue replaces healthy tissue and blocks blood flow.

Colostomy: a procedure that uses the colon to create an artificial opening.

Crohn's disease: inflammation of the GI tract, especially the small and large intestine.

Diverticula: small pouches in the lining of the mucous membranes of an organ.

Edentulism: the complete loss of teeth.

Fundoplication: surgery in which the fundus of the stomach is wrapped around the esophagus.

Gastroenteritis: inflammation of the stomach and intestines.

Hematemesis: vomiting of blood.

Hematochezia: bright red blood in stool.

Hepatitis: an inflammation of the liver.

Hernia: protrusion of an organ or tissue through an abnormal opening in the body.

Herniorrhaphy: repair of a hernia.

Ileostomy: end of small intestine brought out through the abdominal wall.

Ileus: absence of normal movement within the intestine.

Impaction: condition that occurs when stool in the rectum becomes so hard that it cannot be passed normally.

Incidental appendectomy: appendectomy performed at the time of another procedure with no known disease process in the appendix.

Intussusception: bowel becomes obstructed when a portion of the intestine telescopes into another portion.

Lysis: destruction of adhesions.

Mallory-Weiss: bleeding laceration of the esophagogastric junction.

Mastication: chewing of food.

McBurney's point: area of the abdomen that, when touched, causes pain that may be indicative of appendicitis.

Melena: dark blood in stool.

Mucositis: an inflammation/ulceration of the digestive tract commonly occurring in the oral cavity.

Necrotic: dead tissue that lacks a blood supply.

Occult blood: blood only found by laboratory inspection.

Pancreatitis: inflammation of the pancreas often caused by gallstones or chronic heavy alcohol use.

Percutaneous endoscopic gastrostomy: a tube put through the abdominal wall into the stomach with the use of a scope.

Peristalsis: rhythmic muscle contractions that move food down the digestive tract.

Peritonitis: inflammation of the peritoneum usually caused by bacteria or fungus.

Sialolithiasis: stones in the salivary glands.

Stoma: an artificial opening.

TIPS (transjugular intrahepatic portosystemic shunt): a procedure in which the portal vein is connected to one of the hepatic veins and a stent is inserted.

Toxic hepatitis: when the liver is damaged by chemicals or drugs.

Ulcerative colitis: an inflammatory bowel disease.

Volvulus: an abnormal twisting of the intestine that may impair blood flow to the intestine.

Whipple procedure: a procedure that generally involves removal of the gallbladder, common bile duct, part of the duodenum, and the head of the pancreas.

18

Diseases of the Skin and Subcutaneous Tissue

(ICD-10-CM Chapter 12, Codes L00-L99)

LEARNING OBJECTIVES

1. Apply and assign the correct ICD-10-CM/PCS codes in accordance with Official Guidelines for Coding and Reporting

2. Identify major differences between ICD-10-CM and ICD-9-CM related to the skin and subcutaneous tissue

3. Identify pertinent anatomy and physiology of the skin and subcutaneous tissue

4. Identify diseases of the skin and subcutaneous tissue

5. Assign the correct Z codes and procedure codes related to the skin and subcutaneous tissue

6. Identify common treatments, medications, laboratory values, and diagnostic tests

7. Explain the importance of documentation in relation to MS-DRGs for reimbursement

ABBREVIATIONS/ ACRONYMS

CEA cultured epidermal autograft
FTSG full-thickness skin graft
ICD-9-CM *International Classification of Diseases, 9th Revision, Clinical Modification*
ICD-10-CM *International Classification of Diseases, 10th Revision, Clinical Modification*

ICD-10-PCS *International Classification of Diseases, 10th Revision, Procedure Coding System*
I&D incision and drainage
MS-DRG Medicare Severity diagnosis-related group
SJS Stevens-Johnson Syndrome

STSG split-thickness skin graft
TEN toxic epidermal neurolysis

ICD-10-CM
Official Guidelines for Coding and Reporting

Please refer to the companion Evolve website for the most current guidelines.

12. Chapter 12: Diseases of Skin and Subcutaneous Tissue (L00-L99)

a. Pressure ulcer stage codes

1) Pressure ulcer stages

Codes from category L89, Pressure ulcer, are combination codes that identify the site of the pressure ulcer as well as the stage of the ulcer.

The ICD-10-CM classifies pressure ulcer stages based on severity, which is designated by stages 1-4, unspecified stage and unstageable.

Assign as many codes from category L89 as needed to identify all the pressure ulcers the patient has, if applicable.

EXAMPLE

The patient was admitted to the hospital from the nursing home. Upon examination the physician noted a stage II pressure ulcer on the sacrum, L89.152.

2) Unstageable pressure ulcers

Assignment of the code for unstageable pressure ulcer (L89.–0) should be based on the clinical documentation. These codes are used for pressure ulcers whose stage cannot be clinically determined (e.g., the ulcer is covered by eschar or has been treated with a skin or muscle graft) and pressure ulcers that are documented as deep tissue injury but not documented as due to trauma. This code should not be confused with the codes for unspecified stage (L89.–9). When there is no documentation regarding the stage of the pressure ulcer, assign the appropriate code for unspecified stage (L89.–9).

EXAMPLE

Patient is seen in the physician's office for pneumonia. It is noted in the physical exam that the patient was recently treated for a pressure ulcer of the heel by skin graft. The graft looks to be progressing as planned, J18.9, L89.609.

3) Documented pressure ulcer stage

Assignment of the pressure ulcer stage code should be guided by clinical documentation of the stage or documentation of the terms found in the Alphabetic Index. For clinical terms describing the stage that are not found in the Alphabetic Index, and there is no documentation of the stage, the provider should be queried.

EXAMPLE

Patient has stage IV pressure ulcers on both heels, L89.624, L89.614.

EXAMPLE

In a daily inpatient progress note, the physician documents that the patient has a pressure ulcer of the right heel with partial thickness skin loss, L89.612.

4) Patients admitted with pressure ulcers documented as healed
No code is assigned if the documentation states that the pressure ulcer is completely healed.

5) Patients admitted with pressure ulcers documented as healing
Pressure ulcers described as healing should be assigned the appropriate pressure ulcer stage code based on the documentation in the medical record. If the documentation does not provide information about the stage of the healing pressure ulcer, assign the appropriate code for unspecified stage.

    If the documentation is unclear as to whether the patient has a current (new) pressure ulcer or if the patient is being treated for a healing pressure ulcer, query the provider.

EXAMPLE

On the discharge summary, the provider documents the following discharge diagnoses: Exacerbation of COPD, hypertension, hyperlipidemia, and a healed sacral decubitus, J44.1, I10, E78.5.

EXAMPLE

On the discharge summary, the provider documents the following discharge diagnoses: Exacerbation of COPD, hypertension, hyperlipidemia, and a healing sacral decubitus, J44.1, I10, E78.5, L89.159.

6) Patient admitted with pressure ulcer evolving into another stage during the admission
If a patient is admitted with a pressure ulcer at one stage and it progresses to a higher stage, assign the code for the highest stage reported for that site.

EXAMPLE

Patient is admitted to the hospital from the nursing home for aspiration pneumonia. The admitting provider documents that the patient has a stage II sacral ulcer. At the time of transfer back to the nursing home the provider documents the ulcer as stage III, J69.0, L89.153.

Apply the General Coding Guidelines as found in Chapter 5 and the Procedural Coding Guidelines as found in Chapters 6 and 7.

MAJOR DIFFERENCES BETWEEN ICD-10-CM AND ICD-9-CM

- In ICD-9-CM, the coding of decubitus ulcers required two codes, whereas ICD-10-CM uses a combination code.
- ICD-10-CM introduces a new term, "androgenic alopecia."
- In ICD-10-CM, the terms "dermatitis" and "eczema" are used interchangeably.
- Instructions in ICD-10-CM for allergic contact dermatitis state to code first the responsible drug or substance with codes T36-T65.
- Intraoperative and procedural complications of the skin and subcutaneous tissue include:
  - Intraoperative hemorrhage of skin
  - Accidental puncture or laceration of the skin
  - Postprocedural hemorrhage or hematoma of the skin

ANATOMY AND PHYSIOLOGY

The skin and its accessory organs constitute the **integumentary** system (Figure 18-1), whose functions include protection, temperature regulation, sensory reception, and vitamin D synthesis.

The skin is composed of 3 layers: epidermis, dermis, and subcutaneous layers. The outer layer of the skin, or the **epidermis**, serves as a protective barrier and prevents the entrance of disease-causing organisms. The **dermis**, or middle layer, is composed of fibrous connective tissues that make it strong and elastic. This middle layer contains blood vessels, nerve fibers, sebaceous glands, and some hair follicles. The **subcutaneous** layer contains fat, sweat glands, and additional hair follicles.

The integumentary system also has accessory organs; these include hair, glands, and nails. Three types of glands are located in the skin: sweat glands, sebaceous glands, and mammary glands. The sweat glands assist in temperature regulation, and the sebaceous glands secrete an oily substance, **sebum**, which lubricates the hair and skin.

DISEASE CONDITIONS

Diseases of the Skin and Subcutaneous Tissue (L00-L99), Chapter 12 in the ICD-10-CM code book, are divided into the following categories:

CATEGORY	SECTION TITLES
L00-L08	Infections of the skin and subcutaneous tissue
L10-L14	Bullous disorders
L20-L30	Dermatitis and eczema
L40-L45	Papulosquamous disorders
L50-L54	Urticaria and erythema
L55-L59	Radiation-related disorders of the skin and subcutaneous tissue
L60-L75	Disorders of skin appendages
L76	Intraoperative and postprocedural complications of skin and subcutaneous tissue
L80-L99	Other disorders of the skin and subcutaneous tissue

Infections of the Skin and Subcutaneous Tissue (L00-L08)

It is important to note that this section has an Instructional note that advises the user to assign an additional code (B95-B97) to identify the infectious agent if known.

Carbuncle and Furuncle

Another name for a **furuncle** is a boil, and a cluster of boils is known as a **carbuncle** (Figure 18-2). The organism that is responsible for a boil is *Staphylococcus*. This organism enters the body through a hair follicle. An additional code is required to identify the organism responsible.

Cellulitis/Abscess of the Skin

Cellulitis is an acute inflammation of tissue that is characterized by swelling, redness, and tenderness that are most often caused by a bacterial infection. An **abscess** is a localized collection of pus that causes swelling. Cellulitis is generally treated with antibiotics; an abscess may be treated with antibiotics and also may require incision and drainage.

As is noted in these code categories, acute lymphangitis is included and is **NOT** coded separately in a patient with cellulitis or abscess. An additional code is used to identify the organism causing the cellulitis, when documented. In ICD-10-CM, if a patient has an abscess and cellulitis, two codes are required.

Cellulitis associated with a superficial injury, burn, or frostbite requires the use of two codes: one code for the injury/burn/frostbite and one code for the cellulitis. The sequence of these codes is dependent on the focus of treatment. For superficial injuries with cellulitis, it is likely that treatment will be focused on the cellulitis.

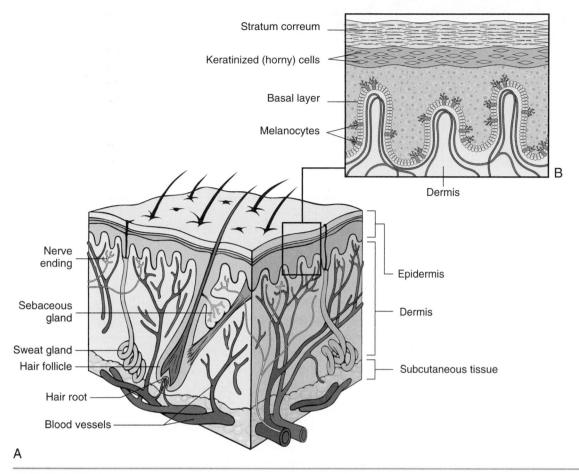

Stratum correum

Keratinized (horny) cells

Basal layer

Melanocytes

Dermis

B

Nerve ending

Sebaceous gland

Sweat gland

Hair follicle

Hair root

Blood vessels

Epidermis

Dermis

Subcutaneous tissue

A

FIGURE 18-1. The skin. **A,** Three layers of the skin. **B,** Epidermis.

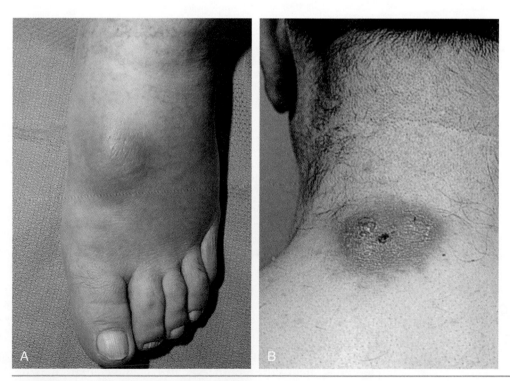

A

B

FIGURE 18-2. A, Furuncle. **B,** Carbuncle.

EXAMPLE | Patient with cat scratch of the right hand with localized cellulitis admitted for treatment of cellulitis, L03.113, S60.511A, W55.03xA.

Cellulitis associated with a traumatic open wound requires the use of two codes: one code for the open wound, complicated, and one code for the cellulitis. The sequence of these codes is dependent on the focus of treatment. If the focus of treatment is the open wound, the code for the wound is sequenced first, followed by the code for cellulitis. If, on the other hand, the focus of the treatment is the cellulitis and the wound is trivial, or if the wound was treated on a separate occasion, the cellulitis would be sequenced first.

EXAMPLE | Patient stepped on a piece of glass and injured his foot 2 days ago. He is now being admitted to the hospital for treatment of cellulitis in the left leg, L03.116, S91.312A, W25.xxxA.

Gangrenous cellulitis is assigned only the code for gangrene—NOT a code for cellulitis. Cellulitis associated with a skin ulcer requires the use of two codes: one for the ulcer and one for the cellulitis. The sequence of codes is dependent on the focus of treatment.

EXAMPLE | Patient has a chronic right leg ulcer with cellulitis. She is admitted to the hospital for treatment of the leg ulcer, L97.919, L03.115.

Cellulitis occurring in areas other than the skin is coded to the chapter that is most appropriate. The coder will find direction in the Alphabetic Index.

EXAMPLE | Patient has cellulitis of the lip, K13.0.

EXERCISE 18-1

Assign codes to the following conditions.

1. Cellulitis of the face
2. Cellulitis with lymphangitis of the breast. *Staphylococcus aureus* infection
3. Cellulitis of the left foot due to patient stepping on a nail with open puncture wound of the foot
4. Gangrenous cellulitis of toe
5. Neck abscess
6. Cellulitis, rectum

Bullous Disorders (L10-L14)

Pemphigus

Pemphigus is a rare autoimmune disorder that causes blistering of the skin and mucous membranes, such as the mouth, eyes, throat, and genitals. In people with this disorder, their immune systems attack cells of the epidermis or mucous membranes. This attack causes blisters to form that do not heal and can cover large areas of skin. This disorder is not contagious and may have a genetic predisposition. This disease often affects people of Mediterranean descent, and there is a particular form that is found in the rainforests of Brazil. Although this disorder can occur at any age, the most common onset is in middle age or older. There is a similar but different disorder that causes blistering in areas below the dermis named pemphigoid.

There are several different types of pemphigus:
- Pemphigus vulgaris—most common in the United States with sores usually starting in the mouth. The blisters form within the deep layer of the epidermis and are very painful
- Pemphigus vegetans—sores are usually found in the groin and under the arms
- Pemphigus foliaceus—sores on the face and scalp. This type of pemphigus is not found in the mouth
- Paraneoplastic pemphigus—this disorder is found in people with certain types of cancer

This disorder is treated by using steroids or a combination of steroids, anti-inflammatory medications, and at times immunosuppressive drugs. It is possible after a number of years of treatment that these patients can go into complete remissions.

Dermatitis and Eczema (L20-L30)

Dermatitis is an inflammation of the skin that is used to describe a variety of skin conditions that can be caused by infections, allergies, and substances either in contact with the skin or ingested. If the dermatitis is caused by contact with a substance, it is **exogenous** and if it is caused by ingestion of a substance, it is **endogenous.** The terms dermatitis and eczema are synonymous and can be used interchangeably. Stasis dermatitis is not included in this chapter and can be found in the chapter on diseases of the circulatory system.

The types of skin symptoms that may be caused by dermatitis include itchiness, reddening, crusting, scaling, and blisters, to name a few. In ICD-10-CM it should be noted that at categories L23.3 (Allergic contact dermatitis), L24-.4 (Irritant contact dermatitis), L25.1 (Unspecified contact dermatitis), and L27 (Dermatitis due to substances taken internally), there is an Instructional note to code first T36-T65 to identify the drug, if this is an adverse effect. An adverse effect can occur as the result of taking a medication as prescribed.

EXAMPLE Patient presents to physician's office with a red, crusty rash on her legs and arms. It is determined that she has irritant contact dermatitis due to using laundry detergent, L24.0.

Intertriginous dermatitis, a type of rash that is found in body folds, is a common condition in the overweight patient, possibly because of skin chafing and the inability of sweat to evaporate. This condition is not found under the Dermatitis heading in the Index but may be located under **Intertrigo.**

Papulosquamous Disorders (L40-L45)

Psoriasis is an inflammation of the skin caused by a fault in the immune system. There are several types of psoriasis, the most common of which is plaque psoriasis. The skin on the elbows, knees, lower back, and scalp are the most common areas plaques are found. Psoriasis usually itches, and the skin may crack and bleed. This is a life-long condition for which there is no cure. Some people develop psoriatic arthritis, which is a systemic rheumatic disease.

EXAMPLE | Patient is admitted for total hip replacement due to psoriatic arthropathy of the left hip, L40.50, 0SRB0JZ.

Urticaria and Erythema (L49-L54)

"**Hives**" and "**urticaria**" are synonymous terms that refer to vascular reactions of the skin that present as wheals, welts, or reddened patches (Figure 18-3) and are associated with **pruritus** (itching). Hives usually occur as an allergic reaction to food, bug bites, or drugs.

Stevens-Johnson Syndrome (SJS) is a rare condition where the skin and mucous membranes react to medication or infection. It is characterized by rash and blisters, which can cause skin necrosis. The cause of this syndrome may be unknown, but a patient may be predisposed to this condition if they have diseases such as HIV or SLE that decrease their immunity. There is a gene called HLA-B12 that may make a patient more susceptible. This can be a life-threatening condition.

EXAMPLE | Patient is treated for hives due to peanuts, L50.0.

EXAMPLE | Patient presented with hives. No cause can be determined, L50.9.

EXAMPLE | Patient is admitted to the hospital with probable SJS-TEN, Stevens-Johnson syndrome, toxic epidermal necrolysis. The patient has a fever, chills, blistering of the mouth and eyes, and large areas on the trunk of the body where skin is peeling off. The patient was recently placed on allopurinol for gout. The attending physician places the patient in the burn unit and documents that 30% of the body is affected by TENS, and the likely cause of this is the allopurinol, L51.3, T50.4x5A, L49.3.

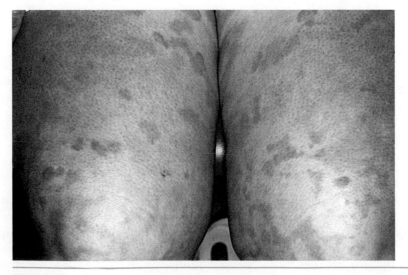

FIGURE 18-3. Urticaria.

EXERCISE 18-2

Assign codes to the following conditions.

1. Contact dermatitis due to mascara _____
2. Contact dermatitis due to tanning bed _____
3. Hives due to penicillin _____
4. Irritant contact dermatitis due to detergent _____
5. Dermatitis, intertriginous _____
6. Fogo selvagem _____
7. Diaper rash _____
8. Patient has dermatitis on the right hand secondary to latex gloves _____
9. Contact urticaria _____

Radiation-Related Disorders of the Skin and Subcutaneous Tissue (L55-L59)

Solar keratosis is also known as actinic keratosis and is a precancerous scaly or crusty growth often found on the areas of the body regularly exposed to sun. These lesions may be treated with medication or cryosurgery. This is a common condition in the United States.

EXAMPLE   A 32-year-old woman presents to dermatologist's office with solar keratosis. The physician documents that this patient has regularly been using tanning beds for the past 10 years, L57.0, W89.1xxA.

Disorders of Skin Appendages (L60-L75)

Alopecia is hair loss. There are many forms of hair loss, but the most common one is androgenic alopecia or male pattern baldness.

EXAMPLE   Physician documents in the record that the patient has male pattern baldness, L64.9.

Rosacea is a skin condition affecting the cheeks, nose, chin, and forehead. It can be characterized by redness, a bulbous nose, or an increased number of blood vessels in the face. Although it is not curable, it can be controlled by avoiding triggers such as alcohol, sun, spicy food, and wind, to name a few.

EXAMPLE   Physician documents that the patient has rhinophyma, L71.1.

Hyperhidrosis is a condition characterized by excessive sweating. It can be secondary to a variety of disorders such as cancer, anxiety, medication, substance abuse, menopause, and Parkinson's disease. It can be treated with drugs, and in severe cases a procedure called an endoscopic thoracic sympathectomy may be performed.

EXAMPLE   Patient with underarm localized primary hyperhidrosis, L74.510.

Other Disorders of Skin and Subcutaneous Tissue (L80-L99)

Skin **ulcers** are open sores of the skin (Figure 18-4). Ulcers may have a variety of causes such as diabetes, skin cancers, venous insufficiency, arteriosclerosis, and pressure sores (**decubitus ulcer**). When coding ulcers, care should be taken to closely follow instructions found under categories L89 and L97.

Pressure Ulcer

A pressure ulcer is more commonly known as a bed sore or decubitus ulcer (Figure 18-5). These ulcers occur over bony areas (e.g., heel, hip, sacrum, ankle, and elbow) of patients who are immobile. Conditions found under this heading are chronic in nature, although the ulcer may be described as infected. The fifth character identifies the site of the ulcer, and sixth character identifies the stage.

An instructional note found under category L89 alerts the coder to code first any associated gangrene (I96). It is also important to note the Excludes2 note found under this section. For classification purposes these ulcers are identified by stages 1–4 and unstageable.

- Stage 1: Red skin with warmth—persistent focal erythema
- Stage 2: Skin swollen with abrasion, blister, and partial thickness skin loss
- Stage 3: Full-thickness skin loss with subcutaneous necrosis
- Stage 4: Necrosis of soft tissues through to underlying muscle/tendon/bone
- Unstageable: Ulcers that have either been previously treated or covered with an eschar and the clinician is unable to determine the stage or they are documented as deep tissue injury not due to trauma

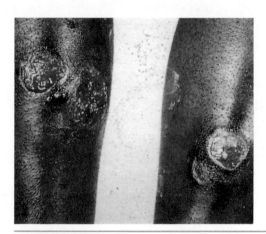

FIGURE 18-4. Ulcers.

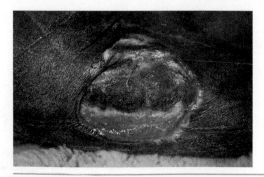

FIGURE 18-5. Decubitus ulcer.

Selecting the stage of the pressure ulcer may be determined by nursing documentation or terms listed in the Index. If a term describing an ulcer is not listed in the Index and there is no documentation of stage, the provider should be queried.

EXAMPLE Patient has a decubitus ulcer on the left buttock with skin loss to bone, L89.324.

If a patient has a healed pressure ulcer, documented no code is assigned. However, if the pressure ulcer is documented as healing, then the ulcer and the stage of the ulcer are assigned codes. Should the documentation be unclear as to whether the patient has a healing or healed pressure ulcer the provider should be queried.

EXAMPLE Patient is admitted with pneumonia. During the physical exam, the physician identifies a decubitus ulcer of the right heel that appears to be healing. The physician cannot give the ulcer a stage as it is covered by a skin graft, J18.9, L89.610.

If a patient has a pressure ulcer on admit that is documented as stage 2 and then during the admission this ulcer progresses to a stage 3, only the most severe stage of the ulcer is assigned.

EXAMPLE Patient is admitted to the hospital with, among other conditions, a stage 1 decubitus ulcer of the left ankle. During this admission, this ankle ulcer progresses to a stage 3, L89.523.

Non–Pressure Chronic Ulcer of the Lower Limb

A code from L97 may be used as the principal or first-listed diagnosis if there is no condition documented as the cause of the ulcer. If there is gangrene associated with the ulcer, the gangrene is to be coded first, which follows the same rule as with decubitus ulcers. This instruction goes on to say that if the ulcer is associated with any of the conditions listed below, the underlying condition should be coded first.

- Atherosclerosis of the lower extremities (I70.23-, J70.24-, I70.00-, I70.34-, I70.43-, I70.44-, I70.53-, I70.54-, I70.63-, I70.64-, I70.73-, I70.74-)
- Chronic venous hypertension (I87.01-, I87.33)
- Diabetic ulcers (E08.621, E08.622, E09.621, E09.622, E10.621, E10.622, E11.621, E11.622, E13.621, E13.622)
- Postphlebitic syndrome (I87.01-, I87.03-)
- Postthrombotic syndrome (I87.01-, I87.03-)
- Varicose ulcer (I83.0-, I83.2-)

EXAMPLE Patient has a chronic stage 2 ulcer of the second toe on the right foot, secondary to type 2 diabetes, E11.621, L97.502.

Assign codes to the following conditions.

1. Decubitus ulcer of the right heel, stage 2 _____

2. Diabetic ulcer of the left toe, skin breakdown only _____

3. Arteriosclerotic ulcer of the left leg with gangrene, of native artery, skin breakdown only _____

4. Ischemic ulcer of the right calf _____

5. Ulcer of the right buttock _____

6. Patient has a sacral stage 4 decubitus ulcer with gangrene _____

7. Patient has pressure ulcers on both buttocks. The buttock on the right has a stage 2 ulcer while the left buttock has a stage 3 ulcer _____

8. Patient is transferred from the nursing home with a fever and infected decubitus ulcers. There is an ulcer of the left hip stage 3 and ulcers of both elbows. The right elbow has a stage 1 ulcer and the left elbow has a stage 2 ulcer _____

9. Patient has a gangrenous ulcer of the left heel; he also has atherosclerosis of the lower extremities _____

FACTORS INFLUENCING HEALTH STATUS AND CONTACT WITH HEALTH SERVICES (Z CODES)

As was discussed in Chapter 8, it is difficult to locate Z codes in the Index. Coders will often say, "I did not know there was a Z code for that." Refer to Chapter 8 for a listing of common main terms used to locate Z codes.

Z codes that may be used with diseases of the skin and subcutaneous tissue include the following:

Z48.817	Encounter for surgical aftercare following surgery on skin and subcutaneous tissue
Z52.10	Skin donor, unspecified
Z52.11	Skin donor, autologous
Z52.19	Skin donor, other
Z84.0	Family history of diseases of the skin and subcutaneous tissue
Z87.2	Personal history of diseases of the skin and subcutaneous tissue
Z94.5	Skin transplant status
Z96.81	Presence of artificial skin

EXAMPLE Patient presents to dermatologist's office for a rash on the cheeks and nose. Patient has a family history of skin disorders, R21, Z84.0.

Assign codes to the following conditions.

1. Patient with a history of eczema _____

2. Patient with a family history of dermatitis _____

COMMON TREATMENTS

CONDITION	MEDICATION
Acne	Tetracycline (Achromycin), isotretinoin (Accutane)
Boils	Bacitracin, Neosporin
Cellulitis	Antibiotics such as nafcillin, oxacillin, cefazolin, vancomycin, linezolid
Psoriasis	Topical corticosteroids

PROCEDURES

Procedures related to the Diseases of the Skin and Subcutaneous Tissue section in ICD-10-PCS may be located in the following tables:

Skin and Breast	0H0-0HY
Subcutaneous Tissue and Fascia	0J0-0JX

Incision and Drainage

Incision and drainage (I&D) is a common form of treatment for abscesses of the skin. The physician cuts into the lining of the abscess, which allows the pus to drain. Usually, the physician cleans the cavity with warm saline. If the abscess is deep, the physician may insert a drainage tube. It is important to be aware that I&D can also be used to describe incision and debridement. In cases in which the documentation is questionable, a physician query may be necessary. In ICD-10-PCS the root operation for incision and drainage is drainage (taking or letting out fluids and/or gases from a body part).

EXERCISE 18-5

Assign codes to the following conditions.

1. Incision and drainage of neck abscess _____

2. I&D of boil on left arm _____

3. Incision and drainage of pilonidal sinus _____

Debridement

Excisional Debridement

Excisional debridement, the surgical removal or cutting away of devitalized tissue, necrosis, or slough. The root operation for debridement in ICD-10-PCS is excision (cutting out or off a portion of a body part) if it is excisional and extraction (pulling or stripping out or off all or a portion of a body part) if it is nonexcisional. Excisional debridements may be performed in a variety of settings (operating room, emergency room, or bedside) and by a variety of healthcare providers (physicians, nurse practitioners, physician assistants, and physical therapists).

Please see the ICD-10-PCS procedural guidelines for overlapping body layers. When an extensive debridement goes beyond the skin and subcutaneous tissue into the muscle, tendon, and/or bone, it is appropriate to assign only a code for the deepest layer of debridement when multiple layers of the same site are debrided. If a patient had a debridement of skin, subcutaneous tissue, muscle and bone, the bone is the deepest layer and debridement of the bone is the only procedure code assigned.

EXAMPLE | Patient with a stage 4 decubitus ulcer of the sacrum is taken to the OR for debridement. The debridement is performed through the skin, muscle, and bone, L89.154, 0QB10ZZ.

Nonexcisional Debridement

Any debridement that does not meet the criteria described earlier for excisional debridement would be coded as nonexcisional. A nonexcisional debridement may be performed by brushing, irrigating, scrubbing, or washing to remove devitalized tissue. Once again, this procedure may be performed in a variety of settings by a variety of healthcare providers.

It is important to remember that if debridement of the skin is performed in preparation for further surgery, the debridement should not be coded separately. For example, prior to reduction of an open fracture, a debridement may be performed.

EXAMPLE | Pulse lavage debridement is performed by wound care nurse on a patient with a stage 3 decubitus ulcer of the right ankle, L89.513, 0HDKXZZ.

EXERCISE 18-6

Assign codes to the following conditions.

1. Excisional debridement of decubitus ulcer of the left heel _____

2. Skin tissue of lower left leg ulcer removed by scrubbing _____

3. Debridement of a fungus of the nail bed of the index finger _____

Skin Grafts

Skin Grafts

Skin grafts are composed of pieces of skin that are removed from one body area (donor) and are used to cover a defect in another body area (recipient).

In ICD-10-PCS skin grafts are coded to the root operation replacement. Replacement is the putting in or on biological (autologous or nonautologous) or synthetic (man-made) material that physically takes the place and/or function of all or a portion of a body part.
- Autologous—donor and recipient are the same person
- Nonautologous—donor and recipient are different people or species
- Synthetic—man-made

EXAMPLE | Patient presents for full-thickness skin graft to the left thigh from the abdomen to repair a skin contracture from third-degree burn of the left thigh. Patient spilled boiling water on himself several months ago, L90.5, T24.312S, X12xxxS, 0HB7XZZ, 0HRJX73.

SECTION: 0 MEDICAL AND SURGICAL
BODY SYSTEM: H SKIN AND BREAST
OPERATION: R REPLACEMENT: *(on multiple pages)*

Putting in or on biological or synthetic material that physically takes the place and/or function of all or a portion of a body part

Body Part	Approach	Device	Qualifier
0 Skin, Scalp 1 Skin, Face 2 Skin, Right Ear 3 Skin, Left Ear 4 Skin, Neck 5 Skin, Chest 6 Skin, Back 7 Skin, Abdomen 8 Skin, Buttock 9 Skin, Perineum A Skin, Genitalia B Skin, Right Upper Arm C Skin, Left Upper Arm D Skin, Right Lower Arm E Skin, Left Lower Arm F Skin, Right Hand G Skin, Left Hand H Skin, Right Upper Leg J Skin, Left Upper Leg K Skin, Right Lower Leg L Skin, Left Lower Leg M Skin, Right Foot N Skin, Left Foot	X External	7 Autologous Tissue Substitute K Nonautologous Tissue Substitute	3 Full Thickness 4 Partial Thickness

FIGURE 18-6. Example of skin graft table from ICD-10-PCS.

Pedicle Grafts or Flaps

Pedicle grafts or **flaps** differ from split-thickness skin graft (STSG) and full-thickness skin graft (FTSG) (Figure 18-7) in that part of the graft or flaps remains attached to the donor site. A pedicle graft is a full-thickness skin and subcutaneous tissue flap/graft that is attached by tissue (Figure 18-8), through which it receives its blood supply.

The ICD-10-PCS root operation for a pedicle graft and for skin transfer flaps is transfer (moving, without taking out, all or a portion of a body part to another location to take over the function of all or a portion of a body part). The body part that is transferred remains connected to its vascular and nervous supply.

EXERCISE 18-7

Assign codes to the following conditions.

1. STSG from patient's left thigh to cover scar contracture due to 2nd degree burn from fire on right forearm _____

2. FTSG to left hand from buttock due to scar from necrotizing fasciitis _____

3. Advancement flap to nose following surgery to remove skin cancer from nose _____

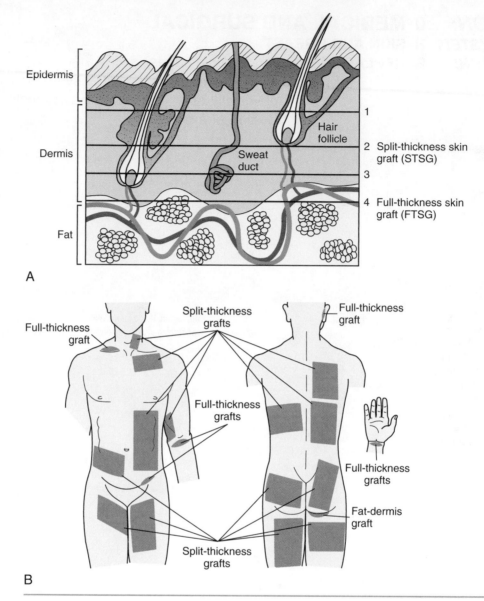

Epidermis

Dermis

Fat

Hair follicle

Sweat duct

1

2 Split-thickness skin graft (STSG)

3

4 Full-thickness skin graft (FTSG)

A

Full-thickness graft

Split-thickness grafts

Full-thickness graft

Full-thickness grafts

Full-thickness grafts

Fat-dermis graft

Split-thickness grafts

B

FIGURE 18-7. Split-thickness and full-thickness skin grafts.

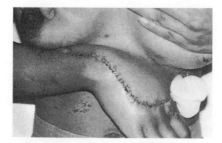

FIGURE 18-8. Pedicle graft.

DOCUMENTATION/REIMBURSEMENT/MS-DRGs

Often, coding difficulties are due to lack of documentation. Sometimes pathology and other test results are not available at the time of discharge or when the physician is dictating the discharge summary or is reporting the final diagnoses.

It is very important for coding to make sure that healthcare providers fully describe the type of debridement that was performed. If sharp instruments were used to cut away devitalized tissue, this must be documented. This can make a significant difference in MS-DRG assignment and reimbursement.

When physicians state that an I&D was performed, it is imperative to identify whether the physician means incision and drainage or incision and debridement. These terms may be used interchangeably. In most cases, the term "I&D" stands for incision and drainage; however, if it seems unlikely that the condition would require this procedure, a query to the physician is warranted.

Frequently missed complications/comorbidities from this chapter include:

- Abscess
- Cellulitis
- Pressure ulcers

Incision and Drainage versus Debridement

EXAMPLE

DIAGNOSES/PROCEDURES	CODES	MS-DRG	RW
Stage 2 decubitus ulcer of right heel	L89.612	594	0.6981
Incision and drainage	0H9KXZZ		
Stage 4 decubitus ulcer of right heel	L89.614	570	2.5158
Excisional debridement	0HBMXZZ		

MS-DRG With and Without MCC/CC

The appropriate assignment of codes to identify the stage of a pressure ulcer may affect MS-DRG assignment.

EXAMPLE

DIAGNOSES/PROCEDURES	CODES	MS-DRG	RW
Patient with pneumonia and decubitus ulcer heel of the right heel	J18.9, L89.609	195	0.7037
Patient with pneumonia and stage 4 decubitus ulcer heel of the right heel	J18.9, L89.604	193	1.4948

CHAPTER REVIEW EXERCISE

Answer the following and assign codes to the following conditions.

1. Abscess of the right leg with cellulitis _____

2. Pressure ulcer of the left heel with cellulitis, stage 3 _____

3. Eczema _____

4. Dermatitis caused by Cipro _____

5. Allergic contact dermatitis due to poison sumac _____

6. Stasis dermatitis with ulcer of the left calf _____

7. Diabetic PVD with left foot ulcer with fat layer exposed _____

8. Incision and drainage of abscess of the right lower leg _____

9. Excision of a pilonidal cyst _____

10. Excisional debridement of decubitus ulcer of the buttock _____
(stage 4) by the attending physician

Write the correct answer(s) in the space(s) provided.

11. What is the difference between a pedicle graft and a split-thickness skin graft?

_____

12. Name one documentation challenge about which coders must be aware in diseases of the skin
and subcutaneous tissue.

_____

13. What are the three accessory organs of the skin?

_____

_____

_____

14. Where in ICD-10-CM would a coder find the skin condition herpes zoster?

_____

15. What is another name for a decubitus ulcer?

_____

16. Name and describe three types of skin grafts.

_____

_____

_____

CHAPTER GLOSSARY

Abscess: a localized collection of pus that causes swelling.

Allograft: graft of tissue between individuals of the same species.

Alopecia: hair loss.

Autograft: graft of tissue from another site on the same individual.

Carbuncle: cluster of boils.

Cellulitis: inflammation of the tissue with possible abscess.

Debridement: removal of devitalized tissue, necrosis, or slough.

Decubitus ulcer: skin ulcer also known as a bed sore.

Dermatitis: inflammation of the skin.

Dermis: layer of skin below the epidermis.

Eczema: type of dermatitis characterized by itching.

Endogenous: type of dermatitis caused by something taken internally, such as medication.

Epidermis: outermost layer of skin.

Excisional: removal by surgical cutting.

Exogenous: type of dermatitis caused by contact with a substance.

Furuncle: a boil.

Heterograft: graft of skin from another species, such as a graft from a pig to a human.

Hives: skin condition also known as urticaria, wherein the skin reacts with welts; characterized by itching.

Homograft: graft from one individual to another of the same species; also known as an allograft.

Hyperhidrosis: excessive sweating.

Integumentary: another name for skin.

Intertrigo: dermatitis in areas where friction may occur.

Pedicle graft or flap: involves identifying a flap that remains attached to its original blood supply and tunneling it under the skin to a particular area such as the breast.

Pemphigus: autoimmune disorder causing blistering of skin and mucous membranes.

Pruritus: itching.

Psoriasis: inflammation of skin caused by a fault in the immune system.

Rosacea: skin condition affecting cheeks, nose, chin, and forehead. It can be characterized by redness, a bulbous nose, or an increased number of blood vessels in the face.

Sebum: substance secreted from the sebaceous gland.

Solar Keratosis: precancerous scaly growth.

Stevens-Johnson Syndrome: skin necrosis caused by a reaction to medication or infection.

Subcutaneous: inner layer of the skin that contains fat and sweat glands.

Ulcer: open sore of skin.

Urticaria: another name for hives.

Xenograft: graft to an individual from another species; also known as a heterograft.

19

Diseases of the Musculoskeletal System and Connective Tissue

(ICD-10-CM Chapter 13, Codes M00-M99)

CHAPTER OUTLINE

ICD-10-CM Official Guidelines for Coding and Reporting

Major Differences Between ICD-10-CM and ICD-9-CM

Anatomy and Physiology

Disease Conditions
Infectious (M00-M02) and Inflammatory Arthropathies (M05-M14)
Osteoarthritis (M15-M19) and Other Joint Disorders (M20-M25)
Systemic Connective Tissue Disorders (M30-M36)
Deforming Dorsopathies (M40-M43), Spondylopathies (M45-M49), and Other Dorsopathies (M50-M54)
Disorders of Muscles (M60-M63), Synovium, Tendon (M65-M67), and Other Soft Tissue (M70-M79)
Disorders of Bone Density and Structure (M80-M85), Other Osteopathies (M86-M90), and Chondropathies (M91-M94)

Factors Influencing Health Status and Contact With Health Services (Z Codes)

Common Treatments

Procedures
Arthroscopic Surgery
Joint Replacement
Vertebroplasty/Kyphoplasty
Fusion Procedures of the Spine

Documentation/Reimbursement/MS-DRGs
Pathologic Fracture versus Traumatic Fracture
Correct Procedure Code

Chapter Review Exercise

Chapter Glossary

LEARNING OBJECTIVES

1. Apply and assign the correct ICD-10-CM/PCS codes in accordance with Official Guidelines for Coding and Reporting
2. Identify major differences between ICD-10-CM and ICD-9-CM related to the musculoskletal system and connective tissue
3. Identify pertinent anatomy and physiology of the musculoskeletal system and connective tissue
4. Identify diseases of the musculoskeletal system and connective tissue

5. Assign the correct Z codes and procedure codes related to the musculoskeletal system and connective tissue

6. Identify common treatments, medications, laboratory values, and diagnostic tests

7. Explain the importance of documentation as it relates to MS-DRGs for reimbursement

ABBREVIATIONS/ACRONYMS

AKA above-knee amputation

DEXA dual-energy x-ray absorptiometry (bone density)

DIC disseminated intravascular coagulation

DJD degenerative joint disease

ICD-9-CM *International Classification of Diseases, 9th Revision, Clinical Modification*

ICD-10-CM *International Classification of Diseases, 10th Revision, Clinical Modification*

ICD-10-PCS *International Classification of Diseases, 10th Revision, Procedure Coding System*

IV intravenous

JRA juvenile rheumatoid arthritis

MAO monoamine oxidase

MRI magnetic resonance imaging

MS-DRG Medicare Severity diagnosis-related group

NSAIDs nonsteroidal anti-inflammatory drugs

OA osteoarthritis

PMR polymyalgia rheumatica

PV percutaneous vertebroplasty

RA rheumatoid arthritis

SLE systemic lupus erythematosus

ICD-10-CM
Official Guidelines for Coding and Reporting

Please refer to the companion Evolve website for the most current guidelines.

13. Chapter 13: Diseases of the Musculoskeletal System and Connective Tissue (M00-M99)

a. Site and laterality

Most of the codes within Chapter 13 have site and laterality designations. The site represents the bone, joint or the muscle involved. For some conditions where more than one bone, joint or muscle is usually involved, such as osteoarthritis, there is a "multiple sites" code available. For categories where no multiple site code is provided and more than one bone, joint or muscle is involved, multiple codes should be used to indicate the different sites involved.

1) Bone versus joint

For certain conditions, the bone may be affected at the upper or lower end, (e.g., avascular necrosis of bone, M87, Osteoporosis, M80, M81). Though the portion of the bone affected may be at the joint, the site designation will be the bone, not the joint.

EXAMPLE

The patient is being evaluated for hip replacement surgery because of idiopathic avascular necrosis of the right hip, M87.051.

b. Acute traumatic versus chronic or recurrent musculoskeletal conditions

Many musculoskeletal conditions are a result of previous injury or trauma to a site, or are recurrent conditions. Bone, joint or muscle conditions that are the result of a healed injury are usually found in chapter 13. Recurrent bone, joint or muscle conditions are also usually found in chapter 13. Any current, acute injury should be coded to the appropriate injury code from chapter 19. Chronic or recurrent conditions should generally be coded with a code from chapter 13. If it is difficult to determine from the documentation in the record which code is best to describe a condition, query the provider.

EXAMPLE

The patient was seen in the ER for recurrent dislocation of left little finger, M24.445.

c. Coding of Pathologic Fractures

7th character A is for use as long as the patient is receiving active treatment for the fracture. Examples of active treatment are: surgical treatment, emergency department encounter, evaluation and treatment by a new physician. 7th character, D is to be used for encounters after the patient has completed active treatment. The other 7th characters, listed under each subcategory in the Tabular List, are to be used for subsequent encounters for treatment of problems associated with the healing, such as malunions, nonunions, and sequelae.

Care for complications of surgical treatment for fracture repairs during the healing or recovery phase should be coded with the appropriate complication codes.

See Section I.C.19. Coding of traumatic fractures.

EXAMPLE | The patient was seen for follow-up after vertebroplasty for pathologic fracture of the L1 vertebra, which is healing. Patient has osteoporosis of vertebrae, M80.08xD.

d. Osteoporosis

Osteoporosis is a systemic condition, meaning that all bones of the musculoskeletal system are affected. Therefore, site is not a component of the codes under category M81, Osteoporosis without current pathological fracture. The site codes under category M80, Osteoporosis with current pathological fracture, identify the site of the fracture, not the osteoporosis.

1) Osteoporosis without pathological fracture

Category M81, Osteoporosis without current pathological fracture, is for use for patients with osteoporosis who do not currently have a pathologic fracture due to the osteoporosis, even if they have had a fracture in the past. For patients with a history of osteoporosis fractures, status code Z87.310, Personal history of (healed) osteoporosis fracture, should follow the code from M81.

2) Osteoporosis with current pathological fracture

Category M80, Osteoporosis with current pathological fracture, is for patients who have a current pathologic fracture at the time of an encounter. The codes under M80 identify the site of the fracture. A code from category M80, not a traumatic fracture code, should be used for any patient with known osteoporosis who suffers a fracture, even if the patient had a minor fall or trauma, if that fall or trauma would not usually break a normal, healthy bone.

EXAMPLE | The patient underwent a percutaneous vertebroplasty (synthetic substitute) for pathologic fracture of the L1 vertebra due to delayed healing. Patient has osteoporosis of vertebrae, M80.08xG, 0QU03JZ.

Apply the General Coding Guidelines as found in Chapter 5 and the Procedural Coding Guideline as found in Chapters 6 and 7.

MAJOR DIFFERENCES BETWEEN ICD-10-CM AND ICD-9-CM

Some of the differences have already been identified in the guidelines section. Other differences include:

- ICD-10-CM identifies three different causes for pathologic fractures:
  - Neoplastic disease
  - Osteoporosis
  - Other specified disease
- The code assigned is a combination code that identifies the pathologic fracture and the cause of the fracture.

- In ICD-10-CM, bacterial organisms are included in some of the infectious arthropathy codes. A code from the infectious disease chapter may still need to be assigned to completely identify the organism.
- Codes for gout have been moved to the Musculoskeletal System chapter in ICD-10-CM from the Endocrine, Nutritional, and Metabolic Disease chapter in ICD-9-CM.
- Most codes in Chapter 13 have site and laterality designations.
- Some codes in Chapter 13 of ICD-10-CM require the seventh-character extension that describes the type of encounter, the stage of the fracture's healing process, and any residual effects or sequelae from the fracture. These extensions are as follows:

  A   Initial encounter for fracture
  D   Subsequent encounter for fracture with routine healing
  G   Subsequent encounter for fracture with delayed healing
  K   Subsequent encounter for fracture with nonunion
  P   Subsequent encounter for fracture with malunion
  S   Sequela

- Procedural complications affecting the musculoskeletal system are included in Chapter 13 of ICD-10-CM. Some of the complications include:
  - Pseudoarthrosis after a fusion or arthrodesis
  - Postlaminectomy syndrome
  - Fractures following insertion of orthopedic implants, prosthesis, or bone plates
  - Intraoperative hemorrhage, hematoma, or accidental laceration

ANATOMY AND PHYSIOLOGY

The musculoskeletal system is made up of muscles, bones, ligaments, tendons, cartilage, and the joints they form. The purposes of the musculoskeletal system are to provide a framework and to protect the internal organs. Bones also are important for hematopoiesis and for storing calcium and phosphate. **Hematopoiesis** is the development of blood cells that occurs in the bone marrow and lymphatic tissue of normal adults.

A good grasp of anatomy is essential in coding conditions of the musculoskeletal system. It is important to know that the femur is the long bone in the thigh area, and that the radius and the ulna are two bones in the forearm. Pictures are best for illustrating the locations of the skeletal structures (Figure 19-1) and muscles (Figure 19-2). It is particularly important to understand the terms used in the musculoskeletal chapter to describe the location of structures relative to the body as a whole or to other body structures (Figure 19-3). **Anterior** or **ventral** describes the front of the body or an organ. **Posterior** or **dorsal** relates to the back of the body or an organ. The terms medial and lateral describe the position of the body or an organ relative to the median sagittal plane that divides the body in half. **Medial** refers to a structure that is closer to the median plane than is another structure in the body. The eyes are medial to the ears. **Lateral** refers to a structure that is to the side of the body. The ears are lateral to the eyes. The terms **superior** (above) and **inferior** (below) describe the position of the body or an organ relative to the vertical axis of the body. The shoulders are superior to the hips, and the ankles are inferior to the knees. Other terms that may be used are **cranial**, which means toward the head, and **caudal**, which means towards the tail. **Proximal** (closer to the point of reference) and **distal** (farther from the point of reference) are often used to describe a location in the limbs. The shoulder is proximal to the elbow, and the wrist is distal to the elbow. **Supine** refers to lying on the back, face up. **Prone** is lying on the stomach, face down.

The **joints** are the means of joining two bones together; they assist with body movement. **Ligaments** are dense fibrous bands of connective tissue that provide stability for the joint. Ligaments can be injured by overstretching or tearing (sprain). **Tendons** are the connective tissue that attaches muscle to bone. Tendons are susceptible to strain injuries. The **fascia** is the tissue just below the skin that covers and separates the underlying layers of muscle.

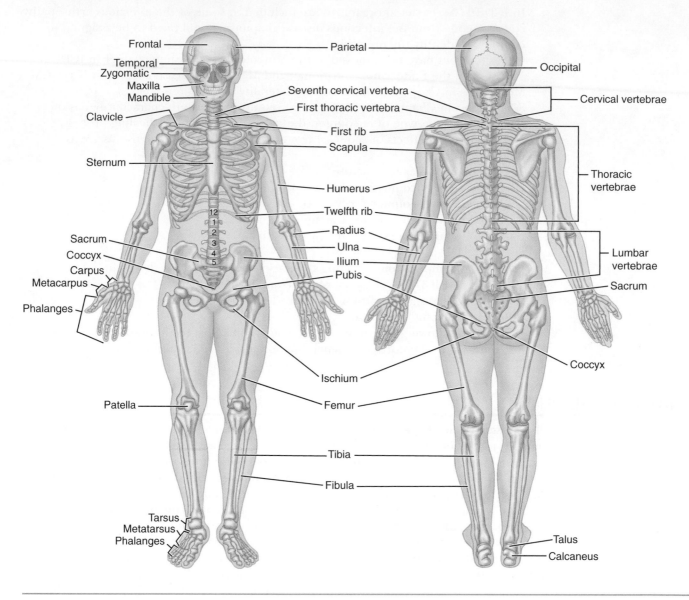

FIGURE 19-1. Anterior and posterior views of the human skeleton.

DISEASE CONDITIONS

Diseases of the Musculoskeletal System and Connective Tissue (M00-M99), Chapter 13 in the ICD-10-CM code book, are divided into the following categories:

CATEGORY	SECTION TITLES
M00-M02	Infectious arthropathies
M05-M14	Inflammatory polyarthropathies
M15-M19	Osteoarthritis
M20-M25	Other joint disorders
M26-M27	Dentofacial anomalies, including malocclusion, and other disorders of the jaw
M30-M36	Systemic connective tissue disorders
M40-M43	Deforming dorsopathies
M45-M49	Spondylopathies
M50-M54	Other dorsopathies
M60-M63	Disorders of muscles
M65-M67	Disorders of synovium and tendon
M70-M79	Other soft-tissue disorders

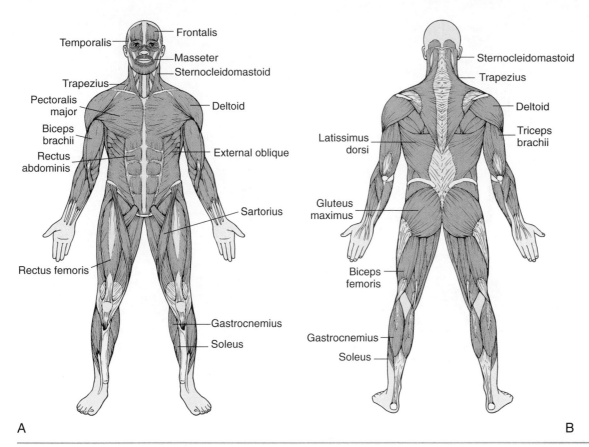

FIGURE 19-2. Normal muscular system. **A,** Anterior view. **B,** Posterior view.

CATEGORY	SECTION TITLES
M80-M85	Disorders of bone density and structure
M86-M90	Other osteopathies
M91-M94	Chondropathies
M95	Other disorders of the musculoskeletal system and connective tissue
M96	Intraoperative and postprocedural complications and disorders of musculoskeletal system, not elsewhere classified
M99	Biomechanical lesions, not elsewhere classified

Infectious (M00-M02) and Inflammatory Arthropathies (M05-M14)

Arthropathy is a disease that affects the joints. The term arthropathy is generic, and symptoms and treatment will depend on the cause of the arthropathy. Common causes include:

- Infectious—due to an infection of the joint
- Crystal—due to diseases such as gout that deposit crystals in the joint
- Diabetic—a manifestation of diabetes
- Neuropathic—a manifestation due to nerve damage around the joint
- Enteropathic—a type of arthritis that is related to colitis such a Crohn's or ulcerative colitis

Rheumatoid arthritis (RA) is a chronic, inflammatory, systemic disease that affects the joints, often causing deformity (Figure 19-4). RA is one of the most severe and disabling forms of arthritis. Damage may extend beyond the joints, affecting the heart and blood vessels and producing damage within the layers of skin.

Juvenile rheumatoid arthritis (JRA) affects children, usually between the ages of 2 and 5 years. Various forms of JRA may affect only a few joints, may affect many joints, or may be systemic in nature (also known as Still's disease).

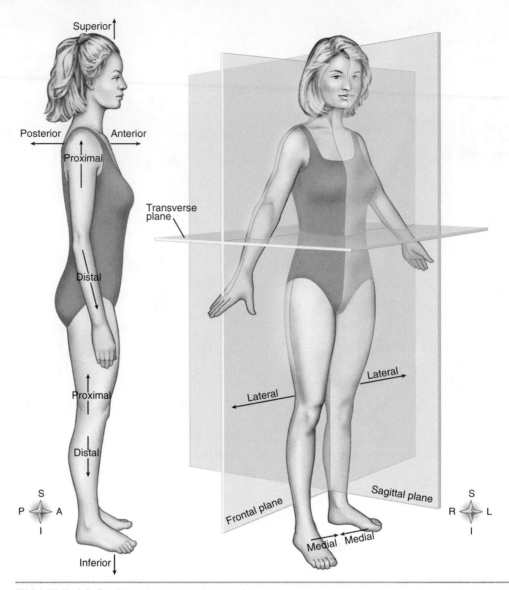

FIGURE 19-3. Directions and planes of the body.

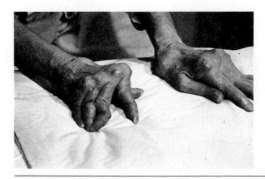

FIGURE 19-4. Joint deformity from rheumatoid arthritis.

EXAMPLE	Fourteen-year-old child is being treated for Still's disease, M08.20.

EXERCISE 19-1

Assign codes to the following conditions.

1. Juvenile RA left knee _____
2. Arthritis bilateral hips due to Crohn's disease _____
3. Rheumatoid lung disease _____
4. Septic arthritis right shoulder due to MRSA _____
5. Idiopathic chronic gout left wrist _____

Osteoarthritis (M15-M19) and Other Joint Disorders (M20-M25)

Osteoarthritis

Osteoarthritis is a type of arthritis that develops as the result of wear and tear on the joints. It occurs because of breakdown and loss of cartilage within the joints (Figure 19-5). Osteoarthritis (OA) or degenerative joint disease (DJD), the most common form of arthritis, is more common in the elderly. Weight-bearing joints such as the knees and hips are often affected. The most common symptoms include sore and stiff joints, particularly in the morning or with changes of weather. Edema and deformity may also be present. Treatment depends on the severity of the condition and the success of conservative medical treatments (i.e., anti-inflammatory medications, exercise, steroid injections). In severe cases, surgery may be required to replace affected joints.

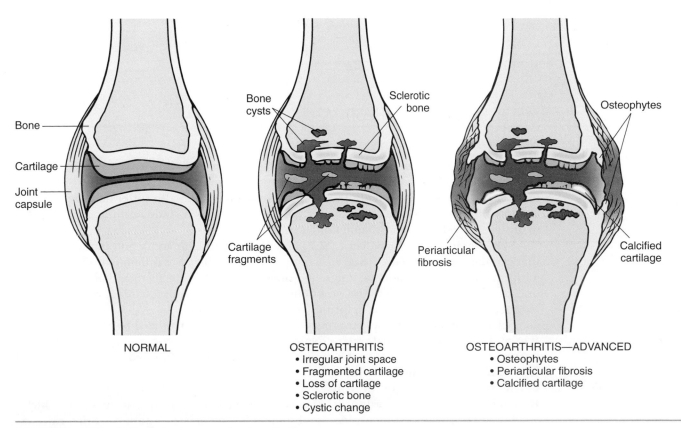

FIGURE 19-5. Pathologic changes of osteoarthritis.

Primary osteoarthritis is an idiopathic condition that occurs in previously intact joints and has no apparent initiating factor. Primary osteoarthritis is related to the aging process and typically occurs in older individuals. **Secondary osteoarthritis** refers to degenerative disease of the joints that results from a predisposing condition such as trauma or disease. Secondary osteoarthritis may occur in relatively young individuals and usually affects the joints of one area.

EXAMPLE | Patient has primary osteoarthritis of both hips, M16.0.

EXAMPLE | Patient is being treated for osteoarthritis hands and wrists, M15.9.

Recurrent dislocations are not coded as an injury even if due to trauma. After the initial dislocation, the joint becomes less stable and requires less force to dislocate the joint again. The most common sites for recurrent dislocation to occur are shoulders, fingers, and knees.

EXAMPLE | Patient was treated in the ER for recurrent dislocation of left shoulder. A closed reduction was performed, M24.412, 0RSKXZZ.

EXERCISE 19-2

Assign codes to the following conditions.

1. Pain both knees due to DJD _____
2. Loose body in left knee joint _____
3. Talipes planus, right (acquired) _____
4. Contracture, left hand _____
5. Osteoarthritis, right shoulder _____

Systemic Connective Tissue Disorders (M30-M36)

Collagen Diseases

The main component of connective tissue is collagen. Collagen diseases result from immune system malfunctions in which the immune system identifies the body's connective tissue as foreign and attacks it. A patient's heart, lungs, and kidneys may also suffer damage. No cure is known for these diseases. The most common conditions include systemic lupus erythematosus, scleroderma, and rheumatoid arthritis.

Systemic lupus erythematosus (SLE) is a chronic, inflammatory autoimmune disease that can damage connective tissue anywhere in the body. It causes inflammation of the skin, joints, nervous system, kidneys, lungs, and other organs. A butterfly rash that spreads from one cheek across the nose to the other cheek is a common symptom (Figure 19-6). Fever, fatigue, weight loss, and joint deformity may also be present.

Scleroderma is a chronic, progressive disease that is characterized by hardening of the skin and scarring of internal organs. No cure is known for scleroderma; treatment is supportive and varies according to the organs that are affected. CREST syndrome is a form of scleroderma that includes the following:

Calcinosis—calcification of the skin

Raynaud's phenomenon—a disorder that is characterized by vasospastic attacks in which blood vessels to the fingers, toes, and sometimes the ears and nose constrict, causing discoloration and pain

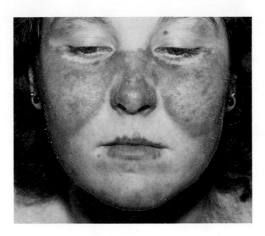

FIGURE 19-6. Butterfly rash that may accompany systemic lupus erythematosus.

Esophageal dysfunction—such as reflux or difficulty in swallowing
Sclerodactyly—hardening of the skin of the fingers or toes
Telangiectasia—dilatation of tiny blood vessels, particularly of the skin

EXAMPLE   Patient is being treated for CREST syndrome, M34.1.

Polymyalgia Rheumatica

Polymyalgia rheumatica, or PMR, is a syndrome that is characterized by severe aching and stiffness in the neck, shoulder girdle, and pelvic girdle. It is classified as a rheumatic disease, although its origin remains undetermined. It has been closely linked to temporal arteritis.

EXERCISE 19-3

Assign codes to the following conditions.

1. Sicca syndrome   _____
2. SLE with nephrotic syndrome   _____
3. Mixed connective tissue disease   _____
4. Kawasaki disease   _____
5. Giant cell arteritis   _____

Deforming Dorsopathies (M40-M43), Spondylopathies (M45-M49), and Other Dorsopathies (M50-M54)

Spinal Deformities

Sometimes, the normal curvatures of the spine are altered. **Lordosis** is an exaggerated inward curvature of the spine that may be caused by increased abdominal girth due to obesity, pregnancy, or abdominal tumor (Figure 19-7, *A*). Improved posture, exercise, and weight loss can often alleviate symptoms. **Kyphosis** is an excessive posterior curvature of the thoracic spine that may not be detected until a hump in the upper back is noticeable (Figure 19-7, *B*). In older people, particularly women, osteoporosis is often the cause. If it occurs in children or adolescents, the exact cause may have to be determined, so that the best

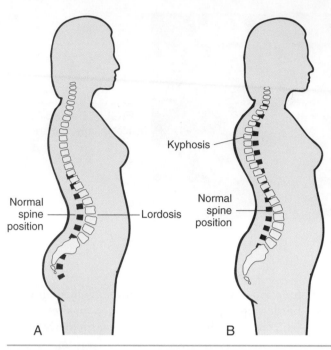

FIGURE 19-7. A, Lordosis. **B,** Kyphosis.

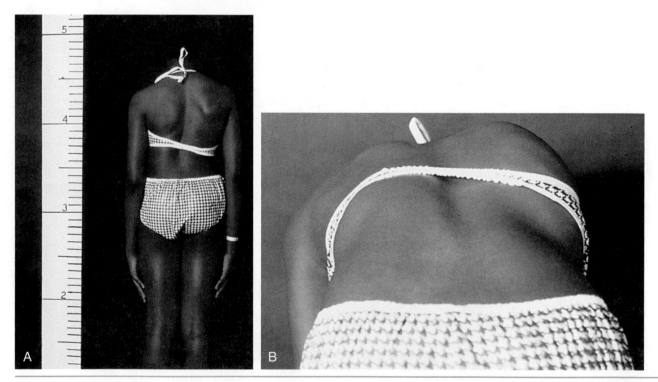

FIGURE 19-8. Scoliosis. **A,** Note scapular asymmetry in the upright position. **B,** Bending forward reveals a mild rib hump deformity.

treatment approach can be selected. **Scoliosis** is a lateral or sideways curvature of the spine (Figure 9-8). School screening programs may detect spinal abnormalities. Varying degrees of abnormality may be observed, and often, conservative medical management is attempted. In severe cases, the performance of procedures that fuse the vertebrae and the application of internal fixation devices such as rods, wires, plates, and/or screws may be necessary to correct the problem.

| **EXAMPLE** | The patient is being treated conservatively for kyphoscoliosis, M41.9. |

| **EXAMPLE** | Patient has back, buttock, and leg pain due to acquired lumbar spondylolisthesis, M43.16. |

Dorsopathies are conditions or diseases that affect the back or spine. Code assignment may depend on the location or region that is affected. The spinal column contains 33 vertebrae, as indicated in Figure 19-9. Seven cervical vertebrae are found in the neck. Twelve thoracic,

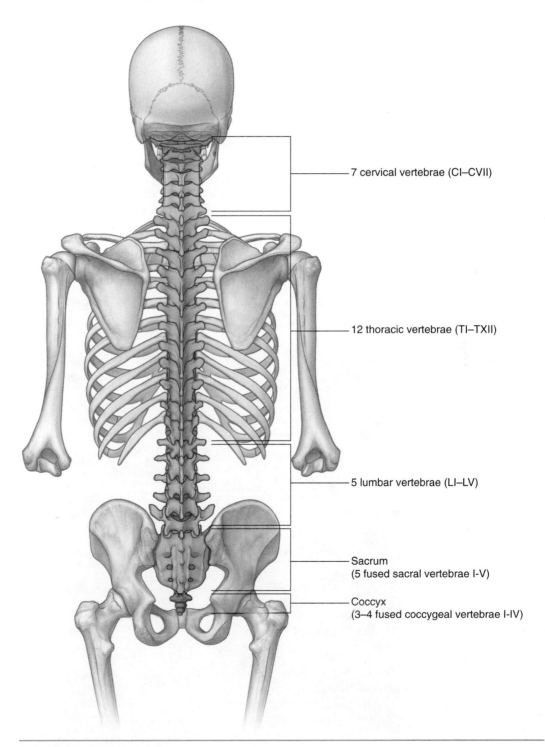

7 cervical vertebrae (CI–CVII)

12 thoracic vertebrae (TI–TXII)

5 lumbar vertebrae (LI–LV)

Sacrum
(5 fused sacral vertebrae I-V)

Coccyx
(3–4 fused coccygeal vertebrae I-IV)

FIGURE 19-9. Vertebrae.

or dorsal, vertebrae are found in the region of the chest, or thorax; these provide attachment for 12 pairs of ribs. Five lumbar vertebrae are located in the lower back. Five fused sacral vertebrae form the sacrum, a solid bone that fits like a wedge between the bones of the hip and the coccyx. The coccyx consists of three or four vertebrae fused together at the bottom of the sacrum. Between each vertebra is a thick, fibrous disc of cartilage known as an intervertebral disc. Intervertebral discs may become displaced, herniated, ruptured, and/or prolapsed with resultant pain.

Spondylosis (spinal osteoarthritis) is a degenerative disorder that may cause loss of normal spinal structure and function. Although aging is the primary cause, the location and rate of degeneration are individualized. The degenerative process of spondylosis may affect the cervical, thoracic, and/or lumbar regions of the spine, including the intervertebral discs and facet joints. **Facet joints** are small, stabilizing joints located between and behind adjacent vertebrae.

Spondylolisthesis occurs when one vertebra slips on another (Figure 19-10). Symptoms usually appear when the spinal nerves are pinched by the vertebrae. Symptoms such as back, buttock, and leg pain are often aggravated by activity and relieved with rest. The amount of slippage is identified by grades.

Spinal stenosis is a narrowing of the central spinal canal, or areas of the spine where the nerve roots exit (neuroforamina). This narrowing is often caused by arthritis and therefore is most often found in persons from older age groups. Spinal stenosis may be caused by other factors such as injury, infection, tumor, or congenital abnormality. Stenosis does not necessarily cause symptoms; if symptoms do appear, they usually indicate the presence of **radiculopathy** (nerve root compression) or **myelopathy** (spinal cord compression).

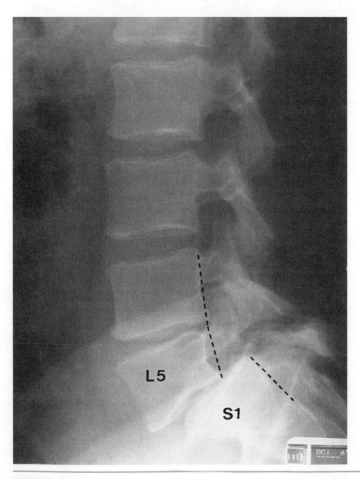

FIGURE 19-10. Spondylolysis with resulting grade 2 spondylolisthesis.

EXAMPLE | The patient's magnetic resonance imaging (MRI) showed stenosis cervical vertebrae, M48.02.

EXAMPLE | Patient's CT shows spondylosis lumbosacral region with myelopathy, M47.17.

EXERCISE 19-4

Assign codes to the following conditions.

1. Cervical spondylosis without myelopathy   _____
2. Degenerative disc disease lumbar spine   _____
3. Right-sided sciatica due to sitting on wallet   _____
4. Chronic low back pain   _____
5. Torticollis   _____
6. Pain in neck   _____
7. OA thoracic spine   _____
8. Stenosis lumbosacral vertebra   _____
9. Lumbago due to disc herniation at L4-L5   _____
10. Sacroiliitis   _____

Disorders of Muscles (M60-M63), Synovium, Tendon (M65-M67), and Other Soft Tissue (M70-M79)

Bursitis

Bursitis is inflammation of a bursa, which is a tiny, fluid-filled sac found between muscles, tendons, and bones designed to reduce friction and facilitate movement. Symptoms of bursitis include pain and tenderness when the affected body part is moved, limited range of motion, and edema or swelling. Areas most affected are the shoulders, elbows, hips, and knees. Bursitis may be caused by trauma, overuse of the joint, infection, or diseases such as gout and RA.

EXAMPLE | Patient is being seen for bursitis left olecranon process, M70.22.

EXAMPLE | Patient is being treated for right prepatellar bursitis, M70.41.

Necrotizing Fasciitis

Necrotizing fasciitis or "**flesh-eating disease**" is a rare but serious condition in which an infection occurs in the tissues below the skin. The tissues may quickly die because of poor blood supply, possibly leading to the death of the patient. Necrotizing fasciitis is usually caused by group A streptococcus (the same bacterium that causes strep throat) and is often preceded by an injury to the skin.

Fibromyalgia

Fibromyalgia, one of the most common diseases affecting the muscles, is characterized by widespread muscle pain associated with chronic fatigue. Other common symptoms of this condition include "brain fog," irritable bowel syndrome, sleep disorders, chronic headaches, anxiety, and depression. Fibromyalgia is a chronic condition that may be aggravated by weather conditions, infection, allergies, hormones, stress, and overexertion. Most available treatments focus on improving sleep and controlling pain.

EXERCISE 19-5

Assign codes to the following conditions.

1. Necrotizing fasciitis due to group A strep with gangrene right leg   _____

2. Pain due to bursitis left shoulder   _____

3. Insomnia due to fibromyalgia   _____

4. De Quervain's disease   _____

Disorders of Bone Density and Structure (M80-M85), Other Osteopathies (M86-M90), and Chondropathies (M91-M94)

Osteoporosis

Osteoporosis is a metabolic bone disorder that results in decreased bone mass and density. Osteoporosis, which is most common in older persons, particularly postmenopausal women, may also occur as the result of other diseases such as hyperparathyroidism or Cushing's syndrome; use of steroids may contribute to bone loss. Individuals with osteoporosis are susceptible for pathologic fractures. These fractures most often occur in the vertebrae of the spine, wrists, and hips (Figure 19-11).

EXAMPLE | Patient is being treated for postmenopausal osteoporosis, M81.0.

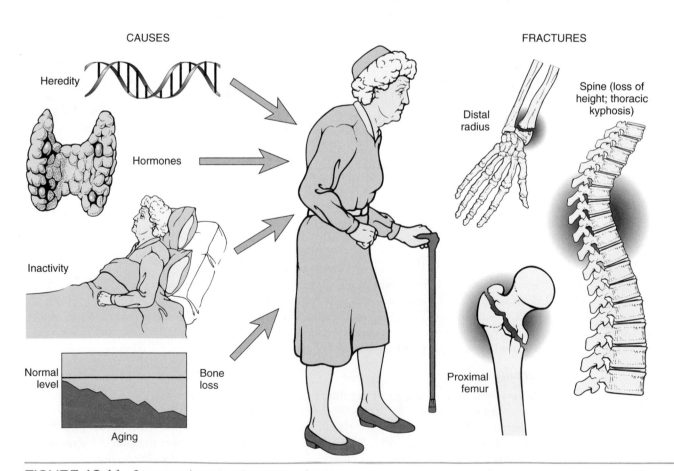

FIGURE 19-11. Causes and results of osteoporosis.

EXAMPLE Patient has osteoporosis due to disuse, M81.8.

Pathologic Fractures and Fracture Aftercare

A **pathologic fracture** is a break in a bone that occurs because of underlying disorders that weaken the bone, including malignancy, benign bone tumors, metabolic disorders, infection, and osteoporosis. A pathologic fracture may result from normal stress placed on an abnormal bone. Fractures may occur spontaneously in individuals with diseased bones as the result of minor exertion or trauma. Because the bone is already diseased, the healing process of the fracture can be complicated by delayed healing, nonunion, pseudarthrosis, necrosis, and infection. A fracture cannot be coded as both a traumatic fracture and a pathologic fracture; it is one or the other. Only a physician can determine whether the severity of trauma corresponds with the injury. Compression fractures of the spine are often pathologic, but a thorough review of the record and/or a physician query may be necessary to determine the appropriate fracture code. Other terms that may indicate a pathologic fracture are stress fracture, fatigue fracture, or insufficiency fracture.

Active treatment for a pathologic fracture includes surgery, an Emergency Room encounter, and/or evaluation and treatment by a new physician. According to the guidelines, when a patient is receiving active treatment, the acute fracture code is assigned with a 7th character A. A 7th character D is used for encounters after the patient has completed active treatment.

EXAMPLE Elderly woman with osteoporosis sustains a spontaneous fracture of the lumbar spine after removing a heavy turkey roaster from the oven, M80.08xA.

EXAMPLE Patient had a cast change for pathologic right radial fracture, M84.433D, 2W0CX2Z.

EXAMPLE Pathologic fracture distal left femur due to osteosarcoma femur, M84.552A, C40.22.

Osteomyelitis

Osteomyelitis is an infection of the bone that often starts in another part of the body and spreads to the bone via the blood (Figure 19-12). In children, the long bones are usually

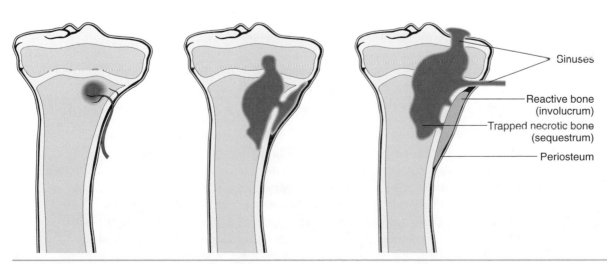

FIGURE 19-12. Progression of osteomyelitis. Bacterial growth results in bone destruction and abscess formation.

affected. In adults, the vertebrae and the pelvis are the most commonly affected areas. *Staphylococcus aureus* bacteria are usually the cause of acute osteomyelitis. This organism may enter the bloodstream through a wound or a contaminated intravenous needle. Chronic osteomyelitis results when bone tissue dies as a result of the lost blood supply. Risk factors include recent trauma, diabetes, hemodialysis, and intravenous (IV) drug abuse. People who have had a splenectomy are also at higher risk for osteomyelitis. Prolonged IV antibiotic therapy may be required.

EXAMPLE Subacute osteomyelitis sacrum with decubitus sacral ulcer, stage III, M46.28, L89.153.

EXAMPLE Chronic osteomyelitis due to *staphylococcus aureus* left tibia, M86.662, B95.61.

EXERCISE 19-6

Assign codes to the following conditions.

1. Thoracic kyphosis due to osteoporosis _____

2. Osteomyelitis with periostitis, right tibia. Cultures did not _____
   grow any organisms.

3. Osteochondritis dissecans _____

4. Pathologic fracture, left wrist, due to osteoporosis _____

5. Stress fracture, right lower leg _____

6. Chest pain due to costochondritis _____

7. Cast change for pathologic fracture, right radius _____

8. Nontraumatic slipped upper left femoral epiphysis _____

FACTORS INFLUENCING HEALTH STATUS AND CONTACT WITH HEALTH SERVICES (Z CODES)

As was discussed in Chapter 8, it may be difficult to locate Z codes in the index. Coders often say, "I did not know there was a Z code for that." Refer to Chapter 8 for a listing of common main terms used to locate Z codes.

It is important for the coder to be familiar with different types and uses of Z codes.

Z13.820	Encounter for screening for osteoporosis
Z13.828	Encounter for screening for other musculoskeletal disorder
Z44.001	Encounter for fitting and adjustment of unspecified right artificial arm
Z44.002	Encounter for fitting and adjustment of unspecified left artificial arm
Z44.009	Encounter for fitting and adjustment of unspecified artificial arm, unspecified arm
Z44.011	Encounter for fitting and adjustment of complete right artificial arm
Z44.012	Encounter for fitting and adjustment of complete left artificial arm
Z44.019	Encounter for fitting and adjustment of complete artificial arm, unspecified arm
Z44.021	Encounter for fitting and adjustment of partial artificial right arm
Z44.022	Encounter for fitting and adjustment of partial artificial left arm
Z44.029	Encounter for fitting and adjustment of partial artificial arm, unspecified arm
Z44.101	Encounter for fitting and adjustment of unspecified right artificial leg
Z44.102	Encounter for fitting and adjustment of unspecified left artifical leg
Z44.109	Encounter for fitting and adjustment of unspecified artificial leg, unspecified leg

Z44.111	Encounter for fitting and adjustment of complete right artificial leg
Z44.112	Encounter for fitting and adjustment of complete left artificial leg
Z44.119	Encounter for fitting and adjustment of complete artificial leg, unspecified leg
Z44.121	Encounter for fitting and adjustment of partial artificial right leg
Z44.122	Encounter for fitting and adjustment of partial artificial left leg
Z44.129	Encounter for fitting and adjustment of partial artificial leg, unspecified leg
Z47.1	Aftercare following joint replacement surgery
Z47.2	Encounter for removal of internal fixation device
Z47.31	Aftercare following explantation of shoulder joint prosthesis
Z47.32	Aftercare following explantation of hip joint prosthesis
Z47.33	Aftercare following explantation of knee joint prosthesis
Z47.81	Encounter for orthopedic aftercare following surgical amputation
Z47.82	Encounter for orthopedic aftercare following scoliosis surgery
Z47.89	Encounter for other orthopedic aftercare
Z52.20	Bone donor, unspecified
Z52.21	Bone donor, autologous
Z52.29	Bone donor, other
Z79.83	Long term (current) use of bisphosphonates
Z82.61	Family history of arthritis
Z82.62	Family history of osteoporosis
Z82.69	Family history of other diseases of the musculoskeletal system and connective tissue
Z87.310	Personal history of (healed) osteoporosis fracture
Z87.311	Personal history of (healed) other pathological fracture
Z87.312	Personal history of (healed) stress fracture
Z87.39	Personal history of other diseases of the musculoskeletal system and connective tissue
Z89.011	Acquired absence of right thumb
Z89.012	Acquired absence of left thumb
Z89.019	Acquired absence of unspecified thumb
Z89.021	Acquired absence of right finger(s)
Z89.022	Acquired absence of left finger(s)
Z89.029	Acquired absence of unspecified finger(s)
Z89.111	Acquired absence of right hand
Z89.112	Acquired absence of left hand
Z89.119	Acquired absence of unspecified hand
Z89.121	Acquired absence of right wrist
Z89.122	Acquired absence of left wrist
Z89.129	Acquired absence of unspecified wrist
Z89.201	Acquired absence of right upper limb, unspecified level
Z89.202	Acquired absence of left upper limb, unspecified level
Z89.209	Acquired absence of unspecified upper limb, unspecified level
Z89.211	Acquired absence of right upper limb below elbow
Z89.212	Acquired absence of left upper limb below elbow
Z89.219	Acquired absence of unspecified upper limb below elbow
Z89.221	Acquired absence of right upper limb above elbow
Z89.222	Acquired absence of left upper limb above elbow
Z89.229	Acquired absence of unspecified upper limb above elbow
Z89.231	Acquired absence of right shoulder
Z89.232	Acquired absence of left shoulder
Z89.239	Acquired absence of unspecified shoulder
Z89.411	Acquired absence of right great toe

Z89.412	Acquired absence of left great toe
Z89.419	Acquired absence of unspecified great toe
Z89.421	Acquired absence of other right toe(s)
Z89.422	Acquired absence of other left toe(s)
Z89.429	Acquired absence of other toe(s), unspecified side
Z89.431	Acquired absence of right foot
Z89.432	Acquired absence of left foot
Z89.439	Acquired absence of unspecified foot
Z89.441	Acquired absence of right ankle
Z89.442	Acquired absence of left ankle
Z89.449	Acquired absence of unspecified ankle
Z89.511	Acquired absence of right leg below knee
Z89.512	Acquired absence of left leg below knee
Z89.519	Acquired absence of unspecified leg below knee
Z89.521	Acquired absence of right knee
Z89.522	Acquired absence of left knee
Z89.529	Acquired absence of unspecified knee
Z89.611	Acquired absence of right leg above knee
Z89.612	Acquired absence of left leg above knee
Z89.619	Acquired absence of unspecified leg above knee
Z89.621	Acquired absence of right hip joint
Z89.622	Acquired absence of left hip joint
Z89.629	Acquired absence of unspecified hip joint
Z89.9	Acquired absence of limb, unspecified
Z94.6	Bone transplant status
Z96.60	Presence of unspecified orthopedic joint implant
Z96.611	Presence of right artificial shoulder joint
Z96.612	Presence of left artificial shoulder joint
Z96.619	Presence of unspecified artificial shoulder joint
Z96.621	Presence of right artificial elbow joint
Z96.622	Presence of left artificial elbow joint
Z96.629	Presence of unspecified artificial elbow joint
Z96.631	Presence of right artificial wrist joint
Z96.632	Presence of left artificial wrist joint
Z96.639	Presence of unspecified artificial wrist joint
Z96.641	Presence of right artificial hip joint
Z96.642	Presence of left artificial hip joint
Z96.643	Presence of artificial hip joint, bilateral
Z96.649	Presence of unspecified artificial hip joint
Z96.651	Presence of right artificial knee joint
Z96.652	Presence of left artificial knee joint
Z96.653	Presence of artificial knee joint, bilateral
Z96.659	Presence of unspecified artificial knee joint
Z96.661	Presence of right artificial ankle joint
Z96.662	Presence of left artificial ankle joint
Z96.669	Presence of unspecified artificial ankle joint
Z96.691	Finger-joint replacement of right hand
Z96.692	Finger-joint replacement of left hand
Z96.693	Finger-joint replacement, bilateral
Z96.698	Presence of other orthopedic joint implants
Z96.7	Presence of other bone and tendon implants
Z97.10	Presence of artificial limb (complete) (partial), unspecified

Z97.11	Presence of artificial right arm (complete) (partial)
Z97.12	Presence of artificial left arm (complete) (partial)
Z97.13	Presence of artificial right leg (complete) (partial)
Z97.14	Presence of artificial left leg (complete) (partial)
Z97.15	Presence of artificial arms, bilateral (complete) (partial)
Z97.16	Presence of artificial legs, bilateral (complete) (partial)
Z98.1	Arthrodesis status

EXAMPLE   Patient is status post bilateral knee replacements 1 year ago, Z96.653.

EXAMPLE   Patient with a family history of rheumatoid arthritis is being screened for rheumatoid arthritis, Z13.828, Z82.61.

EXERCISE 19-7

Assign codes to the following conditions.

1. Status post right knee replacement   _____

2. Dual-energy x-ray absorptiometry (DEXA) scan screening for osteoporosis   _____

3. Amputation status right foot   _____

4. Encounter to remove screw from left tibia. Previous fracture left tibial shaft.   _____

5. Previous amputation, left great toe   _____

COMMON TREATMENTS

Many conditions or diseases of the musculoskeletal system cause pain and inflammation. Anti-inflammatory agents reduce inflammation in joints and muscles, antiarthritics are used to treat arthritic symptoms, and muscle relaxants may be helpful for acute low back pain and muscle spasms. Physical therapy and chiropractic treatment may be beneficial for many conditions. Medical treatment is usually tried before surgical intervention is considered.

CONDITION	MEDICATION/TREATMENT
Rheumatoid arthritis	Celecoxib (Celebrex), gold compounds such as Ridaura and Myochrysine
Osteoarthritis	Analgesics
	Nonsteroidal anti-inflammatory drugs (NSAIDs) for pain and inflammation (aspirin, ibuprofen [Motrin, Advil], nabumetone [Relafen], naproxen [Aleve, Naprosyn], diclofenac [Voltaren], indomethacin [Indocin], etodolac [Lodine], oxaprozin [Daypro], celecoxib [Celebrex])
Fibromyalgia	Analgesics for pain, muscle relaxants, antidepressants, and sleep aids
Bursitis	Rest, immobilization, ice, NSAIDs
Necrotizing fasciitis	Aggressive antibiotic therapy with surgical debridement
Osteomyelitis	Antibiotics depending on causative organism
Osteoporosis	Alendronate (Fosamax), Boniva (ibandronate), calcitonin, calcium with vitamin D

PROCEDURES

Procedures related to the musculoskeletal system and connective tissue in ICD-10-PCS can be located in the following tables:

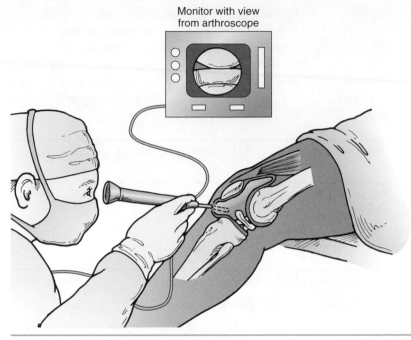

FIGURE 19-13. Arthroscopic examination of a joint.

0K2-0KX	Muscles
0L2-0LX	Tendons
0M2-0MX	Bursae and Ligaments
0N2-0NW	Head and Facial Bones
0P2-0PW	Upper Bones
0Q2-0QW	Lower Bones
0R2-0RW	Upper Joints
0S2-0S2	Lower Joints

Arthroscopic Surgery

Arthroscopic surgery is a minimally invasive surgery that involves the use of highly specialized instruments to perform surgery through very small incisions (½ inch) on joints. Advantages of arthroscopic surgery include small incisions, minimal scar tissue, and less pain after surgery with quicker recovery. Arthroscopic procedures can be performed on any of the joints and joint structures. Occasionally, an arthroscopic procedure is performed for diagnostic purposes, and no additional therapeutic procedures are performed (Figure 19-13). The root operation for a diagnostic arthroscopic examination is inspection (visual/manual exploration).

EXAMPLE Arthroscopic examination of the left knee for chronic pain. All joint structures appear to be intact, M25.562, 0SJD4ZZ.

EXAMPLE Arthroscopic meniscectomy (partial) for torn right medial meniscus (old injury), M23.203, 0SBC4ZZ.

Joint Replacement

Joint replacement consists of removal of an arthritic or damaged joint and replacement with an artificial joint, which is also known as a prosthesis. Materials used in total joint replacement are designed to enable the joint to move similarly to a normal joint. The root operation for a total joint replacement is replacement (putting in or on biologic or synthetic material that replaces a body part). The prosthesis is generally composed of two parts; a

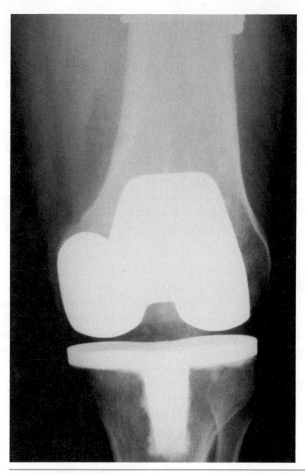

FIGURE 19-14. Total knee replacement for osteoarthritis.

metal piece fits closely into a matching sturdy plastic piece (Figure 19-14). Several metals, including stainless steel, alloys of cobalt and chrome, and titanium, are used. The plastic material is durable and wear-resistant (polyethylene). A plastic bone cement may be used to anchor the prosthesis into the bone. Hip and knee replacements are the most common joint replacements, but other joints, including the ankle, foot, shoulder, elbow, and fingers, can be replaced. In cases in which the disease process does not affect the entire joint, partial joint replacement may be performed. Other options besides total joint replacement procedures are available. A resurfacing procedure may be an option. A surface replacement procedure leaves more of the patient's bone in place with resurfacing of the affected area of the joint. As with replacement procedures, resurfacing can involve partial or total joint resurfacing. The root operation for a resurfacing procedure is supplement (putting in a device that reinforces or augments a body part).

Common complications of joint replacement include infection, blood clot, nerve injury, loosening, dislocation, wear and tear, and breakage of the prosthesis. It may be necessary to remove the prosthesis and insert a new prosthesis.

EXAMPLE | Primary osteoarthritis both knees. Patient is hospitalized for right partial knee replacement (femoral surface) with synthetic substitute, M17.0, OSRTOJZ.

Vertebroplasty/Kyphoplasty

Percutaneous vertebroplasty (PV) is a technique that is used to treat pain caused by compression fractures of the vertebrae. The root operation for a vertebroplasty is supplement (putting in a device that reinforces or augments a body part). Under x-ray guidance, an acrylic cement is injected through a needle into a collapsed or weakened vertebra. This stabilizes the fracture, allowing the patient to resume normal activity and decrease the use of analgesics. PV does not reverse osteoporosis or prevent future compression fractures. This procedure is usually performed by interventional radiologists.

Kyphoplasty, similar to PV, is used to treat fractures of the spine; however, in kyphoplasty, a special balloon device is inserted into the compacted vertebrae in an attempt to restore vertebrae to a more normal state by improving the alignment of the spine. The root operations for a kyphoplasty are reposition (moving to its normal or other suitable location some or all of a body part) and supplement (putting in a device that reinforces or augments a body part). After the balloon has been removed, the cavity is filled with a cement-like material to stabilize the fracture. Kyphoplasty is usually performed under fluoroscopic guidance through a small incision in the back.

EXAMPLE	Compression fractures T11-T12 due to osteoporosis. Percutaneous vertebroplasty (synthetic substitute) was performed in radiology, M80.08xA, 0PU43JZ.

Fusion Procedures of the Spine

Spinal decompression is a surgical procedure that frees space for nerves in the spinal canal. A number of different surgical methods, including laminectomy, laminotomy, laminoplasty, foraminotomy, and anterior discectomy, can be performed to accomplish a decompression. Although in many cases decompression involves removal of tissue that is constricting or compressing nerve structures, in some cases, the spine becomes unstable and spinal fusion is performed at the time of the decompression.

Spinal fusion is the creation of a solid bone bridge between two or more adjacent vertebrae to create stability between levels of the spine. The root operation for spinal fusion or refusion is fusion (rendering a joint immobile). Fusion is a gradual process (6 to 9 months or longer) in which bone is grown across desired areas to form a solid fusion. Bone grafts, interbody fusion, and other devices are used to facilitate and promote the fusion process. If a fusion fails to heal or fuse properly, this is called a nonunion or pseudarthrosis; repeat or refusion procedure may be required. A bone graft may be obtained from a variety of sources. Bone may be harvested from the patient's (autologous) spine or from the iliac crest. Bone graft material can also be obtained from a bone bank (harvested from cadavers [allograft]). Synthetic bone materials made from demineralized bone matrix (DBM) and calcium phosphates or hydroxyapatites (some derived from sea coral) may also be used. The use of metal devices (e.g. screws, rods, plates, cables, wires) can facilitate correction of a deformed spine and may increase the probability of attaining solid spinal fusion. Spinal instrumentation can be placed in the front or in the back portion of the spine. Devices are usually made of metal, commonly stainless steel or titanium. Spinal instrumentation is gradually covered by scar tissue and sometimes by new growth of bone. Even when the spine has healed solidly, the instrumentation is rarely removed. A 360-degree spinal fusion is a spinal fusion of both the anterior and posterior portions of the spine during the same operative episode. Using a lateral transverse approach, both the anterior and posterior vertebral columns can be operated on through a single incision. Sometimes a spinal fusion is performed as a "staged procedure" with a posterior fusion performed one day and an anterior fusion is performed a few days later.

During any spinal fusion procedure, the documentation should be reviewed to ascertain the site of the fusion, the operative approach, any device used, and whether the fusion was on the anterior or posterior column of the spine (Figure 19-15).

There are some PCS guidelines specific to spinal fusions that state:

- The body part coded for a spinal vertebral joint(s) rendered immobile by a spinal fusion procedure is classified by the level of the spine (e.g. thoracic). There are distinct body part values for a single vertebral joint and for multiple vertebral joints at each spinal level.

EXAMPLE:	Body part values specify lumbar vertebral joint, lumbar vertebral joints, 2 or more, and lumbosacral vertebral joint.

SECTION: 0 MEDICAL AND SURGICAL
BODY SYSTEM: S LOWER JOINTS
OPERATION: G FUSION: Joining together portions of an articular body part, rendering the articular body part immobile

Body Part	Approach	Device	Qualifier
0 Lumbar Vertebral Joint 1 Lumbar Vertebral Joint, 2-4 3 Lumbosacral Joint	0 Open 3 Percutaneous 4 Percutaneous Endoscopic	3 Interbody Internal Fixation Device 4 Internal Fixation Device 7 Autologous Tissue Substitute H Interbody Synthetic Substitute J Synthetic Substitute K Nonautologous Tissue Substitute N Interbody Nonautologous Tissue Substitute Z No Device	0 Anterior Approach, Anterior Column 1 Posterior Approach, Posterior Column J Posterior Approach, Anterior Column K Lateral Transverse Process Approach, Posterior Column
5 Sacrococcygeal Joint 6 Coccygeal Joint 7 Sacroiliac Joint, Right 8 Sacroiliac Joint, Left	0 Open 3 Percutaneous 4 Percutaneous Endoscopic	4 Internal Fixation Device 7 Autologous Tissue Substitute J Synthetic Substitute K Nonautologous Tissue Substitute Z No Device	Z No Qualifier
9 Hip Joint, Right B Hip Joint, Left C Knee Joint, Right D Knee Joint, Left F Ankle Joint, Right G Ankle Joint, Left H Tarsal Joint, Right J Tarsal Joint, Left K Metatarsal-Tarsal Joint, Right L Metatarsal-Tarsal Joint, Left M Metatarsal-Phalangeal Joint, Right N Metatarsal-Phalangeal Joint, Left P Toe Phalangeal Joint, Right Q Toe Phalangeal Joint, Left	0 Open 3 Percutaneous 4 Percutaneous Endoscopic	4 Internal Fixation Device 5 External Fixation Device 7 Autologous Tissue Substitute J Synthetic Substitute K Nonautologous Tissue Substitute Z No Device	Z No Qualifier

FIGURE 19-15. Table used to code lumbar fusion.

■   If multiple vertebral joints are fused, a separate procedure is coded for each vertebral joint that uses a different device and/or qualifier.

EXAMPLE: Fusion of lumbar vertebral joint, posterior approach, anterior column, and fusion of lumbar vertebral joint, posterior approach, posterior column, are coded separately.

■   Combinations of devices and materials are often used on a vertebral joint to render the joint immobile. When combinations of devices are used on the same vertebral joint, the device value coded for the procedure is as follows:
  • If an interbody fusion device is used to render the joint immobile (alone or containing other material like bone graft), the procedure is coded with the device value Interbody Fusion Device.

- If bone graft is the only device used to render the joint immobile, the procedure is coded with the device value Nonautologous Tissue Substitute or Autologous Tissue Substitute.
- If a mixture of autologous and nonautologous bone graft (with or without biological or synthetic extenders or binders) is used to render the joint immobile, code the procedure with the device value Autologous Tissue Substitute. Fusion of a vertebral joint using a cage-style interbody fusion device containing morselized bone graft is coded to the device Interbody Fusion Device.
- Fusion of a vertebral joint using a bone dowel interbody fusion device made of cadaver bone and packed with a mixture of local morselized bone and demineralized bone matrix is coded to the device Interbody Fusion Device.
- Fusion of a vertebral joint using both autologous bone graft and bone bank bone graft is coded to the device Autologous Tissue Substitute.

EXAMPLE
> The patient was admitted for surgical intervention for cervical disc herniation with myelopathy. Partial discectomy at C3 and spinal fusion of C3-C4 and C4-C5 were performed via the anterior approach (anterior column) using interbody fusion device, M50.02, 0RG20A0, 0RB30ZZ.

EXERCISE 19-8

Assign codes for all diagnoses and procedures.

1. Open bone biopsy left upper femur, which confirmed acute   _____
   and chronic osteomyelitis
2. Excision Baker's cyst, right   _____
3. Open partial hip replacement (femoral head) for OA right hip   _____
   with metallic prosthesis
4. Removal of fixation device lumbar spine   _____
5. Arthroscopy right knee. Mild osteoarthritis   _____
6. Necrotizing fasciitis with excisional debridement of   _____
   subcutaneous tissue and fascia, right forearm
7. Pathologic fracture T12 due to postmenopausal osteoporosis.   _____
   Percutaneous kyphoplasty with synthetic substitute was
   performed

DOCUMENTATION/REIMBURSEMENT/MS-DRGs

Often, coding difficulties are due to lack of documentation. Sometimes pathology, radiology, and other test results are not available at the time of discharge or when the physician is dictating the discharge summary or is reporting the final diagnoses.

Frequently missed complications/comorbidities from this chapter include:

- Avascular necrosis
- Pathologic fractures
- Malunion/nonunion of fracture

Pathologic Fracture versus Traumatic Fracture

EXAMPLE Patient was admitted from the Emergency Room with a fractured right hip. The patient has severe osteoporosis and had fallen on the morning of admission.

DIAGNOSES	CODES	MS-DRG	RW
Pathologic fracture hip due to osteoporosis	M80.051A	544	0.7660
Traumatic fracture hip in patient with osteoporosis	S72.001A, M81.0, W19.xxxA	536	0.7256

A physician query may be necessary to make sure that the appropriate MS-DRG is assigned for optimal reimbursement.

Correct Procedure Code

EXAMPLE Patient was admitted for resurfacing of left femoral head with resurfacing device due to primary osteoarthritis.

DIAGNOSES	CODES	MS-DRG	RW
Osteoarthritis hip	M16.12	470	2.0866
Resurfacing femoral	0SUS0BZ		
Osteoarthritis hip	M16.12	468	2.5700
Revision hip replacement, femoral component	0QP70JZ, 0QR70JZ		

In this example, an error was made when resurfacing of the femoral head was coded as a revision. This error would have resulted in an overpayment to the facility.

CHAPTER REVIEW EXERCISE

Assign codes for all diagnoses and procedures.

1. Osteitis deformans of skull _____

2. Wry neck _____

3. Hallux valgus, left big toe _____

4. Frozen right shoulder _____

5. Plantar fasciitis _____

6. Recurrent dislocation right thumb _____

7. Osteoporosis due to long-term use of steroids _____

8. Instability left ankle _____

9. Ganglion tendon sheath of the right wrist with removal _____

10. Tennis elbow, right _____

11. Polymyalgia rheumatica _____

12. Myositis _____

13. Pain in both wrists _____

14. Avascular necrosis (left femur) due to sickle cell (hemoglobin SS) disease _____

15. Stiffness, left elbow _____

16. History of right above the knee amputation (AKA) _____

17. Housemaid's knee (right) _____

18. Scleroderma with lung involvement _____

19. Arthropathy due to Crohn's disease _____

20. Felty's syndrome, right hand _____

21. Pyogenic arthritis left knee due to *Staphylococcus aureus* _____

22. Osteoarthritis right shoulder treated with intra-articular steroid injection _____

23. Paget's disease, left femur _____

24. Chondromalacia right patella _____

Write the correct answer(s) in the blank(s) provided.

25. Explain the difference between radiculopathy and myelopathy.

_____

26. Which MS-DRG has higher reimbursement: pathologic fracture or traumatic fracture?

_____

Why? _____

27. Another name for osteoarthritis.

_____

28. List 4 symptoms of SLE.

1. _____

2. _____

3. _____

4. _____

29. Which individuals are at risk for osteoporosis?

_____

30. List 3 examples of aftercare for a pathologic fracture.

1. _____

2. _____

3. _____

CHAPTER GLOSSARY

Anterior: front of the body or an organ.

Arthropathy: disease that affects the joints.

Arthroscopic: minimally invasive surgery that involves the use of highly specialized instruments to perform surgery through very small incisions on joints.

Bursitis: inflammation of a bursa, which is a tiny, fluid-filled sac that is found between muscles, tendons, and bones that reduces friction and facilitates movement.

Caudal: toward the tail.

Cranial: toward the head.

Distal: farther from the median plane; term is often used to describe a location in the limbs.

Dorsal: back of the body or an organ.

Dorsopathies: conditions or diseases that affect the back or spine.

Facet joints: small, stabilizing joints located between and behind adjacent vertebrae.

Fascia: tissue just below the skin that covers and separates the underlying layers of muscle.

Fibromyalgia: one of the most common diseases affecting the muscles; it is characterized by widespread muscle pain associated with chronic fatigue.

Hematopoiesis: development of blood cells that occurs in the bone marrow and lymphatic tissue of normal adults.

Inferior: position of the body or an organ relative to the vertical axis of the body.

Joints: means of joining two bones together.

Juvenile rheumatoid arthritis: type of arthritis that affects children, usually between the ages of 2 and 5 years.

Kyphoplasty: procedure performed to treat and stabilize fractures of the spine.

Kyphosis: excessive posterior curvature of the thoracic spine that may not be detected until a hump in the upper back is noticeable.

Lateral: position of a structure that is to the side of the body.

Ligaments: dense, fibrous bands of connective tissue that provide stability for the joint.

Lordosis: exaggerated inward curvature of the spine that may be caused by increased abdominal girth due to obesity, pregnancy, or abdominal tumor.

Medial: position of a structure closer to the median plane than is another structure in the body.

Myelopathy: compression of the spinal cord.

Necrotizing fasciitis (or "flesh-eating disease"): a rare but serious condition in which an infection occurs in the tissues below the skin.

Osteoarthritis: type of arthritis that develops as the result of wear and tear on the joints.

Osteomyelitis: infection of the bone that often starts in another part of the body and spreads to the bone via the blood.

Osteoporosis: metabolic bone disorder that results in decreased bone mass and density.

Pathologic fracture: break in a bone that occurs because of underlying disorders that weaken the bone, including malignancy, benign bone tumor, metabolic disorder, infection, and osteoporosis.

Percutaneous vertebroplasty: technique in which x-ray guidance is used to inject an acrylic cement through a needle into a collapsed or weakened vertebra; procedure is performed to treat pain caused by compression fractures of the vertebrae.

Polymyalgia rheumatica: syndrome classified as a rheumatic disease that is characterized by severe aching and stiffness in the neck, shoulder girdle, and pelvic girdle.

Posterior: back of the body or an organ.

Primary osteoarthritis: idiopathic degenerative condition that occurs in previously intact joints, with no apparent initiating factor.

Prone: lying on the stomach, face down.

Proximal: closer to the median plane.

Radiculopathy: compression of a nerve root.

Rheumatoid arthritis: chronic, inflammatory systemic disease that affects the joints, often causing deformity.

Scleroderma: chronic, progressive disease characterized by hardening of the skin and scarring of internal organs.

Scoliosis: deviation of the vertical line of the spine.

Secondary osteoarthritis: degenerative disease of the joints that results from some predisposing condition such as trauma or disease.

Spinal decompression: surgical procedure that frees space for the nerves in the spinal canal.

Spinal fusion: the creation of a solid bone bridge between two or more adjacent vertebrae to enhance stability between levels of the spine.

Spinal stenosis: narrowing of the central spinal canal or the areas of the spine where the nerve roots exit (neuroforamina).

Spondylolisthesis: condition in which one vertebra slips on another.

Spondylosis (or spinal osteoarthritis): degenerative disorder that may cause loss of normal spinal structure and function.

Superior: position of the body or an organ relative to the vertical axis of the body.

Supine: lying on the back, face up.

Systemic lupus erythematosus: chronic, inflammatory autoimmune disease that can damage connective tissue anywhere in the body.

Tendons: connective tissue that attaches muscle to bone.

Ventral: front of the body or an organ.

20

Diseases of the Genitourinary System

(ICD-10-CM Chapter 14, Codes N00-N99)

LEARNING OBJECTIVES

1. Apply and assign the correct ICD-10-CM/PCS codes in accordance with Official Guidelines for Coding and Reporting
2. Identify major differences between ICD-10-CM and ICD-9-CM related to the genitourinary system
3. Identify pertinent anatomy and physiology of diseases of the genitourinary system

4. Identify diseases of the genitourinary system
5. Assign the correct Z codes and procedure codes related to the genitourinary system
6. Identify common treatments, medications, laboratory values, and diagnostic tests
7. Explain the importance of documentation in relation to MS-DRGs for reimbursement

**ABBREVIATIONS/
ACRONYMS**

ARF acute renal failure

ARI acute renal insufficiency

AV arteriovenous

BUN blood urea nitrogen

CAPD continuous ambulatory peritoneal dialysis

CC chief complaint

CCPD continuous cycling peritoneal dialysis

CIN cervical intraepithelial neoplasia

CKD chronic kidney disease

CRF chronic renal failure

CRI chronic renal insufficiency

D&C dilatation and curettage

DIEP deep inferior epigastric perforator

ESRD end-stage renal disease

ESWL extracorporeal shock wave lithotripsy

FSG focal segmental glomerulosclerosis

GAP gluteal artery perforator

GFR glomerular filtration rate

GN glomerulonephritis

HSIL high-grade squamous intraepithelial lesion

ICD-9-CM *International Classification of Diseases, 9th Revision, Clinical Modification*

ICD-10-CM *International Classification of Diseases, 10th Revision, Clinical Modification*

ICD-10-PCS *International Classification of Diseases, 10th Revision, Procedure Coding System*

Ig immunoglobulin

LAVH laparoscopically assisted vaginal hysterectomy

LDMF latissimus dorsi musculocutaneous flap

LSIL low-grade squamous intraepithelial lesion

LUTS lower urinary tract symptoms

MRSA methicillin-resistant *Staphylococcus aureus*

MS-DRG Medicare Severity diagnosis-related group

NEC not elsewhere classifiable

NKF National Kidney Foundation

NOS not otherwise specified

OIG Office of the Inspector General

PID pelvic inflammatory disease

PSA prostate-specific antigen

RPGN rapidly progressive glomerulonephritis

SIEA superficial inferior epigastric artery

SIL squamous intraepithelial lesion

TRAM transverse rectus abdominis musculocutaneous

TULIP transurethral ultrasound-guided laser-induced prostatectomy

TUMT transurethral microwave thermotherapy

TUNA transurethral needle ablation of prostate

TURP transurethral resection of the prostate

UHDDS Uniform Hospital Discharge Data Set

UTI urinary tract infection

VIN vulvular intraepithelial neoplasia

VLAP visual laser ablation of the prostate

VUR vesicoureteral reflux

ICD-10-CM

Official Guidelines for Coding and Reporting

Please refer to the companion Evolve website for the most current guidelines.

14. Chapter 14: Diseases of Genitourinary System (N00-N99)

  a. Chronic kidney disease

    1) Stages of chronic kidney disease (CKD)

      The ICD-10-CM classifies CKD based on severity. The severity of CKD is designated by stages 1-5. Stage 2, code N18.2, equates to mild CKD; stage 3, code N18.3, equates to moderate CKD; and stage 4, code N18.4, equates to severe CKD. Code N18.6, End stage renal disease (ESRD), is assigned when the provider has documented end-stage-renal disease (ESRD).

      If both a stage of CKD and ESRD are documented, assign code N18.6 only.

EXAMPLE

Patient was admitted to the hospital for fluid overload due to noncompliance with attending renal dialysis sessions. Patient has stage 5 CKD. Hemodialysis was performed, E87.70, N18.6, Z91.15, 5A1D00Z.

2) Chronic kidney disease and kidney transplant status
Patients who have undergone kidney transplant may still have some form of chronic kidney disease (CKD) because the kidney transplant may not fully restore kidney function. Therefore, the presence of CKD alone does not constitute a transplant complication. Assign the appropriate N18 code for the patient's stage of CKD and code Z94.0, Kidney transplant status. If a transplant complication such as failure or rejection or other transplant complication is documented, see section I.C.19.g for information on coding complications of a kidney transplant. If the documentation is unclear as to whether the patient has a complication of the transplant, query the provider.

EXAMPLE   Patient had a kidney transplant last year but still has mild CKD, stage 2, N18.2, Z94.0.

3) Chronic kidney disease with other conditions
Patients with CKD may also suffer from other serious conditions, most commonly diabetes mellitus and hypertension. The sequencing of the CKD code in relationship to codes for other contributing conditions is based on the conventions in the Tabular List.
See I.C.9. Hypertensive chronic kidney disease.
See I.C.19. Chronic kidney disease and kidney transplant complications.

EXAMPLE   Patient has chronic kidney disease due to hypertension, I12.9, N18.9.

Apply the General Coding Guidelines as found in Chapter 5 and the Procedural Coding Guidelines as found in Chapters 6 and 7.

MAJOR DIFFERENCES BETWEEN ICD-10-CM AND ICD-9-CM

- In ICD-10-CM the various stages of dysplasia of the vagina are identified.
- In ICD-10-CM laterality is used to identify conditions under the N60 category, benign mammary dysplasia.
- Procedural complications affecting the genitourinary system are included in Chapter 14 of ICD-10-CM. Some of the complications include:
  - Postprocedural renal failure
  - Postprocedural urethral stricture
  - Prolapse of the vaginal vault after hysterectomy
  - Complications of urinary tract stoma
  - Intraoperative hemorrhage, hematoma, or accidental laceration

ANATOMY AND PHYSIOLOGY

Urinary Tract

The kidneys, ureters, urinary bladder, and urethra form the urinary tract (Figure 20-1). Its main function involves producing, storing, and excreting urine. The kidneys and ureters make up the upper urinary tract, and the bladder and urethra constitute the lower urinary

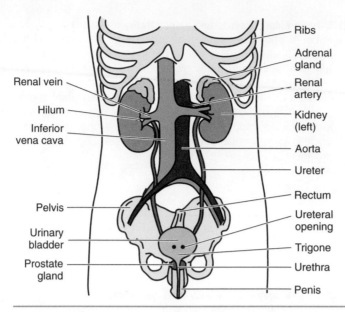

FIGURE 20-1. Gross anatomy of the urinary system (male).

tract. The kidneys are two bean-shaped organs that are located on either side of the spine or retroperitoneally. The kidneys form a complex filtration system that cleanses the blood of waste products that become urine. Each kidney has a ureter that allows the urine to travel to the bladder for storage. The bladder is expandable, and openings into the ureters close so that urine cannot flow backward or reflux into the kidneys. The urine is excreted out of the body through a tube called the urethra. It is easy to confuse the terminology for urethra and ureter. Less than half of a single kidney is needed to do all the work that can be accomplished by two kidneys. The main difference between the male and female urinary tracts is the length of the urethra. The male urethra is 20 cm long; the female urethra measures only 3 cm.

Male Genital Tract

The main parts of the male genital or reproductive tract are the testes, epididymis, vas deferens, seminal vesicles, prostate, and penis (Figure 20-2). Its primary function is the production of sperm. The main diseases related to the male genital tract are infertility, infection, and tumor.

Female Genital Tract

The main parts of the female genital or reproductive tract are the vulva, vagina, uterus, fallopian tubes, and ovaries (Figure 20-3). Reproduction is its primary function. The main diseases and conditions of the female genital tract are related to infection, tumor, hormonal disorders, and pregnancy.

Breast

Male and female breasts are similar in that they are formed embryologically from the same tissues. It is possible for males to have breast disorders also. The female breast (Figure 20-4) will start to develop during puberty due to the hormone estrogen. Female breasts are considered an accessory organ of reproduction and are composed of fat and fibrous tissue with mammary glands for the production of milk (**lactation**).

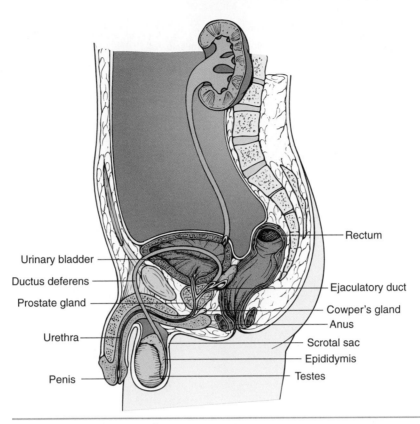

FIGURE 20-2. Normal male reproductive system.

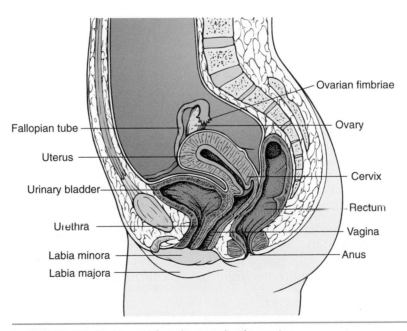

FIGURE 20-3. Normal female reproductive system.

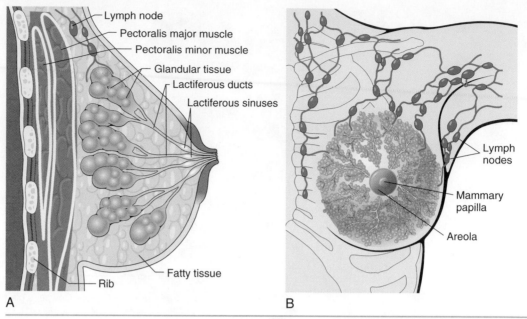

FIGURE 20-4. Views of the breast. **A,** Sagittal. **B,** Frontal. Notice the numerous lymph nodes.

DISEASE CONDITIONS

It is important to note that disorders of the breast are classified as Diseases of the Genitourinary System in ICD-10-CM.

Diseases of the Genitourinary System, Chapter 11 in the ICD-10-CM code book, are divided into the following categories:

CATEGORY	SECTION TITLES
N00-N08	Glomerular diseases
N10-N16	Renal tubulo-interstitial diseases
N17-N19	Acute renal failure and chronic kidney disease
N20-N23	Urolithiasis
N25-N29	Other disorders of the kidney and ureter
N30-N39	Other diseases of the urinary system
N40-N51	Diseases of male genital organs
N60-N65	Disorders of the breast
N70-N77	Inflammatory diseases of female pelvic organs
N80-N98	Noninflammatory disorders of the female genital tract
N99	Intraoperative and postprocedural complications and disorders of genitourinary system, not elsewhere classified

Glomerular Diseases (N00-N08)

Nephritic Syndrome/Nephrotic Syndrome

Nephrotic syndrome is a condition that is marked by **proteinuria** (protein in the urine), low levels of protein in the blood, hypercholesterolemia, and swelling of the eyes, feet, and hands. Damage to the kidneys' glomeruli can result in nephrotic syndrome. Treatment focuses on identifying the underlying cause and reducing cholesterol, blood pressure, and protein in urine through diet and medications.

EXAMPLE Acute nephritic syndrome with extracapillary glomerulonephritis, N00.7.

Glomerulonephritis

Glomerulonephritis (GN) (Figure 20-5) is inflammation of the glomeruli of the kidneys. (See Figure 20-6 for illustration of the anatomy of the kidney.) Glomerulonephritis can be a temporary, reversible condition, or it may be a chronic progressive condition that results in chronic renal failure and end-stage renal disease. GN may cause hypertension and may not be discovered until the hypertension becomes difficult to control. Specific disorders that are associated with glomerulonephritis include the following:

- Focal segmental glomerulosclerosis (FSG)
- Goodpasture's syndrome
- Immunoglobulin (Ig)A nephropathy (Berger's disease)
- IgM mesangial proliferative glomerulonephritis
- Lupus nephritis
- Membranoproliferative glomerulonephritis I
- Membranoproliferative glomerulonephritis II
- Poststreptococcal glomerulonephritis
- Rapidly progressive (crescentic) glomerulonephritis
- Rapidly progressive glomerulonephritis (RPGN)

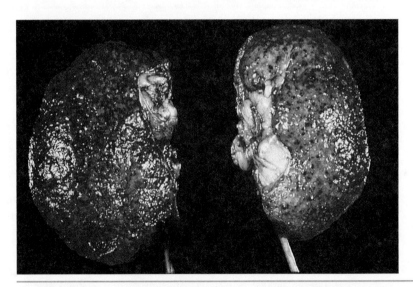

FIGURE 20-5. End-stage glomerulopathy–chronic glomerulonephritis.

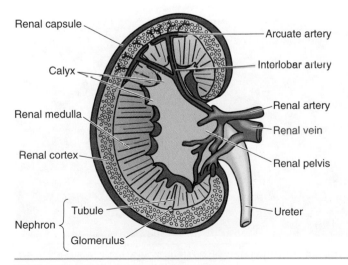

FIGURE 20-6. Anatomy of the kidney.

EXAMPLE | Minimal change glomerulonephritis, N05.0.

EXAMPLE | RPGN, N01.9.

EXERCISE 20-1

Assign codes to the following conditions.

1. Nephrotic syndrome _____

2. Nephritis due to lupus _____

3. Focal segmental glomerulonephritis _____

Renal Tubulo-Interstitial Diseases (N10-N16)

Renal tubulo-interstitial diseases involve the structures in the kidney outside the glomerulus. These conditions generally affect the tubules and/or the interstitium of the kidney and not the glomeruli. Some of the more common conditions in this section include acute pyelo-nephritis, hydronephrosis, and vesicoureteral reflux.

Pyelonephritis involves the kidneys and is an upper urinary tract infection. The most common cause is due to organisms from the intestinal tract (E. coli and *Enterococcus faecalis*) entering the urinary tract. It may initially start out as a lower urinary tract infection such as cystitis or prostatitis. Common symptoms include:

• Dysuria
• Flank pain
• Costovertebral angle tenderness

Chronic, recurrent infections can result in damage and scarring of the kidneys (Figure 20-7). In patients with recurrent infections, it may be necessary to do further testing to determine if there are some structural abnormalities such as vesicoureteral reflux, polycystic disease, or some other cause.

EXAMPLE | Patient was seen in the ER with flank pain and dysuria. Patient was given antibiotics for acute pyelonephritis, N10.

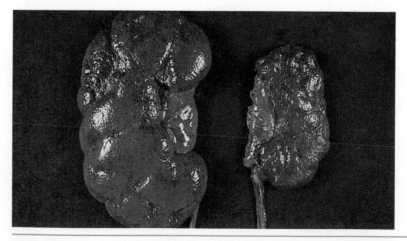

FIGURE 20-7. Small, shrunken, irregularly scarred kidney of a patient with chronic pyelonephritis. The other kidney is of normal size but has scarring on the upper pole.

Vesicoureteral reflux (VUR) is an abnormality in the flow of urine from the bladder into the ureters and/or kidneys. The normal flow is from the kidneys through the ureter into the bladder. In VUR the urine flows backwards. Damage to the kidney(s) may occur depending of the severity of the reflux and other complications such as recurrent urinary tract infections.

EXAMPLE   Patient is being followed by a urologist for VUR with nephropathy of the right kidney, N13.721.

Hydronephrosis is abnormal dilatation of the renal pelvis that is caused by pressure from urine that cannot flow past an obstruction in the urinary tract (Figure 20-8). **Hydroureter** is the accumulation of urine in the ureters. These conditions may be documented in x-ray reports, ultrasound, or other diagnostic tests, but they must be documented by a physician before code assignment. Obstruction can result from a stone, tumor, infection, prostatic hypertrophy, or congenital abnormalities.

EXAMPLE   Hydronephrosis due to ureterolithiasis, N13.2.

EXERCISE 20-2

Assign codes to the following conditions.

1. Acute and chronic pyelonephritis due to *Pseudomonas*   _____
2. Hydronephrosis due to kinking of ureter   _____
3. Bilateral VUR with hydroureter   _____
4. Obstructive uropathy   _____

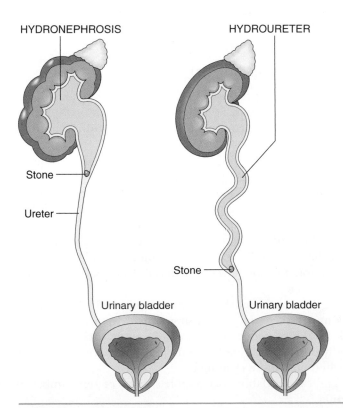

FIGURE 20-8. Hydronephrosis caused by a stone (obstruction) in the proximal part of the ureter and hydroureter with hydronephrosis caused by a stone in the distal part of the ureter.

Acute Renal Failure and Chronic Kidney Disease (N17-N19) and Urolithiasis (N20-N23)

Acute Renal Failure

Acute renal failure (ARF) is sudden and severe impairment in renal function characterized by oliguria, increased serum urea, and acidosis. With treatment, ARF is usually reversible. ARF often occurs in hospitalized patients with serious systemic illness such as infection, low blood pressure, shock, and as an adverse effect of the use of certain antibiotics and drugs. Obstruction of the urinary tract and dehydration may also cause ARF. It is possible for a patient with chronic renal failure or chronic kidney disease to also develop ARF. In this case, codes are assigned for both the acute and chronic renal failure.

If a patient is admitted for multiple reasons including ARF, the guidelines for principal diagnosis selection need to be applied. Often times, the acute renal failure is a result of another condition and should be coded as a secondary diagnosis.

EXAMPLE Patient is admitted with an exacerbation of congestive heart failure. The patient is also in acute renal failure. This physician documents that the ARF is due to the patient's fluid overload, I50.9, N17.9.

When a patient is admitted to the hospital with acute renal failure and dehydration, according to *Coding Clinic for ICD-9-CM* (2002:3Q:p21-22),[1] ARF is the principal diagnosis, and the dehydration is a secondary diagnosis. Patients with both conditions are generally treated with IV fluids, and ARF is more serious than dehydration. A patient who is dehydrated and has no impairment in renal function may be given IV fluids and sent home instead of being admitted to the hospital.

EXAMPLE Acute renal failure due to dehydration, N17.9, E86.0.

Chronic Kidney Disease (CKD)

Codes for chronic kidney disease (CKD) identify the various stages of CKD that were developed by the National Kidney Foundation (NKF) (Table 20-1). In the past, CKD has been documented with imprecise terms such as chronic kidney failure (CRF) and chronic renal insufficiency (CRI).

Using these NKF guidelines, levels of kidney damage and kidney function must be determined to accurately assign the code for CKD. A patient's glomerular filtration rate (GFR) indicates the level of kidney function and indicates the stage of the disease, which may progress slowly over many years. Early detection through laboratory tests and proper treatment can limit the effects of CKD, if the disease is discovered in the early stages.

If CKD is left untreated, a patient will develop end-stage renal disease (ESRD). This condition is characterized by the near or complete failure of kidney function, which leaves the patient unable to process waste material. Dialysis or transplantation may be needed to treat the condition.

CKD can develop from ARF if renal function is not restored through dialysis or treatment. This may take several weeks or months. Documentation in the health record that might indicate the presence of renal failure could include the following:
1. Markedly elevated values of serum creatinine or blood urea nitrogen (BUN), or diminished creatinine clearance
2. Other clinical and laboratory manifestations of renal impairment are as follows:
   * Anemia
   * Hyperphosphatemia
   * Hypocalcemia

TABLE 20-1 FIVE STAGES OF CHRONIC KIDNEY DISEASE

Stage	Description	Glomerular Filtration Rate (GFR)
At increased risk	Risk factors for kidney disease (e.g., diabetes, high blood pressure, family history, older age, ethnic group)	Higher than 90
1	Kidney damage (protein in the urine) and normal GFR	Higher than 90
2	Kidney damage and mild decrease in GFR	60-89
3	Moderate decrease in GFR	30-59
4	Severe decrease in GFR	15-29
5	Kidney failure (dialysis or kidney transplant needed)	Less than 15

Data from the National Kidney Foundation.

- Hyperkalemia
- Renal osteodystrophy
- Uremic symptoms: nausea, vomiting, itching, hemorrhagic conditions, hypertension, edema, dyspnea, lethargy, coma, etc.

EXAMPLE   Hyperkalemia due to chronic kidney disease (CKD), E87.5, N18.9.

Hypertension and Chronic Kidney Disease

ICD-10-CM presumes a cause-and-effect relationship with hypertension and chronic kidney disease. This is addressed in the coding guidelines. Code N18.– has instructions to code first hypertensive chronic kidney disease, if applicable. The physician would have to specifically document that CKD is NOT due to hypertension to negate the cause-and-effect relationship. Hypertension and hypertensive manifestations are discussed more extensively in Chapter 15, Diseases of the Circulatory System.

EXAMPLE   Patient has chronic kidney disease, stage 3, and benign hypertension, I12.9, N18.3.

Diabetic Nephropathy

Diabetes mellitus can have effects on many organs, including the kidneys. If diabetes is not well controlled, it may cause renal complications such as glomerulosclerosis, pyelonephritis, and papillary necrosis. Diabetic patients with renal manifestations may be prone to infections that can cause further damage to the kidneys.

Unlike the relationship between chronic kidney disease and hypertension, diabetes and renal disease must be linked in a manner that denotes a direct relationship. For example, diabetic nephropathy or intercapillary glomerulosclerosis due to diabetes shows a cause-and-effect relationship with diabetes. It is possible for a patient to have nephropathy and diabetes, and no documentation indicates that nephropathy is due to diabetes. In Chapter 12 of this book, diabetes mellitus and manifestations of the disease are discussed in greater depth.

EXAMPLE   Patient is admitted for treatment of diabetes mellitus, type 2. Patient is on hemodialysis for end-stage renal disease, E11.9, N18.6, Z99.2.

EXAMPLE   Patient had intercapillary glomerulosclerosis due to diabetes mellitus type 1, E10.21.

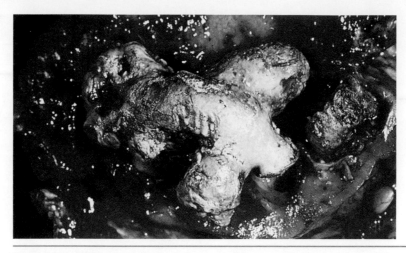

FIGURE 20-9. Irregularly shaped struvite stone in the renal pelvis.

Urolithiasis

Calculi or stones (Figure 20-9) may develop anywhere in the urinary tract and can vary in size. "**Urolithiasis**" describes a stone in the urinary tract. The terms "**nephrolithiasis**" and "**ureterolithiasis**" provide greater specificity with regard to location of the stone. Patients with stones are often asymptomatic unless they result in infection or start to move and obstruct the flow of urine. Obstructions due to stones are very painful and may result in admission to the hospital for pain control, identification, and treatment of the stone. Procedures such as extracorporeal shock wave lithotripsy (ESWL) and laser lithotripsy can be used to break up larger stones. "**Renal colic**" describes the intense pain associated with the body's efforts to try to force the stone through the ureters. Renal colic is not coded separately from a renal or ureteral calculus. Pain or renal colic is integral to the presence of urinary tract calculus.

EXAMPLE	Hematuria due to renal stone, N20.0.

EXERCISE 20-3

Assign codes to the following conditions.

1. Acute on chronic renal failure   _____
2. Essential hypertension; stage 4 CKD   _____
3. Flank pain due to ureteral stone   _____

Other Disorders of the Kidney and Ureter (N25-N29) and Other Diseases of the Urinary System (N30-N39)

Urinary Tract Infections

Urinary tract infection (UTI) is a general term that is used to describe infection of any area of the urinary tract. **Cystitis** is a lower tract infection that affects the bladder (Figure 20-10), and **urethritis** affects the urethra. An upper tract infection that involves the kidneys is called pyelonephritis.

The term "urinary tract infection" is commonly used when referring to cystitis, urethritis, or pyelonephritis. UTIs are assigned codes based on the site of infection, if known,

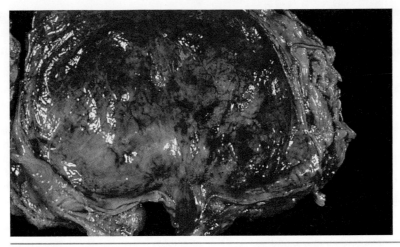

FIGURE 20-10. Acute cystitis. The mucosa of the bladder is red and swollen.

although it is not always possible to distinguish between the three conditions on clinical grounds alone. Only the code for cystitis should be assigned when the physician indicates the bladder as the infection site. Additional sites may be coded if the infection has spread. However, if the documentation includes both UTI and cystitis as diagnoses, only N30.90 should be used. If the site of the UTI is not documented or identified, code N39.0, urinary tract infection, NOS, should be assigned; this code can ONLY be used if the site is not identified and not in combination with any other codes where the site is identified.

EXAMPLE

Urinary tract infection due to acute pyelonephritis, N10.
   The code N39.0 is not assigned because the site of infection has been identified as the kidneys. No bacteria have been identified, so no organism code is assigned.

Most UTIs are due to bacteria. Urinalysis (Table 20-2) and culture and sensitivity tests may be performed to identify the causative organism and to determine which drugs are more effective in treating the infection. Less common are infections caused by viruses, fungi, or parasites. Infections that are due to sexually transmitted disease such as chlamydia or candidiasis are discussed in the infectious and parasitic disease chapter. An instructional note is provided about the use of an additional code to identify the organism as well as the code for the urinary tract infection (Figure 20-11). The following are the most common organisms responsible for UTIs:

- *Escherichia coli (E. coli)*
- *Proteus (mirabilis) (morganii)*
- Methicillin-susceptible *Staphylococcus aureus*
- Methicillin-resistant *Staphylococcus aureus*
- *Staphylococcus saprophyticus*
- Group B *Streptococcus*
- *Klebsiella pneumoniae*

If a causative organism or infectious agent is documented by the physician, this should be coded, in addition to the infection. It would not be appropriate to code an organism on the basis of a urine culture or sensitivity report only. Sometimes the documentation will indicate that the urine grew gram negative bacteria, awaiting sensitivity report. The next progress note will indicate that the urine culture is positive for *Escherichia coli (E. coli)*. The *E. coli* is the gram negative bacteria that was identified and the only code necessary to show the causative organism is B96.2- for the *E. coli*. It would be incorrect to also assign A49.9, other gram negative organisms.

TABLE 20-2 ROUTINE URINALYSIS*[2]

	Normal	Abnormal	Pathology
Characteristics			
Color and clarity	Pale to darker yellow, and clear	Very pale	Excessive water
		Cloudy, milky white blood cells	Pus, urinary tract infection
		Hematuria, red blood cells, reddish to reddish brown	Bleeding in infection, calculi, or cancer
Odor	Aromatic	Fishy	Cystitis
		Fruity	Diabetes mellitus
		Foul	Urinary tract infection
Chemical nature	pH is generally slightly acidic, 6.5	Alkaline	Infections cause ammonia to form
Specific gravity	1.003-1.030—reflects quantity of waste, minerals, and solids in urine	Higher—causes precipitation of solutes Lower—polyuria	Kidney stones, diabetes mellitus, diabetes insipidus
Constituent Compounds			
Protein	None, or small	Albuminuria	Nephritis, renal failure, amount infection
Glucose	None	Glycosuria	Faulty carbohydrate metabolism, as in diabetes mellitus
Ketone bodies	None	Ketonuria	Diabetic acidosis
Bile and bilirubin	None	Bilirubinuria	Hepatic or gallbladder disease
Casts	None—or small number of hyaline casts	Urinary casts composed of red or white blood cells, fat, or pus	Nephritis, renal disease, inflammation, metal poisoning
Nitrogenous wastes	Ammonia, creatinine, urea, and uric acid	Azoturia, creatinine, and urea clearance tests disproportionate to normal BUN/creatinine ratio	Hepatic disease, renal disease
Crystals	None to trace	Acidic urine, alkaline urine, hypercalcemia, metabolism error	Not significant unless the crystals are large (stones); certain types are interpreted by physician
Fat droplets	None	Lipoiduria	Nephrosis

BUN, Blood urea nitrogen.
*Routine urinalysis is the physical, chemical, and microscopic examination of urine for abnormal elements; this may help the clinician to estimate renal function and may provide clues of systemic disease. This table includes some important characteristics and elements that are screened for in basic urinalysis. Other normal constituents of urine that are studied routinely for diagnosis include calcium, potassium, sodium, phosphorus, creatinine, and volume in a 24-hour period.

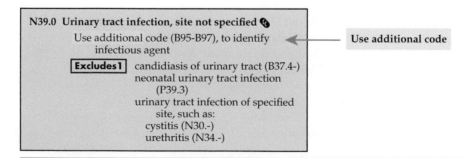

FIGURE 20-11. Instruction is given to use an additional code to identify the organism or infectious agent.

EXAMPLE | Urinary tract infection due to *E. coli,* N39.0, B96.20.

EXAMPLE | Acute cystitis due to *Proteus mirabilis,* N30.00, B96.4.

Some patients are plagued by recurrent and/or chronic UTIs. For this reason, they are sometimes treated with a daily dose of antibiotic to prevent an infection or for prophylactic measures. This should be coded as Z79.2, long-term (current) use of antibiotic, and Z87.41 to identify the personal history of urinary tract infection. It would be inappropriate to assign a code for an infection that is not a current condition.

The term "urosepsis" can cause confusion. Some physicians use the term "urosepsis" to mean an infection of the urinary tract without systemic infection. Other physicians may document urosepsis and mean that the patient has a UTI that has progressed to sepsis. In the Alphabetic Index of ICD-10-CM the term "urosepsis" does not have a code listed but does have an instruction to code to the condition. A physician query may be necessary to determine what that condition is.

EXAMPLE | Urosepsis in patient with UTI due to *Proteus mirabilis,* N39.0. B96.4; ICD-10-CM Alphabetic Index entry for urosepsis instructs to code to condition. According to the guidelines, the physician should be queried.

EXAMPLE | Sepsis due to *Staphylococcus aureus* with urinary tract infection as the source, A41.01, N39.0.

Urinary Incontinence

Urinary incontinence can be a significant health problem that interferes with a patient's activities of daily living. This problem is more common among women because of specific features of their anatomy and as the result of childbearing. Incontinence often occurs after radical prostatectomy but usually resolves in time.

Types of incontinence include stress, urge, mixed, and overflow incontinence. **Stress incontinence** is the involuntary loss of small amounts of urine due to increased pressure from coughing, sneezing, or laughing. **Urge incontinence** is the sudden and involuntary loss of large amounts of urine. **Mixed incontinence** is a combination of stress and urge incontinence. **Overflow incontinence** is the constant dribbling of urine. Treatments include diet, Kegel exercises, biofeedback, and bladder training.

EXAMPLE | Neurogenic bladder with stress incontinence, N31.9, N39.3.

EXERCISE 20-4

Assign codes to the following conditions.

1. Neurogenic bladder _____
2. Stricture of the urethra _____
3. UTI due to *Klebsiella pneumoniae* _____
4. Overflow incontinence associated with overactive bladder _____

Diseases of the Male Genital Organs (N40-N51)

Prostate

The most common diseases of the male genitourinary tract are those that affect the prostate. The prostate gland can become inflamed or enlarged, causing urinary problems. The prostate surrounds the urethra, through which urine flows. The flow of urine can be obstructed by the prostate. **Benign prostatic hyperplasia** and **benign prostatic hypertrophy** are conditions that result in enlargement of the prostate gland; these conditions usually occur in men who are older than 50 years of age (Figure 20-12). Symptoms may include frequency, nocturia, difficulty starting urination, a weak stream of urine, and inability to completely empty the bladder. Within the N40.1 code category there are special instructions for coding lower urinary tract symptoms (LUTS) (Figure 20-13). This corresponds with the general coding guideline that signs and symptoms that are integral to the disease process should not be assigned as additional codes, *unless otherwise instructed by the classification.*

    Prostatitis or inflammation of the prostate may be acute and/or chronic in nature and may be due to bacteria or to inflammation that is not caused by a bacterial infection. Bacterial infections can be easily treated with antibiotics. Nonbacterial prostatitis involves treatment of urinary symptoms, which may be ongoing. There is an instructional note to use an additional code to identify the infectious agent. Use the Index and the Tabular to verify the accuracy of organism codes as referenced in the Tabular instructional note.

EXAMPLE   Chronic prostatitis due to staphylococcus N41.1, B95.8.

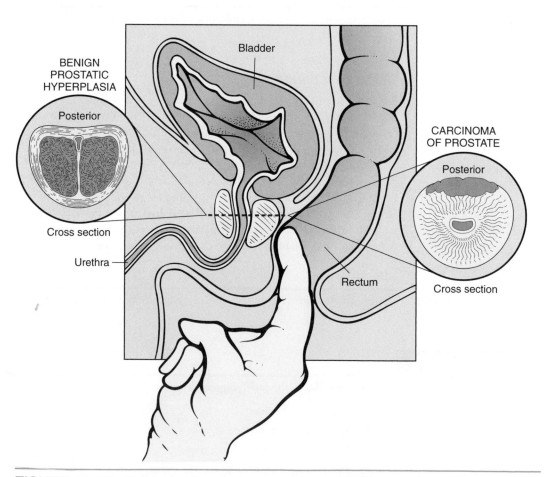

FIGURE 20-12. Digital prostate or rectal examination to identify prostatic abnormalities.

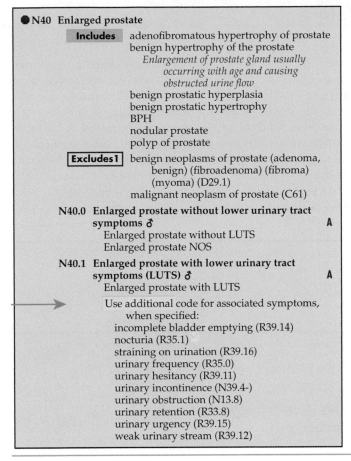

● N40 **Enlarged prostate**

| Includes | adenofibromatous hypertrophy of prostate |

benign hypertrophy of the prostate
Enlargement of prostate gland usually
occurring with age and causing
obstructed urine flow
benign prostatic hyperplasia
benign prostatic hypertrophy
BPH
nodular prostate
polyp of prostate

| Excludes1 | benign neoplasms of prostate (adenoma, benign) (fibroadenoma) (fibroma) (myoma) (D29.1) |

malignant neoplasm of prostate (C61)

N40.0 **Enlarged prostate without lower urinary tract**
symptoms ♂   A
Enlarged prostate without LUTS
Enlarged prostate NOS

N40.1 **Enlarged prostate with lower urinary tract**
symptoms (LUTS) ♂   A
Enlarged prostate with LUTS

Use additional code for associated symptoms,
when specified:
incomplete bladder emptying (R39.14)
nocturia (R35.1)
straining on urination (R39.16)
urinary frequency (R35.0)
urinary hesitancy (R39.11)
urinary incontinence (N39.4-)
urinary obstruction (N13.8)
urinary retention (R33.8)
urinary urgency (R39.15)
weak urinary stream (R39.12)

FIGURE 20-13. Instructions to use additional code(s) for lower urinary tract symptoms (LUTS).

Prostate-specific antigen (PSA) is a protein produced by the prostate gland. A blood test to measure PSA is a means of screening for prostate cancer. The risk of cancer is based on the following:

- PSA levels under 4 ng/mL: "normal"
- 4 to 10 ng/mL: 20% to 30% risk
- 10 to 20 ng/mL: 50% to 75% risk
- Above 20 ng/mL: 90%

Elevated levels do not always indicate cancer but may be elevated due to other prostate problems such as BPH or prostatitis.

EXAMPLE   Patient was seen in the clinic for an elevated PSA. It was determined that the patient's severe benign prostatic hypertrophy was the cause, N40.0.

EXAMPLE   Patient was referred to a urologist for elevated PSA, R97.2.

EXERCISE 20-5

Assign codes to the following conditions.

1. Nocturia due to benign prostatic hypertrophy   _____
2. Acute prostatitis due to *Escherichia coli*   _____
3. Scrotal pain and swelling due to epididymitis   _____
4. Hydrocele   _____
5. Phimosis   _____

Disorders of Breast (N60-N65)

Breast

Many conditions of the breast described in this chapter are treated in the outpatient setting. Conditions of the breast in a pregnant woman are coded in the obstetrical chapter, or Chapter 15, of the ICD-10-CM code book. Male patients can also have conditions that are classified to the breast. **Mastitis** is inflammation or infection of the breast (Figure 20-14). Swelling, redness, tenderness, and pain may be noted. A breast abscess may form if mastitis is not treated. An abscess may require incision and drainage.

Some patients undergo prophylactic breast removal because they have a strong family history of breast cancer and/or genetic susceptibility or a personal history of breast cancer. After breast reconstruction is performed, complications such as infection, pain, and malfunction or failure of the implant or tissue expander, may occur.

EXAMPLE	Patient has diffuse fibroadenosis of both breasts, N60.21, N60.22.

EXERCISE 20-6

Assign codes to the following conditions.

1. Fibrocystic disease of breast, bilateral _____
2. Nipple discharge, right breast _____
3. Male patient with gynecomastia _____
4. Mastodynia _____

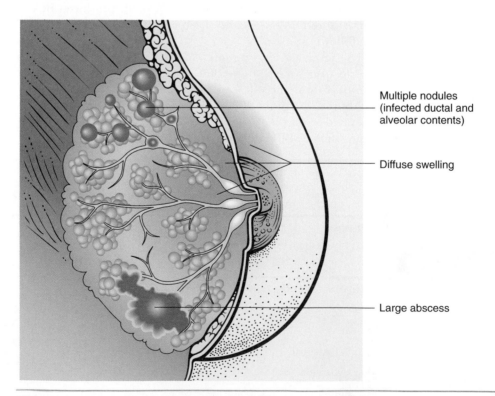

Multiple nodules (infected ductal and alveolar contents)

Diffuse swelling

Large abscess

FIGURE 20-14. Acute mastitis typically occurs during lactation.

Inflammatory Diseases of Female Pelvic Organs (N70-N77)

Pelvic Inflammatory Disease

Pelvic inflammatory disease (PID) occurs when vaginal or cervical infection spreads and involves the uterus, fallopian tubes, ovaries, and surrounding tissues. **Salpingitis** is inflammation of the fallopian tubes, which are the most common sites of pelvic inflammation. **Endometritis** is inflammation of the uterus, and **oophoritis** is inflammation of the ovaries. The most prevalent symptoms of these infections include vaginal discharge, pain, and possibly a fever. Complications that may result include infertility, chronic pain, tubal pregnancy, recurrent inflammation, and abscess.

EXAMPLE | Acute and chronic right salpingo-oophoritis, N70.03, N70.13.

EXERCISE 20-7

Assign codes to the following conditions.

1. Tubo-ovarian abscess   _____
2. Cervicitis   _____
3. Bartholin's cyst   _____
4. Pelvic adhesions, female   _____
5. PID   _____

Noninflammatory Disorders of Female Genital Tract (N80-N98)

Endometriosis

Endometriosis is a chronic condition in which endometrial material, the tissue that lines the inside of the uterus, grows outside the uterus and attaches to other organs in the pelvic cavity. Code assignment is based on site of implantation (Figure 20-15). The most common sites are the ovaries and fallopian tubes. Although it is uncommon, endometrial tissue can spread to sites throughout the body to areas such as the lungs. Pain and infertility are the two most common symptoms.

EXAMPLE | Endometriosis of the uterus, N80.0.

Genital Prolapse

Genital prolapse occurs when pelvic organs such as the uterus, bladder, and rectum shift from their normal anatomic positions and protrude into the vagina or press against the wall of the vagina (Figure 20-16). Weakening or damage to the ligaments, muscles, and connective tissues that support these organs is the cause of genital prolapse. It occurs commonly in postmenopausal women who have had children. Other contributing factors include genetics, pelvic surgery, and pressures within the abdomen that would weaken the pelvic floor. Different types of prolapse are usually graded on the basis of severity. **Uterine prolapse** is the descent of the uterus and cervix into the vaginal canal. **Cystocele** occurs when the bladder descends and presses into the wall of the vagina. **Urethrocele** results when the urethra presses into the vagina; it usually is reported in conjunction with a cystocele, which is then called a **cystourethrocele**. **Rectocele** is the descent of the rectum and pressing of the rectum against the vaginal wall. **Vaginal vault prolapse** may occur after a hysterectomy has been performed, when the top of the vagina descends into the vault.

EXAMPLE | Examination of the patient showed a second degree uterine prolapse, N81.2.

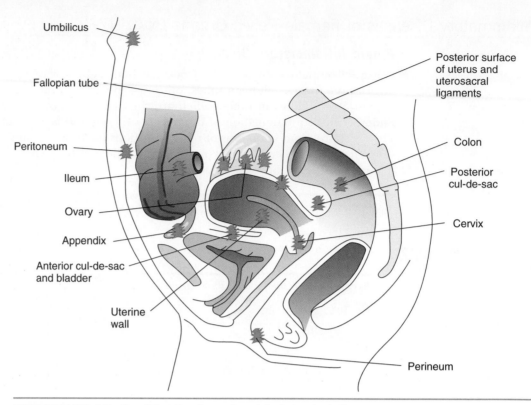

FIGURE 20-15. Possible sites for endometriosis implantation.

Fistulas

A **fistula** is an abnormal passage or communication between two internal organs, or leading from an organ to the surface of the body (Figure 20-17). A **urethrovaginal fistula** is an abnormal passage between the urethra and the vagina. The bladder has the potential to communicate with the uterus, vagina, and rectum, forming a **vesicouterine fistula**, **vesicovaginal fistula**, and/or **rectovesical fistula**, respectively.

EXAMPLE   Rectovesicovaginal fistula, N82.3.

Cervical and Vulvular Dysplasia

Cervical dysplasia is the abnormal growth of cells on the surface of the cervix. Although not cancer, it is considered a precancerous condition. Cervical dysplasia usually has no symptoms and is discovered on a Pap smear. Dysplasia that is identified on a Pap smear is described using the term **squamous intraepithelial lesion (SIL)**. These abnormal Pap smear changes may be graded as:

- Low-grade (LSIL)
- High-grade (HSIL)
- Possibly cancerous (malignant)

Dysplasia that is seen on a biopsy of the cervix uses the term **cervical intraepithelial neoplasia (CIN)** and is grouped into the following three categories:

- CIN I—mild dysplasia
- CIN II—moderate to marked dysplasia
- CIN III—severe dysplasia to carcinoma in situ

Vulvar intraepithelial neoplasia (VIN) refers to certain changes that can occur in the skin that covers the vulva. It is similar to CIN or dysplasia of the cervix and can be diagnosed with a biopsy. VIN is grouped into the following three categories:

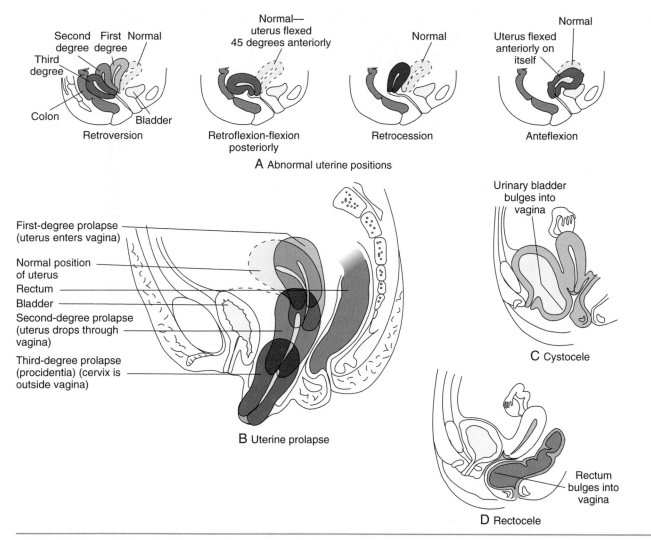

FIGURE 20-16. Structural abnormalities of the uterus.

- VIN I—mild dysplasia
- VIN II—moderate to marked dysplasia
- VIN III—severe dysplasia to carcinoma in situ

If either of these conditions (CIN or VIN) are left untreated, it may result in invasive cancer.

EXAMPLE   Patient was seen in the clinic, and her cervical biopsy results showed CIN II, N87.1.

EXERCISE 20-8

Assign codes to the following conditions.

1. Endometriosis of fallopian tube _____
2. Cystocele with female stress incontinence _____
3. Corpus luteum cyst _____
4. Chocolate cyst of the ovary _____
5. Vaginal stenosis _____

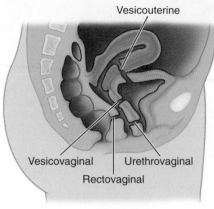

Vesicouterine

Vesicovaginal   Urethrovaginal

Rectovaginal

A

FIGURE 20-17. Various types of fistulas, designated according to site or to organs with which they communicate. **A,** Genitourinary fistulas. **B,** Anal fistulas.

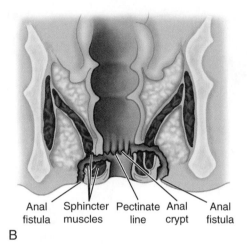

Anal   Sphincter   Pectinate   Anal   Anal
fistula   muscles   line   crypt   fistula

B

FACTORS INFLUENCING HEALTH STATUS AND CONTACT WITH HEALTH SERVICES (Z CODES)

As was discussed in Chapter 8, it may be difficult to locate Z codes in the Index. Coders often say, "I did not know there was a Z code for that." Refer to Chapter 8 for a listing of common main terms used to locate Z codes.

Z codes that may be used with diseases of the genitourinary system include the following:

Z01.411	Encounter for gynecological examination (general)(routine) with abnormal findings
Z01.419	Encounter for gynecological examination (general)(routine) without abnormal findings
Z01.42	Encounter for cervical smear to confirm findings of recent normal smear following initial abnormal smear
Z13.89	Encounter for screening of other disorder
Z41.2	Encounter for routine and ritual male circumcision
Z43.5	Encounter for attention to cystostomy
Z43.6	Encounter for attention to other artificial openings of urinary tract
Z43.7	Encounter for attention to artificial vagina

Z44.30	Encounter for fitting and adjustment of external breast prosthesis, unspecified breast
Z44.31	Encounter for fitting and adjustment of external right breast prosthesis
Z44.32	Encounter for fitting and adjustment of external left breast prosthesis
Z45.811	Encounter for adjustment or removal of right breast implant
Z45.812	Encounter for adjustment or removal of left breast implant
Z45.819	Encounter for adjustment or removal of unspecified breast implant
Z46.6	Encounter for fitting and adjustment of urinary device
Z49.01	Encounter for fitting and adjustment of extracorporeal dialysis catheter
Z49.02	Encounter for fitting and adjustment of peritoneal dialysis catheter
Z49.31	Encounter for adequacy testing for hemodialysis
Z49.32	Encounter for adequacy testing for peritoneal dialysis
Z52.4	Kidney donor
Z52.810	Egg (Oocyte) donor under age 35, anonymous recipient; Egg donor under age 35 NOS
Z52.811	Egg (Oocyte) donor under age 35, designated recipient
Z52.812	Egg (Oocyte) donor age 35 and over, anonymous recipient; Egg donor age 35 and over NOS
Z52.813	Egg (Oocyte) donor age 35 and over, designated recipient
Z52.819	Egg (Oocyte) donor, unspecified
Z78.0	Asymptomatic menopausal state
Z79.890	Hormone replacement therapy (postmenopausal)
Z82.71	Family history of polycystic kidney
Z84.1	Family history of disorders of kidney and ureter
Z84.2	Family history of other diseases of the genitourinary system
Z87.410	Personal history of cervical dysplasia
Z87.411	Personal history of vaginal dysplasia
Z87.412	Personal history of vulvar dysplasia
Z87.430	Personal history of prostatic dysplasia
Z87.438	Personal history of other disease of male genital organs
Z87.440	Personal history of urinary (tract) infections
Z87.441	Personal history of nephrotic syndrome
Z87.442	Personal history of urinary calculi
Z87.448	Personal history of other diseases of the urinary system
Z90.10	Acquired absence of unspecified breast and nipple
Z90.11	Acquired absence of right breast and nipple
Z90.12	Acquired absence of left breast and nipple
Z90.13	Acquired absence of bilateral breasts and nipples
Z90.5	Acquired absence of kidney
Z90.6	Acquired absence of other parts of urinary tract
Z90.710	Acquired absence of both cervix and uterus
Z90.711	Acquired absence of uterus with remaining cervical stump
Z90.712	Acquired absence of cervix with remaining uterus
Z90.721	Acquired absence of ovaries, unilateral
Z90.722	Acquired absence of ovaries, bilateral
Z90.79	Acquired absence of other genital organ(s)
Z91.15	Patient's noncompliance with renal dialysis
Z93.50	Unspecified cystostomy status
Z93.51	Cutaneous-vesicostomy status
Z93.52	Appendico-vesicostomy status
Z93.59	Other cystostomy status
Z93.6	Other artificial openings of urinary tract status

Z94.0	Kidney transplant status
Z96.0	Presence of urogenital implants
Z98.51	Tubal ligation status
Z98.52	Vasectomy status
Z98.82	Breast implant status
Z98.86	Personal history of breast implant removal
Z98.870	Personal history of in utero procedure during pregnancy
Z98.871	Personal history of in utero procedure while a fetus
Z99.2	Dependence on renal dialysis

EXAMPLE

Adult male is admitted for elective routine circumcision, Z41.2, 0VTTXZZ.
 The Z code indicates that a procedure is going to be performed, but it is not the procedure code. A diagnosis code is not assigned because no medical condition is present.

EXAMPLE

Patient is admitted for kidney donation. A laparoscopic left nephrectomy is performed, Z52.4, 0TT14ZZ.

EXERCISE 20-9

Assign codes to the following conditions.

1. Status post kidney transplant   _____
2. Personal history of kidney stones   _____
3. Family history of polycystic kidney disease   _____
4. Acquired absence of uterus and cervix   _____

COMMON TREATMENTS

CONDITION	MEDICATION/TREATMENT
Glomerulonephritis	If due to infection, antibiotics
	Diuretics, antihypertensives, and diet
	Serious cases may be treated with corticosteroids and/or Cytoxan
Acute renal failure	Fluid management and treat the underlying cause
	Dialysis, if necessary
Chronic renal failure	Determine cause. Control blood pressure and diet
Cystitis	Fluids and possibly antibiotics
Urethritis	Antibiotics
Pyelonephritis	Antibiotics
Calculus of urinary tract	Fluids, pain control, blood pressure control, and antibiotics, if associated infection
Urinary incontinence	Kegel exercises, biofeedback, and medications such as Detrol
Prostatitis	Antibiotics
Benign prostatic hyperplasia	Medications such as tamsulosin hydrochloride (Flomax) and terazosin hydrochloride (Hytrin)
Mastitis	Compresses, massage, fluids, and possibly antibiotics
PID	Antibiotics
Endometriosis	Pain medication and/or hormonal therapy

PROCEDURES

Procedures related to the genitourinary system in ICD-10-PCS can be located in the following tables:

0H0-0HY	Skin and Breast
0T1-0TY	Urinary System
0U1-0UY	Female Reproductive System
0V1-0VW	Male Reproductive System
302-3E1	Administration
5A0-5A2	Extracorporeal Assistance and Performance

Cystoscopy is an endoscopic approach used for many procedures involving the urinary tract (Figure 20-18). Often, another diagnostic or therapeutic procedure, such as biopsy, removal of a stone, dilatation of a stricture, or control of hemorrhage, is performed during a cystoscopic examination.

EXAMPLE | Bladder lesion with diagnostic transurethral biopsy of the bladder via cystoscope, N32.9, 0TBB8ZX.

Dialysis

Dialysis is needed when the kidneys can no longer filter the blood and form urine. Two basic types of dialysis are available. **Hemodialysis** uses a machine called a hemodialyzer to remove wastes from the blood (Figure 20-19). Access is obtained through a surgically created internal (arteriovenous [AV]) fistula that allows blood to pass from the body to the machine for cleansing. Sometimes, an AV graft (Figure 20-20) is used for permanent access. The root operation for creation of an AV fistula is bypass (altering the route of passage of the contents of a tubular body). If treatment must be begun before permanent access is ready or available, temporary access can be obtained through a catheter. Usually, hemodialysis is conducted at dialysis centers, and it is often scheduled 3 times per week. A dialysis session may take 3 to 5 hours to complete. The root operation for hemodialysis is performance (completely taking over a physiological function by extracorporeal means).

If the encounter is for dialysis, a Z code is assigned as the principal diagnosis. In cases where the patient is receiving treatment in preparation for dialysis (e.g., creation of an arteriovenous fistula), the principal diagnosis will be the medical condition for which the dialysis is required.

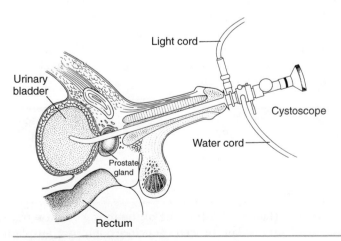

FIGURE 20-18. Cystoscopy.

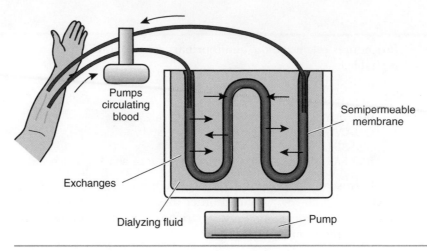

FIGURE 20-19. Hemodialysis.

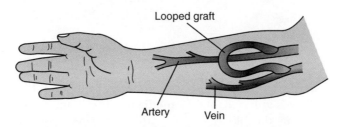

FIGURE 20-20. Arteriovenous graft for dialysis.

EXAMPLE | Patient with ESRD is admitted for hemodialysis, Z99.2, N18.6, 5A1D00Z.

EXAMPLE | Patient with ESRD and hypertension is admitted for creation of an AV fistula (left radiocephalic fistula using a synthetic graft). Patient has dialysis on M, W, and F. I12.0, N18.6, Z99.2, 031C0JF.

Peritoneal dialysis uses the peritoneal membrane in the patient's own body along with a dialysate solution to filter out wastes and excess fluid (Figure 20-21). Dialyzing fluid passes into the peritoneal cavity through a permanent indwelling peritoneal catheter (Tenckhoff catheter) and is then drained from the peritoneal cavity. **Continuous ambulatory peritoneal dialysis** (CAPD) takes about 15 minutes and is performed 3 to 4 times per day and once at night. **Continuous cycling peritoneal dialysis** (CCPD) uses a cycling machine and is performed while the patient sleeps. In some cases, a combination of the two may be needed to achieve the best results. The root operation for peritoneal dialysis is irrigation (putting in or on a cleansing substance).

EXAMPLE | Patient with end-stage renal failure has peritoneal dialysis while hospitalized for acute prostatitis, N41.0, N18.6, Z99.2, 3E1M39Z.

Kidney Transplantation

A kidney transplant (Figure 20-22) is one of the most common transplant operations. Prior to performance of a transplant procedure, a thorough pretransplant evaluation is necessary to assess the patient's overall health and identify potential problems to increase the chances

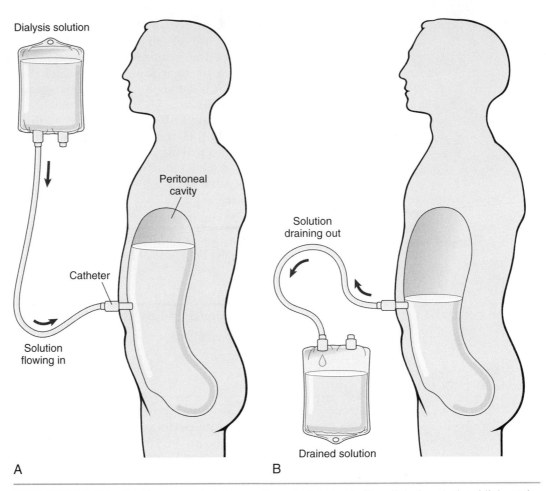

FIGURE 20-21. Continuous ambulatory peritoneal dialysis. **A,** The dialysis solution (dialysate) flows from a collapsible plastic bag through a Tenckhoff catheter into the patient's peritoneal cavity. The empty bag is folded and inserted into undergarments. **B,** After 4 to 8 hours, the bag is unfolded, and the fluid is allowed to drain into it with the help of gravity. The full bag is discarded, and a new bag of fresh dialysate is attached.

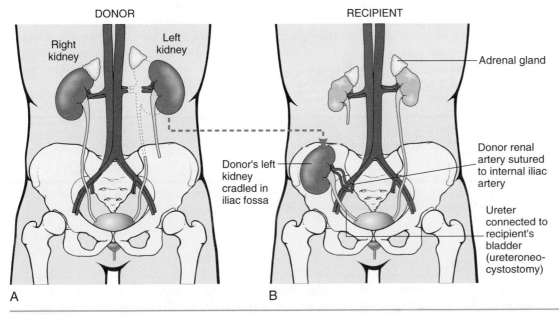

FIGURE 20-22. Kidney transplantation. **A,** Left kidney of the donor is removed for transplant. **B,** The kidney is transplanted to the right pelvis of the recipient.

of a successful transplant. A couple of different types of kidney transplants may be performed—transplant from a live related donor, transplant from a live nonrelated donor, and transplant from a cadaver. Transplants from a living donor are generally scheduled in advance, and the kidney may be transplanted immediately following removal from the donor. The root operation for a kidney transplant is transplantation (putting in a living body part from a person/animal).

Patients who are on a waiting list for a kidney are notified when a kidney becomes available that is a good match; they must report to the hospital immediately. The transplanted kidney will usually start making urine as soon as the blood starts to flow through it, and most patients feel much better after their surgery has been completed. In most cases, only one kidney is necessary to take over for two failed kidneys. Most of the time, the diseased kidneys are left in place.

| EXAMPLE | Patient was admitted for kidney transplant. Patient has CKD, stage 5 due to hypertension. Patient never did receive dialysis. The transplant was performed using the spouse's left kidney, I12.0, N18.5, 0TY10Z0. |

| EXAMPLE | Patient is admitted for kidney donation. A laparoscopic left nephrectomy is performed, Z52.4, 0TT14ZZ. |

Prostate Procedures

Prostate procedures are most often performed for benign prostatic hypertrophy or for prostate cancer. A biopsy is usually performed prior to a prostatectomy. Correct procedural code assignment depends on the method of the procedure performed. When **transurethral resection of the prostate** (TURP) is performed, it is not necessary to code the cystoscopy that is performed in the course of the surgical procedure. Cystoscopy is the approach that is used in transurethral procedures. Transurethral ultrasound-guided laser-induced prostatectomy (TULIP) and visual laser ablation of the prostate (VLAP) are two types of laser treatments used for ablation of prostatic tissue. Transurethral microwave thermotherapy (TUMT) and transurethral needle ablation (TUNA) of the prostate use radiofrequency energy to ablate obstructive prostatic tissue; these procedures can be performed in the physician's office. For the prostate procedures, if a biopsy is performed, the root operation is excision (cutting out or off without replacement some of a body part). If a prostatectomy with complete removal of the prostate gland is performed, resection is the root operation (cutting out or off without replacement all of a body part). If an ablation is done, destruction is the root operation (eradicating without replacement some or all of a body part [none of the body part is physically taken out]).

| EXAMPLE | Cancer of the prostate with radical prostatectomy (including bilateral seminal vesicles) with diagnostic pelvic lymph node sampling, C61, 0VT00ZZ, 0VT30ZZ, 07BC0ZX. |

| EXAMPLE | Benign prostatic hypertrophy with urinary obstruction. Endoscopic transurethral ultrasound-guided laser-induced prostatectomy, N40.1, N13.8, 0VB08ZZ. |

Breast Biopsies and Reconstruction

Breast biopsies are performed for diagnostic purposes to determine the nature of a breast abnormality or mass. The root operation for biopsy is excision (cutting out or off some of a body part without replacement). In a biopsy of the breast, a tissue sample is taken for diagnostic examination.

At times, breast biopsy is performed during the same operative episode as a therapeutic procedure or more definitive treatment such as a mastectomy. In these cases, the biopsy is coded in addition to the mastectomy.

Breast reconstructions are often performed following a mastectomy. Reconstruction may be done immediately or as a delayed procedure. The type of reconstruction and the timing of when it is done vary according to the patient's need for radiation and the type of mastectomy that is performed. Reconstruction may also be performed in stages. Implants and tissue expanders are sometimes used to create the breast. Tissue expanders are removed after the skin and muscles have been expanded to accommodate the breast implant or further reconstruction.

Tissue flap procedures use tissue from the abdomen, back, thighs, or buttocks to reconstruct the breast. Several flap procedures are currently used (Figure 20-23); these include the following:

- Transverse rectus abdominis musculocutaneous (TRAM)
- Latissimus dorsi musculocutaneous flap (LDMF)
- Lateral transverse thigh flap
- Nipple—Areola reconstruction
- Deep inferior epigastric perforator (DIEP) flap free
- Superficial inferior epigastric artery (SIEA) flap free
- Gluteal artery perforator (GAP) flap free

A **pedicle flap** involves a flap that remains attached to its original blood supply and tunneling it under the skin to the breast area. A **free flap** involves the cutting of skin, fat, blood vessels, and muscle free from their locations and moving them to the chest area. Blood vessels are connected with the use of a microscope. A free flap takes more time to

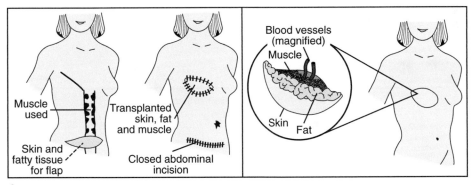

A

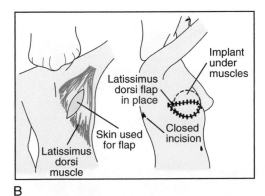

B

FIGURE 20-23. Various flaps used for breast reconstruction.

complete. The root operation for free flap reconstruction is replacement (putting in or on biologic or synthetic material that replaces a body part). The root operation for pedicle flap reconstruction is transfer (moving a body part with taking out to another location to take over the function of another body part).

EXAMPLE Patient admitted for bilateral breast reduction due to hypertrophy, N62, 0HBV0ZZ.

Removal of Stones

Extracorporeal shock wave lithotripsy (ESWL) is used to break up kidney stones into small particles that can then pass through the urinary tract in the urine. Different devices can be used to transmit shock waves, and usually, x-ray or ultrasound is used to reveal the exact location of the stone. The root operation for ESWL is fragmentation (breaking solid matter into pieces).

If the stone is quite large, or the location is such that ESWL is not very effective, a **percutaneous nephrolithotomy** is performed. The root operation for nephrolithotomy is extirpation (taking or cutting out solid matter). The stone is removed by the surgeon with the use of a nephroscope. At times, an ultrasonic or electrohydraulic probe is used to break up the stone, and the fragments are then removed. A nephrostomy tube may have to remain within the kidney during the postoperative phase.

Ureteroscopic stone removal is necessary when a kidney stone has traveled into one of the ureters. The ureteroscope is inserted through the urethra and bladder and into the ureter until the stone can be removed or is broken into pieces.

EXAMPLE Patient was treated with percutaneous nephrostomy with removal of left kidney stone, N20.0, 0TC13ZZ.

EXERCISE 20-10

Assign codes for all diagnoses and procedures.

1. Right solitary renal cyst (acquired) with right partial laparoscopic nephrectomy _____

2. Endoscopic transurethral needle ablation of prostate (TUNA) in patient with benign prostatic hyperplasia _____

3. Laparoscopically assisted vaginal hysterectomy (LAVH) in patient with endometriosis of the uterus _____

4. Extracorporeal shock wave lithotripsy bladder stone _____

5. Bilateral modified radical mastectomy, and breast reconstruction with latissimus dorsi musculocutaneous flap (LDMF) following prophylactic removal due to strong family history of breast cancer _____

6. Peritoneal dialysis in patient with ESRD and anemia of chronic renal disease _____

7. Left kidney transplant in patient with hypertensive renal disease and end-stage renal failure. The patient's spouse was the donor. _____

8. Left breast cyst with percutaneous breast aspiration _____

DOCUMENTATION/REIMBURSEMENT/MS-DRGs

Often, coding difficulties are due to lack of documentation. Sometimes pathology and other test results are not available at the time of discharge, or when the physician is dictating the discharge summary or is reporting the final diagnoses.

Definitions and ways a physician uses terms such as "urosepsis" versus "sepsis," and "acute renal insufficiency" versus "acute renal failure" can be problematic and may require a physician query.

Frequently missed complications/comorbidities from this chapter include the following:

- Acute renal failure
- CKD, stages 4 and 5
- ESRD
- Secondary hyperparathyroidism of renal origin
- Hydronephrosis
- Calculus of ureter
- Genital tract fistulas

Urosepsis versus Sepsis

EXAMPLE

Urosepsis due to urinary tract infection compared with sepsis as the principal diagnosis

DIAGNOSES	CODES	MS-DRG	RW
UTI	N39.0	690	0.7870
Sepsis due to UTI	A41.9, N39.0	872	1.1339

MS-DRG With and Without MCC/CC

The presence of a complication and/or comorbidity (CC) can make a difference in reimbursement, depending on the principal diagnosis and the MS-DRG assigned. The code for acute renal failure is a CC, and the code for acute renal insufficiency is not an MCC/CC when it is used as a secondary diagnosis.

EXAMPLE

Patient with pneumonia and acute renal failure (ARF) compared with patient with pneumonia and acute renal insufficiency (ARI)

DIAGNOSES	CODES	MS-DRG	RW
Pneumonia with ARF	J18.9, N17.9	194	1.0026
Pneumonia with ARI	J18.9, N28.9	195	0.7037

CHAPTER REVIEW EXERCISE

Assign codes for all diagnoses and procedures.

1. Pelvic pain due to interstitial cystitis _____

2. Benign hyperplasia of the prostate with urinary obstruction _____

3. Patient with benign prostatic hypertrophy with urinary obstruction and history of renal calculi is admitted for TURP (endoscopic). After the procedure, the patient has slight hematuria. _____

4. Complete ureterovaginal prolapse _____

5. Prerenal azotemia _____

6. Vesicoureteral reflux _____

7. Menometrorrhagia with chronic blood loss anemia _____

8. Infertility due to tubal endometriosis   _____

9. Hematuria with diagnostic cystoscope performed to inspect bladder   _____

10. Acute tubular necrosis in patient with labile hypertension   _____

11. Berger's disease   _____

12. Rectovesical fistula   _____

13. Chronic glomerulonephritis due to amyloidosis   _____

14. Multinodular prostate   _____

15. Infertility due to azoospermia   _____

16. Incision and drainage of Bartholin's abscess   _____

17. Total abdominal hysterectomy with right salpingo-oophorectomy for symptomatic uterine fibroids and follicular cyst right ovary. Family history of cervical cancer   _____

18. Infertility due to dysmucorrhea   _____

19. Urethroscrotal fistula   _____

20. Nonfunctioning right kidney with laparoscopic nephrectomy   _____

21. Postmenopausal bleeding. Diagnostic dilatation and curettage (D&C) of uterus   _____

22. Patient with ESRD following transplant nephrectomy who is noncompliant with dialysis sessions   _____

23. Descensus of uterus   _____

24. Left ureteral stent was placed (percutaneous endoscopic approach) due to obstruction of the ureter due to stone   _____

25. Bilateral laparoscopic oophorectomy with salpingectomy due to polycystic ovarian syndrome   _____

Write the correct answer(s) in the space(s) provided.

26. Which MS-DRG is reimbursed at a higher rate: MS-DRG 690 or MS-DRG 872?

_____

27. Define fistula.

_____

28. Pyelonephritis involves what organ?

_____

29. Describe the main difference in the female and male genitourinary tract.

_____

30. Define ARF.

_____

CHAPTER GLOSSARY

Acute renal failure: sudden and severe impairment of renal function characterized by oliguria, increased serum urea, and acidosis.

Benign prostatic hyperplasia: condition resulting in enlargement of the prostate gland; usually occurs in men older than 50 years of age.

Benign prostatic hypertrophy: condition resulting in enlargement of the prostate gland; usually occurs in men older than 50 years of age.

Calculus: a stone. Calculi, which vary in size, can develop anywhere in the urinary tract.

Cervical dysplasia: abnormal growth of cells on the surface of the cervix.

Cervical intraepithelial neoplasia (CIN): dysplasia that is seen on a biopsy of the cervix.

Continuous ambulatory peritoneal dialysis: type of peritoneal dialysis that takes about 15 minutes and is performed 3 to 4 times per day and once at night.

Continuous cycling peritoneal dialysis: type of peritoneal dialysis that uses a cycling machine and is performed while the patient sleeps.

Cystitis: lower tract infection that affects the bladder.

Cystocele: when the bladder descends and presses into the wall of the vagina.

Cystoscopy: approach used for many procedures of the urinary tract.

Cystourethrocele: a urethrocele in conjunction with a cystocele.

Endometriosis: a chronic condition in which endometrial material, the tissue that lines the inside of the uterus, grows outside the uterus and attaches to other organs in the pelvic cavity.

Endometritis: inflammation of the uterus.

Extracorporeal shock wave lithotripsy: used to break up kidney stones into small particles that can then pass through the urinary tract into the urine.

Fistula: abnormal passage or communication between two internal organs, or leading from an organ to the surface of the body.

Free flap: involves the cutting of skin, fat, blood vessels, and muscle free from its location and moving it to the chest area.

Genital prolapse: when pelvic organs such as the uterus, bladder, and rectum shift from their normal anatomic positions and protrude into the vagina or press against the wall of the vagina.

Glomerulonephritis: inflammation of the glomeruli of the kidneys.

Hematuria: the presence of blood in the urine.

Hemodialysis: process that uses a machine called a hemodialyzer to remove wastes from the blood.

Hydronephrosis: abnormal dilatation of the renal pelvis caused by pressure from urine that cannot flow past an obstruction in the urinary tract.

Hydroureter: accumulation of urine in the ureters.

Lactation: the secretion of milk from mammary glands.

Mastitis: inflammation or infection of the breast.

Mixed incontinence: combination of stress and urge incontinence.

Nephrolithiasis: kidney stone.

Nephrotic syndrome: condition marked by proteinuria (protein in the urine), low levels of protein in the blood, hypercholesterolemia, and swelling of the eyes, feet, and hands.

Oophoritis: inflammation of the ovaries.

Overflow incontinence: the constant dribbling of urine.

Pedicle flap: involves identifying a flap that remains attached to its original blood supply and tunneling it under the skin to a particular area such as the breast.

Pelvic inflammatory disease: when vaginal or cervical infections spread and involve the uterus, fallopian tubes, ovaries, and surrounding tissues.

Percutaneous nephrolithotomy: procedure in which the surgeon uses a nephroscope to remove a stone. At times, an ultrasonic or electrohydraulic probe is used to break up the stone, and the fragments are then removed.

Peritoneal dialysis: when the peritoneal membrane in the patient's own body is used with a dialysate solution to filter out the wastes and excess fluids.

Prostate-specific antigen (PSA): protein produced by the prostate gland.

Prostatitis: inflammation of the prostate that can be acute and/or chronic in nature and is due to a bacterium or inflammation that is not caused by a bacterial infection.

Proteinuria: protein in urine.

Pyelonephritis: upper tract infection that involves the kidneys.

Rectocele: descent of the rectum and pressing of the rectum against the vaginal wall.

Rectovesical fistula: a communication between the bladder and the rectum.

Renal colic: intense pain associated with the body's efforts to try to force the stone through the ureters.

Salpingitis: inflammation of the fallopian tubes, which are the most common site of pelvic inflammation.

Squamous intraepithelial lesion (SIL): dysplasia of the cervix that is identified on a Pap smear.

Stress incontinence: involuntary loss of small amounts of urine due to increased pressure resulting from coughing, sneezing, or laughing.

Transurethral resection of the prostate: endoscopic removal of prostate tissue.

Ureterolithiasis: ureter stone.

Urethritis: infection of the urethra.

Urethrocele: when the urethra presses into the vagina.

Urethrovaginal fistula: abnormal passage between the urethra and the vagina.

Urge incontinence: sudden and involuntary loss of large amounts of urine.

Urinary tract infection: general term used to describe infection in any area of the urinary tract.

Urolithiasis: a stone in the urinary tract.

Uterine prolapse: descent of the uterus and the cervix into the vaginal canal.

Vaginal vault prolapse: condition that may occur following a hysterectomy, when the top of the vagina descends.

Vesicoureteral reflux: abnormality in the flow of urine from the bladder into the ureters and/or kidneys.

Vesicouterine fistula: communication between the bladder and the uterus.

Vesicovaginal fistula: communication between the bladder and the vagina.

Vulvar intraepithelial neoplasia (VIN): certain changes that can occur in the skin that covers the vulva.

REFERENCES

1. American Hospital Association. *Coding Clinic for ICD-9-CM* 2002:3Q:p21-22. ARF due to dehydration and treated with IV hydration only.

2. From Frazier ME, Drzymkowski JW. *Essentials of Human Diseases and Conditions*, 3rd ed. St. Louis: Saunders, 2004, Table 11-1, p 504.

21

Pregnancy, Childbirth, and the Puerperium

(ICD-10-CM Chapter 15, Codes O00-O9A)

LEARNING OBJECTIVES

1. Apply and assign the correct ICD-10-CM/PCS codes in accordance with Official Guidelines for Coding and Reporting
2. Identify major differences between ICD-10-CM and ICD-9-CM related to complications of pregnancy, childbirth, and the puerperium
3. Identify pertinent anatomy and physiology of pregnancy, childbirth, and the puerperium
4. Recognize conditions and complications of pregnancy, childbirth, and the puerperium

5. Assign the correct Z codes and procedure codes related to pregnancy, childbirth, and the puerperium

6. Identify common treatments, medications, laboratory values, and diagnostic tests

7. Explain the importance of documentation in relation to MS-DRGs for reimbursement

ABBREVIATIONS/ ACRONYMS

AROM artificial rupture of membranes

CPD cephalopelvic disproportion

D&C dilatation and curettage

EDC estimated date of confinement

EMS emergency medical services

GBS group B strep

GDM gestational diabetes mellitus

hCG human chorionic gonadotropin

HELLP hemolysis, elevated liver enzymes, and low platelet count

ICD-9-CM *International Classification of Diseases,*

9th Revision, Clinical Modification

ICD-10-CM *International Classification of Diseases, 10th Revision, Clinical Modification*

ICD-10-PCS *International Classification of Diseases, 10th Revision, Procedure Coding System*

IOL induction of labor

LGA large for gestational age

LTCS low transverse cesarean section

MS-DRG Medicare Severity diagnosis-related group

NRFHT nonreassuring fetal heart rate

NST nonstress test

OB obstetrics

PIH pregnancy-induced hypertension

POCs products of conception

PPROM preterm premature rupture of membranes

PROM premature rupture of membranes

PTA prior to admission

PTL preterm labor

SVD spontaneous vaginal delivery

UTI urinary tract infection

VBAC vaginal birth after cesarean section

ICD-10-CM

Official Guidelines for Coding and Reporting

Please refer to the companion Evolve website for the most current guidelines.

15. Chapter 15: Pregnancy, Childbirth, and the Puerperium (O00-*O9A*)

   a. General Rules for Obstetric Cases

   1) Codes from chapter 15 and sequencing priority

   Obstetric cases require codes from chapter 15, codes in the range O00-O9A, Pregnancy, Childbirth, and the Puerperium. Chapter 15 codes have sequencing priority over codes from other chapters. Additional codes from other chapters may be used in conjunction with chapter 15 codes to further specify conditions. Should the provider document that the pregnancy is incidental to the encounter, then code Z33.1, Pregnant state, incidental, should be used in place of any chapter 15 codes. It is the provider's responsibility to state that the condition being treated is not affecting the pregnancy.

In most cases, when a patient is pregnant, a code from Chapter 15 must be assigned regardless of what condition the patient presents with. The exception to this rule would occur when a physician documents that the pregnancy is incidental to the reason for this encounter. Almost ALWAYS, codes from the pregnancy chapter are to be assigned. This does not mean that codes from other chapters cannot be used to more fully describe a condition. The codes from Chapter 15 have sequencing priority.

EXAMPLE

Patient presents to physician office with pain and burning on urination. The physician documents that the patient is 26 weeks pregnant and has a UTI. Codes would be as follows: Infections of the genitourinary tract in pregnancy, O23.42, N39.0, Z3A.26.

EXAMPLE

A patient with gastroenteritis is seen in the emergency room (ER). The ER physician documents that the pregnancy is incidental to her gastroenteritis. Codes would be as follows: Gastroenteritis, K52.9, Pregnancy state, incidental, Z33.1.

2) Chapter 15 codes used only on the maternal record
Chapter 15 codes are to be used only on the maternal record, never on the record of the newborn.

It can be confusing as to what can be reported on the mother's chart and what can be reported on the newborn's chart. If possible it may be helpful to code both charts at the same time.

In the example above, if a pregnant woman has a UTI that in turn affects the care of the newborn, the code O23.42 would not be used on the newborn chart. The code P00.1 would be assigned to the newborn chart and is found in the index. See Figure 22-1 for an example of a condition that may complicate pregnancy.

Codes that are assigned to the newborn are discussed in Chapter 22.

3) Final character for trimester
The majority of codes in Chapter 15 have a final character indicating the trimester of pregnancy. The timeframes for the trimesters are indicated at the beginning of the chapter. If trimester is not a component of a code it is because the condition always occurs in a specific trimester, or the concept of trimester of pregnancy is not applicable. Certain codes have characters for only certain trimesters because the condition does not occur in all trimesters, but it may occur in more than just one.

Assignment of the final character for trimester should be based on the provider's documentation of the trimester (or number of weeks) for the current admission/ encounter. This applies to the assignment of trimester for pre-existing conditions as well as those that develop during or are due to the pregnancy. The provider's documentation of the number of weeks may be used to assign the appropriate code identifying the trimester.

Whenever delivery occurs during the current admission, and there is an "in childbirth" option for the obstetric complication being coded, the "in childbirth" code should be assigned.

4) Selection of trimester for inpatient admissions that encompass more than one trimesters
In instances when a patient is admitted to a hospital for complications of pregnancy during one trimester and remains in the hospital into a subsequent trimester, the trimester character for the antepartum complication code should be assigned on the basis of the trimester when the complication developed, not the trimester of the discharge. If the condition developed prior to the current admission/encounter or represents a pre-existing condition, the trimester character for the trimester at the time of the admission/encounter should be assigned.

5) Unspecified trimester
Each category that includes codes for trimester has a code for "unspecified trimester." The "unspecified trimester" code should rarely be used, such as when the documentation in the record is insufficient to determine the trimester and it is not possible to obtain clarification.

EXAMPLE   Patient in the third trimester of pregnancy is admitted with oligohydramnios, O41.03X0.

6) *7th character for Fetus Identification*
Where applicable, a 7th character is to be assigned for certain categories (O31, O32, O33.3–O33.6, O35, O36, O40, O41, O60.1, O60.2, O64, and O69) to identify the fetus for which the complication code applies.
Assign 7th character "0":
- For single gestations
- When the documentation in the record is insufficient to determine the fetus affected and it is not possible to obtain clarification.
- When it is not possible to clinically determine which fetus is affected.

Pregnancy *(Continued)*
  complicated by *(Continued)*
    hyperemesis (gravidarum) (mild)
        O21.0 - *see also* Hyperemesis,
        gravidarum
    hypertension - *see* Hypertension, com-
        plicating pregnancy
    hypertensive
        heart and renal disease, pre-
            existing – *see* Hypertension,
            complicating, pregnancy, pre-
            existing, with, heart disease,
            with renal disease
        heart disease, pre-existing – *see*
            Hypertension, complicating,
            pregnancy, pre-existing, with,
            heart disease
        renal disease, pre-existing – *see*
            Hypertension, complicating,
            pregnancy, pre-existing, with,
            renal disease
    hypotension O26.5-
    immune disorders NEC (conditions in
        D80-D89) O99.11-
    incarceration, uterus O34.51-
    incompetent cervix O34.3-
    infection(s) O98.91-
        amniotic fluid or sac O41.10-
        bladder O23.1-
        carrier state NEC O99.830
            streptococcus B O99.820
        genital organ or tract O23.9-
            specified NEC O23.59-
        genitourinary tract O23.9-
        gonorrhea O98.21-
        hepatitis (viral) O98.41-
        HIV O98.71-
        human immunodeficiency [HIV]
            O98.71-
        kidney O23.0-
        nipple O91.01-
        parasitic disease O98.91-
            specified NEC O98.81-
        protozoal disease O98.61-
        sexually transmitted NEC O98.31-
        specified type NEC O98.81-
        syphilis O98.11-
        tuberculosis O98.01-
        urethra O23.2-
        urinary (tract) O23.4-
            specified NEC O23.3-

FIGURE 21-1. A urinary tract infection is an example of a condition that may complicate pregnancy.

b. Selection of OB Principal or First-listed Diagnosis

1) Routine outpatient prenatal visits

For routine outpatient prenatal visits when no complications are present, a code from category Z34, Encounter for supervision of normal pregnancy, should be used as the first-listed diagnosis. These codes should not be used in conjunction with chapter 15 codes.

2) Prenatal outpatient visits for high-risk patients

For routine prenatal outpatient visits for patients with high-risk pregnancies, a code from category O09, Supervision of high-risk pregnancy, should be used as the first-listed diagnosis. Secondary chapter 15 codes may be used in conjunction with these codes if appropriate.

| EXAMPLE | The patient is seen in her first trimester at 13 weeks for a routine prenatal visit. She also has a 2-year-old daughter, Z34.81, Z3A.13. |

| EXAMPLE | The patient is seen at 11 weeks for a routine prenatal visit. The physician documents that she has iron deficiency anemia, O99.011, D50.9, Z3A.11. |

For a patient at high risk, first-listed diagnoses should be selected from the O09 category for outpatient prenatal visits. ICD-10-CM has separate codes for different high-risk categories such as infertility, history of abortion, multiparity, history of preterm labor, poor reproductive history, insufficient prenatal care, elderly primigravida or multigravida, and young primigravida or multigravida. The *Merck Manual* reports that "high-risk" pregnancy has no formal or universally accepted definition, but it goes on to list the following risk factors:

- Weight of mother less than 100 lb
- Obese mother
- Short stature of mother
- Structural abnormalities such as double uterus or incompetent cervix
- Disorders of a mother that are present prior to pregnancy, such as heart disease, high blood pressure, and seizure

| EXAMPLE | A pregnant patient at 10 weeks presents for a routine prenatal visit. During her previous pregnancy, she had early pregnancy vomiting and the physician documents high-risk pregnancy, O09.891. |

| EXAMPLE | A gravid patient at 12 weeks presents for a routine prenatal visit. This patient had preeclampsia on her previous pregnancy and the physician documents high-risk pregnancy. She has blood work taken on this visit and is found to be anemic. The physician prescribes an iron supplement, O09.891, O99.011, D64.9, Z3A.10. |

> **3) Episodes when no delivery occurs**
> In episodes when no delivery occurs, the principal diagnosis should correspond to the principal complication of the pregnancy which necessitated the encounter. Should more than one complication exist, all of which are treated or monitored, any of the complications codes may be sequenced first.

At times, a pregnant woman may have to be admitted to the hospital prior to delivery and sent home before delivery occurs. In these cases, the principal diagnosis is the reason the patient was admitted to the hospital.

| EXAMPLE | A pregnant patient at 13 weeks presents to the ER with dehydration related to **hyperemesis gravidarum**. The physician in the ER discovers that the patient has pregnancy-induced hypertension. The patient is admitted, O21.1, O13.1, Z3A.13. |

> **4) When a delivery occurs**
> When a delivery occurs, the principal diagnosis should correspond to the main circumstances or complication of the delivery. In cases of cesarean delivery, the selection of the principal diagnosis should be the condition established after study that was responsible for the patient's admission. If the patient was admitted with a condition that resulted in the performance of a cesarean procedure, that condition should be selected as the principal diagnosis. If the reason for the admission/encounter was unrelated to the condition resulting in the cesarean delivery, the condition related to the reason for the admission/encounter should be selected as the principal diagnosis.

EXAMPLE | A patient is admitted to the hospital in labor at 40 weeks. She is 40 years old, and labor proceeds uneventfully. This is her sixth pregnancy, and the baby weighs 11 lb. She is delivered by a physician, who performs a midline episiotomy. Physician documents LGA, O36.63x0, O09.523, Z3A.40, Z37.0, 0W8NXZZ.

EXAMPLE | A patient is admitted to the hospital for severe preeclampsia. She is 36 weeks pregnant. A low transverse cervical cesarean section (LTCS) is performed immediately, and she delivers a healthy baby boy, O14.13, O60.14x0, Z3A.36, Z37.0, 10D00Z1.

> **5) Outcome of delivery**
> A code from category Z37, Outcome of delivery, should be included on every maternal record when a delivery has occurred. These codes are not to be used on subsequent records or on the newborn record.

EXAMPLE | Healthy 40-year-old primigravida presents to the hospital at 37 weeks and delivers twins vaginally, O30.003, O09.513, Z3A.37, Z37.2, 10E0XZZ.

EXAMPLE | A pregnant woman at 39 weeks presents to the hospital for delivery of known quadruplets. She is taken to the operating room for a cesarean section (LTCS). As the babies are delivered, it is discovered that one has died in utero, O30.203, O36.4xx0, Z3A.39, Z37.62, 10D00Z1.

> **c. Pre-existing conditions versus conditions due to the pregnancy**
> Certain categories in Chapter 15 distinguish between conditions of the mother that existed prior to pregnancy (pre-existing) and those that are a direct result of pregnancy. When assigning codes from Chapter 15, it is important to assess if a condition was pre-existing prior to pregnancy or developed during or due to the pregnancy in order to assign the correct code.
> Categories that do not distinguish between pre-existing and pregnancy-related conditions may be used for either. It is acceptable to use codes specifically for the puerperium with codes complicating pregnancy and childbirth if a condition arises postpartum during the delivery encounter.
>
> **d. Pre-existing hypertension in pregnancy**
> Category O10, Pre-existing hypertension complicating pregnancy, childbirth and the puerperium, includes codes for hypertensive heart and hypertensive chronic kidney disease. When assigning one of the O10 codes that includes hypertensive heart disease or hypertensive chronic kidney disease, it is necessary to add a secondary code from the appropriate hypertension category to specify the type of heart failure or chronic kidney disease.
> *See Section I.C.9. Hypertension.*

If a condition existed prior to the pregnancy, it is considered pre-existing, as opposed to a condition that develops as a direct result of a pregnancy. If there are categories that do not make a distinction between pre-existing and pregnancy-related, then it is acceptable to use them for either. If a condition arises postpartum, it is acceptable to assign codes specifically for the puerperium.

EXAMPLE | Patient is seen by the obstetrician at 30 weeks for lab work related to her diabetes. The patient has had diabetes type 1 since childhood, O24.013, Z3A.30.

EXAMPLE | Patient delivered baby 2 weeks ago. She is feeling very shaky and her blood sugars are extremely high. Physician documents gestational diabetes, O24.439.

EXAMPLE | Patient has had varicose veins in her legs for years. She is now in the 22nd week of her pregnancy and complaining of pain in her lower extremities. Physician documents varicose veins, O22.02, Z3A.22.

e. Fetal Conditions Affecting the Management of the Mother

1) Codes from categories O35 and O36

Codes from categories O35, Maternal care for known or suspected fetal abnormality and damage, and O36, Maternal care for other fetal problems, are assigned only when the fetal condition is actually responsible for modifying the management of the mother, i.e., by requiring diagnostic studies, additional observation, special care, or termination of pregnancy. The fact that the fetal condition exists does not justify assigning a code from this series to the mother's record.

2) In utero surgery

In cases when surgery is performed on the fetus, a diagnosis code from category O35, Maternal care for known or suspected fetal abnormality and damage, should be assigned identifying the fetal condition. Assign the appropriate procedure code for the procedure performed.

No code from Chapter 16, the perinatal codes, should be used on the mother's record to identify fetal conditions. Surgery performed in utero on a fetus is still to be coded as an obstetric encounter.

EXAMPLE | Fetal chromosomal abnormality with elective termination of pregnancy at 14 weeks, with insertion of laminaria and aspiration curettage of uterus, with complete extraction of products of conception, Z33.2, O35.1xx0, Z3A.14, 10A07ZW, 10A07Z6.

EXAMPLE | Mother presents for delivery at 40 weeks. The physician documents that the baby appears large for dates (LGA [large for gestational age]). The mother vaginally delivers a 7 lb baby girl without any complications, O80, Z3A.40, Z37.0.

In this case, the LGA code would not be used because it does not affect the management of the mother.

EXAMPLE | A fetus is known to have spina bifida. The parents find a surgeon trained in operating in utero and have this problem corrected at 20 weeks. Central nervous system malformation in fetus O35.0xx0, Z3A.20, 10Q00ZE, Open correction of fetal defect.

f. HIV Infection in Pregnancy, Childbirth and the Puerperium

During pregnancy, childbirth or the puerperium, a patient admitted because of an HIV-related illness should receive a principal diagnosis from subcategory O98.7-, Human immunodeficiency [HIV] disease complicating pregnancy, childbirth and the puerperium, followed by the code(s) for the HIV-related illness(es).

Patients with asymptomatic HIV infection status admitted during pregnancy, childbirth, or the puerperium should receive codes of O98.7- and Z21, Asymptomatic human immunodeficiency virus [HIV] infection status.

EXAMPLE | A 32-year-old female who is 23 weeks pregnant with known AIDS is admitted with severe diarrhea determined to be caused by cryptosporidium. She is treated with IV fluids, O98.712, B20, A07.2, Z3A.23.

EXAMPLE | A 23-year-old gravid female is admitted in preterm labor at 35 weeks. She has had an uneventful pregnancy, except for the fact that she has an asymptomatic human immunodeficiency virus (HIV) infection. She vaginally delivers a 7 lb 2 oz baby, O60.14x0, O98.713, Z37.0, Z21, Z3A.35, 10E0XZZ.

g. **Diabetes mellitus in pregnancy**
   Diabetes mellitus is a significant complicating factor in pregnancy. Pregnant women who are diabetic should be assigned a code **from category** O24, Diabetes mellitus in pregnancy, childbirth, and the puerperium, first, followed by the appropriate diabetes code(s) (E08-E13) from Chapter 4.

h. **Long term use of insulin**
   Code Z79.4, Long-term (current) use of insulin, should also be assigned if the diabetes mellitus is being treated with insulin.

EXAMPLE   Patient is admitted to hospital in diabetic ketoacidosis. The admitting physician documents that the patient is 12 weeks pregnant with a history of type I diabetes. She is treated with sliding scale insulin, O24.011, E10.10, Z79.4, Z3A.12.

i. **Gestational (pregnancy induced) diabetes**
   Gestational (pregnancy induced) diabetes can occur during the second and third trimester of pregnancy in women who were not diabetic prior to pregnancy. Gestational diabetes can cause complications in the pregnancy similar to those of pre-existing diabetes mellitus. It also puts the woman at greater risk of developing diabetes after the pregnancy. Codes for gestational diabetes are in subcategory O24.4, Gestational diabetes mellitus. No other code from category O24, Diabetes mellitus in pregnancy, childbirth, and the puerperium, should be used with a code from O24.4

   The codes under subcategory O24.4 include diet controlled and insulin controlled. If a patient with gestational diabetes is treated with both diet and insulin, only the code for insulin-controlled is required. Code Z79.4, Long-term (current) use of insulin, should not be assigned with codes from subcategory O24.4.

   An abnormal glucose tolerance in pregnancy is assigned a code from subcategory O99.81, Abnormal glucose complicating pregnancy, childbirth, and the puerperium.

EXAMPLE   A patient is admitted to the hospital in labor at 39 weeks. She has had a relatively uneventful pregnancy except for gestational diabetes which was diet controlled. She vaginally delivers a healthy 7 lb baby girl, O24.410, Z3A.39, Z37.0, 10E0XZZ.

j. **Sepsis and septic shock complicating abortion, pregnancy, childbirth and the puerperium**
   When assigning a chapter 15 code for sepsis complicating abortion, pregnancy, childbirth, and the puerperium, a code for the specific type of infection should be assigned as an additional diagnosis. If severe sepsis is present, a code from subcategory R65.2, Severe sepsis, and code(s) for associated organ dysfunction(s) should also be assigned as additional diagnoses.

k. **Puerperal sepsis**
   Code O85, Puerperal sepsis, should be assigned with a secondary code to identify the causal organism (e.g., for a bacterial infection, assign a code from category B95-B96, Bacterial infections in conditions classified elsewhere). A code from category A40, Streptococcal sepsis, or A41, Other sepsis, should not be used for puerperal sepsis. If applicable, use additional codes to identify severe sepsis (R65.2-) and any associated acute organ dysfunction.

EXAMPLE   A 38-week primagravida spontaneously delivers an SGA baby. Following delivery the obstetrician manually removes fragments of the retained placenta. On the second day after delivery the patient develops a fever and foul smelling discharge. Antibiotics are initiated and puerperal sepsis is documented, O73.1, O85, Z3A.38, Z37.0, 10D17ZZ, 10E0XZZ.

l. **Alcohol and tobacco use during pregnancy, childbirth and the puerperium**

1) **Alcohol use during pregnancy, childbirth and the puerperium**

Codes under subcategory O99.31, Alcohol use complicating pregnancy, childbirth, and the puerperium, should be assigned for any pregnancy case when a mother uses alcohol during the pregnancy or postpartum. A secondary code from category F10, Alcohol related disorders, should also be assigned to identify manifestations of the alcohol use.

2) **Tobacco use during pregnancy, childbirth and the puerperium**

Codes under subcategory O99.33, Smoking (tobacco) complicating pregnancy, childbirth, and the puerperium, should be assigned for any pregnancy case when a mother uses any type of tobacco product during the pregnancy or postpartum. A secondary code from category F17, Nicotine dependence, or code Z72.0, Tobacco use, should also be assigned to identify the type of nicotine dependence.

EXAMPLE Patient reports to the emergency room in labor. She is 30 weeks pregnant and admits to drinking daily during this pregnancy. She is admitted for administration of terbutaline. Physician documents early labor due to alcohol abuse, O60.03, O99.313, F10.10, Z3A.30.

m. **Poisoning, toxic effects, adverse effects and underdosing in a pregnant patient**

A code from subcategory O9A.2, Injury, poisoning and certain other consequences of external causes complicating pregnancy, childbirth, and the puerperium, should be sequenced first, followed by the appropriate poisoning, toxic effect, adverse effect or underdosing code, and then the additional code(s) that specifies the condition caused by the poisoning, toxic effect, adverse effect or underdosing.

See Section I.C.19. Adverse effects, poisoning, underdosing and toxic effects.

EXAMPLE Patient is 18 weeks pregnant. She presents to the ED in an altered mental state after taking a whole bottle of Valium. She was trying to kill herself after an argument with her mother, O9A.212, T42.4x2A, R41.82, Z3A.18.

n. **Normal Delivery, Code O80**

1) **Encounter for full term uncomplicated delivery**

Code O80 should be assigned when a woman is admitted for a full-term normal delivery and delivers a single, healthy infant without any complications antepartum, during the delivery, or postpartum during the delivery episode. Code O80 is always a principal diagnosis. It is not to be used if any other code from chapter 15 is needed to describe a current complication of the antenatal, delivery, or perinatal period. Additional codes from other chapters may be used with code O80 if they are not related to or are in any way complicating the pregnancy.

2) **Uncomplicated delivery with resolved antepartum complication**

Code O80 may be used if the patient had a complication at some point during the pregnancy, but the complication is not present at the time of the admission for delivery.

3) **Outcome of delivery for O80**

Z37.0, Single live birth, is the only outcome of delivery code appropriate for use with O80.

EXAMPLE Patient is admitted to the hospital in labor. She is 40 weeks pregnant. She has had an uneventful pregnancy and vaginally delivers a 7 lb 2 oz baby boy. The doctor performs an episiotomy followed by suturing during delivery, O80, Z37.0, Z3A.40, 0W8NXZZ.

EXAMPLE Patient is admitted to the hospital in labor. She is 40 weeks pregnant. She has had an uneventful pregnancy and vaginally delivers a 7 lb 2 oz baby boy. The doctor performs an episiotomy and the baby is delivered with the use of a vacuum extractor, O75.9, Z3A.40, Z37.0, 10D07Z6, 0W8NXZZ.

The use of a vacuum extractor in the above example prohibits the use of code O80 for this delivery.

EXAMPLE Patient is admitted to the hospital in labor. She is 40 weeks pregnant, has had an uneventful pregnancy, and vaginally delivers a 7 lb 2 oz baby boy. The doctor performs an episiotomy with a first-degree extension with repair, O70.0, Z3A.40, Z37.0, 0HQ9XZZ.

As in the previous example, the first-degree extension in this example prohibits the use of O80. When an extension of an episiotomy occurs, both the episiotomy and laceration repair are coded.

EXAMPLE Patient is admitted to the hospital in labor. She is 40 weeks pregnant. She had a UTI early on in her pregnancy and was treated appropriately. She delivers a 7 lb 2 oz baby boy by spontaneous vaginal delivery, O80, Z3A.40, Z37.0, 10E0XZZ.

o. The Peripartum and Postpartum Periods
1) Peripartum and Postpartum periods
The postpartum period begins immediately after delivery and continues for six weeks following delivery. The peripartum period is defined as the last month of pregnancy to five months postpartum.

EXAMPLE Patient is admitted to hospital for mastitis. She is 5 weeks postpartum and is given a course of intravenous (IV) antibiotics, O91.22.

2) Peripartum and postpartum complication
A postpartum complication is any complication occurring within the six-week period.

EXAMPLE Patient is admitted to the hospital 3 weeks postpartum. She is having pain in her lower right leg and is given a diagnosis of deep vein thrombosis. The patient is treated with IV heparin, O87.1, I82.4Z1.

3) Pregnancy-related complications after 6 week period
Chapter 15 codes may also be used to describe pregnancy-related complications after the peripartum or postpartum period if the provider documents that a condition is pregnancy related.

EXAMPLE Patient is admitted to the hospital with postpartum cholecystitis. She delivered 12 weeks prior to this presentation, O99.63, K81.9.
In this case, the physician documented that this was a postpartum condition; therefore, it was coded as such even though it occurred beyond the 6-week time period.

4) Admission for routine postpartum care following delivery outside hospital
When the mother delivers outside the hospital prior to admission and is admitted for routine postpartum care and no complications are noted, code Z39.0, Encounter for care and examination of mother immediately after delivery, should be assigned as the principal diagnosis.

EXAMPLE
Patient delivers baby at 38 weeks in the car on the way to the hospital. She is admitted through the ER for examination, Z39.0, Z3A.38.

5) Pregnancy associated cardiomyopathy
Pregnancy associated cardiomyopathy, code O90.3, is unique in that it may be diagnosed in the third trimester of pregnancy but may continue to progress months after delivery. For this reason, it is referred to as peripartum cardiomyopathy. Code O90.3 is only for use when the cardiomyopathy develops as a result of pregnancy in a woman who did not have pre-existing heart disease.

EXAMPLE
Patient is 2 weeks postpartum. She presents to physician's office complaining of shortness of breath, swollen ankles, and frequent awakening to urinate. The physician performs chest CT. His diagnosis is postpartum cardiomyopathy, O90.3.

p. Code O94, Sequelae of complication of pregnancy, childbirth, and the puerperium
1) Code O94
Code O94, Sequelae of complication of pregnancy, childbirth, and the puerperium, is for use in those cases when an initial complication of a pregnancy develops a sequelae requiring care or treatment at a future date.
2) After the initial postpartum period
This code may be used at any time after the initial postpartum period.
3) Sequencing of Code O94
This code, like all **sequela** codes, is to be sequenced following the code describing the sequelae of the complication.

EXAMPLE
The patient presents to the physician's office complaining of painful intercourse.
She is 6 months postpartum. The obstetrician determines that the patient is suffering from a late effect of the repair of the perineum, N94.1, O94, Y83.8.

q. Abortions
1) Abortion with Liveborn Fetus
When an attempted termination of pregnancy results in a liveborn fetus, assign a code from subcategory O60.1, Preterm labor with preterm delivery, and a code from category Z37, Outcome of Delivery. The procedure code for the attempted termination of pregnancy should also be assigned.

EXAMPLE
A woman is admitted at 22 weeks for insertion of a laminaria for termination of pregnancy. She delivers a liveborn fetus, O60.12x0, Z3A.22, Z37.0, 10E0XZZ, 10A07ZW.

2) Retained Products of Conception following an abortion
Subsequent encounters for retained products of conception following a spontaneous abortion or elective termination of pregnancy are assigned the appropriate code from category O03, Spontaneous abortion, or codes O07.4, Failed attempted termination of pregnancy without complication and Z33.2, Encounter for elective termination of pregnancy. This advice is appropriate even when the patient was discharged previously with a discharge diagnosis of complete abortion.

EXAMPLE
Retained products of conception after spontaneous abortion at 8 weeks' gestation. The products of conception were initially passed at home 2 days ago. D&C was performed, O03.4, Z3A.08, 10D17ZZ.

> **r. Abuse in a pregnant patient**
> For suspected or confirmed cases of abuse of a pregnant patient, a code(s) from subcategories O9A.3, Physical abuse complicating pregnancy, childbirth, and the puerperium, O9A.4, Sexual abuse complicating pregnancy, childbirth, and the puerperium, and O9A.5, Psychological abuse complicating pregnancy, childbirth, and the puerperium, should be sequenced first, followed by the appropriate codes (if applicable) to identify any associated current injury due to physical abuse, sexual abuse, and the perpetrator of abuse.
> *See Section I.C.19.f. Adult and child abuse, neglect and other maltreatment.*

EXAMPLE Pregnant woman is admitted at 37 weeks in active labor after being physically abused by her spouse. She goes on to have a normal vaginal delivery, O9a.32, Z3A.37, Z37.0, Y07.01, 10E0XZZ.

MAJOR DIFFERENCES BETWEEN ICD-10-CM AND ICD-9-CM

- The final character in most codes in this chapter of ICD-10-CM indicates the trimester of pregnancy, not the episode of care. Trimesters are defined at the beginning of Chapter 15. They are as follows:
  - First Trimester—less than 14 weeks 0 days
  - Second Trimester—14 weeks 0 days to less than 28 weeks 0 days
  - Third Trimester—28 weeks 0 days until delivery
- Supervision of care for high-risk pregnancy has been moved to this chapter.
- Guidelines added for preexisting conditions versus conditions due to the pregnancy have been added to ICD-10-CM.
- Guidelines for the use of alcohol and tobacco in pregnancy have been added to ICD-10-CM.
- Guidelines for adverse effects and underdosing in a pregnant patient have been added to ICD-10-CM.
- A guideline for pregnancy-associated cardiomyopathy has been added to ICD-10-CM.
- Many of the guidelines for abortion have been removed from ICD-10-CM due to either episode-of-care issues or due to the fact that elective, legal, and therapeutic abortions are no longer classified here.
- Characters have been added to identify a specific fetus affected by obstetric conditions.
- The reason for obstruction is incorporated into obstructed labor codes.

ANATOMY AND PHYSIOLOGY

The organs of the female reproductive system include the ovaries, fallopian tubes, uterus, vagina, and cervix (Figure 21-2). These organs aid in reproduction and supply hormones that aid in the development of secondary female sex characteristics such as body hair and breasts.

The **vulva** is the external covering to the vagina. The **labia** surround the vaginal opening. The vagina is a muscular tube that extends from the vaginal opening to the uterus. The **vagina** serves three purposes: It is the receptacle for sperm during intercourse, it serves as the birth canal for childbirth, and it rids the body of menstrual blood during menstruation.

The **cervix** is the neck of the uterus and serves as an outlet from the uterus. The **uterus** is a muscular organ that serves as an incubator for the developing fetus. The wall of the uterus is composed of three layers. The inner layer, the endometrium, is where an egg grows if fertilized.

The **ovaries** produce female hormones and eggs. If the egg is fertilized and becomes a fetus, all the other female organs assist in development and expulsion of the fetus. When an egg becomes mature and is ready for fertilization, it travels through the **fallopian tube** to the uterus. The purpose of the fallopian tube is to deliver the mature egg to the uterus for fertilization. See Figure 21-3 for the anatomy of a normal uterine pregnancy.

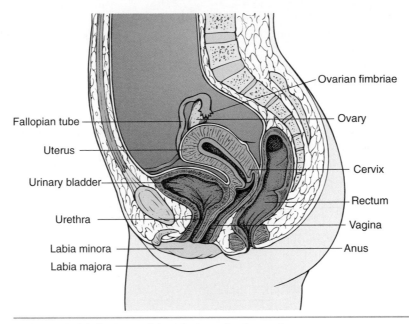

FIGURE 21-2. Normal female reproductive system.

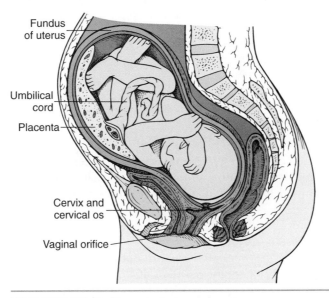

FIGURE 21-3. Normal uterine pregnancy.

To confirm a pregnancy, a woman's blood or urine may be tested for human chorionic gonadotropin (hCG). In the early months of pregnancy, secretion of hCG occurs at a high level.

Common Pregnancy Definitions

Antepartum: before delivery
Elderly obstetric patient: 35 years or older at date of delivery
Gravid: pregnant
Habitual aborter: a woman who miscarries at least three consecutive times
Lactation: process of milk production
Multigravida or **multiparity:** two or more pregnancies

Postpartum: after delivery

Postterm pregnancy: pregnancy longer than 40 weeks up to 42 weeks

Precipitate labor: rapid labor and delivery

Pregestational: condition present prior to pregnancy

Prenatal: before birth

Primigravida: first pregnancy

Prolonged pregnancy: beyond 42 weeks of pregnancy

Puerperium: time from delivery through first 6 weeks post partum

Stillbirth: dead at birth

Young obstetric patient: younger than 16 years at date of delivery

CONDITIONS OF PREGNANCY, CHILDBIRTH, AND PUERPERIUM

Pregnancy, Childbirth, and the Puerperium (O00-O9A), Chapter 15 in the ICD-10-CM code book, is divided into the following categories:

CATEGORY	SECTION TITLES
O00-O08	Pregnancy with abortive outcome
O09	Supervision of high-risk pregnancy
O10-O16	Edema, proteinuria, and hypertensive disorders in pregnancy, childbirth, and the puerperium
O20-O29	Other maternal disorders predominantly related to pregnancy
O30-O48	Maternal care related to the fetus and amniotic cavity and possible delivery problems
O60-O77	Complications of labor and delivery
O80-O82	Encounter for delivery
O85-O92	Complications predominantly related to the puerperium
O94-O9A	Other obstetric conditions, not elsewhere classified

Coding of Pregnancy

A normal pregnancy (Figure 21-4) usually lasts anywhere from 37 to 40 weeks. These weeks are counted from the beginning of the last menstrual cycle. A normal pregnancy has three trimesters, counted from the first day of the last menstrual period. They are defined as follows:

- First trimester—less than 14 weeks 0 days
- Second trimester—14 weeks 0 days to less than 28 weeks 0 days
- Third trimester—28 weeks 0 days until delivery

When a pregnancy lasts longer than 40 weeks (post-term), complications can occur; and therefore this is no longer considered a normal pregnancy. Documentation of weeks/ trimester should be made by the provider.

Labor is the process of expelling the products of conception from the uterus through the vagina to the outside world. There are four stages of labor:

- First Stage—Dilation

  Begins with cervical dilation and regular uterine contraction and ends when the patient is completely dilated and **effaced** (shortening or thinning of the cervix has occurred). The average length of time for this process is 10 to 14 hours.

- Second Stage—Expulsion

  Begins with complete dilation and effacement of the cervix and ends with the birth of the baby. The average length of time for this process is 1 to 4 hours.

- Third Stage—Placenta

  Begins with the birth of the baby and ends with the delivery of the placenta. The average length of time for this process is from 5 to 15 minutes.

- Fourth Stage—Return to normal

  Begins with the delivery of the placenta and ends 1 to 2 hours after delivery, when uterine tone is established.

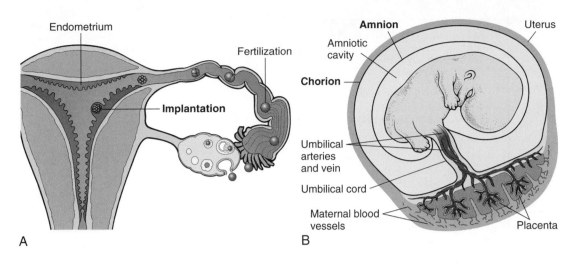

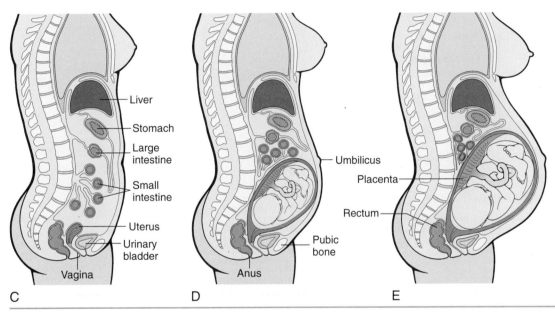

FIGURE 21-4. A, Implantation of the embryo in the endometrium. **B,** The placenta and membranes (chorion and amnion). **C–E,** Sagittal sections of pregnancy. **C,** Nonpregnant woman. **D,** Woman who is 20 weeks pregnant. **E,** Woman who is 30 weeks pregnant.

All deliveries require an outcome of delivery code on the mother's record. The outcome of delivery is the code used to describe the number of newborns delivered and their status, i.e., live or stillborn. The outcome of delivery code is found in the Alphabetic Index under the main term "outcome of delivery." **It is important to note that if code O80 is selected, it cannot be used with any other code in Chapter 15.**

When codes are selected for complications of pregnancy, childbirth, and the puerperium, a variety of main terms in the index may be accessed. If the condition is affecting the pregnancy, the index term is pregnancy. Likewise if the condition is affecting labor, the index directs the coder to see delivery. The Alphabetic Index may be checked directly for a condition (Figure 21-5).

Other main terms in the Alphabetic Index that may be used to locate pregnancy-related codes include the following:

- Failure
- Laceration
- Puerperal
- Pregnancy
- Delivery
- Outcome

Hypertension, hypertensive *(Continued)*
  with *(Continued)*
    kidney involvement - *see* Hyper-
      tension, kidney
    renal sclerosis (conditions in N26) -
      see Hypertension, kidney
  benign, intracranial G93.2
  cardiorenal (disease) I13.10
    with heart failure I13.0
      with stage I through stage IV
        chronic kidney disease
        I13.0
      with stage V or end stage renal
        disease I13.2
    without heart failure I13.10
      with stage I through stage IV
        chronic kidney disease
        I13.10
      with stage V or end stage renal
        disease I13.11
  cardiovascular
    disease (arteriosclerotic) (sclerotic) -
      see Hypertension, heart
    renal (disease) (sclerosis) - *see*
      Hypertension, cardiorenal
  chronic venous - *see* Hypertension,
    venous (chronic)
  complicating
    childbirth (labor) O10.92
      with
        heart disease O10.12
        with renal disease
          O10.32
        renal disease O10.22
        with heart disease
          O10.32
      essential O10.02
      secondary O10.42
    pregnancy O16.-

FIGURE 21-5. Alphabetic Index entry for hypertension complicating pregnancy.

EXERCISE 21-1

Answer the following questions.

1. The duration of a normal pregnancy is

    _____

2. Can code O80 be used with O66.5xx0?

    _____

3. What are the three most common areas of the Alphabetic Index to look under for codes related to Chapter 15?

  1. _____

  2. _____

  3. _____

4. What are the organs of the female reproductive system? _____

5. To confirm a pregnancy, what is tested for from a woman's blood or urine?

    _____

6. If a woman is pregnant for the first time at age 36, what would be another term for her?

    _____

7. If a woman delivers at 41 weeks, what would this be considered? _____

8. How long does the puerperium last? _____

Identify the main term(s) that would be used to locate the following in the Alphabetic Index.

9. Obstructed labor _____

10. First-degree perineal laceration delivered single liveborn vaginally _____

11. Arrested labor _____

12. Fever due to amnionitis during labor _____

13. Twin pregnancy _____

14. Oligohydramnios _____

15. Premature rupture of membranes _____

16. Primary uterine inertia _____

17. Postpartum hemorrhage _____

18. Breech delivery _____

19. Prolonged labor _____

20. Precipitous delivery _____

Pregnancy With Abortive Outcome (O00-O08)

Ectopic and Molar Pregnancy

Ectopic pregnancies usually occur when the egg is implanted outside the cavity of the uterus, most commonly in the fallopian tube (Figure 21-6). This type of pregnancy occurs in 1 of every 50 pregnancies. Pelvic infections may predispose a woman to having ectopic pregnancies.

EXAMPLE Patient presents to physician's office with abdominal pain and vaginal bleeding. She is 10 weeks pregnant. An ultrasound performed in the office determines that the patient has an ectopic pregnancy of the fallopian tubes. She is scheduled for emergency surgery, O00.1, Z3A.10.

Molar pregnancies are rare and occur in 1 in 1000 pregnancies. In a **molar pregnancy** the embryo does not form at all or is malformed. The early placenta develops into a mass of cysts within a hydatidiform mole (Figure 21-7). Occasionally, a molar pregnancy can turn into a rare pregnancy-related form of cancer.

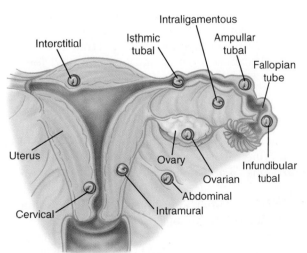

FIGURE 21-6. Diagram showing locations of ectopic (extrauterine) pregnancy.

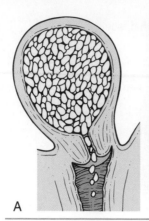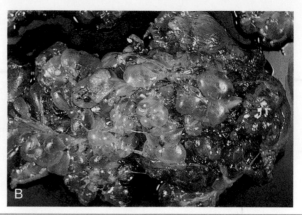

FIGURE 21-7. Hydatidiform mole.

EXAMPLE

> Patient presents to her physician's office with a pregnancy in the 10th week. She comes in because she is experiencing dark brown vaginal bleeding. The physician identifies a molar pregnancy. The patient is admitted to the hospital for vacuum curettage to remove the molar tissue.
>
> Codes: Hydatidiform mole O0.19
>
> 10 weeks gestation of pregnancy Z3A.10
>
> Extraction of products conception, vacuum, via natural or artificial opening 10A07Z6.

It is appropriate to use codes from O08.– to describe any complications that may occur during an ectopic or molar pregnancy. According to the general rule for obstetric cases, additional codes from other chapters may be used in conjunction with Chapter 15 codes to further specify conditions.

EXAMPLE

> Patient is admitted to the hospital at 18 weeks with a tubal pregnancy without intrauterine pregnancy. After the tubal pregnancy is removed, the patient develops a urinary tract infection (UTI).
>
> Codes: Tubal pregnancy without intrauterine pregnancy O00.1
>
> Urinary tract infection following an ectopic and molar pregnancy O08.83
>
> 18 weeks gestation of pregnancy Z3A.18.

Abortion is the termination of a pregnancy by natural causes or medical intervention. Abortions occurring either naturally (spontaneously) or those performed with medical intervention (induced termination of pregnancy or elective abortion) may have complications such as hemorrhage, lacerations, and sepsis. ICD-10-CM contains codes that include two types of abortions: spontaneous/complete or incomplete with or without complications, and induced or elective abortions (abortions with medical intervention) with complications. If a patient is admitted for an elective termination of pregnancy and there are no complications, the code Z33.2 (Encounter for elective termination of pregnancy) is the principal diagnosis. In some instances a patient may be admitted for an elective abortion and the attempt to abort the fetus is unsuccessful, resulting in an incomplete elective abortion. In these cases a code from category O07 would be assigned.

Types of Abortion

Complete abortion is an abortion in which all the products of conception are expelled.

Elective abortion is the elective termination of pregnancy.

Incomplete abortion is an abortion in which not all of the products of conception are expelled.

Inevitable abortion occurs when symptoms are present, and a miscarriage will happen.

Miscarriage is spontaneous termination of a pregnancy before the fetus has reached 20 weeks.

Missed abortion is a pregnancy with fetal demise before 20 weeks, when no products of conception are expelled.

Spontaneous abortion is the loss of a fetus due to natural causes; it is also known as a
 miscarriage.

Therapeutic abortion is an abortion performed when the pregnancy is endangering the
 mother's health, or when the fetus has a condition that is incompatible with life.

Threatened abortion occurs when symptoms are present that indicate that a miscarriage
 is possible.

EXAMPLE	Patient presents to the hospital with known pregnancy. She is in her 11th week and is now complaining of severe back pain and vaginal bleeding. The physician examines the patient and determines that she has suffered an incomplete abortion. A dilation and curettage (D&C) is performed, and the patient is discharged, O03.4, Z3A.11, 10D17ZZ.
EXAMPLE	Pregnant patient at 9 weeks presents to the hospital with vaginal bleeding and abdominal cramps. She is evaluated in the ER and is found to have a UTI. It is also determined that she has suffered a complete miscarriage. The patient is monitored for several hours and is discharged on a course of antibiotics, O03.88, Z3A.09.
EXAMPLE	Spontaneous abortion at 12 weeks, incomplete, in patient with gestational hypertension. D&C was performed, O03.4, O13.1, Z3A.12, 10D17ZZ.
EXAMPLE	Patient had a spontaneous abortion 2 weeks ago. She presents to the hospital with a high fever, hypotension, and chills. Sepsis is suspected and she is admitted, O03.87.

EXERCISE 21-2

Assign codes to the following conditions.

1. Ruptured ectopic pregnancy of the fallopian tube at 6 weeks _____

2. Vesicular mole _____

3. Ectopic pregnancy of the fallopian tube followed by oliguria _____

4. Woman is admitted to the hospital after having a miscarriage. The physician performs a suction curettage to remove the products of conception. It is believed that the miscarriage occurred in association with placenta previa. _____

5. Patient presents to the hospital at 8 weeks for an elective abortion. After the abortion is performed by suction curettage, she spikes a high fever and is diagnosed with endometritis. _____

6. Patient with missed abortion at 10 weeks was admitted to the hospital for a therapeutic abortion by D&C. _____

7. Patient presents to the hospital for an elective abortion at 20 weeks because the fetus is hydrocephalic. An aspiration curettage is performed. _____

8. Patient presents to the hospital with hemorrhage after a self-induced abortion at 6 weeks. Physician performs a D&C to control hemorrhage. _____

Supervision of High-Risk Pregnancy (O09)

These codes were moved from the V code section in ICD-9-CM to the pregnancy chapter in ICD-10-CM. Every pregnancy contains some risk of problems. Pregnancies that are high-risk mean there is a greater chance of problems. Some of the codes in this category include previous pregnancies with history of molar pregnancy, ectopic pregnancy, pre-term labor, elderly obstetric patient, and history of in utero procedures.

Patient presents today at 32 weeks. Patient is being seen weekly during this pregnancy secondary to a previous neonatal death, O09.293, Z3A.32.

Edema, Proteinuria, and Hyperlensive Disorders in Pregnancy, Childbirth, and the Puerperium (O10-O16)

Hypertension in Pregnancy

Pregnancy can be complicated by high blood pressure. In the United States, approximately 6%–8% of pregnancies are complicated by high blood pressure. A patient may have had high blood pressure prior to conceiving or may develop high blood pressure (gestational) during the pregnancy. When it develops during the pregnancy, this may be referred to as pregnancy-induced hypertension (PIH). The effects of high blood pressure can cause low birth weight or early delivery and may affect the mother's kidneys. High blood pressure in pregnancy may lead to preeclampsia or eclampsia.

Preeclampsia is related to increased blood pressure and protein in the mother's urine that occurs in the second or third trimester of pregnancy. Preeclampsia may be referred to as **toxemia** of pregnancy. Risk factors for developing preeclampsia include obesity, multiple pregnancies, first pregnancy, under the age of 20 or over the age of 40, or women with chronic diseases such as diabetes, chronic hypertension, and lupus. Preeclampsia is detected by high blood pressure, protein in the urine, swelling of the hands and feet, and weight gain of more than 2 lbs per week. The only treatment for preeclampsia is delivery of the baby. Preeclampsia can be monitored in the early stages but should it develop into seizures (eclampsia) or HELLP (hemolytic anemia, elevated liver enzymes, low platelet count) syndrome, this becomes a life-threatening condition.

EXAMPLE | Patient presents to her doctors office for routine check up at 24 weeks of pregnancy. Blood pressure is elevated and patient's hands and feet are quite swollen. The physician performs a lab test to look for protein in the urine. The test is positive. The physician documents PIH, O13.2, Z3A.24.

Other Maternal Disorders Predominantly Related to Pregnancy (O20-O29)

Hyperemesis gravidarum is a severe form of morning sickness, which presents with persistent vomiting and nausea. Many pregnant women develop morning sickness during the first 3 months of pregnancy. This is attributed to the rising blood levels of HCG, which is secreted by the placenta. When the vomiting gets severe, it can lead to metabolic disturbances such as electrolyte imbalance.

EXAMPLE | Patient in her 8th week presents to obstetrician's office with terrible nausea and vomiting. He diagnoses her with hyperemesis gravidarium and dehydration, O21.1, E86.0, Z3A.08.

Another condition that occurs in about 5% of the pregnancies in the United States is gestational diabetes. Gestational diabetes (GDM) is diabetes brought on by the patient's pregnant condition and typically occurs in the second trimester of pregnancy. GDM can affect the baby in several ways; the baby may be large for its gestational age, the baby can have hypoglycemia, and the baby may develop jaundice. Sometimes women have diabetes prior to becoming pregnant and in that case, it may also complicate the pregnancy.

EXAMPLE | Patient is in her 24th week of pregnancy and has pre-existing type 1 diabetes, O24.012, Z3A.24.

Maternal Care Related to the Fetus and Amniotic Cavity and Possible Delivery Problems (O30-O48)

In ICD-10-CM there are certain codes that require a seventh character that identifies which fetus is affected in multiple gestations by the condition code assigned. Categories using the 7th character are O31, O32, O33.3–O33.6, O35, O36, O40, O41, O60.1, O60.2, O64, and O69.

Assign 7th character "0" in the following cases:

- For single gestations
- When the documentation in the record is not sufficient to determine the fetus affected and it is not possible to obtain clarification
- When it is not clinically possible to determine the fetus affected

---

EXAMPLE

If a patient was being delivered by cesarean section for a breech presentation for a single gestation, code O32.1xx0 would be assigned.

EXAMPLE

However, if the patient was being delivered by cesarean section at 39 weeks for a breech presentation for a twin pregnancy with Twin A in the vertex position and Twin B in the breech position, code O32.1xx2 would be assigned along with the code for twin pregnancy O30.003 and Z3A.39 for weeks of gestation.

7th Character Identifying Fetus Affected	
0	not applicable or unspecified
1	fetus 1
2	fetus 2
3	fetus 3
4	fetus 4
5	fetus 5
9	other fetus

It is important to note that if there is a fetal problem and it does not affect the care of the mother, then a code is not assigned. It is also important to assign a code when the management of the mother is affected by the fetal condition. For example, if there are diagnostic studies required, observation, termination, or care this would affect the management of the mother.

Malpresentation of the fetus would include any presentation other than vertex. Malpresentation would include breech, face, brow, and shoulder. The most common malpresentation is breech, and it occurs in around 4% of deliveries. Malpresentation may be the reason a cesarean section is performed. Sometimes labor becomes obstructed due to fetal presentation. Figure 21-8 shows some examples of fetal presentation.

EXAMPLE

Pregnant patient at 20 weeks is tested for spina bifida with a maternal serum alpha-fetoprotein (MSAFP) test. The test is positive so the physician performs an amniocentesis, which is positive for spinal bifida, O35.0xx0, Z3A.20, 10903ZU.

Premature rupture of the membranes (PROM) is a condition that occurs when the membranes rupture more than an hour before the onset of labor. Usually labor will ensue; however, if left to go on too long, there becomes a high risk of infection.

EXAMPLE

Patient in the 35th week of pregnancy is seen in obstetrician's office in early labor. She reports that the evening before while making dinner, she suspected her water may have broken. She is sent to the hospital with a diagnosis of PROM, O42.013, Z3A.35.

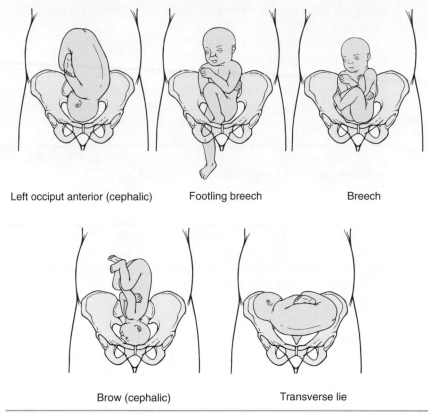

Left occiput anterior (cephalic)   Footling breech   Breech

Brow (cephalic)   Transverse lie

FIGURE 21-8. Fetal presentations.

EXERCISE 21-3

Answer the questions and assign codes to the following conditions.

1. Patient vaginally delivered at 35 weeks; single liveborn infant _____

2. Patient presents with PIH at 32 weeks; she is treated and sent home. _____

3. Patient presents at 39 weeks in labor; she had a previous cesarean section and delivered on this admit with no complications; vaginal delivery of single liveborn _____

4. Patient is given pitocin to induce labor for post-dates (41 weeks); induction is unsuccessful and she is sent home. _____

5. Patient presents at 35 weeks with premature rupture of membranes and delivers a healthy newborn vaginally. _____

6. Patient with a history of preterm labor is seen in the OB office for a routine pregnancy visit. She is in her 18th week. _____

7. An obese pregnant woman at 20 weeks presents to the hospital with extremely high blood pressure. The physician documents mild preeclampsia. She is put on medications and sent home. _____

8. A pregnant woman at 40 weeks presents to the hospital with gestational diabetes; she delivers a single liveborn vaginally. _____

9. A pregnant woman presents to the hospital in labor with a diagnosis of severe preeclampsia. She has smoked this entire pregnancy. She is 35 weeks pregnant and delivers a baby girl vaginally. _____

10. A pregnant woman at 30 weeks presents to the hospital in labor; she has a twin pregnancy and vaginally delivers two baby girls. _____

11. A 15-year-old girl at 37 weeks presents to the hospital in labor. She has a known twin pregnancy. A low cervical cesarean section is performed. One of the twins is stillborn. _____

12. The patient at 39 weeks had a low transverse cesarean section due to the baby being large for dates. _____

13. The patient was induced at 39 weeks as the baby was suspected to have spina bifida; she vaginally delivered a 5 lb baby boy. _____

14. The patient presents for delivery at 40 weeks. She is a known type 2 diabetic, treated with insulin at the onset of pregnancy. She delivers a large for dates baby via cesarean section. _____

15. Pregnant woman at 20 weeks presents to doctor's office with complaints of blurred vision. Testing is done, and the diagnosis of gestational diabetes is made. _____

Complications of Labor and Delivery (O60-O77)

A completely normal vaginal delivery is not all that common. There are many conditions that may complicate either or both labor and delivery. Some of the more common are listed below:

- Preterm labor—occurs when the onset of labor is before 37 completed weeks of pregnancy
- Precipitate labor—very rapid labor
- Failure to progress—labor does not progress as expected, slow cervical dilatation, or lack of descent
- Obstructed labor—could be due to malposition or malpresentation of fetus, pelvic abnormality, or fetopelvic disproportion
- Cord complications, such as entanglement, compression or cord around the neck of the fetus
- Lacerations during delivery (Figure 21-9).

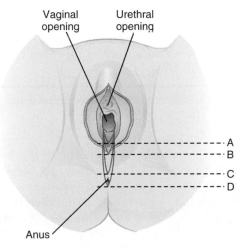

FIGURE 21-9. Perineal lacerations:
A, First-degree is laceration of artificial tissues.
B, Second-degree is limited to the pelvic floor and may involve the perineal or vaginal muscles.
C, Third-degree involves the anal sphincter.
D, Fourth-degree involves anal or rectal mucosa.

- First degree—perineal laceration and could involve the labia, skin, vagina, or vulva
- Second degree—perineal laceration of the pelvic floor, perineal muscles, or vaginal muscles
- Third degree—perineal laceration of the anal sphincter or rectovaginal septum
- Fourth degree—perineal laceration involving the anal or rectal mucosa
- Retained placenta—when the placenta is not totally expulsed
- Non reassuring fetal heart rate—abnormal fetal heart rate or rhythm (i.e., bradycardia, decelerations, irregularity)

Encounter for Delivery (O80, O82)

When a delivery occurs where minimal or no assistance is required, a code from this category is assigned along with the code for outcome of delivery (Z37.0). Minimal assistance would include episiotomy, but otherwise the delivery would be spontaneous, cephalic, vaginal, full-term, single, liveborn fetus. This code is never used with any other codes from Chapter 15.

Code O82 is used when there is no indication for the reason a cesarean delivery is being performed. This case scenario would be highly unlikely.

EXAMPLE	Patient is admitted to the hospital at 39 weeks in labor. Labor progresses and patient goes on to spontaneously deliver a normal newborn, O80, Z3A.39, Z37.0

Complications Predominantly Related to the Puerperium (O85-O92)

The definition of puerperium is from the time of delivery through the first 6 weeks postpartum. This code category does include postpartum infections, complications of anesthesia occurring postpartum, complications of cesarean delivery, and issues with lactation.

EXAMPLE	Patient is 2 weeks post normal vaginal delivery. She presents to the physician's office with painful cracked nipples due to nursing, O92.13.

Other Obstetric Conditions, Not Elsewhere Classified (O94-O9a)

This category contains codes for sexually transmitted diseases, infections and viral conditions, as well as AIDS. There are codes for smoking, alcohol, and drug abuse that complicate pregnancy.

Group B strep (GBS) is a type of bacterial infection that can be found in the vagina and/or lower intestine of up to 30% of all healthy women. If a person has this bacteria but has no signs or symptoms of disease, it is called a colonization (carrier). The problem with being a carrier is that this infection can be passed on to the baby. Usually a woman is tested late in her pregnancy for group B strep, and if the culture is positive she will be given antibiotics during labor to help prevent the spread of this bacteria to the baby.

EXAMPLE	Patient with asymptomatic HIV infection is seen in obstetrician's office at 16 weeks for a check-up, O98.712, Z21, Z3A.16.

Due to the fact that there is no known safe amount of alcohol to drink while pregnant, any pregnancy case where the mother uses alcohol during pregnancy should be assigned a code from subcategory O99.31. Use of alcohol in pregnancy can cause disorders ranging from miscarriage and stillbirth to low birth weight and lifelong disorders such as learning disabilities, poor memory, difficulty paying attention, low IQ, and speech or language delays to name a few.

Answer the questions and assign codes to the following conditions.

1. Patient presents with acute sinusitis. She is 8 weeks pregnant. Physician documents that the pregnancy is incidental to her acute sinusitis.

    _____

2. Patient has a postpartum hemorrhage; she delivered 5 days PTA.

    _____

3. A pregnant woman presents to the hospital in preterm labor at 34 weeks; she is treated with tocolysis for 3 days and is sent home on bed rest.

    _____

4. A pregnant woman presents to the hospital in labor at 32 weeks. After 2 weeks of treatment with tocolytics, she goes into heavy labor. Her cervix has failed to dilate, and a low transverse cesarean section is performed. She delivers a healthy baby boy.

    _____

5. Pregnant woman at 20 weeks is admitted to the hospital with *Pneumocystis carinii* pneumonia and known AIDS; she is treated with high-dose antibiotics and is discharged.

    _____

6. The patient has been dependent on methadone for the entire pregnancy. She delivers a baby girl on this admit at 38 weeks. She has no complications during delivery and has a normal spontaneous vaginal birth.

    _____

7. Pregnant woman had pneumonia early in her pregnancy. She presents to the hospital in labor at 39 weeks with no other complaints. She vaginally delivers a healthy baby.

    _____

8. Can code O80 be used as a secondary diagnosis?

    _____

9. What is the only outcome of delivery that can be used with O80?

    _____

10. If surgery is performed in utero, is this coded on the baby's chart or on the mother's chart?

    _____

11. A woman delivers a 5-lb baby in her home at 39 weeks. She is brought by paramedics to the hospital, where they find that she has a first-degree perineal laceration. This is repaired, and the patient is admitted.

    _____

12. A woman is admitted 6 weeks after a cesarean delivery with infection of the cesarean wound.

    _____

13. A woman delivered 5 weeks ago. She is admitted for an abscess of the breast.

    _____

14. A patient presents with abdominal pain 3 months after the birth of her first baby. The physician documents that she has cholelithiasis that is related to her pregnancy.

    _____

15. Two weeks after delivery, a woman has terrible pain in her leg. Her physician diagnoses her with a superficial thrombophlebitis of the leg.

    _____

16. Five months after delivery of her first born, an obese woman is diagnosed with postpartum cardiomyopathy.

    _____

FACTORS INFLUENCING HEALTH STATUS AND CONTACT WITH HEALTH SERVICES (Z CODES)

As was discussed in Chapter 8, it is difficult to locate Z codes in the Index. Coders will often say, "I did not know there was a Z code for that."

Refer to Chapter 8 for a listing of common main terms used to locate Z codes. Z codes that may be used during pregnancy, childbirth, and the puerperium include the following:

Z codes are often used for encounters relating to pregnancy, childbirth, and the puerperium. Normal encounters for routine prenatal visits will use category Z34, Encounter for supervision of a normal pregnancy. These codes are first-listed and are not used with any other code from the OB chapter. Codes from category Z3A, Weeks of gestation, may be used to provide additional information about the pregnancy.

Z02.81	Encounter for paternity testing
Z02.82	Encounter for adoption services
Z03.71	Encounter for suspected problem with amniotic cavity and membrane ruled out
Z03.72	Encounter for suspected placental problem ruled out
Z03.73	Encounter for suspected fetal anomaly ruled out
Z03.74	Encounter for suspected problem with fetal growth ruled out
Z03.75	Encounter for suspected cervical shortening ruled out
Z03.79	Encounter for other suspected maternal and fetal conditions ruled out
Z30.011	Encounter for initial prescription of contraceptive pills
Z30.012	Encounter for prescription of emergency contraception
Z30.013	Encounter for initial prescription of injectable contraceptive
Z30.014	Encounter for initial prescription of intrauterine contraceptive device
Z30.018	Encounter for initial prescription of other contraceptive
Z30.019	Encounter for initial prescription of contraceptives, unspecified
Z30.02	Counseling and instruction in natural family planning to avoid pregnancy
Z30.09	Encounter for other general counseling and advice on contraception
Z30.2	Encounter for sterilization
Z30.40	Encounter for surveillance of contraceptives, unspecified
Z30.41	Encounter for surveillance of contraceptive pills
Z30.42	Encounter for surveillance of injectable contraceptive
Z30.43	Encounter for surveillance of intrauterine contraceptive device
Z30.49	Encounter for surveillance of other contraceptives
Z30.8	Encounter for other contraceptive management
Z30.9	Encounter for contraceptive management, unspecified
Z31.0	Encounter for reversal of previous sterilization
Z31.41	Encounter for fertility testing
Z31.42	Aftercare following sterilization reversal
Z31.430	Encounter of female for testing for genetic disease carrier status for procreative management
Z31.438	Encounter for other genetic testing of female for procreative management
Z31.440	Encounter of male for testing for genetic disease carrier status for procreative management
Z31.441	Encounter for testing of male partner of habitual aborter
Z31.448	Encounter for other genetic testing of male for procreative management
Z31.49	Encounter for other procreative investigation and testing
Z31.5	Encounter for genetic counseling
Z31.61	Procreative counseling and advice using natural family planning
Z31.62	Encounter for fertility preservation counseling
Z31.69	Encounter for other general counseling and advice on procreation

Z31.81	Encounter for male factor infertility in female patient
Z31.82	Encounter for Rh incompatibility status
Z31.83	Encounter for assisted reproductive fertility procedure cycle
Z31.84	Encounter for fertility preservation procedure
Z31.89	Encounter for other procreative management
Z31.9	Encounter for procreative management, unspecified
Z32.00	Encounter for pregnancy test, result unknown
Z32.01	Encounter for pregnancy test, result positive
Z32.02	Encounter for pregnancy test, result negative
Z32.2	Encounter for childbirth instruction
Z32.3	Encounter for childcare instruction
Z33.1	Pregnant state, incidental
Z33.2	Encounter for elective termination of pregnancy
Z34.00	Encounter for supervision of normal first pregnancy, unspecified trimester
Z34.01	Encounter for supervision of normal first pregnancy, first trimester
Z34.02	Encounter for supervision of normal first pregnancy, second trimester
Z34.03	Encounter for supervision of normal first pregnancy, third trimester
Z34.80	Encounter for supervision of other normal pregnancy, unspecified trimester
Z34.81	Encounter for supervision of other normal pregnancy, first trimester
Z34.82	Encounter for supervision of other normal pregnancy, second trimester
Z34.83	Encounter for supervision of other normal pregnancy, third trimester
Z34.90	Encounter for supervision of normal pregnancy, unspecified, unspecified trimester
Z34.91	Encounter for supervision of normal pregnancy, unspecified, first trimester
Z34.92	Encounter for supervision of normal pregnancy, unspecified, second trimester
Z34.93	Encounter for supervision of normal pregnancy, unspecified, third trimester
Z36	Encounter for antenatal screening of mother
Z3A	Weeks of gestation

Note: Codes from category Z3A are for use, only on the maternal record, to indicate the weeks of gestation of the pregnancy.

Code first	complications of pregnancy, childbirth and the puerperium (O00-O9A)
Z3A.0	Weeks of gestation of pregnancy, unspecified or less than 10 weeks

	Z3A.00	Weeks of gestation of pregnancy not specified
	Z3A.01	Less than 8 weeks gestation of pregnancy
	Z3A.08	8 weeks gestation of pregnancy
	Z3A.09	9 weeks gestation of pregnancy
Z3A.1		Weeks of gestation of pregnancy, weeks 10-19
	Z3A.10	10 weeks gestation of pregnancy
	Z3A.11	11 weeks gestation of pregnancy
	Z3A.12	12 weeks gestation of pregnancy
	Z3A.13	13 weeks gestation of pregnancy
	Z3A.14	14 weeks gestation of pregnancy
	Z3A.15	15 weeks gestation of pregnancy
	Z3A.16	16 weeks gestation of pregnancy
	Z3A.17	17 weeks gestation of pregnancy
	Z3A.18	18 weeks gestation of pregnancy
	Z3A.19	19 weeks gestation of pregnancy
Z3A.2		Weeks of gestation of pregnancy, weeks 20-29
	Z3A.20	20 weeks gestation of pregnancy
	Z3A.21	21 weeks gestation of pregnancy
	Z3A.22	22 weeks gestation of pregnancy
	Z3A.23	23 weeks gestation of pregnancy
	Z3A.24	24 weeks gestation of pregnancy

	Z3A.25	25 weeks gestation of pregnancy
	Z3A.26	26 weeks gestation of pregnancy
	Z3A.27	27 weeks gestation of pregnancy
	Z3A.28	28 weeks gestation of pregnancy
	Z3A.29	29 weeks gestation of pregnancy
Z3A.3		Weeks of gestation of pregnancy, weeks 30-39
	Z3A.30	30 weeks gestation of pregnancy
	Z3A.31	31 weeks gestation of pregnancy
	Z3A.32	32 weeks gestation of pregnancy
	Z3A.33	33 weeks gestation of pregnancy
	Z3A.34	34 weeks gestation of pregnancy
	Z3A.35	35 weeks gestation of pregnancy
	Z3A.36	36 weeks gestation of pregnancy
	Z3A.37	37 weeks gestation of pregnancy
	Z3A.38	38 weeks gestation of pregnancy
	Z3A.39	39 weeks gestation of pregnancy
Z3A.4		Weeks of gestation of pregnancy, weeks 40 or greater
	Z3A.40	40 weeks gestation of pregnancy
	Z3A.41	41 weeks gestation of pregnancy
	Z3A.42	42 weeks gestation of pregnancy
	Z3A.49	Greater than 42 weeks gestation of pregnancy
Z37.0		Single live birth
Z37.1		Single stillbirth
Z37.2		Twins, both liveborn
Z37.3		Twins, one liveborn and one stillborn
Z37.4		Twins, both stillborn
Z37.50		Multiple births, unspecified, all liveborn
Z37.51		Triplets, all liveborn
Z37.52		Quadruplets, all liveborn
Z37.53		Quintuplets, all liveborn
Z37.54		Sextuplets, all liveborn
Z37.59		Other multiple births, all liveborn
Z37.60		Multiple births, unspecified, some liveborn
Z37.61		Triplets, some liveborn
Z37.62		Quadruplets, some liveborn
Z37.63		Quintuplets, some liveborn
Z37.64		Sextuplets, some liveborn
Z37.69		Other multiple births, some liveborn
Z37.7		Other multiple births, all stillborn
Z37.9		Outcome of delivery, unspecified
Z39.0		Encounter for care and examination of mother immediately after delivery
Z39.1		Encounter for care and examination of lactating mother
Z39.2		Encounter for routine postpartum follow-up
Z76.81		Expectant parent(s) prebirth pediatrician visit
Z79.3		Long-term (current) use of hormonal contraceptives
Z86.32		Personal history of gestational diabetes
Z87.51		Personal history of pre-term labor
Z87.59		Personal history of other complications of pregnancy childbirth, and the puerperium
Z92.0		Personal history of contraception
Z97.5		Presence of (intrauterine) contraceptive device

| EXAMPLE | Primigravida seen in OB office at 25 weeks for routine postpartum care, Z34.02, Z3A.25. |

| EXAMPLE | Patient missed a period and is seen in physician office for a pregnancy test. The test is positive, Z32.01. |

COMMON TREATMENTS

CONDITION	MEDICATION/TREATMENT
Narcotics for Labor Pain	Stadol (butorphanol), fentanyl Demerol (meperidine) Nubain (nalbuphine) Used for decreasing pain
Anesthesia for Labor Pain	Epidural is a regional anesthetic injected into the epidural space Spinal is also a regional anesthetic which is injected into the cerebrospinal fluid
Drugs for Inducing Labor	Pitocin is a synthetic oxytocin which is a natural hormone produced by a woman's body to cause the uterus to contract Cervidil (dinoprostone) is vaginally inserted and used for ripening of the cervix
Drugs Used to Inhibit Labor	Beta agonists (terbutaline, ritodrine, isoxsuprine), magnesium sulfate

PROCEDURES

Procedures that may be related to complications of pregnancy, childbirth, and the puerperium in ICD-10-PCS may be found in the following tables:

Obstetrics	102-10Y
Female Reproductive System	0U1-0UY

The obstetric procedure codes have a first character value of "1" and a second character value of "0" for the body system of pregnancy. There are 12 root operations in the obstetric section making up the third character:

- Change "2"
- Drainage "9"
- Abortion "A"
- Extraction "D"
- Delivery "E"
- Insertion "H"
- Inspection "J"
- Removal "P"
- Repair "Q"
- Reposition "S"
- Resection "T"
- Transplantation "Y"

The fourth character in the obstetrics section is the body part, of which there are three:

- Products of conception
- Products of conception, retained
- Products of conception, ectopic. Products of conception consist of fetus, embryo, amnion, umbilical cord, and placenta.

The fifth character is the approach and follows similar definitions from the med/surg chapter.

The sixth character is for devices such as fetal monitoring electrodes, and the seventh character is for qualifiers and represents:

- Types of extraction (i.e., forceps, or type of cesarean section)
- Type of fluid removed (i.e., amniotic fluid, fetal cerebrospinal fluid)
- Body system of the products of conception on which the repair was done

Seven Characters of an Obstetrics Code						
CHARACTER 1	**CHARACTER 2**	**CHARACTER 3**	**CHARACTER 4**	**CHARACTER 5**	**CHARACTER 6**	**CHARACTER 7**
Section	Body System	Root Operation	Body Part	Approach	Device	Qualifier

Labor

Labor can be induced in a variety of ways. Often, artificial rupture of the membranes (AROM) is performed to start labor. Pitocin induction may also be used. Pitocin is a drug used for medical induction of labor.

A nonstress test (NST) is performed to confirm the health of the baby. A mother is hooked up to a fetal monitor and the test is performed without giving the mother medications. The test records the baby's heart rate while moving. This test may be performed throughout the pregnancy if the mother has medical conditions or if the pregnancy is considered high risk. Results of these tests are recorded as "reactive," meaning the baby moved and the heart rate increased appropriately, or "nonreactive," which means that either the baby did not move or the heart rate did not increase enough when the baby did move.

When the NST is abnormal, another test is performed. This test is called a CST, or a contraction stress test. In this test, which is done during fetal monitoring, a drug (Pitocin) may be administered to initiate contractions. The purpose is to see how the baby will handle the stress of labor. The baby's heart should speed up during a contraction; if this does not happen during this test, problems may occur during labor.

Amnioinfusion (administration of a substance) is the insertion of normal saline or lactated Ringer's solution into the amniotic sac. The injection may be done transabdominally or transcervically. This procedure is performed for a variety of reasons, such as oligohydramnios, variable decelerations, and thick meconium. The volume of amniotic fluid is increased, which increases the likelihood of better outcomes of delivery.

Delivery

In a normal pregnancy with no complications, a code of 10E0XZZ may be assigned for manually assisted delivery (Figure 21-10). This code should not be assigned if any other procedures were performed to assist in delivery. Forceps and vacuum extraction may be used in cases in which the baby does not spontaneously deliver and assistance is needed (Figure 21-11).

Episiotomy is performed to facilitate delivery. The root operation in ICD-10-PCS for an episiotomy is division of the female perineum. This is not assigned a code from the obstetric

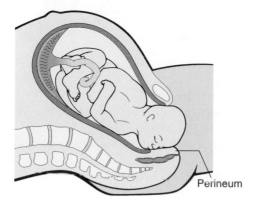

Perineum

FIGURE 21-10. Cephalic presentation ("crowning") of the fetus during delivery from the vaginal (birth) canal during a normal delivery.

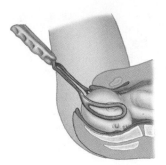

FIGURE 21-11. Forceps delivery.

table, but from the female reproductive system tables. The physician makes a cut in the perineum to make room for the baby's head to emerge. Repair of an episiotomy is included in the code for episiotomy. Sometimes, an episiotomy will extend and will become a laceration. If this happens, codes for both episiotomy and laceration repair are required. The degree of perineal laceration is coded under the diagnostic category of O70. If more than one degree is mentioned, only the highest degree should be assigned.

Cesarean Section

A cesarean section (C-section) is an operation that is performed to deliver a baby through an incision in the abdomen. The root operation for a cesarean section is extraction of products of conception. This procedure is performed for a variety of reasons:

- *Cephalopelvic disproportion (CPD):* This is when the baby's head is too large to fit through the birth canal.
- *Prolapsed cord:* The cord is being delivered before the baby.
- *Fetal distress:* Distress of the fetus during labor or before, noted by low oxygen levels or the presence of meconium
- *Conditions of the mother:* Such as hypertension or active herpes

Three main types of cesarean operations are performed: 1) classical, which involves a vertical incision in the main body of the uterus; 2) low cervical or low transverse, which is the most common and is done via a horizontal incision in the lower uterus; and 3) extraperitoneal, which is an incision in the lower part of the uterus without entering the peritoneal cavity, which is performed to prevent infection.

Vaginal birth after cesarean section (VBAC) occurs when a woman delivers vaginally after having delivered previously via cesarean section. At one point in time, it was believed that it was unsafe for a woman who had delivered via C-section to deliver vaginally. Many variables go into deciding whether a VBAC is a safe option; however, it is being performed more and more frequently.

EXERCISE 21-5

Assign codes for all diagnoses and procedures.

1. Patient is induced by pitocin for postdate pregnancy (41 weeks). She delivers a 6 lb 4 oz baby vaginally. _____

2. Elderly multigravida at 39 weeks presents in labor. After 20 hours of labor, an LTCS is performed because of failure to progress. She delivers a normal newborn. _____

3. A 22-year-old primigravida at 40 weeks presents for induction. She is known to have oligohydramnios. Pitocin is administered, and she goes on to vaginally deliver an SGA normal newborn. The physician performs an episiotomy to facilitate delivery, and a second-degree extension is repaired. _____

4. Patient presents in active labor. She is in her 38th week of
pregnancy. She labors for 8 hours, after which the physician
decides to perform a low cervical C-section because of CPD.
A normal newborn is delivered. _____

5. Patient presents with severe preeclampsia. She is in her 39th
week of pregnancy. She is taken directly to the operating
room, where an LTCS is performed. She delivers a normal
newborn. _____

DOCUMENTATION/REIMBURSEMENT/MS-DRGs

Often, coding difficulties are due to lack of documentation. Sometimes pathology and other
test results are not available at the time of discharge or when the physician is dictating the
discharge summary or is reporting the final diagnoses.

The most common MS-DRGs for deliveries include the following:

MS-DRG	RW
766 C-Section without CC/MCC	0.8497
765 C-Section with CC/MCC	1.1269
775 Vaginal Delivery without complicating dx	0.5286
774 Vaginal Delivery with complicating dx	0.7406
767 Vaginal Delivery with Sterilization or D&C	0.8547

CHAPTER REVIEW EXERCISE

Assign codes for all diagnoses and procedures.

1. Breech presentation with obstructed labor at 39 weeks; delivery
by cesarean section (LTCS); single liveborn _____

2. Patient admitted 2 weeks post delivery with postpartum
depression _____

3. Patient at 40 weeks delivers 12 lb baby (LGA), requiring an
episiotomy. _____

4. Patient at 37 weeks is admitted to the hospital for delivery; she is
being treated with methadone for heroin dependence; vaginal
delivery of single liveborn _____

5. Patient with a history of preterm labor and previous cesarean
section is admitted in labor at 39 weeks; she has a vaginal birth
after cesarean (VBAC) of single liveborn. _____

6. Patient at 36 weeks is admitted to hospital for HELLP (hemolytic
anemia, elevated liver enzymes, and low platelet count) syndrome;
she is taken to the operating room for delivery by cesarean section
(LTCS) of single liveborn. _____

7. Patient is admitted to the hospital in preterm labor; she is 35
weeks pregnant; 3 days after admission, the patient vaginally
delivers a small for gestational age (SGA) baby. _____

8. Patient presents to physician's office for a routine obstetric visit;
she is in her 30th week of pregnancy; she had a stillborn 1 year
ago. _____

9. Patient is admitted to the hospital at 33 weeks; she has a twin pregnancy and has a spontaneous vaginal delivery (SVD) of liveborn twins; the evening after delivery, she hemorrhages.   _____

10. Patient is 8 weeks pregnant and has known uterine fibroids; the fibroids are so large that the physician recommends an abortion; patient presents to hospital for abortion to be performed by aspiration curettage.   _____

11. The patient was treated for a right sprained wrist. Incidentally, the patient is 10 weeks pregnant.   _____

12. Urinary tract infection in patient who delivered 1 week ago   _____

13. This mother delivered liveborn twins vaginally at 36 weeks during her hospital stay. What outcome of delivery is coded on the mother's record?   _____

14. The patient was admitted for treatment of hyperemesis gravidarum. The patient is 12 weeks pregnant.   _____

15. The patient has a high-risk pregnancy and two previous miscarriages. She is currently at 28 weeks.   _____

16. The patient is 16 weeks pregnant, and her condition is complicated by diabetes mellitus, type 2, which is uncontrolled.   _____

17. The patient is admitted with HIV and *Pneumocystis carinii* pneumonia (PCP) and is 35 weeks pregnant.   _____

18. The patient is 19 weeks pregnant and has hypothyroidism.   _____

19. The patient delivered a baby 6 days ago. She is now being admitted because of dehiscence of her cesarean wound. The wound was sutured.   _____

20. Urinary tract infection in a patient who is 30 weeks pregnant   _____

21. A 33-year-old presents at 40 weeks in labor. She has had an uneventful pregnancy, except for slight anemia which is still being treated with iron. She has an uncomplicated vaginal delivery of a 6 lb baby girl.   _____

22. A 15-year-old pregnant female presents at 39 weeks in active labor. She has no past history, except for several bouts of asthma as a toddler. She had an uncomplicated delivery of a healthy baby boy.   _____

23. A patient is admitted in labor at 39 weeks and delivers a 7 lb baby boy vaginally. The physician requests a social work consult because this mother has struggled with depression prior to and during this pregnancy.   _____

24. Patient is 40 weeks pregnant. The physician documents that chlamydia was discovered early on in the pregnancy, and the patient now tests negative. Patient has a spontaneous vaginal delivery of an 8 lb baby girl.   _____

25. Patient is admitted to the hospital in labor at 39 weeks. She has had an uneventful pregnancy and goes on to a spontaneous vaginal delivery of twin boys.   _____

26. A patient is admitted to the hospital 4 weeks post partum with a high fever. The physician suspects endometritis. The patient is treated with IV antibiotics.   _____

27. A patient is admitted in labor at 39 weeks and she delivers a 7 lb baby boy. After vaginal delivery, she hemorrhages. The physician documents that the hemorrhage is due to a retained placenta. Physician manually removes the retained placenta.   _____

CHAPTER GLOSSARY

Abortion: termination of a pregnancy by natural causes or by medical intervention.

Amnioinfusion: the insertion of normal saline or lactated Ringer's solution into the amniotic sac.

Antepartum: time from conception until delivery or childbirth with regard to the mother.

Cervix: the neck of the uterus that serves as an outlet from the uterus.

Complete abortion: abortion in which all the products of conception are expelled.

Ectopic: type of pregnancy that occurs when the egg is implanted outside the cavity of the uterus.

Effaced: cervical thinning.

Elderly obstetric patient: 35 years or older at date of delivery.

Elective abortion: the elective termination of pregnancy.

Endometritis: inflammation of the uterus.

Fallopian tube: delivers the mature egg to the uterus for fertilization.

Gravid: pregnant.

Habitual aborter: a woman who miscarries at least three consecutive times.

Hyperemesis gravidarum: excessive vomiting in pregnancy.

Incomplete abortion: abortion in which not all of the products of conception are expelled.

Inevitable abortion: abortion that occurs when symptoms are present and a miscarriage will happen.

Labia: surrounds the vaginal opening.

Labor: process by which the products of conception are expelled from the uterus.

Lactation: process of milk production.

Miscarriage: spontaneous termination of pregnancy before the fetus has reached 20 weeks.

Missed abortion: pregnancy with fetal demise before 20 weeks; products of conception are not expelled.

Molar pregnancy: fertilized ovum is converted to a mole.

Multigravida: a woman with two or more pregnancies.

Multiparity: a woman with two or more pregnancies.

Ovaries: produce female hormones and eggs.

Postpartum: after delivery or childbirth.

Postterm pregnancy: pregnancy longer than 40 weeks up to 42 weeks.

Precipitate labor: rapid labor and delivery.

Preeclampsia: pregnancy complication characterized by hypertension, edema, and/or proteinuria.

Pregestational: condition present prior to pregnancy.

Prenatal: before birth.

Primigravida: first pregnancy.

Prolonged pregnancy: beyond 42 weeks of pregnancy.

Puerperium: time from delivery through the first 6 weeks postpartum.

Spontaneous abortion: loss of a fetus due to natural causes; also known as *miscarriage*.

Stillbirth: born dead.

Therapeutic abortion: abortion performed when the pregnancy is endangering the mother's health, or when the fetus has a condition that is incompatible with life.

Threatened abortion: abortion that occurs when symptoms are present that indicate the possibility of a miscarriage.

Toxemia: another term for preeclampsia, which is pregnancy complicated by hypertension, edema, or proteinuria.

Uterus: a muscular organ that serves as an incubator for the developing fetus.

Vagina: a muscular tube that extends from the vaginal opening to the uterus.

Vulva: the external covering to the vagina.

Young obstetric patient: younger than 16 years at date of delivery.

REFERENCES

1. From Chabner D. *The Language of Medicine*, 8th ed. St. Louis: Saunders, 2007, Table 19-2, p 776.
2. From Chabner D. *The Language of Medicine*, 8th ed. St. Louis: Saunders, 2007, Table 19-3, p 777.
3. Modified from *Harrison's Manual of Medicine*, 15th ed. New York: McGraw-Hill Professional, 2002, p 284.

22

Certain Conditions Originating in the Perinatal Period and Congenital Malformations, Deformations, and Chromosomal Abnormalities

(ICD-10-CM Chapter 16, Codes P00-P96 and Chapter 17, Codes Q00-Q99)

Factors Influencing Health Status and Contact With Health Services (Z Codes)
Documentation/Reimbursement/MS-DRGs
Chapter Review Exercise
Chapter Glossary

LEARNING OBJECTIVES

1. Apply and assign the correct ICD-10-CM/PCS codes in accordance with Official Guidelines for Coding and Reporting
2. Identify major differences between ICD-10-CM/PCS and ICD-9-CM related to perinatal conditions and congenital malformations, deformations, and chromosomal abnormalities
3. Identify perinatal conditions and congenital malformations, deformations, and chromosomal abnormalities
4. Assign the correct Z codes and procedure codes to perinatal conditions and congenital malformations, deformations, and chromosomal abnormalities
5. Identify common treatments, medications, laboratory values, and diagnostic tests
6. Explain the importance of documentation as it relates to MS-DRGs for reimbursement

ABBREVIATIONS/ ACRONYMS

AGA appropriate for gestational age

BPD bronchopulmonary dysplasia

CAP community acquired pneumonia

CHD congenital heart disease

CVS chorionic villus sampling

ICD-9-CM *International Classification of Diseases, 9th Revision, Clinical Modification*

ICD-10-CM *International Classification of Diseases, 10th Revision, Clinical Modification*

ICD-10-PCS *International Classification of Diseases, 10th Revision, Procedure Coding System*

IUGR intrauterine growth retardation

LGA large for gestational age

MSAFP maternal serum alpha-fetoprotein

MS-DRG Medicare severity diagnosis-related group

NICU neonatal intensive care unit

OI osteogenesis imperfecta

PDA patent ductus arteriosus

PKU phenylketonuria

PPH primary pulmonary hypertension

PWS Prader-Willi syndrome

RDS respiratory distress syndrome

SGA small for gestational age

TOF tetralogy of Fallot

TTN transitory tachypnea of the newborn

VSD ventricular septal defect

ICD-10-CM

Official Guidelines for Coding and Reporting

Please refer to the companion Evolve website for the most current guidelines.

16. Chapter 16: Newborn (Perinatal) Guidelines (P00-P96)

For coding and reporting purposes the perinatal period is defined as before birth through the 28th day following birth. The following guidelines are provided for reporting purposes

a. General Perinatal Rules

1) Use of Chapter 16 Codes

Codes in this chapter are <u>never</u> for use on the maternal record. Codes from Chapter 15, the obstetric chapter, are never permitted on the newborn record. Chapter 16 codes may be used throughout the life of the patient if the condition is still present.

2) Principal Diagnosis for Birth Record

When coding the birth episode in a newborn record, assign a code from category Z38, Liveborn infants according to place of birth and type of delivery, as the principal diagnosis. A code from category Z38 is assigned only once, to a newborn at the time of birth. If a newborn is transferred to another institution, a code from category Z38 should not be used at the receiving hospital.

A code from category Z38 is used only on the newborn record, not on the mother's record.

3) Use of Codes from other Chapters with Codes from Chapter 16

Codes from other chapters may be used with codes from chapter 16 if the codes from the other chapters provide more specific detail. Codes for signs and symptoms may be assigned when a definitive diagnosis has not been established. If the reason for the encounter is a perinatal condition, the code from chapter 16 should be sequenced first.

EXAMPLE | An infant was delivered in the hospital via cesarean section. On discharge, the infant was examined and appeared completely healthy with the exception of neonatal jaundice. A bilirubin count should be performed in 2 days, Z38.01, P59.9.

4) Use of Chapter 16 Codes after the Perinatal Period

Should a condition originate in the perinatal period, and continue throughout the life of the patient, the perinatal code should continue to be used regardless of the patient's age.

EXAMPLE | A 3-year-old child is seen in the pediatrician's office with a diagnosis of bronchopulmonary dysplasia (BPD), P27.1.

5) Birth process or community acquired conditions

If a newborn has a condition that may be either due to the birth process or community acquired and the documentation does not indicate which it is, the default is due to the birth process and the code from Chapter 16 should be used. If the condition is community-acquired, a code from Chapter 16 should not be assigned.

EXAMPLE | A 3-week-old baby is admitted for cough and fever, and on the discharge summary the physician documents pneumonia, P23.9.

EXAMPLE | A 3-week-old baby is admitted for cough and fever, and on the discharge summary the physician documents congenital pneumonia, P23.9.

EXAMPLE | A 3-week-old baby is admitted for cough and fever, and on the discharge summary the physician documents community acquired pneumonia, J18.9.

6) Code all clinically significant conditions

If a newborn has a condition that may be either due to the birth process or community acquired and all the clinically significant conditions noted on routine newborn examination should be coded. A condition is clinically significant if it requires:

■ clinical evaluation; or
■ therapeutic treatment; or
■ diagnostic procedures; or
■ extended length of hospital stay; or
■ increased nursing care and/or monitoring; or
■ has implications for future health care needs

Note: The perinatal guidelines listed above are the same as the general coding guidelines for "additional diagnoses", except for the final point regarding implications for future health care needs. Codes should be assigned for conditions that have been specified by the provider as having implications for future health care needs.

EXAMPLE   The infant was born via vaginal delivery and suffered a fractured clavicle caused by the delivery, Z38.00, P13.4.

b. Observation and Evaluation of Newborns for Suspected Conditions not Found
Assign a code from categories P00-P04 to identify those instances when a healthy newborn is evaluated for a suspected condition that is determined after study not to be present. Do not use a code from categories P00-P04 when the patient has identified signs or symptoms of a suspected problem; in such cases, code the sign or symptom.

EXAMPLE   A male infant was born by a precipitous vaginal delivery and was observed for a spontaneous pneumothorax. Chest x-ray was negative, Z38.00, P03.9.

c. Coding Additional Perinatal Diagnoses
1) Assigning codes for conditions that require treatment
Assign codes for conditions that require treatment or further investigation, prolong the length of stay, or require resource utilization.
2) Codes for conditions specified as having implications for future health care needs
Assign codes for conditions that have been specified by the provider as having implications for future health care needs.
Note: This guideline should not be used for adult patients.

EXAMPLE   A male infant was born via vaginal delivery. The clinician will evaluate and review treatment options for his undescended right testicle at the 6-week appointment, Z38.00, Q53.10.

d. Prematurity and Fetal Growth Retardation
Providers utilize different criteria in determining prematurity. A code for prematurity should not be assigned unless it is documented. Assignment of codes in categories P05, Disorders of newborn related to slow fetal growth and fetal malnutrition, and P07, Disorders of newborn related to short gestation and low birth weight, not elsewhere classified, should be based on the recorded birth weight and estimated gestational age. Codes from category P05 should not be assigned with codes from category P07.
When both birth weight and gestational age are available, two codes from category P07 should be assigned, with the code for birth weight sequenced before the code for gestational age.
A code from P05 and codes from P07.2 and P07.3 may be used to specify weeks of gestation as documented by the provider in the record.

EXAMPLE   A premature infant was born in the hospital via vaginal delivery. The infant weighed 4 pounds and was 33 weeks' gestational age, Z38.00, P07.17, P07.32.

e. Low birth weight and immaturity status
Codes from category P07, Disorders of newborn related to short gestation and low birth weight, not elsewhere classified, are for use for a child or adult who was premature or had a low birth weight as a newborn and this is affecting the patient's current health status. *See Section I.C.21. Factors influencing health status and contact with health services, Status.*
f. Bacterial Sepsis of Newborn
Category P36, Bacterial sepsis of newborn, includes congenital sepsis. If a perinate is documented as having sepsis without documentation of congenital or community acquired, the default is congenital and a code from category P36 should be assigned. If the P36 code includes the causal organism, an additional code from category B95,

Streptococcus, Staphylococcus, and Enterococcus as the cause of diseases classified elsewhere, or B96, Other bacterial agents as the cause of diseases classified elsewhere, should not be assigned. If the P36 code does not include the causal organism, assign an additional code from category B96. If applicable, use additional codes to identify severe sepsis (R65.2-) and any associated acute organ dysfunction.

EXAMPLE

A 2-week-old infant is admitted to the hospital with high fever. The infant is diagnosed with group B strep sepsis, P36.0.

g. Stillbirth

Code P95, Stillbirth, is only for use in institutions that maintain separate records for stillbirths. No other code should be used with P95. Code P95 should not be used on the mother's record.

17. Chapter 17: Congenital malformations, deformations, and chromosomal abnormalities (Q00-Q99)

Assign an appropriate code(s) from categories Q00-Q99, Congenital malformations, deformations, and chromosomal abnormalities when a malformation/deformation or chromosomal abnormality is documented. A malformation/deformation/or chromosomal abnormality may be the principal/first-listed diagnosis on a record or a secondary diagnosis.

When a malformation/deformation/or chromosomal abnormality does not have a unique code assignment, assign additional code(s) for any manifestations that may be present.

When the code assignment specifically identifies the malformation/deformation/or chromosomal abnormality, manifestations that are an inherent component of the anomaly should not be coded separately. Additional codes should be assigned for manifestations that are not an inherent component.

Codes from Chapter 17 may be used throughout the life of the patient. If a congenital malformation or deformity has been corrected, a personal history code should be used to identify the history of the malformation or deformity. Although present at birth, malformation/deformation/or chromosomal abnormality may not be identified until later in life. Whenever the condition is diagnosed by the physician, it is appropriate to assign a code from codes Q00-Q99.

For the birth admission, the appropriate code from category Z38, Liveborn infants, according to place of birth and type of delivery, should be sequenced as the principal diagnosis, followed by any congenital anomaly codes, Q00-Q99.

EXAMPLE

Infant delivered vaginally was discovered to have a supernumerary finger of the left hand, Z38.00, Q69.0.

EXAMPLE

Infant delivered via C-section with known tetralogy of Fallot, Z38.01, Q21.3.

EXAMPLE

Patient is a 40-year-old male complaining of nausea, vomiting, and abdominal pain. He is admitted to the hospital, and it is determined that he has Meckel's diverticulum, Q43.0.

Apply the General Coding Guidelines as found in Chapter 5 and the Procedural Coding Guidelines as found in Chapters 6 and 7.

MAJOR DIFFERENCES BETWEEN ICD-10-CM AND ICD-9-CM

The following code changes have occurred in ICD-10-CM:
- Different codes are used for "light for gestational age" and "small for gestational age."
- Birth weight should be sequenced before gestational age.
- Codes for assigning birth trauma have been expanded.

- Code changes identify slow fetal growth and malnutrition.
- Codes identify low birth weight not due to slow fetal growth or malnutrition.
- The term "fetus" has been removed from many titles.
- Stillbirth code P95 cannot be used with any additional codes and is only used in hospitals that maintain separate records for stillborns.

EXERCISE 22-1

Answer the questions and assign codes to the following conditions.

1. A congenital anomaly is always listed second on a newborn record.
   A. True
   B. False

2. A congenital anomaly code can be assigned to an adult record.
   A. True
   B. False

3. Codes from Chapter 15 can be used on the newborn record.
   A. True
   B. False

4. Chapter 16 codes can be used anytime throughout the life of the patient.
   A. True
   B. False

5. Code P02.7 belongs on the mother's record.
   A. True
   B. False

6. If a newborn has a condition that has implications for future health care needs, that condition may be coded. The same is true for the adult population.
   A. True
   B. False

7. When a newborn is transferred to another hospital, the principal diagnosis should be a code from the Z38 series.
   A. True
   B. False

8. Codes in category P00 can be assigned as a principal diagnosis.
   A. True
   B. False

9. A coder should assign a code for prematurity on the basis of weeks and/or weight in grams.
   A. True
   B. False

10. If the mother of a newborn has hypertension, code P00.0 is assigned.
    A. True
    B. False

11. When the code P74.1 is used would it also be appropriate _____ to use code E86.0?

12. If it is not clearly documented on the infant's chart whether _____ a condition is community acquired or is due to the birth process, which is the default?

13. What makes a condition clinically significant?

    _____

14. What category of codes is used as the principal diagnosis _____ for newborns?

15. When a baby is born extremely prematurely at 25 weeks' gestation and has a birth weight of 950 grams, and physician documents extreme immatunity, what code or codes are assigned? _____

16. When a newborn has a diagnosis of sepsis, what code or codes are assigned? _____

17. What is the definition of "congenital"?

_____

18. The principal diagnosis code for a single newborn who is delivered by a cesarean section is _____

19. How long does the perinatal period last? _____

20. It is permissible to use codes from other chapters with codes from Chapter 16. _____
    A. True
    B. False

DISEASE CONDITIONS

Certain Conditions Originating in the Perinatal Period (P00-P96), Chapter 16 in the ICD-10-CM code book, and Congenital Malformations, Deformations, and Chromosomal Abnormalities (Q00-Q99), Chapter 17, is divided into the following categories:

CATEGORY	SECTION TITLES
P00-P04	Newborn affected by maternal factors and by complications of pregnancy, labor, and delivery
P05-P08	Disorders of the newborn related to length of gestation and fetal growth
P09	Abnormal findings on neonatal screening
P10-P15	Birth trauma
P19-P29	Respiratory and cardiovascular disorders specific to the perinatal period
P35-P39	Infections specific to the perinatal period
P50-P61	Hemorrhagic and hematological disorders of newborn
P70-P74	Transitory endocrine and metabolic disorders specific to newborn
P76-P78	Digestive system disorders of newborn
P80-P83	Conditions involving the integument and temperature regulation of newborn
P84	Other problems with newborn
P90-P96	Other disorders originating in the perinatal period
Q00-Q07	Congenital malformations of the nervous system
Q10-Q18	Congenital malformations of the eye, ear, face, and neck
Q20-Q28	Congenital malformations of the circulatory system
Q30-Q34	Congenital malformations of the respiratory system
Q35-Q37	Cleft lip and cleft palate
Q38-Q45	Other congenital malformations of the digestive system
Q50-Q56	Congenital malformations of genital organs
Q60-Q64	Congenital malformations of the urinary system
Q65-Q79	Congenital malformations and deformations of the musculoskeletal system
Q80-Q89	Other congenital malformations
Q90-Q99	Chromosomal abnormalities, not elsewhere classified

Coding the Birth of an Infant

All newborn charts must contain a code from Z38.- for the principal diagnosis on the baby's birth record. In ICD-10-CM the Z codes for the birth of an infant describe the place of birth as well as the type of delivery and the number of infants delivered. This Z code is only used one time. If the baby is transferred to another facility, these sets of Z codes are not used and the reason for admission at that facility is the principal diagnosis.

EXAMPLE | Single liveborn, born in hospital, via cesarean section, Z38.01.

EXAMPLE | Twin, mate liveborn, delivered vaginally in hospital, Z38.30.

EXAMPLE | Single liveborn delivered by cesarean section at Hospital A. The infant was transferred to Hospital B because of bladder exstrophy.
Hospital A   Z38.01, Q64.10
Hospital B   Q64.10

The guidelines state that all clinically significant conditions noted on routine newborn examination should be coded. These follow the same general guidelines for assigning secondary diagnoses except for the guideline regarding implications for future healthcare needs.

A condition is clinically significant if it requires the following:

- Clinical evaluation, or
- Therapeutic treatment, or
- Diagnostic procedures, or
- Extended length of hospital stay, or
- Increased nursing care and/or monitoring; or if it has
- Implications for future healthcare needs (applies to newborn only)

Apgar Scores

Most babies are assessed after birth by what is known as an **Apgar** test (Figure 22-1). This test is usually given twice—once at 1 minute and again at 5 minutes. If problems are noted with the baby, the test may be done a third time. It is good to be familiar with this test because a low Apgar score is often indicative of problems.

Five factors are used for evaluation; the baby is given a score of 0 to 2 for each factor. These consist of the following:

1. Heart (pulse)
2. Breathing (rate and effort)
3. Activity and muscle tone
4. Grimace (reflex irritability)
5. Appearance (skin coloration)

If a baby scores 7 or above at 1 minute after birth, the baby is considered healthy. If a score between 4 and 6 is recorded at 1 minute, usually the baby needs immediate care with oxygen or suctioning.

APGAR SCORING CHART

SIGN	0	1	2
Heart rate	**Absent**	**Below 100**	**Over 100**
Respiratory effort	**Absent**	**Slow, irregular**	**Good, crying**
Muscle tone	**Limp**	**Some flexion of extremities**	**Active motion**
Response to catheter in nostril (tested after oropharynx is clear)	**No response**	**Grimace**	**Cough or sneeze**
Color	**Blue, pale**	**Body pink, extremities blue**	**Completely pink**

FIGURE 22-1. Apgar scoring chart.

Newborn Affected by Maternal Factors and by Complications of Pregnancy, Labor, and Delivery (P00-P04)

The codes in these categories are used when a maternal condition is specified as the cause for a confirmed or potential morbidity or if a newborn is suspected of having a condition resulting from exposure from the mother or birth process without signs or symptoms and after examination and observation this condition is found not to exist. Sometimes, a mother is running a fever during labor, and the physician must make sure that the infant does not have an infection. The physician orders tests, observation, and/or treatment until this condition can be ruled out. If the newborn is experiencing signs or symptoms, then a code from category P00.- is not to be used. Likewise, a P00.- code may be assigned as the principal diagnosis code for readmission when a condition is suspected and is subsequently ruled out. It is important to remember that this code can be used only during the neonatal period (the first 28 days of life). These codes are used even if treatment is begun for a suspected condition that is ruled out. As is stated in the guidelines, these conditions are assigned only if and when the maternal condition has actually affected the fetus or the newborn. Just because a mother has a condition does not necessarily mean that it affects the newborn.

EXAMPLE During the third trimester of pregnancy, mother develops shingles. After vaginal delivery baby is isolated for suspected shingles, Z38.00, P00.2.

Disorders of the Newborn Related to Length of Gestation and Fetal Growth (P05-P08)

Prematurity must be documented by the provider in order to assign a code for this condition. Codes for (P05) Newborns light for gestational age should not be assigned with codes (P07) disorders of the newborn related to short gestation and low birth weight, NEC. If both birth weight and gestational age are available, both should be coded with the birth weight sequenced first. Sometimes in later admissions or on later visits, a physician may document something such as "ex-25 week preemie," and in this case, even if the child is older, this code can be assigned as the fact that the child is a preemie may account for or contribute to the current condition. This also follows the rule that Chapter 16 codes may be used throughout a patient's life.

EXAMPLE Infant delivered vaginally is premature as documented by provider. The baby is delivered at 28 weeks and weighs 1720 grams, Z38.00, P07.16, P07.31.

EXAMPLE The physician documented that the baby was small for gestational age (SGA). The baby weighed 1850 grams. The infant was born in the hospital by vaginal delivery, Z38.00, P05.17.

Birth Trauma (P10-P15)

Cephalhematoma is a condition of blood between the skull and periosteum of a newborn. This condition is often caused by either a prolonged second stage of labor or injury to the skull during birth caused by instrumentation. In most cases this is a benign condition that requires no treatment, and the hematoma resolves on its own.

EXAMPLE Newborn delivered via difficult vaginal birth. Infant suffered a cephalhematoma secondary to the use of a forceps delivery, Z38.00, P12.0.

Respiratory and Cardiovascular Disorders Specific to the Perinatal Period (P19-P29)

Respiratory Problems After Birth

If a baby is born by cesarean section, a pediatrician may be asked to be present for the birth. If an abnormal heart rate occurs during labor, or any indications suggest that the baby might be in trouble, a pediatrician may be called and is asked to be present for the delivery. Documentation by the physician should note any abnormal conditions.

Transitory Tachypnea of Newborn (TTN). This is a respiratory problem that is likely due to retained lung fluid. It usually resolves in 24 to 48 hours. The baby may be treated with oxygen.

Apnea of the Newborn. This tends to occur in premature infants and is defined as a pause in breathing for longer than 15 seconds that can result in cyanosis.

Respiratory Distress Syndrome (RDS). This syndrome rarely affects full-term infants. It is caused by lack of lung surfactant. Surfactant is a chemical that keeps the air sacs from collapsing. The more premature the baby is, the greater is the chance of RDS. Treatment for mild cases consists of oxygen. Patients with more severe disease must be ventilated; sometimes, an artificial lung surfactant is placed in the lungs of an infant who is at high risk, to try to prevent RDS.

EXAMPLE Respiratory distress syndrome in liveborn infant that was delivered vaginally, Z38.00, P22.0.

Meconium Aspiration Syndrome

Meconium is the fecal matter within a baby's intestines before birth. Normally, it is expelled after birth, but if problems occur during labor, the baby may expel meconium into the amniotic fluid. Meconium may be inhaled by the baby while within the uterus or during birth. Inhalation of meconium occurs most often in postterm babies.

A physician may suspect aspiration if the newborn is covered with meconium, or if thick meconium is found in the amniotic fluid. Aspiration of meconium can result in major problems for the newborn.

A variety of codes may be used to indicate the different ways in which meconium may be found.

- Meconium staining P96.83
- Meconium passage during delivery P03.82
- Meconium aspiration without respiratory symptoms P24.00
- Meconium aspiration with respiratory symptoms P24.01
- Fetal and newborn aspiration, unspecified P24.9

Bronchopulmonary Dysplasia (BPD)

Bronchopulmonary dysplasia (BPD) is a chronic lung disease that develops in babies during the first 4 weeks after birth. It occurs most often in premature babies, that is, those weighing less than 1500 grams. Sometimes, the ventilator that is keeping a baby alive may cause BPD. BPD may also be caused by infections, such as pneumonia.

EXAMPLE A 4-week old infant is diagnosed with bronchopulmonary dysplasia. Infant was on a ventilator following birth, P27.1.

Infections Specific to the Perinatal Period (P35-P39)

Infection in the Perinatal Period

Newborn Sepsis. To locate infections of the newborn in the index, it is best to look under the main term for the infection, and then to look for a subterm of newborn, fetal, or congenital.

For example, newborn sepsis codes to P36.-. It is also important to assign a code from category B96 to identify the organism responsible for the infection if not identified by another code in this category. Additional codes for severe sepsis (R65.2-) and any associated acute organ dysfunction should be assigned if applicable.

The guidelines also state that if a newborn has a condition that may be due to the birth process or may be community acquired, and the documentation is not clear regarding the underlying cause, the default is to the congenital condition.

EXAMPLE   A 7-day-old infant presents to the physician's office with pneumonia, P23.9.

Hemorrhagic and Hematological Disorders of Newborn (P50-P61)

Many newborns have jaundice. Jaundice results from too many red blood cells and the breakdown of these cells into bilirubin. A large amount of bilirubin causes the skin to take on a yellow color. The most common types of jaundice are:

Physiological (normal) jaundice: this occurs in most newborns. It is a mild form of jaundice that is due to the immaturity of the baby's liver. This type of jaundice usually occurs 2 to 4 days following birth and is gone by 2 weeks of age. It is the most common type of jaundice.

Jaundice of prematurity: this type of jaundice occurs in newborns that are born premature. Their systems are even more immature and, therefore, they are more likely to get jaundice.

Breastfeeding jaundice: this occurs when a breastfeeding baby is not getting enough breast milk because of difficulty with breastfeeding or because the mother's milk isn't in yet. This is not caused by a problem with the breast milk itself but by the baby not getting enough to drink.

Other factors may cause jaundice, but the next most common cause is Rh or ABO incompatibility. ABO incompatibility affects newborns who have mothers with a blood type of O and babies whose blood type is A, B, or AB.

A Coombs' test may be performed on newborns who are jaundiced. This is done to look for possible causes of **hemolysis** (the breaking down of red blood cells). Two common forms of hemolysis in the newborn are Rh incompatibility and ABO incompatibility. Rh incompatibility occurs when an Rh-negative (anti-Rh antibodies in blood) mom gives birth to an Rh-positive baby. If any maternal and fetal blood gets mixed during pregnancy or the birth process, the mother's Rh-negative antibodies will attack the baby's Rh-positive RBCs and destroy them. ABO incompatibility is very similar in mechanism.

Most often, jaundice is treated by putting a baby under "bili" lights. Phototherapy code 6A600ZZ is used for this treatment. In very mild cases, a mother is instructed to put the baby in a sunlit window. In very severe cases, a transfusion may be required.

EXAMPLE   Newborn with Rh incompatibility. Infant was delivered vaginally, Z38.00, P55.0.

Other Problems With the Newborn (P84)

Fetal Distress

Fetal distress occurs when the fetus develops a problem before or during labor. No exact consensus has been reached as to what constitutes fetal distress, but the term often refers to **hypoxia** (insufficient oxygen in blood), **bradycardia** (slow heartbeat), **tachycardia** (fast heartbeat), fetal acidosis, and/or the presence of thick meconium.

EXAMPLE   Fetal distress first noted during labor, infant born vaginally, Z38.00, P84.

EXAMPLE	Fetal hypoxia in infant born by C-Section, Z38.01, P84.

EXAMPLE	Abnormal fetal heart rate or rhythm during labor, infant delivered by C-Section, Z38.01, P03.811.

Other Disorders Originating in the Perinatal Period (P90-P96)

Feeding Problems in Newborns

Newborns are prone to a variety of minor feeding problems. Most newborns spit up, but if spitting up interferes with feeding and growing, it may be GERD. Vomiting could be the result of a more serious infectious condition. Projectile vomiting can occur because of a blockage in the stomach. Overfeeding infants can cause spitting up and diarrhea. Overfeeding is usually done in response to crying. Underfeeding may lead to failure to thrive. Underfeeding usually occurs when an infant has difficulty sucking or swallowing. Sometimes infants have a problem with breastfeeding. When they are not growing at the suspected rate for their age, they may be considered to have failure to thrive or if their weight is disproportionately low compared to their height and head circumference.

EXAMPLE	Newborn delivered vaginally has lost more weight than usual at discharge. Physician documents that a lactation consult should be ordered as there seems to be problems with breastfeeding, Z38.00, P92.5.

EXERCISE 22-2

Answer the following questions.

1. Should the first-listed code on newborn charts be from category Z37? _____

2. If a baby has a low Apgar score it would be indicative of no problems. T or F? _____

3. Mother had a urinary tract infection (UTI) during the pregnancy; this was treated, and no effect on the fetus was observed. Should code P00.1 be added to the baby's chart? _____

4. Mother had an automobile accident. She needed to undergo immediate surgery to correct the open fracture of her arm. It was decided that a cesarean section should be performed and the baby delivered prior to repair of the fracture. Should code P00.5 be added to the baby's chart? _____

5. A baby is born with spina bifida, and the mother had taken statins during pregnancy. Should code P04.1 be used on the baby's chart? _____

6. A baby is born to a mother who used cocaine during the pregnancy. The baby experiences no signs of withdrawal but has a positive drug screen. Should P04.41 be used on this baby's chart? _____

7. A newborn is delivered via vacuum extractor. A large hematoma is located on the scalp. Should P03.3 be coded? _____

Assign codes to the following.

8. Preterm baby born via vaginal delivery at 27 weeks at a weight of 2100 grams _____

9. Baby was delivered via a difficult vaginal delivery at 40 weeks. _____
   Upon delivery the pediatrician noted a fractured clavicle

10. Mother used heroin during this pregnancy. Upon vaginal _____
    delivery, it is noted that the baby is jittery and is
    experiencing symptoms of withdrawal

11. Meconium aspiration syndrome _____

12. Neonatal bradycardia _____

13. Sepsis of the newborn due to group B strep _____

14. Neonatal jaundice due to preterm delivery _____

15. Anemia of the newborn due to prematurity _____

16. Hypomagnesemia of the newborn _____

17. Hypoxia of the newborn _____

18. Meconium staining _____

19. Neonatal abstinence syndrome _____

20. Floppy baby syndrome _____

Congenital Malformations of the Nervous System (Q00-Q07)

Chapter 17
Congenital Malformations, Deformation, and Chromosomal Abnormalities

A **congenital anomaly** is an abnormal condition that is present at birth. Sometimes, conditions that a person is born with do not appear until later in life. Some conditions are congenital by definition, such as Meckel's diverticulum. This condition is present at birth but may not manifest until later in life. Congenital anomalies may be located in the Alphabetic Index under the specific condition or anomaly and/or deformity.

Spina bifida is a disorder that involves incomplete development of the brain, spinal cord, and/or their protective coverings (Figure 22-2). It occurs in 1 in every 2000 births in the United States. Pregnant women can be tested with a blood test called MSAFP (maternal serum alpha-fetoprotein) to screen for spina bifida. This disorder occurs during the first month of pregnancy and is caused by the spine of the fetus not closing properly. This results

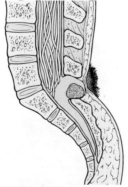

SPINA BIFIDA
Posterior vertebral arches
have not fused; there is no
herniation of the spinal cord
or meninges

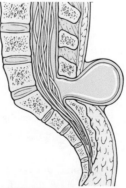

MENINGOCELE
External protruding sac
contains meninges and CSF

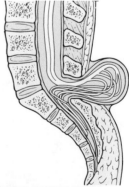

MYELOMENINGOCELE
External sac contains
meninges, CSF, and the
spinal cord

FIGURE 22-2. Congenital spinal cord defects.

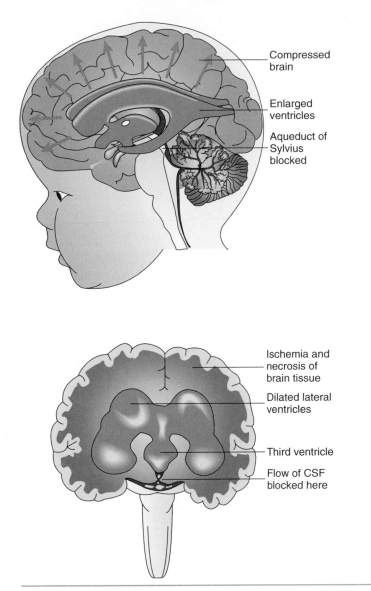

Compressed brain

Enlarged ventricles

Aqueduct of Sylvius blocked

Ischemia and necrosis of brain tissue

Dilated lateral ventricles

Third ventricle

Flow of CSF blocked here

FIGURE 22-3. Hydrocephalus.

in permanent nerve damage to various degrees, even though the opening can be closed in utero or after birth. Three types of spina bifida have been identified: (1) myelomeningocele, which is the most severe form; the spinal cord and the meninges protrude from the opening in the spine; (2) meningocele, which is the most rare form; the spinal cord is normally developed, but the meninges protrudes through the opening; and (3) occulta, which is the mildest form; one or more vertebrae are malformed; this type usually involves no treatment.

Children with spina bifida often have bowel and bladder complications and hydro-cephalus (Figure 22-3). Spina bifida has no cure because nerve tissue cannot be repaired. Treatment is rendered according to the severity of the condition. Children born with spina bifida are usually treated through surgery that is performed to close the opening within 24 hours of birth. If a child is born with the most severe type, he or she often has **hydrocepha-lus**; this is treated by inserting a **ventriculoperitoneal shunt** into the brain to drain accumu-lating fluid (Figure 22-4). Another complication of a severe case of spina bifida is a tethered spinal cord. A tethered spinal cord is a cord that does not move up and down during move-ment, as it is designed to do. If a child has severe pain, surgery may be performed to unte-ther the spinal cord.

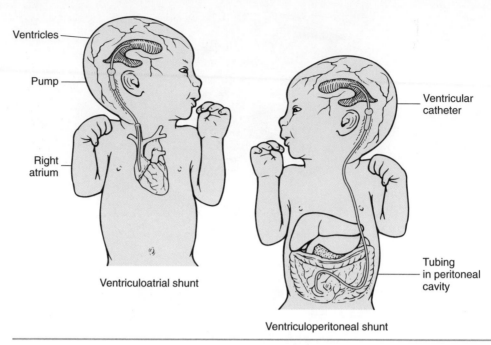

FIGURE 22-4. Shunting procedures for hydrocephalus. **Ventriculoperitoneal shunt** is the preferred procedure.

EXAMPLE | A child with Cockayne's Syndrome is seen by a physician who documents that the patient has mental retardation, retinal atrophy, and microcephaly, Q87.1, H35.89, F79, Q02.

EXAMPLE | Baby born by cesarean section is found to have spina bifida with hydrocephalus, Z38.01, Q05.4.

Congenital Malformations of the Circulatory System (Q20-Q28)

Tetralogy of Fallot

Tetralogy of Fallot (Figure 22-5) is a congenital heart defect that manifests with four key features: (1) a hole between the ventricles (ventral septal defect [VSD]); (2) pulmonary stenosis; (3) aorta lying directly over the hole; and (4) thick, muscled right ventricle (hypertrophy). Treatment recommended for this condition is surgery. Often, surgery requires two stages. The first stage occurs when the infant is first born; a little later, after growth has occurred, the second stage is performed. Patients who have undergone repair often are at greater risk for arrhythmia; sometimes, additional surgery is required later in life. The operation performed to treat this condition is called the **Blalock-Taussig procedure.**

EXAMPLE | VSD is diagnosed in a newborn along with pulmonary stenosis and hypertrophy of the right ventricle, as well as dextroposition of the aorta. The baby is seen by a cardiac surgeon who diagnoses Tetralogy of Fallot. The surgeon recommends surgery, Q21.3.

Cleft Lip and Cleft Palate (Q35-Q37)

A **cleft lip/palate** is an opening in the lip or palate of an infant that occurs in utero. Three different types of clefts can occur on one or both sides of the mouth:

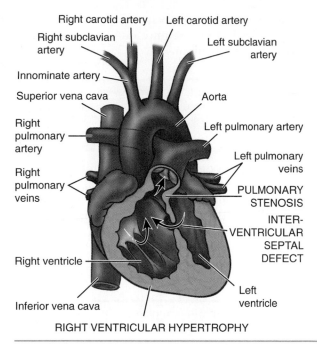

FIGURE 22-5. Tetralogy of Fallot.

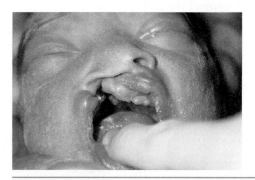

FIGURE 22-6. Unilateral cleft lip.

1. Cleft lip without a cleft palate (Figure 22-6)
2. Cleft palate without a cleft lip
3. Cleft lip and cleft palate together

Approximately 1 in 600 babies is born with a cleft. Surgery is performed to repair the cleft; often, surgery is completed in several stages. The first surgery is usually done when a baby is 10 weeks of age or older and weighs at least 10 pounds.

EXAMPLE   The child was admitted for repair of unilateral upper cleft lip and soft and hard palate. A repair of both the hard and soft palate and lip is performed by external approach, Q37.5, 0CQ0XZZ, 0CQ2XZZ, 0CQ3XZZ.

Other Congenital Malformations of the Digestive System (Q38-A45)

Meckel's Diverticulum

Meckel's diverticulum occurs during the fifth week of fetal development. This is a small pouch on the wall of the small bowel that contains ectopic tissue. It occurs in about 2% of the population, and most people who have this condition have no problems. Complications of Meckel's diverticulum include hematochezia in children and obstruction or diverticulitis in adults. Treatment varies but may require only observation and treatment of symptoms or surgery to remove the diverticulum.

| EXAMPLE | A 60-year-old woman presents to the hospital with severe abdominal pain. A scan is performed, and Meckel's diverticulum is discovered. The surgeon is called in and performs an open ileal resection, Q43.0, 0DTB0ZZ. |

Hirschsprung's disease is a disease of the large intestine and causes intestinal obstruction or severe constipation. Infants with this disease are lacking in nerve cells in the large intestine. These nerve cells signal the muscles to push out the fecal matter in the intestine. If these cells are not present, then the stool remains in the intestine. The symptoms of this disease usually occur shortly after birth and include lots of gas, bloody diarrhea, and green or brown vomit. In order to correct this problem, sometimes surgery is performed to remove the part of the intestine that has no nerve cells.

| EXAMPLE | Newborn is brought to pediatrician with symptoms of fussiness and gas. After examination, the doctor documents congenital megacolon, Q43.1. |

Congenital Malformations of Genital Organs (Q50-Q56)

Undescended testes, also known as cryptorchism, is a common condition occurring in approximately 3% of full term births and 30% of premature births. An undescended testicle is a condition where one of the testes is located outside of the scrotum; this may also be referred to as an ectopic testicle. Risk factors for this condition occurring include family with a history of this condition, premature birth, or low birth weight. In 80% of the cases, the testicle will travel to the correct position within the first year of birth. In some cases surgery termed orchipexy will need to be performed.

| EXAMPLE | At birth the pediatrician examining the baby found that he had bilateral undescended testicles. He recommended that this be watched by the pediatrician, Q53.20. |

Hypospadias is a condition where the opening of the urethra is not in the normal position at the end of the penis. Most often the opening can be found at the underside of the penis (Figure 22-7). Depending on how close or far the opening is from the normal anatomic position will determine the symptoms. Some of the symptoms are abnormal spraying of urine and having to sit when urinating. When infants are diagnosed with hypospadias, they should not be circumcised as the foreskin can be used when surgical repair is performed. Often infants that have hypospadias also have chordee (downward curve of the penis). Surgery to repair these defects is usually performed before a child turns 2 years old.

| EXAMPLE | Baby was born with hypospadias and chordee, Q54.1. |

Congenital Malformations of the Urinary System (Q60-Q64)

Exstrophy of the urinary bladder is a condition where a child is born with part of the urinary bladder outside of the body. This condition is a rare condition that most often occurs in males. It generally occurs with other urinary issues such as epispadias, undescended testicles, and a widening of the pubic symphysis. Surgery is used to repair this birth defect and most often requires more than one surgery.

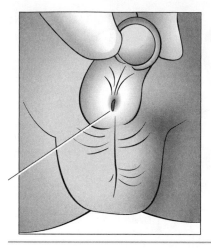

FIGURE 22-7. Hypospadias, urethral opening underside.

EXAMPLE Baby is born with exstrophy of the urinary bladder, Q64.10.

Congenital Malformations and Deformations of the Musculoskeletal System (Q65-Q79)

Congenital malformations of the musculoskeletal system are not uncommon. Some common deformities are:

- Clubfoot—foot turns inward and downward. It is the most common congenital disorder of the legs and can be repaired with a series of casts or in extreme cases with surgery
- Hip dislocations—often occur in breech births
- Funnel chest—chest appears sunken as breast bone is pushed abnormally inward
- Polydactyly—extra digits
- Syndactyly—webbed digits
- Oteogenesis imperfecta—congenital disease causing weak bones

EXAMPLE Baby born by C-section is diagnosed with pigeon chest, Z38.01, Q67.7.

Other Congenital Malformations (Q80-Q89)

Prader-Willi Syndrome is a congenital condition caused by an abnormality of the 15th chromosome. The child with this condition will often be short in stature and have uncontrollable hunger. They never feel full, and they require fewer calories because they have less muscle mass. This is a disorder of the hypothalmus and has symptoms such as stubborness, temper tantrums, learning disabilities, hoarding, low sex hormone levels, and repetitive thoughts and verbalizations. People with this disorder can live a normal lifespan if the obesity can be controlled.

Marfan's Syndrome

Marfan's syndrome (Figure 22-8), which is caused by a gene mutation, is an inherited condition that affects the connective tissue. Because connective tissue is found throughout the body, Marfan's may affect many body systems. Often, patients with Marfan's have skeletal defects, such as spider-like fingers, pectus excavatum, and curvature of the spine. They also may have cardiovascular problems such as aortic regurgitation or prolapse of the mitral valve.

EXAMPLE Aortic regurgitation in a patient with Marfan's syndrome, Q87.418.

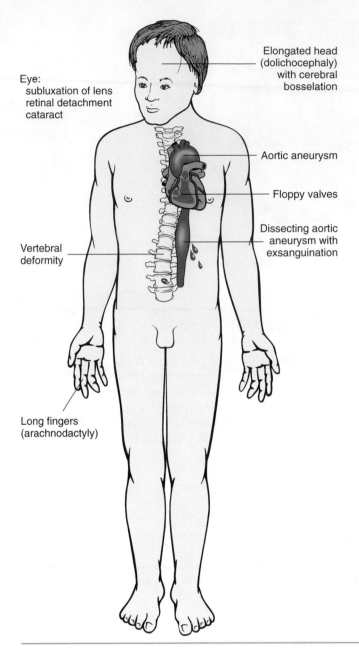

Eye:
subluxation of lens
retinal detachment
cataract

Elongated head
(dolichocephaly)
with cerebral
bosselation

Aortic aneurysm

Floppy valves

Dissecting aortic
aneurysm with
exsanguination

Vertebral
deformity

Long fingers
(arachnodactyly)

FIGURE 22-8. Typical features of Marfan's syndrome.

Chromosomal Abnormalities, Not Elsewhere Classified (Q90-Q99)

One in 200 babies is born with a chromosomal abnormality. Each egg and sperm cell contains 23 chromosomes. When they unite, 23 pairs or 46 chromosomes are created. If a baby is born with too many, too few, or broken or rearranged chromosomes, birth defects may occur. A chromosomal abnormality with three instead of two of a specific chromosome is called a **trisomy.** In most cases, when this occurs, the pregnancy ends in a miscarriage.

Down's syndrome (Figure 22-9), the most common chromosomal abnormality, is also known as trisomy 21. Babies with Down's syndrome have an extra chromosome 21. Children with Down's syndrome can have a combination of birth defects. Some of these are characteristic facial features, mental retardation, and heart defects. No cure is known for Down's syndrome; however, the older the mother is, the greater is the risk; research suggests that

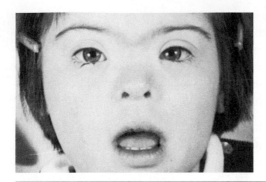

FIGURE 22-9. Photograph of 3½-year-old girl with typical facial appearance of Down's syndrome.

folic acid can help to prevent this condition. Physicians can test for this condition during pregnancy with a test called chorionic villus sampling (CVS). A tiny sample of tissue is taken from the placenta of the mother for this test, which is performed transcervically or transvaginally. CVS can also be used to test for other disorders.

EXAMPLE   Patient with Down's syndrome, Q90.9.

Klinefelter's syndrome is a sex chromosome disorder which occurs only in males; the individual has an extra X chromosome. Most commonly, the child is born with 47 chromosomes in each cell, rather than 46. Symptoms of this condition generally do not appear until puberty. Individuals have low levels of testosterone and small testicles and may exhibit behavior problems.

EXAMPLE   Patient diagnosed with Klinefelter's syndrome, Q98.4.

EXERCISE 22-3

Assign codes to the following conditions.

1. Unilateral, complete cleft lip _____
2. Tongue tie _____
3. Patent ductus arteriosus (PDA) of the newborn _____
4. Ventricular septal defect (VSD) of the newborn _____
5. Preauricular cyst _____
6. Transposition of the great vessels _____
7. Ptosis of the eyelid present at birth _____
8. Microcephalus _____
9. Arnold-Chiari syndrome type II _____
10. Cerebral cyst present at birth _____
11. Supernumerary ear _____
12. Branchial cleft cyst _____
13. Hypospadia _____
14. Micro-penis _____
15. Conjoined twins _____

FACTORS INFLUENCING HEALTH STATUS AND CONTACT WITH HEALTH SERVICES (Z CODES)

As was discussed in Chapter 8, it may be difficult to locate Z codes in the Index. Coders often say, "I did not know there was a Z code for that."

Refer to Chapter 8 for a listing of common main terms used to locate Z codes.

Z00.110	Health examination for newborn under 8 days old
Z00.111	Health examination for newborn 8 to 28 days old
Z13.71	Encounter for nonprocreative screening for genetic disease carrier status
Z13.79	Encounter for other screening for genetic and chromosomal anomalies
Z28.01	Immunization not carried out because of acute illness of patient
Z28.02	Immunization not carried out because of chronic illness or condition of patient
Z28.03	Immunization not carried out because of immune-compromised state of patient
Z28.04	Immunization not carried out because of patient allergy to vaccine or component
Z28.09	Immunization not carried out because of other contraindication
Z28.1	Immunization not carried out because of patient decision for reasons of belief or group pressure
Z28.20	Immunization not carried out because of patient decision for unspecified reason
Z28.21	Immunization not carried out because of patient refusal
Z28.29	Immunization not carried out because of patient decision for other reason
Z28.3	Underimmunization status
Z28.81	Immunization not carried out due to patient having had the disease
Z28.82	Immunization not carried out because of caregiver refusal
Z28.89	Immunization not carried out for other reason
Z28.9	Immunization not carried out for unspecified reason
Z38.00	Single liveborn infant, delivered vaginally
Z38.01	Single liveborn infant, delivered by cesarean
Z38.1	Single liveborn infant, born outside hospital
Z38.2	Single liveborn infant, unspecified as to place of birth
Z38.30	Twin liveborn infant, delivered vaginally
Z38.31	Twin liveborn infant, delivered by cesarean
Z38.4	Twin liveborn infant, born outside of hospital
Z38.5	Twin liveborn infant, unspecified as to place of birth
Z38.61	Triplet liveborn infant, delivered vaginally
Z38.62	Triplet liveborn infant, delivered by cesarean
Z38.63	Quadruplet liveborn infant, delivered vaginally
Z38.64	Quadruplet liveborn infant, delivered by cesarean
Z38.65	Quadruplet liveborn infant, delivered vaginally
Z38.66	Quadruplet liveborn infant, delivered by cesarean
Z38.68	Other multiple liveborn infant, delivered vaginally
Z38.69	Other multiple liveborn, delivered by cesarean
Z38.7	Other multiple liveborn infant, born outside hospital
Z38.8	Other multiple liveborn infant, unspecified as to place of birth
Z41.2	Encounter for routine and ritual male circumcision
Z82.71	Family history of polycystic kidney
Z82.79	Family history of other congenital malformations, deformations, and chromosomal abnormalities
Z87.71	Personal history of hypospadias
Z87.79	Personal history of other congenital malformations and deformations

EXAMPLE Newborn is seen at 5 days for well baby check up, Z00.110.

DOCUMENTATION/REIMBURSEMENT/MS-DRGs

Often, coding difficulties are due to lack of documentation. Sometimes pathology and other test results are not available at the time of discharge or when the physician is dictating the discharge summary or is reporting the final diagnoses.

Frequently missed complications/comorbidities from congenital anomalies and perinatal conditions include:

- Congenital deformities of the brain
- Tetralogy of Fallot
- Congenital anomalies of the pulmonary artery
- Congenital pneumonia
- Meconium aspiration with respiratory symptoms
- Necrotizing enterocolitis
- Chronic respiratory disease arising in the perinatal period
- Convulsions of the newborn
- Ventricular septal defect
- Renal agenesis and dysgenesis
- Polycystic kidney disease
- Exstrophy of urinary bladder
- Osteogenesis imperfect
- Apnea of the newborn
- Congenital anemia
- Drug withdrawal syndrome in newborn

NEWBORN MS-DRGS	RW	DRG TITLE
789	1.4933	Died or transferred
790	4.9243	Extreme immaturity or RDS
791	3.3631	Premature with major problems
792	2.0293	Premature without major problems
793	3.4547	Full-term neonate with major problems
794	1.2227	Neonate with other significant problems
795	0.1656	Normal newborn

As is evident from the MS-DRGs listed here, correct capture of the discharge disposition is very important, as is following the perinatal guidelines to capture all newborn conditions. It also is important to watch for documentation of prematurity and low birth weight.

	CODE	MS-DRGS	RW
Normal newborn	Z38.00	795	0.1656
Newborn with meconium during delivery	Z38.00 P03.82	794	1.2227
Newborn with aspiration of clear amniotic fluid with respiratory symptoms	Z38.00 P24.10	793	3.4547
Premature newborn	Z38.00	792	2.0293
Delivered at 29 weeks weighing 1500 grams	P07.16 P07.31		
Newborn with respiratory distress syndrome	Z38.00 P22.0	790	4.9243

CHAPTER REVIEW EXERCISE

Where applicable, assign codes for diagnoses, procedures, Z codes, and external cause codes.

1. Newborn delivered by cesarean section   _____

2. Twins born in the parking lot of the hospital   _____

3. Baby was born at 2200 grams; physician documented "small for dates"; delivered vaginally   _____

4. Newborn at 43 weeks' gestation, vaginal delivery. Birthweight is listed as 3500 grams   _____

5. Newborn with IUGR (intrauterine growth retardation); delivered vaginally. _____
   Baby weighed 2200 grams and physician documented light for gestational age

6. Newborn fractured clavicle during birth process; vaginal delivery _____

7. TTN (transitory tachypnea of the newborn); infant delivered by emergency _____
   C-section

8. 7-day-old with thrush; seen in physician office _____

9. Transfer from community hospital for treatment of interstitial pulmonary _____
   fibrosis of prematurity in a newborn

10. Baby is admitted 5 days after birth for jaundice due to breast feeding _____

11. 7-day-old infant with infection of the navel cord _____

12. Newborn with a hydrocele following vaginal delivery _____

13. Baby delivered by cesarean section in respiratory failure and immediately _____
    transferred to NICU (neonatal intensive care unit)

14. Newborn aspirated meconium during vaginal delivery _____

15. Neonatal bradycardia following C-section _____

16. Newborn with fetal alcohol syndrome delivered vaginally _____

17. Newborn delivered vaginally to a mother with chorioamnionitis. The _____
    newborn has a fever and is being monitored for a suspected infection
    related to the mother's condition

18. Newborn with hypoglycemia, whose mother has diabetes, delivered vaginally _____

19. Newborn with apnea following vaginal delivery _____

20. Newborn delivered vaginally in the hospital; failed hearing test _____

CHAPTER GLOSSARY

Anomaly: a deviation from normal standards (e.g., as in congenital defects).

Apgar: test used to measure the condition of a newborn at birth.

Blalock-Taussig procedure: procedure used to treat patients with Tetralogy of Fallot who have insufficient pulmonary arterial flow.

Bradycardia: slow heart rate.

Bronchopulmonary dysplasia: chronic lung disease that develops in babies during the first 4 weeks after birth.

Cephalhematoma: a condition of blood between the skull and periosteum of a newborn.

Cleft lip/palate: opening in the lip or palate of an infant that occurs in utero.

Congenital anomaly: an abnormal condition present at birth.

Hemolysis: the breaking down of red blood cells.

Hydrocephalus: cerebrospinal fluid collection in the skull.

Hypoxia: insufficient oxygen in the blood.

Klinefelter's syndrome: a sex chromosome disorder that occurs in males and is caused by an extra X chromosome.

Marfan's syndrome: an inherited condition that affects connective tissue and is caused by gene mutation.

Meconium: material in the intestine of a fetus.

Perinatal period: before birth through the first 28 days of life.

Prader-Willi Syndrome: a congenital condition caused by an abnormality of the 15th chromosome.

Tachycardia: fast heartbeat.

Tachypnea: fast breathing.

Trisomy: extra chromosome.

Ventriculoperitoneal shunt: procedure used to treat patient with hydrocephalus in whom drainage of the ventricle occurs through an artificial channel between the ventricle and the peritoneum.

23

Injury and Certain Other Consequences of External Causes and External Causes of Morbidity

(ICD-10-CM Chapter 19, Codes S00-T88 and Chapter 20, Codes V00-Y99)

LEARNING OBJECTIVES

1. Apply and assign the correct ICD-10-CM/PCS codes in accordance with Official Guidelines for Coding and Reporting
2. Identify major differences between ICD-10-CM and ICD-9-CM related to injuries and E codes
3. Identify the various types of injuries
4. Assign the correct Z codes, External cause codes, and procedure codes related to injuries
5. Identify common treatments, medications, and diagnostic tests
6. Explain the importance of documentation in relation to MS-DRGs for reimbursement

ABBREVIATIONS/ ACRONYMS

AKA above-knee amputation
ATV all-terrain vehicle
CHI closed head injury
CT computerized tomography
FB foreign body
ICD-9-CM *International Classification of Diseases, 9th Revision, Clinical Modification*
ICD-10-CM *International Classification of Diseases,*

10th Revision, Clinical Modification
ICD-10-PCS *International Classification of Diseases, 10th Revision, Procedure Coding System*
LOC loss of consciousness
MRI magnetic resonance imaging
MS-DRG Medicare Severity diagnosis-related group

MVA motor vehicle accident
OIG Office of the Inspector General
OR Operating Room
ORIF open reduction with internal fixation
SCI spinal cord injury
SLAP superior labrum anterior-posterior
TBI traumatic brain injury

ICD-10-CM

Official Guidelines for Coding and Reporting

Please refer to the companion Evolve website for the most current guidelines.

19. Chapter 19: Injury, poisoning, and certain other consequences of external causes (S00-T88)

   a. *Application of 7th Characters in Chapter 19*

   Most categories in chapter 19 have a 7th character requirement for each applicable code. Most categories in this chapter have three **7th character values** (with the exception of fractures): A, initial encounter, D, subsequent encounter and S, sequela. **Categories for traumatic fractures have additional 7th character values**.

   7th character "A", initial encounter is used while the patient is receiving active treatment for the **condition**. Examples of active treatment are: surgical treatment, emergency department encounter, and evaluation and treatment by a new physician.

   7th character "D" subsequent encounter is used for encounters after the patient has received active treatment of the **condition** and is receiving routine care for the condition during the healing or recovery phase. Examples of subsequent care are: cast change or removal, removal of external or internal fixation device, medication adjustment, other aftercare and follow up visits following **treatment of the injury or condition**.

   The aftercare Z codes should not be used for aftercare for **conditions such as injuries or poisonings, where 7th characters are provided to identify subsequent care. For example,** for aftercare of an injury, assign the acute injury code with the 7th character "D" (subsequent encounter).

   7th character "S", sequela, is for use for complications or conditions that arise as a direct result of a **condition**, such as scar formation after a bum. The scars are sequelae of the bum. When using **7th character "S"**, it is necessary to use both the injury code that precipitated the sequela and the code for the sequela itself. The "S" is added only to the injury code, not the sequela code. The **7th character** "S" identifies the injury responsible for the sequela. The specific type of sequela (e.g. scar) is sequenced first, followed by the injury code.

EXAMPLE | Injury left wrist and dislocation right elbow from fall on escalator in public building. Dislocation was reduced, S53.104A, S69.92xA, W10.0xxA, Y92.29, 0RSLXZZ.

EXAMPLE | The patient is seen in follow-up for healing blow-out fracture, S02.3xxD, X58.xxxD.

EXAMPLE | Left wrist with keloid scar due to previous burns from fire (accidental), L91.0, T23.072S, X08.8xxS.

b. Coding of Injuries

When coding injuries, assign separate codes for each injury unless a combination code is provided, in which case the combination code is assigned. Code T07, Unspecified multiple injuries should not be assigned **in the inpatient setting** unless information for a more specific code is not available. Traumatic injury codes (S00-T14.9) are not to be used for normal, healing surgical wounds or to identify complications of surgical wounds.

The code for the most serious injury, as determined by the provider and the focus of treatment, is sequenced first.

1) Superficial injuries

Superficial injuries such as abrasions or contusions are not coded when associated with more severe injuries of the same site.

EXAMPLE | Abrasion with laceration to the left knee, S81.012A, X58.xxxA.

2) Primary injury with damage to nerves/blood vessels

When a primary injury results in minor damage to peripheral nerves or blood vessels, the primary injury is sequenced first with additional code(s) for injuries to nerves and spinal cord (such as category S04), and/or injury to blood vessels (such as category S15). When the primary injury is to the blood vessels or nerves, that injury should be sequenced first.

EXAMPLE | Minor laceration of splenic artery and fracture of right little finger due to trauma from being kicked and falling during a football game. Suture of laceration of splenic artery, S35.291A, S62.606A, W50.1xxA, Y92.321, 04Q40ZZ.

c. Coding of Traumatic Fractures

The principles of multiple coding of injuries should be followed in coding fractures. Fractures of specified sites are coded individually by site in accordance with both the provisions within categories S02, S12, S22, S32, S42, S49, S52, S59, S62, S72, S79, S82, S89, S92 and the level of detail furnished by medical record content.

A fracture not indicated as open or closed should be coded to closed. A fracture not indicated whether displaced or not displaced should be coded to displaced.

EXAMPLE | Closed fracture of right surgical neck of humerus and left open fracture of anatomic neck of humerus, S42.292D, S42.211A, X58.xxxA.

More specific guidelines are as follows:

1) Initial vs. Subsequent Encounter for Fractures

Traumatic fractures are coded using the appropriate 7th character extension for initial encounter (A, B, C) while the patient is receiving active treatment for the fracture. Examples of active treatment are: surgical treatment, emergency department encounter, and evaluation and treatment by a new physician. The appropriate 7th character for initial encounter should also be assigned for a patient who delayed seeking treatment for the fracture or nonunion.

Fractures are coded using the appropriate 7th character extension for subsequent care for encounters after the patient has completed active treatment of the fracture and is receiving routine care for the fracture during the healing or recovery phase. Examples of fracture aftercare are: cast change or removal, removal of external or internal fixation device, medication adjustment, and follow-up visits following fracture treatment.

Care for complications of surgical treatment for fracture repairs during the healing or recovery phase should be coded with the appropriate complication codes.

Care of complications of fractures, such as malunion and nonunion, should be reported with the appropriate 7th character extensions for subsequent care with nonunion (K, M, N,) or subsequent care with malunion (P, Q, R).

A code from category M80, not a traumatic fracture code, should be used for any patient with known osteoporosis who suffers a fracture, even if the patient had a minor fall or trauma, if that fall or trauma would not usually break a normal, healthy bone.

See Section I.C.13. Osteoporosis.

The aftercare Z codes should not be used for aftercare for traumatic fractures. For aftercare of a traumatic fracture, assign the acute fracture code with the appropriate 7th character.

EXAMPLE

The patient suffered a blow-out fracture 1 week ago and is now being referred to a specialist for consultation, S02.3xxA, X58.xxxA.

EXAMPLE

Subsequent encounter for malunion fracture of right tibia from motor vehicle accident, S82.201P, V89.2xxS.

---

2) Multiple fractures sequencing

Multiple fractures are sequenced in accordance with the severity of the fracture.

EXAMPLE

The patient had a fractured parietal bone of the skull and fracture of the left fifth rib, S02.0xxA, S22.32xA, X58.xxxA.

EXAMPLE

Fractures of multiple metacarpal bones of the right hand, S62.309A, X58.xxxA.

As with Z codes, detailed guidelines have been put forth for the use of external cause codes. The Alphabetic Index for these codes is located prior to the Tabular List and after the Table of Neoplasms and Table of Drugs and Chemicals. Codes are located by using the Alphabetic Index and then verifying the appropriate code in the Tabular List. The assignment of external cause codes may depend on facility policy, particular state requirements, and the following guidelines. For example, the assignment of external cause codes may be useful in determining the number of head injuries that occur as a result of bicycle accidents. This data may be used to support bicycle helmet programs in a particular city or state. Codes for external causes are never used as a principal or first-listed diagnosis. External cause codes are always assigned as an additional code(s). External cause codes are used to identify the cause, the intent, the place of occurrence, the activity, and the status at the time of the event.

The External cause guidelines are used for injuries, poisonings, adverse effects, and complications of surgical and medical care, which are covered in the next three chapters. Some of the external cause guidelines may be addressed in subsequent chapters so the numbering/lettering may not be sequential.

20. Chapter 20: External Causes of Morbidity (V01-Y99)

Introduction: These guidelines are provided for the reporting of external causes of morbidity codes in order that there will be standardization in the process. These codes are secondary codes for use in any health care setting.

External cause codes are intended to provide data for injury research and evaluation of injury prevention strategies. These codes capture how the injury or health condition happened (cause), the intent (unintentional or accidental; or intentional, such as suicide or assault), the place where the event occurred the activity of the patient at the time of the event, and the person's status (e.g., civilian, military).

a. General External Cause Coding Guidelines

1) Used with any code in the range of A00.0-T88.9, Z00-Z99

An external cause code may be used with any code in the range of A00.0-T88.9, Z00-Z99, classification that is a health condition due to an external cause. Though they are most applicable to injuries, they are also valid for use with such things as infections or diseases due to an external source, and other health conditions, such as a heart attack that occurs during strenuous physical activity.

EXAMPLE Concussion due to accidental fall down steps at home, S06.0x9A, W10.9xxA, Y92.009, Y99.8.

EXAMPLE Patient was admitted and treated for an ST elevation myocardial infarction due to shoveling snow in the driveway of his single-family house, I21.3, Y92.014, Y93.h1, Y99.8.

2) External cause code used for length of treatment

Assign the external cause code, with the appropriate 7th character (initial encounter, subsequent encounter or sequela) for each encounter for which the injury or condition is being treated.

3) Use the full range of external cause codes

Use the full range of external cause codes to completely describe the cause, the intent, the place of occurrence, and if applicable, the activity of the patient at the time of the event, and the patient's status, for all injuries, and other health conditions due to an external cause.

4) Assign as many external cause codes as necessary

Assign as many external cause codes as necessary to fully explain each cause. If only one external code can be recorded, assign the code most related to the principal diagnosis.

5) The selection of the appropriate external cause code

The selection of the appropriate external cause code is guided by the Alphabetic Index of External Causes and by Inclusion and Exclusion notes in the Tabular List.

6) External cause code can never be a principal diagnosis

An external cause code can never be a principal (first-listed) diagnosis

7) Combination external cause codes

Certain of the external cause codes are combination codes that identify sequential events that result in an injury, such as a fall which results in striking against an object. The injury may be due to either event or both. The combination external cause code used should correspond to the sequence of events regardless of which caused the most serious injury.

8) No external cause code needed in certain circumstances

No external cause code from Chapter 20 is needed if the external cause and intent are included in a code from another chapter (e.g. T36.0x1- Poisoning by penicillins, accidental (unintentional)).

b. Place of Occurrence Guideline

Codes from category Y92, Place of occurrence of the external cause, are secondary codes for use after other external cause codes to identify the location of the patient at the time of injury or other condition.

A place of occurrence code is used only once, at the initial encounter for treatment. No 7th characters are used for Y92. Only one code from Y92 should be recorded on a medical record. A place of occurrence code should be used in conjunction with an activity code, Y93.

Do not use place of occurrence code Y92.9 if the place is not stated or is not applicable.

EXAMPLE

Injury to the left wrist occurred on the playground at the public park. Patient fell off slide, S69.92xA, W09.0xxA, Y92.830, Y93.59, Y99.8.

c. Activity Code

Assign a code from category Y93, Activity code, to describe the activity of the patient at the time the injury or other health condition occurred.

An activity code is used only once, at the initial encounter for treatment. Only one code from Y93 should be recorded on a medical record. An activity code should be used in conjunction with a place of occurrence code, Y92.

If a patient is a student but is injured while performing an activity for income, use 7th character "2", work related activity. A work related activity is any activity for which payment or income is received.

The activity codes are not applicable to poisonings, adverse effects, misadventures or **sequela**.

Do not assign Y93.9, Unspecified activity, if the activity is not stated.

A code from category Y93 is appropriate for use with external cause and intent codes if identifying the activity provides additional information about the event.

EXAMPLE

Injury left knee due to twisting movement while playing basketball at the YMCA gym, S89.92xA, Y93.67, Y92.310, Y99.8.

d. Place of Occurrence, Activity, and Status Codes Used with other External Cause Code

When applicable, place of occurrence, activity, and external cause status codes are sequenced after the main external cause code(s). Regardless of the number of external cause codes assigned, there should be only one place of occurrence code, one activity code, and one external cause status code assigned to an encounter.

e. If the Reporting Format Limits the Number of External Cause Codes

If the reporting format limits the number of external cause codes that can be used in reporting clinical data, report the code for the cause/intent most related to the principal diagnosis. If the format permits capture of additional external cause codes, the cause/intent, including medical misadventures, of the additional events should be reported rather than the codes for place, activity, or external status.

f. Multiple External Cause Coding Guidelines

More than one external cause code is required to fully describe the external cause of an illness **or** injury. The assignment of external cause codes should be sequenced in the following priority:

If two or more events cause separate injuries, an external cause code should be assigned for each cause. The first-listed external cause code will be selected in the following order:

External codes for child and adult abuse take priority over all other external cause codes.

See Section I.C.19., Child and Adult abuse guidelines.

External cause codes for terrorism events take priority over all other external cause codes except child and adult abuse.

External cause codes for cataclysmic events take priority over all other external cause codes except child and adult abuse and terrorism.

External cause codes for transport accidents take priority over all other external cause codes except cataclysmic events, child and adult abuse and terrorism.

Activity and external cause status codes are assigned following all causal (intent) external cause codes.

The first-listed external cause code should correspond to the cause of the most serious diagnosis due to an assault, accident, or self-harm, following the order of hierarchy listed above.

EXAMPLE

Laceration left wrist from sharp glass, suspected suicide attempt, S61.512A, Y28.0xxA.

h. Unknown or Undetermined Intent Guideline

If the intent (accident, self-harm, assault) of the cause of an injury or other condition is unknown or unspecified, code the intent as accidental intent. All transport accident categories assume accidental intent.

1) Use of undetermined intent

External cause codes for events of undetermined intent are only for use if the documentation in the record specifies that the intent cannot be determined.

EXAMPLE

Laceration left wrist from sharp glass, intent unknown, S61.512A, Y28.0xxA.

i. *Sequelae* (Late Effects) of External Cause Guidelines

1) *Sequelae* external cause codes

Sequela are reported using the external cause code with the 7th character "S" for sequela. These codes should be used with any report of a late effect or sequela resulting from a previous injury.

2) *Sequela* external cause code with a related current injury

A **sequela** external cause code should never be used with a related current nature of injury code.

3) Use of *sequela* external cause codes for subsequent visits

Use a late effect external cause code for subsequent visits when a late effect of the initial injury is being treated. Do not use a late effect external cause code for subsequent visits for follow-up care (e.g., to assess healing, to receive rehabilitative therapy) of the injury when no late effect of the injury has been documented.

j. Terrorism Guidelines

1) Cause of injury identified by the Federal Government (FBI) as terrorism

When the cause of an injury is identified by the Federal Government (FBI) as terrorism, the first-listed external cause code should be a code from category Y38, Terrorism. The definition of terrorism employed by the FBI is found at the inclusion note at the beginning of category Y38. Use additional code for place of occurrence (Y92.-). More than one Y38 code may be assigned if the injury is the result of more than one mechanism of terrorism.

2) Cause of an injury is suspected to be the result of terrorism

When the cause of an injury is suspected to be the result of terrorism a code from category Y38 should not be assigned. Suspected cases should be classified as assault.

3) Code Y38.9, Terrorism, secondary effects

Assign code Y38.9, Terrorism, secondary effects, for conditions occurring subsequent to the terrorist event. This code should not be assigned for conditions that are due to the initial terrorist act.

It is acceptable to assign code Y38.9 with another code from Y38 if there is an injury due to the initial terrorist event and an injury that is a subsequent result of the terrorist event.

EXAMPLE | The patient (civilian) had a head injury due to a terrorist explosion, S09.90xA, Y38.2x2A, Y99.8.

EXAMPLE | The patient (civilian) has chronic posttraumatic stress syndrome following a terrorist attack, subsequent encounter, F43.12, Y38.9x2S.

k. External cause status

A code from category Y99, External cause status, should be assigned whenever any other external cause code is assigned for an encounter, including an Activity code, except for the events noted below. Assign a code from category Y99, External cause status, to indicate the work status of the person at the time the event occurred. The status code indicates whether the event occurred during military activity, whether a non-military person was at work, whether an individual including a student or volunteer was involved in a non-work activity at the time of the causal event.

A code from Y99, External cause status, should be assigned, when applicable, with other external cause codes, such as transport accidents and falls. The external cause status codes are not applicable to poisonings, adverse effects, misadventures or late effects.

Do not assign a code from category Y99 if no other external cause codes (cause, activity) are applicable for the encounter.

An external cause status code is used only once, at the initial encounter for treatment. Only one code from Y99 should be recorded on a medical record.

Do not assign code Y99.9, Unspecified external cause status, if the status is not stated.

Apply the General Coding Guidelines as found in Chapter 5 and the Procedural Coding Guidelines as found in Chapters 6 and 7.

Remember that External cause codes identify how an injury occurred and the intent. External cause codes also identify the place that an injury occurred and describe the activity that caused the injury or other health condition. At the beginning of Chapter 19 in the ICD-10-CM code book, special instructions state that codes from this chapter should be used as secondary codes and that a code from another chapter of the Classification should be assigned indicating the nature of the injury or health condition (Figure 23-1). Also remember, do NOT use code Y92.9 if the place of occurrence is not stated or Y93.9 if the activity was not stated. Physician documentation may not include the detail required to assign the place of occurrence, activity, and the patient's status at the time of the event.

CHAPTER 20

EXTERNAL CAUSES OF MORBIDITY (V00-Y99)

Note: This chapter permits the classification of environmental events and circumstances as the cause of injury, and other adverse effects. Where a code from this section is applicable, it is intended that it shall be used secondary to a code from another chapter of the Classification indicating the nature of the condition. Most often, the condition will be classifiable to Chapter 19, Injury, poisoning and certain other consequences of external causes (S00-T88). Other conditions that may be stated to be due to external causes are classified in Chapters I to XVIII. For these conditions, codes from Chapter 20 should be used to provide additional information as to the cause of the condition.

FIGURE 23-1. Instructional note regarding the use of External cause codes.

MAJOR DIFFERENCES BETWEEN ICD-10-CM AND ICD-9-CM

- ICD-10-CM has more notes with instructions to code also any associated injuries.
- Laterality is specified in ICD-10-CM.
- In ICD-9-CM, there is a fourth digit to identify a laceration that is infected or "complicated." In ICD-10-CM, there are instructional notes under the open-wound categories to code also any associated wound infection.
- In ICD-10-CM, fractures are classified as nondisplaced or displaced. If a fracture is not specified, it should be coded to displaced.
- Most of the codes in Chapter 19 utilize the seventh character. Most of the codes use at least the following extensions:
  - A   Initial encounter
  - D   Subsequent encounter
  - S   Sequela
- Complications such as malunion and nonunion of a fracture are reported with the appropriate seventh-character extensions for subsequent care with nonunion (K, M, N) or subsequent care with malunion (P, Q, R).
- In ICD-9-CM, the guidelines state that if the intent of the cause of an injury is unknown or questionable, code the intent as undetermined. ICD-10-CM guidelines state that if the cause of an injury or other condition is unknown or unspecified, the intent is coded accidental. Undetermined intent is only coded if the documentation in the record indicates that the intent cannot be determined.

EXERCISE 23-1

Assign only the External cause codes to the following. Remember that External cause codes provide information about the cause and intent of an injury. If the place of occurrence, the status of the patient at the time, and/or an activity code is applicable, assign the appropriate codes. Assume initial episode of care, unless otherwise specified.

1. Patient is employed doing data entry and has carpal tunnel syndrome from using computer keyboard   _____
2. Patient fell from a ladder while working as an employee at church   _____
3. Patient was bitten by a dog while jogging at the public park   _____
4. Patient was injured in a motorcycle accident. Patient was the driver and lost control due to wet interstate highway   _____
5. Patient accidentally lacerated hand with hunting knife while hunting in the woods   _____
6. Patient fell out of bed at the nursing home and was injured   _____
7. Patient was injured during an assault with a baseball bat in public parking garage   _____
8. Patient was injured while playing in NHL hockey game. Patient was checked into the boards by another player and fell to the ice   _____
9. Patient was the victim of accidental drowning in lake   _____
10. Patient was the driver and was injured during a motor vehicle collision with a train   _____

ANATOMY AND PHYSIOLOGY

The musculoskeletal chapter outlines the anatomy and physiology that is pertinent to injury. Internal organs and the blood vessels may also be involved in an injury. These are outlined in their respective body system chapters.

DISEASE CONDITIONS

Injury, Poisoning, and Certain Other Consequences of External Causes (S00-T88), Chapter 19 in the ICD-10-CM code book, covers a wide range of codes that will be discussed in the next three chapters of this textbook. Categories marked with an asterisk (*) are covered in this chapter. Chapter 24 discusses burns, adverse effects, and poisonings and Chapter 25 is dedicated to complications associated with surgical and medical care.

The S section is for coding different types of injuries related to single body regions, and the T section is for injuries to unspecified body regions, poisonings, and certain other consequences of external causes. Chapter 19 in the ICD-10-CM code book—Injury, Poisoning, and Certain Other Consequences of External Causes (S00-T88)—is divided into the following categories:

SECTION	SECTION TITLES
*S00-S09	Injuries to the head
*S10-S19	Injuries to the neck
*S20-S29	Injuries to the thorax
*S30-S39	Injuries to the abdomen, lower back, lumbar spine, pelvis, and external genitalia
*S40-S49	Injuries to the shoulder and upper arm
*S50-S59	Injuries to the elbow and forearm
*S60-S69	Injuries to the wrist and hand
*S70-S79	Injuries to the hip and thigh
*S80-S89	Injuries to the knee and lower leg
*S90-S99	Injuries to the ankle and foot
*T07	Injuries involving multiple body regions
*T14	Injury of unspecified body region
*T15-T19	Effects of foreign body entering through natural orifice
T20-T32	Burns and corrosions
T33-T34	Frostbite
T36-T50	Poisoning by, adverse effect of, and underdosing of drugs, medicaments, and biological substances
T51-T65	Toxic effects of substances chiefly nonmedicinal as to source
T66-T78	Other and unspecified effects of external causes
*T79	Certain early complications of trauma
T80-T88	Complications of surgical and medical care, not elsewhere classified

Chapter 20 is divided into the following categories:

V00-V09	Pedestrian injured in transport accident
V10-V19	Pedal cycle rider injured in transport accident
V20-V29	Motorcycle rider injured in transport accident
V30-V39	Occupant of three-wheeled motor vehicle injured in transport accident
V40-V49	Car occupant injured in transport accident
V50-V59	Occupant of pick-up truck or van injured in transport accident
V60-V69	Occupant of heavy transport vehicle injured in transport accident
V70-V79	Bus occupant injured in transport accident
V80-V89	Other land transport accidents
V90-V94	Water transport accidents
V95-V97	Air and space transport accidents
V98-V99	Other and unspecified transport accidents
W00-W19	Slipping, tripping, stumbling, and falls
W20-W49	Exposure to inanimate mechanical forces
W50-W64	Exposure to animate mechanical forces
W65-W74	Accidental non-transport drowning and submersion
W85-W99	Exposure to electric current, radiation and extreme ambient air temperature and pressure
X00-X08	Exposure to smoke, fire, and flames

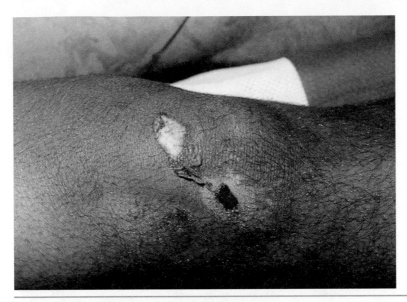

FIGURE 23-2. Abrasion wound of kneecap.

X10-X19	Contact with heat and hot substances
X30-X39	Exposure to forces of nature
X52-X58	Accidental exposure to other specified factors
X71-X83	Intentional self-harm
X92-Y09	Assault
Y21-Y33	Event of undetermined intent
Y35-Y38	Legal intervention, operations of war, military operations, and terrorism
Y62-Y69	Misadventures to patients during surgical and medical care
Y70-Y82	Medical devices associated with adverse incidents in diagnostic and therapeutic use
Y83-Y84	Surgical and other medical procedures as the cause of abnormal reaction of the patient, or of later complication, without mention of misadventure at the time of the procedure
Y90-Y99	Supplementary factors related to causes of morbidity classified elsewhere

Superficial Injuries

Superficial injuries may manifest in the form of contusions, abrasions (Figure 23-2), non-thermal blisters, nonvenomous insect bites, and superficial foreign bodies or splinters and external constriction (Figure 23-3). The physician may not document the term "superficial," so supporting documentation must be used to determine whether the injury fits into the superficial categories. It is not necessary to code superficial injuries when a more serious injury has occurred at the same site.

EXAMPLE

Corneal abrasion due to being struck by tree branch while hiking in the forest, S05.00xA, W22.8xxA, Y92.821, Y93.01, Y99.8.

EXAMPLE

Laceration and abrasion right elbow due to fall from scooter at the lake, S51.011A, V00.141A, Y92.828, Y99.8. The abrasion is not coded separately because it occurred at the same site as a more severe injury.

EXAMPLE

Sprain right ankle and abrasions left knee due to being knocked down while playing basketball during phy-ed in gym, S93.401A, S80.212A, W03.xxxA, Y92.310, Y99.8. Abrasions are coded because they occurred at a different site from the sprain.

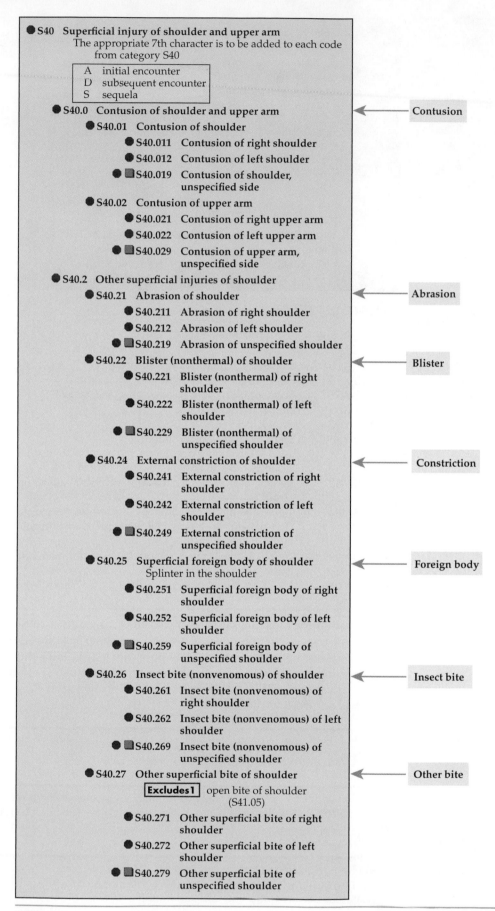

FIGURE 23-3. Superficial injuries.

EXERCISE 23-2

Assign codes to the following conditions. Assume initial episode of care, unless otherwise specified. Do not assign external cause codes.

1. Blister left heel due to rubbing of shoe _____
2. Mosquito bites both legs _____
3. Abrasions right hand and right knee _____
4. Superficial wood splinter right thumb _____
5. Abrasions and deep laceration of left elbow _____

Contusion With Intact Skin Surface

A **contusion** is any injury that results in hemorrhage beneath unbroken skin. Other terms for contusion include "bruise" and "hematoma." Contusions associated with more severe or serious injuries at the same site would not be coded. Occasionally, if a hematoma does not absorb on its own, it may have to be evacuated or aspirated.

EXAMPLE   Contusion right quadriceps after tackle in college football game, S70.11xA, W03.xxxA, Y92.321, Y93.61.

EXAMPLE   Contusion and severe sprain of left ankle after falling into a hole while hiking in the mountains, S93.402A, W17.2xxA, Y92.828, Y93.01, Y99.8.

EXERCISE 23-3

Assign codes to the following conditions. Assume initial episode of care, unless otherwise specified. Do not assign external cause codes.

1. Blackeye (right) _____
2. Subungual hematoma left thumb (traumatic) _____
3. Bruise left ankle _____
4. Hematoma right breast (traumatic) _____
5. Contusion right shin _____

Laceration/Open Wounds

An open wound or **laceration** is an injury that results in a tear in the skin (Figure 23-4). Bruising and swelling can occur around the wound site. Common sites of laceration are body areas with underlying bony support, such as above the eyebrows, on the scalp and face, and over the knees. Traumatic injury codes should not be used to identify surgical wounds, nontraumatic wounds or ulcers, decubitus ulcers, and stasis ulcers. Laceration or open wound codes are assigned by location. Other factors that may make a difference in the code assignment include:

- If there is damage to nail (i.e., thumb nail damaged)
- If the wound is described as a puncture wound
- If the wound is a bite wound that is not classified as superficial
- The presence of a foreign body
- Penetration into a body cavity (i.e., laceration abdominal wall with penetration into peritoneal cavity)

An additional code would be assigned to identify any associated wound infection and any responsible organism.

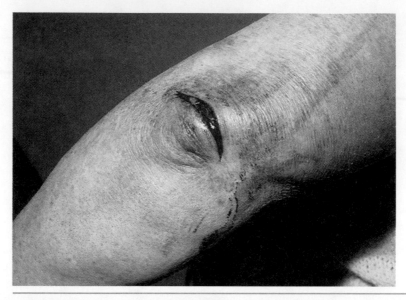

FIGURE 23-4. Laceration of elbow.

EXAMPLE	The patient cut his right eyebrow during fall while downhill skiing; patient fell while skiing at resort, S01.111A, V00.321A, Y92.838, Y93.23, Y99.8.

EXAMPLE	Patient presented to the emergency room with gravel embedded in laceration of left knee. Patient fell while hiking in the mountains 2 days ago. The wound was cleaned and dressing applied, S81.022A, W19.xxxA, Y92.828, Y93.01, Y99.8.

EXERCISE 23-4

Assign codes to the following conditions. Assume initial episode of care, unless otherwise specified. Do not assign external cause codes.

1. Puncture wound left forearm   _____
2. Laceration right calf which occurred 3 days ago, and no   _____
   medical attention has been sought until now
3. Wound left foot with glass pieces in wound   _____

Fractures

A **fracture** is a break in a bone. Bones are rigid but will bend. However, if the impact or force is too great, the bone will break. There are different types of fractures (Figure 23-5) with varying degrees of complexity. In a minor injury, the bone may just crack and may not break all the way through. In a more severe injury, the bone may shatter, or it may break through the skin. Treatment provided for a fracture depends on the specific bone broken, the severity of the break, and whether it is an "open" or a "closed" fracture. If a fracture is not documented as displaced or not displaced, it should be assigned a displaced fracture code.

Fractures fall into two categories:

1. **Closed fracture** or **simple fracture** is diagnosed when the bone is broken, but the skin remains intact. Descriptive words used for a closed fracture include the following:
   - Comminuted—broken, splintered, or crushed into a number of pieces
   - Depressed—portion of the skull that is broken and driven inward

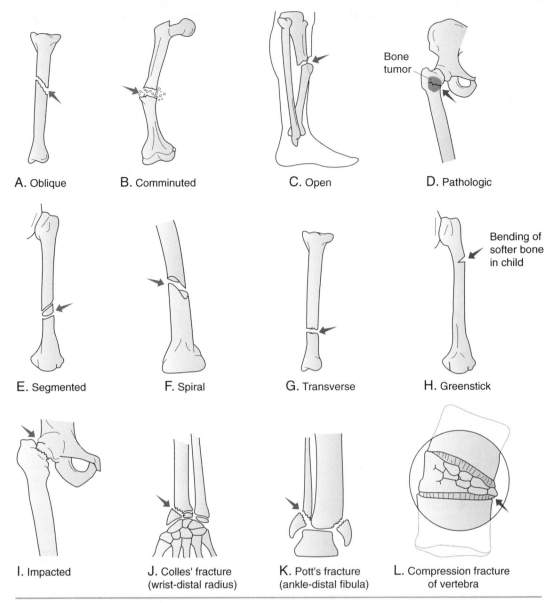

A. Oblique   B. Comminuted   C. Open   D. Pathologic

E. Segmented   F. Spiral   G. Transverse   H. Greenstick

I. Impacted   J. Colles' fracture (wrist-distal radius)   K. Pott's fracture (ankle-distal fibula)   L. Compression fracture of vertebra

Bone tumor

Bending of softer bone in child

FIGURE 23-5. Types of fractures.

- Fissured—incomplete fracture that does not split the bone
- Fracture NOS—not otherwise specified
- Greenstick—the bone is somewhat bent and is partially broken; occurs in children
- Impacted—one fractured bone end is wedged into another broken end
- Linear—straight line fracture
- Simple—fracture that remains in alignment with little damage to surrounding tissue
- Slipped epiphysis—separation of the growing end of the bone (epiphysis) from the shaft of the bone; occurs in children and young adults
- Spiral—occurs when a bone has been twisted apart

2. **Open fracture** or **compound fracture** occurs when the bone exits and is visible through the skin, or a deep wound exposes the bone through the skin. If the wound is superficial and the fracture site is not exposed, the injury is coded as a closed fracture—not an open fracture. Some descriptive words used for an open fracture include the following:

- Compound—fracture in which the bone is sticking through the skin
- Infected—condition in which the bone becomes infected by bacteria
- Missile—penetrating injuries resulting in fractures caused by bullets or stab wounds
- Puncture—a puncture wound is present. The wound may be related to the injury or to bone fragments
- Foreign body—presence of a foreign body within the fracture site

If a fracture is not specified as open or closed, it is coded as a closed fracture. If documentation in the record reveals an open wound around the fracture site, it may be necessary to query the physician as to whether this is an open or a closed fracture. In some instances, a fracture is documented as both open and closed. This usually occurs with a severe fracture with fracture fragments, and it should be coded as an open fracture. A **complicated fracture** is a fracture that causes injury to surrounding tissues; it may be open or closed.

Open fractures may be identified by the **Gustilo open fracture classification**, which is based on the mechanism of the injury and the amount of soft tissue and skeletal injury. This classification system is useful in assessing risk of infection and possible amputation.

- Type I: clean wound smaller than 1 cm in diameter, appears clean, simple fracture pattern, minimal soft tissue injury
- Type II: a laceration greater than 1 cm but with moderate soft tissue injury. Fracture pattern may be more complex
- Type III: an open segmental fracture or a single fracture with extensive soft tissue injury. Also included are injuries older than 8 hours. Type III injuries are subdivided into three types:
  - Type IIIA: adequate soft tissue coverage of the fracture despite high energy trauma or extensive laceration or skin flaps
  - Type IIIB: inadequate soft tissue coverage with periosteal stripping and bone exposure. Soft tissue reconstruction is necessary. Wound is contaminated
  - Type IIIC: any open fracture that is associated with vascular (major arterial) injury that requires repair

See Figure 23-6 for the 7th character extensions applicable to fracture of femur S72. The Gustilo classification is identified for the open fracture 7th character extension.

S72   Fracture of femur

Note: A fracture not indicated as displaced or nondisplaced should be coded to displaced
A fracture not indicated as open or closed should be coded to closed
The open fracture designations are based on the Gustilo open fracture classification

Excludes1: traumatic amputation of hip and thigh (S78.-)
Excludes2: fracture of lower leg and ankle (S82.-)
fracture of foot (S92.-)
periprosthetic fracture of prosthetic implant of hip (T84.040, T84.041)

The appropriate 7th character is to be added to all codes from category S72
A - initial encounter for closed fracture
B - initial encounter for open fracture type I or II
initial encounter for open fracture NOS
C - initial encounter for open fracture type IIIA, IIIB, or IIIC
D - subsequent encounter for closed fracture with routine healing
E - subsequent encounter for open fracture type I or II with routine healing
F - subsequent encounter for open fracture type IIIA, IIIB, or IIIC with routine healing
G - subsequent encounter for closed fracture with delayed healing
H - subsequent encounter for open fracture type I or II with delayed healing
J - subsequent encounter for open fracture type IIIA, IIIB, or IIIC with delayed healing
K - subsequent encounter for closed fracture with nonunion
M - subsequent encounter for open fracture type I or II with nonunion
N - subsequent encounter for open fracture type IIIA, IIIB, or IIIC with nonunion
P - subsequent encounter for closed fracture with malunion
Q - subsequent encounter for open fracture type I or II with malunion
R - subsequent encounter for open fracture type IIIA, IIIB, or IIIC with malunion
S - sequela

FIGURE 23-6. Seventh character extension characters for category S72.

If a physician does not document the exact location of a fracture, *Coding Clinic for ICD-9-CM* (1999:1Q:p5)[1] says it is acceptable to review the entire recording including the radiology report to identify the exact location of the fracture. If there is any question as to the appropriate diagnosis, the physician should be queried before assigning a diagnosis code.

EXAMPLE

> The physician documents closed fracture right femur. The x-ray report indicates a fracture of the shaft of the right femur, S72.301A, X58.xxxA.

It is acceptable to use the more specific code S72.301A instead of S72.91xA as documented by the physician.

EXAMPLE

> The physician documents closed fracture right tibia. The x-ray report indicates a fracture through the shaft of the right tibia and fibula.
>   In this instance, the physician would need to be queried regarding the fracture of the fibula is assigned, S82.201A, S82.401A, X58.xxxA.

Specific coding guidelines assist with sequencing and coding of fractures. The most severe fracture is sequenced first. When a patient presents with multiple fractures, all fractures must be coded. It may be necessary to query the physician for more specific information.

A **pathologic fracture** is a break in a bone that occurs because of underlying disorders that weaken the bone, including malignancy, benign bone tumor, metabolic disorders, infection, and osteoporosis. A fracture can result from normal stress placed on an abnormal bone. Minor trauma can cause fracture. It is important to determine whether a fracture is pathologic or traumatic, so the appropriate code can be assigned. Coding of pathologic fractures is discussed in Chapter 19. Fractures that are due to a birth injury are classified as perinatal conditions.

Skull Fractures

Skull fracture may be associated with traumatic head injury. Injury to the brain may also occur. In most skull fractures, there is no displacement of broken bones. This is a closed or simple fracture. In severe cases, bone fragments are displaced, resulting in an open and/or depressed skull fracture. Fractures of the skull are frequently encountered after falls, crushing injuries, direct blows to the head, or motor vehicle accidents. A simple skull fracture may have little impact on eventual neurologic outcomes of head trauma. Neurological outcomes of a skull fracture are determined by the nature of the brain injury. Some trauma patients can have severe neurologic impairment without having a skull fracture. The cranium, which protects the brain, consists of eight bones: occipital, frontal, sphenoidal, ethmoidal, two parietal, and two temporal bones (Figure 23-7). There is an Instructional note at the beginning of category S02 to code also any associated intracranial injury (S06.-). The level of consciousness is identified within the S06.- codes. **Loss of consciousness** (LOC) occurs when a patient is unable to respond to people or to other stimuli. Unconsciousness and other sudden changes in mental status should be treated as a medical emergency.

EXAMPLE

> Fracture frontal skull bone due to motor vehicle accident involving head-on collision with pick-up truck, unbelted car passenger. The patient did not lose consciousness, S02.0xxA, V43.63xA, Y92.410.

Spine Fractures

As was discussed in Chapter 19, vertebral fractures are often pathologic fractures, particularly in older women with osteoporosis. This chapter focuses on traumatic spinal fractures, which usually occur as the result of motor vehicle accidents, falls, acts of violence, or

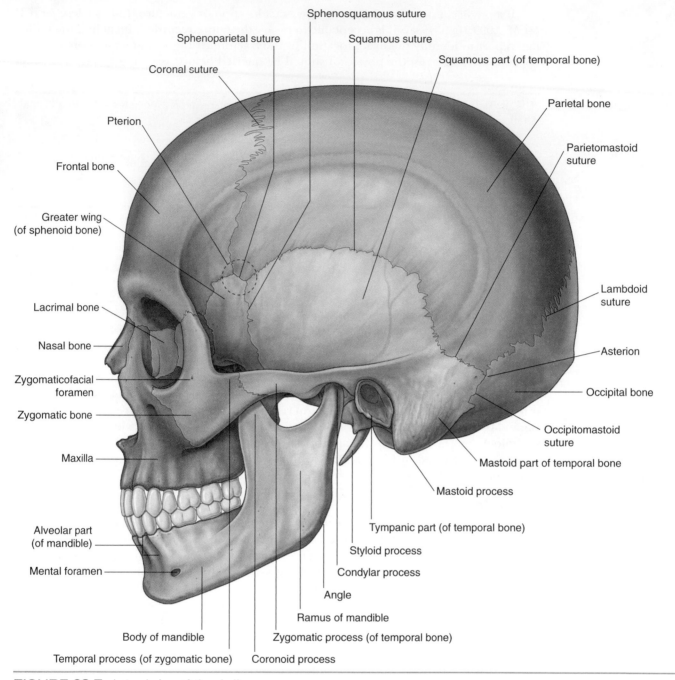

FIGURE 23-7. Lateral view of the skull.

recreational and sporting activities. Spinal fracture does not necessarily indicate damage to the spinal cord, and a spinal cord injury can occur without a spinal fracture (Figure 23-8).

EXAMPLE | Clay shoveler's fracture C7 (nondisplaced) due to strain injury from shoveling while working at construction site, S12.601A, Y93.h1, Y92.69, Y99.0.

Upper Limb Fractures

Shoulder and upper arm (Figure 23-9) injuries, including fractures of the clavicle or the upper part of the humerus, are fairly common. Fractures of the scapula are less common. A **Colles' fracture** is a common fracture in adults. In this type of fracture, the lower end of the radius is fractured, and the wrist and the hand are displaced backward. Fractures of the

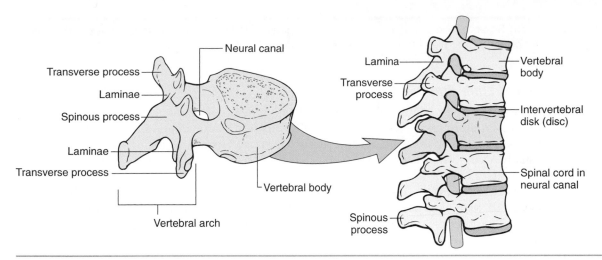

FIGURE 23-8. Lateral view of vertebrae.

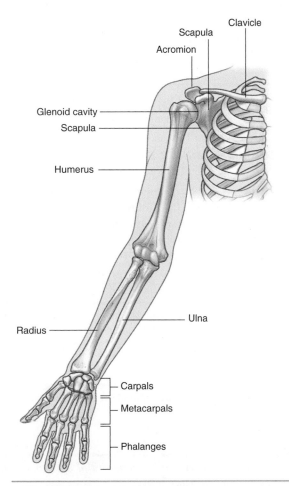

FIGURE 23-9. Bones of the upper limb.

ulna typically occur across the shaft or at the tip of the elbow. Sometimes, the radius is fractured at the same time. Fractures of the radius, which are among the most common of fractures, usually are caused by a fall on an outstretched hand. The disc-shaped head of the bone just below the elbow joint is one of the most common sites of fracture in young adults. Fingers often sustain lacerations, fractures, and tendon ruptures. Fractures are particularly common at the knuckles, usually in the little finger, as the result of a blow.

EXAMPLE | Right Boxers' fracture (neck of the fifth metacarpal) due to brawl at nightclub. The patient was employed at the nightclub as a bouncer, S62.336A, Y04.0xxA, Y99.0.

Lower Limb Fractures

A fractured hip is usually a fracture of the head or neck of the femur. The nature, symptoms, treatment, and possible complications of a fractured femur depend on whether the bone has been broken across its neck or across the shaft. A fracture in the shaft of the femur usually occurs when the femur is subjected to extreme force, as occurs in a motor vehicle accident.

In most cases, the bone ends are considerably displaced, causing severe pain, tenderness, and swelling. The patella is the triangular bone that protects the knee joint. Fracture is usually caused by a direct blow. The tibia is one of the most commonly fractured bones. It may break across the shaft as the result of a direct blow to the front of the leg, or at the upper end from a blow to the outside of the leg below the knee. The fibula, a very common site of fracture, usually breaks just above the ankle as the result of a harsh twisting motion, such as occurs in severe ankle sprain. Injury to the foot commonly results in fractures of the bones in the toes, caused by stubbing or twisting them or as the result of a falling or crushing injury. The calcaneus may fracture after a fall from a height onto a hard surface (Figures 23-10 and 23-11).

EXAMPLE | Left Dupuytren's fracture due to fall from horse while riding in meadow, S82.62xA, V80.010A, Y92.828, Y93.52, Y99.8.

Traumatic Fractures and Fracture Aftercare

Active treatment of a traumatic fracture includes surgery, an emergency room encounter, and/or evaluation and treatment by a new physician. According to the guidelines, when a patient is receiving active treatment, the acute fracture code is assigned.

Following the period of active treatment of a traumatic fracture, other encounters may be necessary. Aftercare may include a cast change or removal, removal of a fixation device, medication adjustments, and other follow-up visits. The fracture code is assigned with the appropriate 7th character extension for subsequent care encounters.

EXAMPLE | Patient is admitted for open reduction of right orbital floor fracture. Patient was involved in a fight at a bar last week, and this was the initial encounter for treatment, S02.3xxA, Y04.0xxA, Y92.29, 0NSP0ZZ.

EXAMPLE | Patient had a cast change for traumatic radial shaft fracture, S52.309D, 2W0CX2Z.

EXERCISE 23-5

Assign codes to the following conditions. Assume initial episode of care, unless otherwise specified. Do not assign external cause codes.

1. Type II Salter Harris fracture left fifth proximal phalanx of the hand _____

2. Nondisplaced right lateral malleolus fracture _____

3. Comminuted left calcaneal fracture _____

4. Open fracture distal right tibia and fibula _____

5. Avulsion fracture of the medial aspect of the left patella _____

6. LeFort I fracture _____

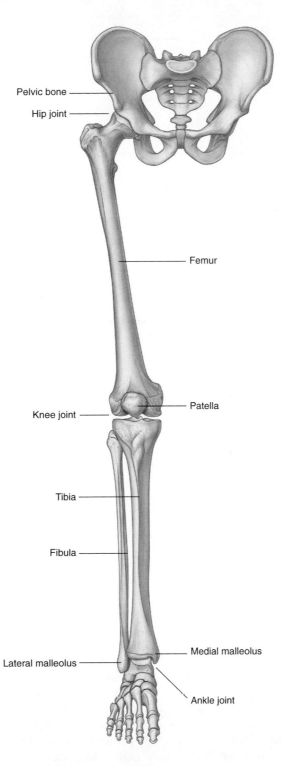

Pelvic bone

Hip joint

Femur

FIGURE 23-10. Bones and joints of the lower limb.

Patella

Knee joint

Tibia

Fibula

Medial malleolus

Lateral malleolus

Ankle joint

7. Fracture cervical spine C1 and C2 _____

8. Compound fracture midshaft of right femur _____

9. Fracture midshaft left clavicle _____

10. Temporal skull fracture with intracerebral hemorrhage _____

11. Patient was seen for removal of internal fixation device from previous right traumatic tibial fracture _____

12. Follow-up visit for traumatic pelvic fracture _____

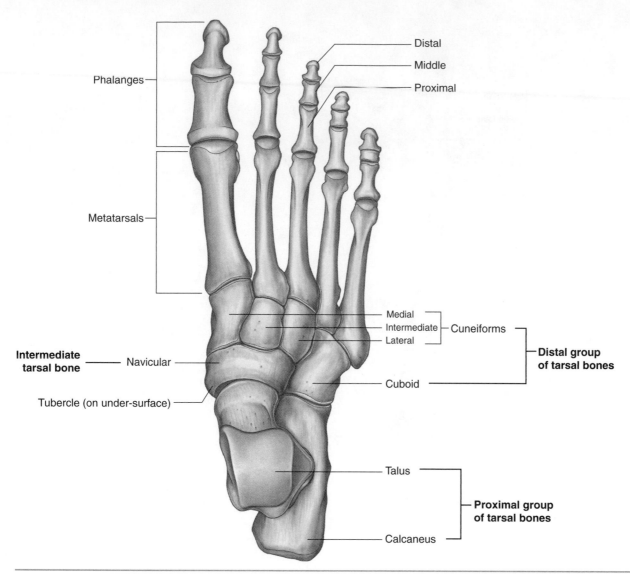

FIGURE 23-11. Dorsal view of right foot.

Dislocations

Dislocation is the displacement of the bones that form a joint. It is the separation of the end of a bone and the joint it meets. A partial or incomplete dislocation is called a **subluxation.** Dislocations may occur as the result of traumatic injury, or they may result from diseases such as rheumatoid arthritis, congenital joint defects, or weakened joints due to previous injury. The shoulder is especially prone to dislocation. The elbow is a common site of dislocation in toddlers. Other sites include fingers, hips, jaws, and spine. Soft tissues such as ligaments, tendons, muscles, and cartilage in and around the joint may stretch or tear as a result of the dislocation. Nerves and blood vessels may also be injured by the dislocated bone.

It is possible for a fracture and dislocation/subluxation to occur at the same anatomic site. In these instances, the index gives the coder instructions under the main term "Dislocation": It says, "with fracture—*see* Fracture" (Figure 23-12). This means that only the fracture code is assigned for fractures/dislocations at the same site. Reduction of fracture/dislocation is coded to reduction of fracture. No additional code is assigned for reduction of a dislocation.

> **Dislocation** (articular)
>   with fracture - *see* Fracture
>   acromioclavicular (joint) S43.10-
>   with displacement
>   100%-200% S43.12-
>   more than 200% S43.13-
>   inferior S43.14-
>   posterior S43.15-
>   ankle S93.0-

FIGURE 23-12. Instruction for dislocation with fracture—see Fracture.

Once a joint has been dislocated, it is not unusual for it to dislocate again; with each recurrence, less force is required to sustain a dislocation. Only the initial occurrence of the dislocation is coded with an injury code, and all subsequent dislocations of the same joint are coded as recurrent dislocations.

EXAMPLE

The patient sustained an open dislocation distal interphalageal joint right little finger during tackle on school football field during game, S63.296A, S61.206A, W03.xxxA, Y92.321, Y93.61, Y99.8.

EXERCISE 23-6

Assign codes to the following conditions. Assume initial episode of care, unless otherwise specified. Do not assign external cause codes.

1. Dislocation right patella   _____
2. Dislocation proximal interphalangeal joint left index finger   _____
3. Recurrent dislocation right shoulder   _____
4. Subluxation left elbow   _____

Sprains and Strains

A **sprain** is a stretch and/or tear of a ligament. The severity of the injury depends on whether a tear is partial or complete and on the number of ligaments involved. A **strain** is an injury to a muscle or a tendon. Depending on the severity of the injury, a strain may be the result of an overstretched muscle or tendon, or it can be caused by a partial or complete tear. Often, the patient is unaware of any specific injury. Strains can be acute or chronic. Chronic strains usually result from overuse or prolonged repetitive movement.

EXAMPLE

The patient has an anterior cruciate ligament sprain due to injury S83.519A, X58.xxxA.

EXERCISE 23-7

Assign codes to the following conditions. Assume initial episode of care, unless otherwise specified. Do not assign external cause codes.

1. Sprain left hand   _____
2. Strain lumbosacral spine   _____
3. Rupture of left Achilles tendon   _____
4. SLAP (superior labrum anterior-posterior) lesion on right   _____
    shoulder

Injury to Nerves/Spinal Cord and Blood Vessel

Spinal cord injury (SCI) is damage to the spinal cord that causes loss of sensation and motor control. The most common causes of SCI include MVAs, falls, acts of violence, and sporting accidents. SCIs tend to occur where the spine is most flexible, in the regions C5-C7 of the neck and T10-L2 at the base of the rib cage. If SCI is suspected, a computed tomography (CT) scan, magnetic resonance imaging (MRI), or a myelogram may be used as a diagnostic tool. Immediate medical treatment should focus on stabilizing the spine and providing aggressive treatment with corticosteroid drugs to limit damage. Surgery may also be necessary to stabilize the spine or fuse the spine with metal plates or pins. Once the initial injury heals, functional improvements may continue for at least 6 months. After this time, any remaining disability is likely to be permanent. Any nerve damage or injury should be coded, in addition to other injuries.

EXAMPLE Spinal cord injury at C2 level due to tackle during NFL football game, S14.102A, W03.xxxA, Y92.321, Y93.61, Y99.0.

Often, injuries to the blood vessels occur in conjunction with other injuries such as fractures, dislocations, open wounds, or lacerations. It is appropriate to assign codes that identify injury to the blood vessels, in addition to fractures and dislocations. Sequencing of codes according to Coding Guidelines depends on which is the primary injury.

EXAMPLE Injury to the thoracic aorta due to MVA involving collision with train. Patient was the driver of the car, S25.00xA, V45.5xxA, Y92.410.

EXERCISE 23-8

Assign codes to the following conditions. Assume initial episode of care, unless otherwise specified. Do not assign external cause codes.

1. Injury to ulnar nerve due to laceration left wrist _____
2. Radial nerve injury due to fracture of right humerus _____
3. Injury to sciatic nerve due to dislocation of left hip _____
4. Spinal cord injury T10 _____
5. Injury to abdominal aorta _____
6. Injury to internal left jugular _____
7. Rupture of right anterior tibial artery _____
8. Dislocation of left femoral neck. Minor damage to the left femoral artery was noted _____

Internal Injuries

Intracranial Injury, Excluding Those With Skull Fracture

A **concussion** is an injury to the brain that results from a significant blow to the head. Length of unconsciousness may relate to severity of the concussion (Figure 23-13). Most people recover with no ill effects. A patient may have to be admitted to the hospital for observation. It may be necessary to review the emergency room and ambulance records to determine the time that the patient was unconscious.

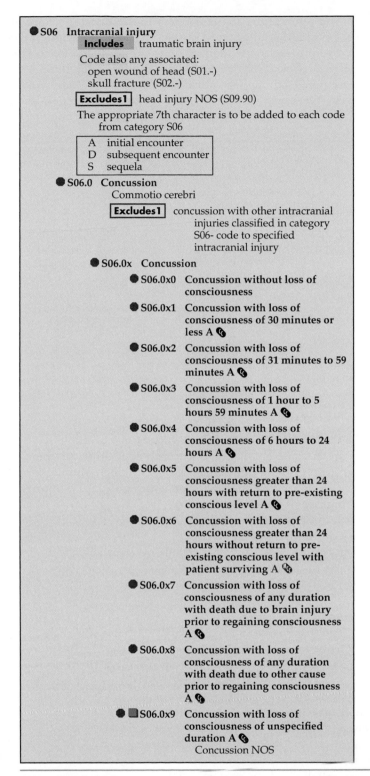

FIGURE 23-13. Concussion codes that include level of consciousness.

Traumatic brain injury (TBI) is injury to the brain that may affect the brain's normal functions. Penetrating injuries are injuries in which a foreign object such as a bullet enters the brain. Symptoms vary depending on the areas of the brain that are damaged.

Closed head injury (CHI) results from a blow to the head. Primary brain damage may occur at the time of the injury or accident. Secondary brain damage may result from complications of the injury such as brain swelling, increased intracranial pressure, seizure, infection, fever, hematoma, high or low blood pressure, anemia, and metabolic changes.

EXAMPLE	Patient was hospitalized with a concussion due to tripping while jumping rope at school. Unconscious for 5 minutes S06.0x1A, W01.0xxA, Y92.219, Y93.56, Y99.8.

EXERCISE 23-9

Assign codes to the following conditions. Assume initial episode of care, unless otherwise specified. Do not assign external cause codes.

1. Cerebral contusion due to fall. Positive for loss of consciousness _____

2. Laceration cerebral (left side) with loss of consciousness for 2 hours _____

3. Subdural hemorrhage due to fall 1 week ago _____

4. Subarachnoid hemorrhage without regaining consciousness. Patient died after 2 days _____

Internal Injury of Thorax, Abdomen, and Pelvis

Injury to the internal organs can occur with or without an open wound. Laceration of the spleen may result from blunt trauma without an open wound; injury to the spleen can occur from an open wound due to a gunshot. Types of internal injuries are as follows:

- Blast injuries of internal organs
- Blunt trauma of internal organs
- Bruise of internal organs
- Concussion injuries (except cerebral) of internal organs
- Crushing of internal organs
- Hematoma of internal organs
- Laceration of internal organs
- Puncture of internal organs
- Traumatic rupture of internal organs

The Organ Injury Scaling was developed by the Organ Injury Scaling Committee of the American Association for the Surgery of Trauma. This scale is graded from I through VI for each organ, with I being least severe and V the most severe injury from which the patient may survive. Grade VI injuries are by definition not salvageable. Scales are available for the following organ injuries:

- Thoracic vascular
- Lung
- Heart
- Chest wall
- Diaphragm
- Spleen
- Liver
- Abdominal vascular
- Kidney
- Ureter
- Bladder
- Urethra

TABLE 23-1 ORGAN INJURY SCALING—LIVER²

Grade	Injury Description	
I	Hematoma	Subscapular, <10% surface area
	Laceration	Capsular tear, <1 cm parenchymal depth
II	Hematoma	Subscapular, 10%-50% surface area
		Intraparenchymal, <10 cm diameter
	Laceration	1-3 cm parenchymal depth, <10 cm length
III	Hematoma	Subscapular, >50% surface area or expanding. Ruptured subscapular or parenchymal hematoma
		Intraparenchymal hematoma >10 cm or expanding
	Laceration	>3 cm parenchymal depth
IV	Laceration	Parenchymal disruption involving 25%-75% of hepatic lobe, or 1-3 Coinaud's segments in a single lobe
V	Laceration	Parenchymal disruption involving >75% of hepatic lobe or >3 Coinaud's segments within a single lobe
	Vascular	Juxtahepatic venous injuries (i.e., retrohepatic vena cava/central major hepatic veins)
VI	Vascular	Hepatic avulsion

Advance one grade for multiple injuries to same organ up to grade III.

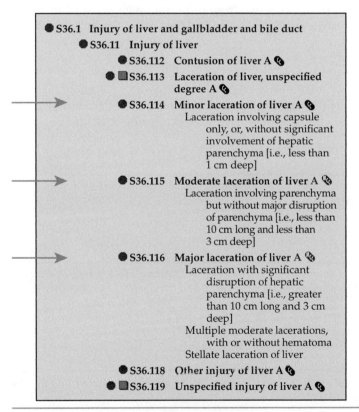

FIGURE 23-14. Types of liver laceration.

Table 23-1 shows the organ injury scale for liver injuries.

These scales can be helpful in coding internal injuries more accurately. They may also be useful for querying the physician about the extent of an internal injury. See Figure 23-14 for liver laceration codes that are specified as minor, moderate, and major.

EXAMPLE
Patient had laceration of right lung due to stab wound (laceration) right chest wall during fight at nightclub, S27.331A, S21.311A, X99.9xxA, Y92.29.

Assign codes to the following conditions. Assume initial episode of care, unless otherwise specified. Do not assign external cause codes.

1. Pneumothorax due to stab wound puncture of the right chest wall   _____

2. A superficial 5-cm laceration spleen due to blunt trauma   _____

3. Grade III laceration liver (involving parenchyma)   _____

4. Minor contusion of the left kidney   _____

5. Mediastinal hematoma due to trauma   _____

Crush Injuries and Amputations

A **crush injury** occurs when a body part is subjected to a high degree of force or pressure, usually after it has been squeezed between two heavy or immobile objects. A crush injury can be more serious than other types of injury such as a fracture or a laceration. In a severe crush, the force of the trauma can damage the underlying tissues, bones, blood vessels, and nerves. Increased pressure from tissue swelling can also damage muscles, blood vessels, and nerves. Instructions say to use additional codes to identify all associated injuries such as the following:

- ▪ Fractures
- ▪ Internal organs injury
- ▪ Intracranial injury

In the Tabular List there is an instructional note under the crush injury codes to "use additional code for any/all associated injuries."

EXAMPLE | Crush injury left foot with metatarsal fractures due to dropping car battery on foot at industrial factory, S97.82xA, S92.302A, W20.8xxA, Y92.63, Y99.0.

EXAMPLE | Employee sustained a crush injury right pointer finger with 3-cm laceration which happened while fixing combine on the farm, S67.190A, S61.210A W30.0xxA, Y92.79, Y99.0.

Assign codes to the following conditions. Assume initial episode of care, unless otherwise specified. Do not assign external cause codes.

1. Crush injury left fingers with fractures of distal phalanges   _____

2. Crush injury to abdomen with injury to bladder and pelvic fracture   _____

3. Crush injury right foot   _____

4. Crush injury left great toe   _____

5. Crush injury right ankle with 4-cm laceration   _____

6. Crush injury abdomen with minor injury to splenic artery   _____

7. Partial traumatic amputation right little toe   _____

Certain Early Complications of Trauma

A variety of complications may occur as the result of injury. An **air embolism** is formed when air or gas bubbles get into the bloodstream and obstruct the circulation. Trauma to the lungs can cause an air embolism, as may occur in divers from rapid changes of pressure.

A **fat embolism** can occur when fat enters the circulatory system after long bone or pelvic fracture. It usually presents 12 to 48 hours after the injury with symptoms such as tachycardia, tachypnea, elevated temperature, hypoxemia, hypocapnia, thrombocytopenia, and occasionally with mild neurologic symptoms. A petechial rash also appears on the upper portions of the body, including the chest, neck, upper arm, axilla, shoulder, oral mucous membranes, and conjunctivae. Infection, shock, anuria, and subcutaneous emphysema are other examples of complications of trauma.

EXAMPLE   Patient was hospitalized for treatment of an open traumatic fracture, right femur (shaft) and developed a fat embolism, S72.301B, T79.1xxA, X58.xxxA.

EXERCISE 23-12

Assign codes to the following conditions. Assume initial episode of care, unless otherwise specified. Do not assign external cause codes.

1. Pain due to twisting injury to left knee _____

2. Patient injured head _____

3. Shoulder injury _____

4. Injury to left hip _____

5. Subcutaneous emphysema due to pneumothorax from a stab wound into thorax _____

6. Infection due to second-degree burn on left thigh _____

7. Traumatic shock due to blunt intraabdominal injury _____

Effects of Foreign Body Entering Through Orifice

A foreign body (FB) can enter the body through natural openings or orifices such as eyes, ears, nose, and mouth. In some cases it may be necessary to seek emergency medical attention for possible removal. One of the most common sites that foreign bodies enter are the eyes. Young children and elderly patients, particularly those with neurologic disorders and/or decreased gag reflexes, are at risk for aspiration and food can become lodged in the esophagus.

EXAMPLE   Small piece of grass from mowing lawn at a single family house stuck on right cornea. Grass was removed, T15.01xA, Y92.017, 08C8XZZ.

EXERCISE 23-13

Assign codes to the following conditions. Assume initial episode of care, unless otherwise specified. Do not assign external cause codes.

1. Hot dog lodged in distal esophagus of patient with dysphagia. _____
   EGD with removal of hot dog

2. 1-year-old swallowed a penny, and x-rays showed that it was _____
   in the stomach

3. Child put sunflower seed in right nostril; removed with forceps _____

4. Patient with cough and hemoptysis was found to have a chicken bone lodged in right main stem bronchus of the lung; bronchoscopy with removal of chicken bone _____

5. Malodorous vaginal discharge due to retained tampon in vagina; manually removed _____

FACTORS INFLUENCING HEALTH STATUS AND CONTACT WITH HEALTH SERVICES (Z CODES)

As was discussed in Chapter 8, it may be difficult to locate Z codes in the index. Coders often say, "I did not know there was a Z code for that." Refer to Chapter 8 for a listing of common main terms used to locate Z codes.

Z codes that may be used with injuries include the following:

Z04.1	Encounter for examination and observation following transport accident
Z04.2	Encounter for examination and observation following work accident
Z04.3	Encounter for examination and observation following other accident
Z13.850	Encounter for screening for traumatic brain injury
Z18.10	Retained metal fragments, unspecified
Z18.11	Retained magnetic metal fragments
Z18.12	Retained nonmagnetic metal fragments
Z18.2	Retained plastic fragments
Z18.31	Retained animal quills or spines
Z18.32	Retained tooth
Z18.33	Retained wood fragments
Z18.39	Other retained organic fragments
Z18.81	Retained glass fragments
Z18.83	Retained stone or crystalline fragments
Z18.89	Other specified retained foreign body fragments
Z18.9	Retained foreign body fragments, unspecified material
Z42.8	Encounter for other plastic and reconstructive surgery following medical procedure or healed injury
Z48.00	Encounter for change or removal of nonsurgical wound dressing
Z48.02	Encounter for removal of sutures
Z87.81	Personal history of (healed) traumatic fracture
Z87.820	Personal history of traumatic brain injury
Z87.821	Personal history of retained foreign body fully removed
Z87.828	Personal history of other (healed) physical injury and trauma
Z91.81	History of falling

EXAMPLE   Patient was seen for suture removal from the left leg, Z48.02, 8EOYXY8.

Admission for Observation Following an Injury

According to the Guidelines, the observation codes should only be used in very limited circumstances, such as when a person is being observed for a suspected condition that is ruled out. The observation codes are not for use if an injury or illness or any signs or symptoms related to the suspected condition are present. In such cases the diagnosis/symptom code is used with the corresponding external cause code. If a patient has minor cuts, bruises, or other superficial injuries, these are coded as secondary diagnoses and the appropriate observation code as the principal.

This Z04.– code category is used for patients who are suspected of having an abnormal condition without a sign or a symptom that requires study. After examination and observation, no condition is determined to exist.

EXAMPLE

Patient has a minor contusion of the right chest wall and is admitted for observation to rule out a concussion. Patient was the driver of a motor vehicle that lost control while taking a curve on a state road and collided with a tree. Patient was discharged when they were able to rule out any type of head injury. Z04.1, S20.211A, V47.52xA, Y92.413.

EXERCISE 23-14

Assign codes to the following conditions. Assume initial episode of care, unless otherwise specified. Do not assign external cause codes.

1. Observation following work accident _____

2. Previous right knee joint replacement _____

3. Observation after MVA for internal abdominal injuries. Internal injuries were ruled out, and patient was discharged with a diagnosis of contusion abdominal wall _____

4. Encounter for removal of screw used to stabilize left tibial fracture; fracture is well healed, and no complications of the fixation device or infections are reported _____

5. Patient had a previous amputation of the left great toe _____

COMMON TREATMENTS

Many injuries are diagnosed with the use of imaging procedures such as x-ray, MRI, CT scans, and ultrasound. Treatment depends on the severity of the injury. For very severe injuries, patients may have to be transferred to hospitals that specialize in the care of trauma patients. Surgical intervention may also be required to repair the specific injury or trauma. Pain medications, anti-inflammatories, corticosteroids, and antibiotics may be necessary to alleviate pain and inflammation and to prevent or fight infection.

PROCEDURES

Procedures related to injuries in ICD-10-PCS can be located in many tables depending on the procedure performed and the body system involved.

Fracture Treatment

A fracture is classified as "open" or "closed." Treatments for fracture are also classified as "open" or "closed," and the coder should not confuse the type of fracture with the type of procedure. An open fracture may not require open treatment, and a closed fracture may need open reduction. The root operation for reduction of a fracture is reposition. The treatment provided will depend on other injuries and the type and location of the fracture. Reduction or manipulation of bone fragments to their proper anatomic position is necessary for appropriate healing. The root operation for reduction of a fracture is reposition (moving to its normal location or other suitable location some or all of a body part). For fractures that are not displaced, stabilization or immobilization may be all that is necessary to promote healing.

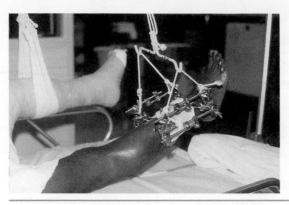

FIGURE 23-15. Example of an external fixation service on the right leg. The left is in a splint.

Reductions may be performed in the operating room or other areas of the hospital, such as the emergency room, fracture treatment room, and/or in radiology.

Closed reduction of a fracture occurs when the surgeon manipulates or reduces fractured bones into anatomic alignment without making an incision through the skin and subcutaneous tissue. The approach for a closed reduction without internal fixation is external. Closed reduction may include internal fixation. Small incision(s) may be made for placement of internal fixation device(s) such as pins, wires, screws, plates, and intramedullary nails. As long as the fracture is not exposed, it is considered a percutaneous fixation. Fixation devices are used to immobilize the fracture, but they do not manipulate or reduce the fracture. Sometimes radiologic guidance is needed for placement of the fixation device(s). It is also possible for a closed reduction to be performed prior to having an open reduction and fixation.

Open reduction of a fracture occurs when the surgeon makes an incision at the fracture site to reduce or manipulate the fracture into anatomic position. Open reduction and internal fixation (ORIF) is a procedure that is very commonly performed for fractures.

External skeletal fixation is another form of fracture treatment (Figure 23-15). This involves insertion of percutaneous pins proximal and distal to the fracture and application of a frame that connects the pins externally. The pins are located internally, except for the portion to which the frame is connected. The frame is located outside the body. These devices can be used to hold a reduced fracture or to assist the surgeon in reducing a fracture.

Repair of Lacerations

Suture is a method used to close cutaneous lacerations. The root operation for suture of skin and subcutaneous tissue is repair (restoring a body part to its normal structure to the extent possible). The risks of bleeding and infection are reduced by approximating skin edges for an aesthetically pleasing and functional result. Routine debridement of wound edges prior to suturing of the wound is considered part of the suturing and should not be coded separately.

Sometimes, a combination of adhesive and sutures is used for wound repair.

EXAMPLE

Laceration left wrist due to suicidal attempt with razor. Laceration was repaired, S61.512A, X78.8xxA, 0HQEXZZ. No place of occurrence was given, so no External cause code is assigned, per guidelines.

EXAMPLE

Laceration nose due to being hit in nose by surfboard while at beach. Laceration of the skin was repaired, S01.21xA, W21.89xA, Y92.832, Y99.8, 0HQ1XZZ.

EXERCISE 23-15

Assign codes for all diagnoses and procedures. Assume initial episode of care, unless otherwise specified. Do not assign external cause codes.

1. Laceration to spleen with parenchymal disruption with total splenectomy _____

2. Coco Puff in left ear (auditory canal); removed by physician _____

3. Closed reduction and percutaneous fixation of left supracondylar fracture elbow _____

4. Manipulation of right shoulder dislocation _____

5. Suture deep laceration of the right hand _____

6. Suture of laceration of the left eyelid _____

7. Open reduction and internal fixation of left hip fracture (traumatic) _____

8. Open manipulation and internal fixation of left acetabular fracture _____

9. Healing traumatic fracture right tibia/fibula with application of short leg cast _____

10. Closed reduction and percutaneous internal fixation of right Bennett's fracture _____

DOCUMENTATION/REIMBURSEMENT/MS-DRGs

Often coding difficulties are due to lack of documentation. Sometimes radiology and other test results are not available at the time of discharge or when the physician is dictating the discharge summary or is reporting the final diagnoses. Documentation may be lacking for how and where an injury happened, so it is difficult to assign appropriate External cause codes.

Identification and accurate coding of all procedures and diagnoses may be instrumental in MS-DRG assignment. It is also important to code associated chronic conditions that may qualify as comorbid conditions. A thorough review of the record is necessary to identify complications that may occur during the stay. In cases of injury, it is very important to pick up all associated procedures. Often, in trauma cases, surgeons are busy trying to save the life of the patient, and documentation is not their top priority. The record should be reviewed for suturing of arteries or lacerations of internal organs, mechanical ventilation, and debridements. Sometimes, in the repair of fractures resulting from trauma, joint replacement may be necessary.

It is difficult to pinpoint any particular codes that may be frequently missed complications/comorbidities from this chapter. There are numerous injury codes on the CC/MCC listing. It is important to code all injuries with the most serious injury as the principal diagnosis.

Correct Orthopedic Procedure Code

EXAMPLE An elderly patient falls and fractures right hip (femoral neck) and undergoes ORIF procedure. An error is made in assigning or entering the procedure code in the second case.

DIAGNOSES	CODES	MS-DRG	RW
Fracture hip	S72.001A, W19.xxxA	482	1.5498
ORIF	0QS604Z		
Fracture hip	S72.001A, W19.xxxA	536	0.7256
Closed reduction without fixation	0QS6XZZ		

Two Diagnoses That Equally Meet the Definition for Principal Diagnosis

EXAMPLE   A patient is admitted with a skull fracture and a right hip fracture. Designation of the principal diagnosis can make a difference in reimbursement. In this case, it may be necessary to query the physician as to which injury is the most serious. If a procedure was performed, that may also help the coder to determine which diagnosis is principal.

DIAGNOSES	CODES	MS-DRG	RW
Fracture hip and skull	S72.001A, S02.91xA, X58.xxxA	536	0.7256
Fracture skull and hip	S02.91xA, S72.001A, X58.xxxA	085	2.1483

Coding Specificity and MS-DRG With and Without MCC/CC

EXAMPLE   Patient is admitted with fractured rib. X-ray report reveals fractures of the right fifth and sixth ribs. No procedures were performed. Patient was also treated for a urinary tract infection.

DIAGNOSES	CODES	MS-DRG	RW
Rib fractures, UTI	S22.31xA, N39.0, X58.xxxA	206	0.7565
Rib fracture, 4 ribs, UTI	S22.41xA, N39.0, X58.xxxA	184	1.0086

In this example, reimbursement is affected by the more specific fracture code, which indicates that two ribs were fractured, and by the assignment of the UTI code (N39.0), which is a CC for MS-DRG 184.

CHAPTER REVIEW EXERCISE

Assign codes for all diagnoses and procedures. Assume initial episode of care, unless otherwise specified. Do not assign external cause codes.

1. Fracture/dislocation right femur with contusion right hip _____

2. Closed reduction of recurrent left shoulder dislocation _____

3. Inversion injury right ankle with severe sprain _____

4. Grade III laceration to the bladder due to gunshot wound (abdominal wall). Exploratory laparotomy with repair of the bladder laceration. _____

5. Crush injury with fracture of the right hand (multiple metacarpals) _____

6. Wound left calf due to dog bite. Wound was cleansed and Steri-Strips applied _____

7. Closed head injury with concussion and brief loss of consciousness (10 minutes) _____

8. Pain caused by anterior dislocation of left shoulder _____

9. Tear of right ulnar collateral ligament of the left thumb–metacarpophalangeal joint _____

10. Sprain right foot _____

11. Crush injury with laceration of left foot _____

12. Hemiarthroplasty due to displaced right femoral neck fracture (traumatic) _____

13. Rib fractures on the left due to child abuse by foster mother   _____

14. Open fractures of left tibial shaft with the fibula. Laceration calf,   _____
which exposes the tibia

15. Flail chest   _____

16. Lacerations of right upper arm with embedded gravel. Skin and   _____
subcutaneous tissue were repaired with sutures

17. Contusions chest and forehead with 2-cm laceration of forehead.   _____
Skin on forehead was sutured

18. Bilateral fractures of the radius. Right upper end and left distal   _____
end. Closed reductions bilaterally

19. Dislocation of left little finger. This is the third time the patient   _____
has dislocated this finger. Closed reduction was performed

20. Intertrochanteric fracture left hip with ORIF   _____

21. Fracture temporal bone   _____

22. Injury to right eye   _____

23. Hangman's fracture (C2)   _____

24. Laceration scalp repaired with staples   _____

25. Fracture of L3 (traumatic)   _____

26. Closed head injury with brain contusion and LOC   _____

27. Subdural hematoma with brief loss of consciousness. Hematoma   _____
was evacuated in the OR through burr hole

28. Peroneal nerve injury due to left fibular fracture (shaft)   _____

29. Shattered C1-C2 vertebra with spinal cord injury   _____

Write the correct answer(s) in the space(s) provided.

30. Define open fracture. _____

CHAPTER GLOSSARY   **Air embolism:** when air or gas bubbles get into the bloodstream and obstruct the circulation.

Closed fracture: injury in which the bone is broken, but the skin remains intact.

Closed head injury: injury that results from a blow to the head.

Closed reduction: the surgeon manipulates or reduces fractured bones into anatomic alignment without making an incision through the skin and subcutaneous tissue.

Colles' fracture: common fracture in adults in which the lower end of the radius is fractured and the wrist and hand are displaced backward.

Complicated fracture: fracture that causes injury to surrounding tissues.

Compound fracture: when the broken bone exits and is visible through the skin, or a deep wound exposes the broken bone through the skin.

Concussion: injury to the brain that results from a significant blow to the head.

Contusion: any mechanical injury that results in hemorrhage beneath unbroken skin.

Crush injury: when a body part is subjected to a high degree of force or pressure, usually after it has been squeezed between two heavy or immobile objects.

Dislocation: displacement of the bones that form a joint; separation of the end of a bone from the joint it meets.

External skeletal fixation: form of fracture treatment that involves insertion of percutaneous pins proximal and distal to the fracture and application of a frame that connects the pins externally.

Fat embolism: when fat enters the circulatory system after long bone or pelvic fracture.

Fracture: break in a bone.

Gustilo open fracture classification: based on the mechanism of the injury and the amount of soft tissue and skeletal injury and is useful in assessing risk of infection and possible amputation.

Laceration: an injury that results in a tear in the skin.

Loss of consciousness: when a patient is unable to respond to people or other stimuli.

Open fracture: when the broken bone exits and is visible through the skin, or a deep wound exposes the broken bone through the skin.

Open reduction: when the surgeon makes an incision at the fracture site to reduce or manipulate the fracture into anatomic position.

Pathologic fracture: break in a bone that occurs because of underlying disorders that weaken the bone, including malignancy, benign bone tumor, metabolic disorder, infection, and osteoporosis.

Simple fracture: injury in which the bone is broken, but the skin remains intact.

Spinal cord injury: damage to the spinal cord that causes loss of sensation and motor control.

Sprain: stretch and/or tear of a ligament.

Strain: injury to a muscle or a tendon.

Subluxation: partial or incomplete dislocation.

Suture: method for closing cutaneous wounds.

Traumatic brain injury: injury to the brain that may result in interference with the brain's normal functions.

REFERENCES

1. American Hospital Association. *Coding Clinic for ICD-9-CM* 1999:1Q:p5. Fracture site specified in radiology report.
2. From American Association for the Surgery of Trauma, Chicago, Illinois.
3. American Hospital Association. *Coding Clinic for ICD-9-CM* 1987:M-A:p1-5. Observation and evaluation for suspected conditions—Guidelines.

24

Burns, Adverse Effects, and Poisonings

(ICD-10-CM Chapters 19 and 20, Codes S00-Y99)

CHAPTER OUTLINE

ICD-10-CM Official Guidelines for Coding and Reporting

Major Differences Between ICD-10-CM and ICD-9-CM

Anatomy and Physiology

Disease Conditions

    Burns and Corrosions (T20-T32) and Frostbite (T33-T34)

    Poisoning by, Adverse Effect of, and Underdosing of Drugs, Medicaments, and Biological Substances (T36-T50)

    Toxic Effects of Substances Chiefly Nonmedicinal as to Source (T51-T65)

    Other and Unspecified Effects of External Causes (T66-T78)

    Late Effects of Injuries, Poisonings, Toxic Effects, and Other External Causes

Factors Influencing Health Status and Contact With Health Services (Z Codes)

Common Treatments

Procedures

    Debridement

    Hyperbaric Oxygen Therapy

Documentation/Reimbursement/MS-DRGs

    Correct Procedure Code

    Adverse Effect versus Poisoning

Chapter Review Exercise

Chapter Glossary

LEARNING OBJECTIVES

1. Apply and assign the correct ICD-10-CM/PCS codes in accordance with Official Guidelines for Coding and Reporting

2. Identify major differences between ICD-10-CM and ICD-9-CM related to burns, adverse effects, and poisonings

3. Identify the various types of burns

4. Differentiate between an adverse effect and a poisoning

5. Assign the correct Z codes, External cause codes, and procedure codes related to burns, adverse effects, and poisonings

6. Identify common treatments

7. Explain the importance of documentation in relation to MS-DRGs for reimbursement

ABBREVIATIONS/ ACRONYMS

AKA above-knee amputation

CC complication/comorbidity

CHF congestive heart failure

COPD chronic obstructive pulmonary disease

HBOT Hyperbaric oxygen therapy

ICD-9-CM *International Classification of Diseases, 9th Revision, Clinical Modification*

ICD-10-CM *International Classification of Diseases, 10th Revision, Clinical Modification*

ICD-10-PCS *International Classification of Diseases, 10th*

ABBREVIATIONS/ ACRONYMS—*cont'd*

Revision, Procedure Coding System

MS-DRG Medicare Severity diagnosis-related group

MVA motor vehicle accident
OR Operating Room

SIRS systemic inflammatory response syndrome
UTI urinary tract infection

ICD-10-CM

Official Guidelines for Coding and Reporting

Please refer to the companion Evolve website for the most current guidelines.

19. Chapter 19: Injury, poisoning, and certain other consequences of external causes (S00-T88)

    d. Coding of Burns and Corrosions

        The ICD-10-CM **makes a distinction** between burns and corrosions. The burn codes are for thermal burns, except sunburns, that come from a heat source, such as a fire or hot appliance. The burn codes are also for burns resulting from electricity and radiation. Corrosions are burns due to chemicals. The guidelines are the same for burns and corrosions.

        Current burns (T20-T25) are classified by depth, extent and by agent (X code). Burns are classified by depth as first degree (erythema), second degree (blistering), and third degree (full-thickness involvement). Burns of the eye and internal organs (T26-T28) are classified by site, but not by degree.

        1) Sequencing of burn and related condition codes

            Sequence first the code that reflects the highest degree of burn when more than one burn is present.

            a. When the reason for the admission or encounter is for treatment of external multiple burns, sequence first the code that reflects the burn of the highest degree.

            b. When a patient has both internal and external burns, the circumstances of admission govern the selection of the principal diagnosis or first-listed diagnosis.

            c. When a patient is admitted for burn injuries and other related conditions such as smoke inhalation and/or respiratory failure, the circumstances of admission govern the selection of the principal or first-listed diagnosis.

EXAMPLE

Second-degree burns of the left hand and first-degree burns of the left forearm, T23.202A, T22.112A.

        2) Burns of the same local site

            Classify burns of the same local site (three-**character** category level, T20-T28) but of different degrees to the subcategory identifying the highest degree recorded in the diagnosis.

EXAMPLE

Second- and third-degree burns of the right thigh, T24.311A.

        3) Non-healing burns

            Non-healing burns are coded as acute burns.

            Necrosis of burned skin should be coded as a non-healed burn.

EXAMPLE

Active treatment for necrosis of third-degree burn on the buttock, T21.35xA.

        4) Infected Burn

            For any documented infected burn site, use an additional code for the infection.

EXAMPLE Active treatment of infected burn right foot, T25.021A, T79.8xxA, L08.9.

5) Assign separate codes for each burn site
When coding burns, assign separate codes for each burn site. Category T30, Burn and corrosion, body region unspecified is extremely vague and should rarely be used.

EXAMPLE Multiple burns over the entire body. The patient expired before he could be admitted, T30.0.

6) Burns and Corrosions Classified According to Extent of Body Surface Involved
Assign codes from category T31, Burns classified according to extent of body surface involved, or T32, Corrosions classified according to extent of body surface involved, when the site of the burn is not specified or when there is a need for additional data. It is advisable to use category T31 as additional coding when needed to provide data for evaluating burn mortality, such as that needed by burn units. It is also advisable to use category T31 as an additional code for reporting purposes when there is mention of a third-degree burn involving 20 percent or more of the body surface.

Categories T31 and T32 are based on the classic "rule of nines" in estimating body surface involved: head and neck are assigned nine percent, each arm nine percent, each leg 18 percent, the anterior trunk 18 percent, posterior trunk 18 percent, and genitalia one percent. Providers may change these percentage assignments where necessary to accommodate infants and children who have proportionately larger heads than adults, and patients who have large buttocks, thighs, or abdomen that involve burns.

EXAMPLE The patient has second-degree (3%) and third-degree (5%) burns of the trunk and first-degree burns (2%) of the right arm, T21.30xA, T22.10xA, T31.10.

7) Encounters for treatment of *sequela* of burns
Encounters for the treatment of the late effects of burns or corrosions (i.e., scars or joint contractures) should be coded with a burn or corrosion code with the 7th character "S" **for** sequela.

8) Sequelae with a late effect code and current burn
When appropriate, both a code for a current burn or corrosion with 7th character "A" or "D" and a burn or corrosion code with **7th character** "S" may be assigned on the same record (when both a current burn and sequelae of an old burn exist). Burns and corrosions do not heal at the same rate and a current healing wound may still exist with sequela of a healed burn or corrosion.

EXAMPLE Contracture of the skin of the right index finger due to burn from fire injury 6 months ago, L90.5, T23.021S.

9) Use of an external cause code with burns and corrosions
An external cause code should be used with burns and corrosions to identify the source and intent of the burn, as well as the place where it occurred.

e. Adverse Effects, Poisoning, Underdosing and Toxic Effects

Codes in categories T36-T65 are combination codes that include the substance **that was taken** as well as the **intent**. No additional external cause code is required for poisonings, toxic effects, adverse effects and underdosing codes.

A code from categories T36-T65 is sequenced first, followed by the code(s) that specify the nature of the adverse effect, poisoning, or toxic effect. Note: This sequencing instruction does not apply to underdosing codes (fifth or sixth character "6", for example T36.0x6-).

1) Do not code directly from the Table of Drugs

Do not code directly from the Table of Drugs and Chemicals. Always refer back to the Tabular List.

2) Use as many codes as necessary to describe

Use as many codes as necessary to describe completely all drugs, medicinal or biological substances.

3) If the same code would describe the causative agent

If the same code would describe the causative agent for more than one adverse reaction, poisoning, toxic effect or underdosing, assign the code only once.

4) If two or more drugs, medicinal or biological substances

If two or more drugs, medicinal or biological substances are reported, code each individually unless **a** combination code is listed in the Table of Drugs and Chemicals.

5) The occurrence of drug toxicity is classified in ICD-10-CM as follows:

(a) Adverse Effect

When coding an adverse effect of a drug that has been correctly prescribed and properly administered, assign the appropriate code for **the nature of the adverse effect followed by the appropriate code for the** adverse effect **of the drug** (T36-T50). **The code for the drug should have a 5th or 6th character "5" (for example T36.0X5-)** Examples of **the nature of an adverse effect** are tachycardia, delirium, gastrointestinal hemorrhaging, vomiting, hypokalemia, hepatitis, renal failure, or respiratory failure.

EXAMPLE Patient was treated for epistaxis which is likely due to the patient's long term use of Coumadin for atrial fibrillation. Patient was taking the Coumadin as prescribed, R04.0, T45.515A, I48.91, Z79.01.

EXAMPLE Hypokalemia due to Lasix therapy for congestive heart failure, E87.6, T50.1x5A, I50.9.

(b) Poisoning

When coding a poisoning or reaction to the improper use of a medication (e.g., overdose, wrong substance given or taken in error, wrong route of administration), **first** assign the appropriate code from categories T36-T50. **The p**oisoning codes have an associated intent **as their 5th or 6th character (**accidental, intentional self-harm, assault and undetermined. Use additional code(s) for all manifestations of poisonings.

If there is also a diagnosis of abuse or dependence **of** the substance, the abuse or dependence is **assigned** as an additional code.

EXAMPLE Chest pain due to accidental poisoning from cocaine. The patient uses cocaine on a daily basis, T40.5x1A, R07.9, F14.10.

Examples of poisoning include:

(i) Error was made in drug prescription

Errors made in drug prescription or in the administration of the drug by provider, nurse, patient, or other person.

<table>
<tr><td>EXAMPLE</td><td>While in the hospital, the nurse accidentally gave the patient 40 mg of Lasix instead of the ordered 20-mg dosage. The patient suffered no ill effects, T50.1x1A, Y92.230.</td></tr>
</table>

(ii) Overdose of a drug intentionally taken
If an overdose of a drug was intentionally taken or administered and resulted in drug toxicity, it would be coded as a poisoning.

<table>
<tr><td>EXAMPLE</td><td>The patient intentionally overdosed with 20 Valium tablets. The patient is in a coma, T42.4x2A, R40.20.</td></tr>
</table>

(iii) Nonprescribed drug taken with correctly prescribed and properly administered drug
If a nonprescribed drug or medicinal agent was taken in combination with a correctly prescribed and properly administered drug, any drug toxicity or other reaction resulting from the interaction of the two drugs would be classified as a poisoning.

(iv) Interaction of drug(s) and alcohol
When a reaction results from the interaction of a drug(s) and alcohol, this would be classified as poisoning.
See Section I.C.4. if poisoning is the result of insulin pump malfunctions.

<table>
<tr><td>EXAMPLE</td><td>A patient combined prescription Percodan with beer and became stuporous and drowsy, T40.2x1A, T51.0x1A, R40.1, R40.0.</td></tr>
</table>

(c) Underdosing
Underdosing refers to taking less of a medication than is prescribed by a provider or a manufacturer's instruction. For underdosing, assign the code from categories T36-T50 (fifth or sixth character "6").

Codes for underdosing should never be assigned as principal or first-listed codes. If a patient has a relapse or exacerbation of the medical condition for which the drug is prescribed because of the reduction in dose, then the medical condition itself should be coded.

Noncompliance (Z91.12-, Z91.13-) or complication of care (Y63.61, Y63.8-Y63.9) codes are to be used with an underdosing code to indicate intent, if known.

<table>
<tr><td>EXAMPLE</td><td>Patient was admitted to the hospital with an exacerbation of asthma. Patient has not been using Flovent inhaler on a daily basis as prescribed due to financial issues, J45.901, T49.1x6A, Z91.120.</td></tr>
</table>

(d) Toxic Effects
When a harmful substance is ingested or comes in contact with a person, this is classified as a toxic effect. The toxic effect codes are in categories T51-T65.

Toxic effect codes have an associated intent: accidental, intentional self-harm, assault and undetermined.

EXAMPLE   A 2-year-old accidentally drank lye, causing burns to the mouth and throat, T54.3x1A, T28.5xxA.

f. Adult and child abuse, neglect and other maltreatment

Sequence first the appropriate code from categories T74.- (Adult and child abuse, neglect and other maltreatment, confirmed) or T76.- (Adult and child abuse, neglect and other maltreatment, suspected) for abuse, neglect and other maltreatment, followed by any accompanying mental health or injury code(s).

If the documentation in the medical record states abuse or neglect it is coded as confirmed (T74.-). It is coded as suspected if it is documented as suspected (T76.-).

For cases of confirmed abuse or neglect an external cause code from the assault section (X92-Y08) should be added to identify the cause of any physical injuries. A perpetrator code (Y07) should be added when the perpetrator of the abuse is known. For suspected cases of abuse or neglect, do not report external cause or perpetrator code.

If a suspected case of abuse, neglect or mistreatment is ruled out during an encounter code Z04.71, **Encounter for examination and observation following alleged physical adult abuse,** ruled out, or code Z04.72, **Encounter for examination and observation following alleged child physical abuse,** ruled out, should be used, not a code from T76.

If a suspected case of alleged rape or sexual abuse is ruled out during an encounter code Z04.41, Encounter for examination and observation following alleged physical adult abuse, ruled out, or code Z04.42, Encounter for examination and observation following alleged rape or sexual abuse, ruled out, should be used, not a code from T76.

See Section I.C.15. Abuse in a pregnant patient.

EXAMPLE   A wife was seen with head and face injuries due to spousal abuse. The patient had been struck repeatedly in the face and head, T74.11xA, S09.93xA, S09.90xA, Y04.2xxA, Y07.01.

20. Chapter 20: External Causes of Morbidity (V01-Y99)

g. Child and Adult Abuse Guideline

Adult and child abuse, neglect and maltreatment are classified as assault. Any of the assault codes may be used to indicate the external cause of any injury resulting from the confirmed abuse.

For confirmed cases of abuse, neglect and maltreatment, when the perpetrator is known, a code from Y07, Perpetrator of maltreatment and neglect, should accompany any other assault codes.

See Section I.C.19. Adult and child abuse, neglect and other maltreatment

Apply the General Coding Guidelines as found in Chapter 5 and the Procedural Coding Guidelines as found in Chapters 6 and 7.

At the beginning of Chapter 19 in the ICD-10-CM code book, special instructions say, "Use secondary code(s) from Chapter 20 to indicate cause of injury" (Figure 24-1).

CHAPTER 19

INJURY, POISONING AND CERTAIN OTHER CONSEQUENCES OF EXTERNAL CAUSES (S00-T88)

Note: Use secondary code(s) from Chapter 20, External causes of morbidity, to indicate cause of injury. Codes within the T section that include the external cause do not require an additional external cause code.

Use additional code to identify any retained foreign body, if applicable (Z18.-)

Excludes1 birth trauma (P10-P15)
obstetric trauma (O70-O71)

FIGURE 24-1. Instructional note regarding the use of External cause code(s).

MAJOR DIFFERENCES BETWEEN ICD-10-CM AND ICD-9-CM

- In ICD-10-CM, there are specific codes for corrosive burns, which are burns due to a chemical. A code to identify the chemical and intent is sequenced before the corrosive burn code.
- ICD-10-CM does not have a code to identify posttraumatic wound infection. An infected burn site is coded with an additional code for the infection.
- Late effects for burns are coded differently in ICD-10-CM. The burn code is assigned with the seventh character *S,* for *sequela.* A code to identify the sequela is also assigned (e.g., contracture, scar, etc.).
- In ICD-10-CM, there are combination codes (T36-T65) that include the substances related to adverse effects, poisonings, toxic effects, and underdosing as well as the external cause. So no additional external cause code is necessary. In ICD-9-CM, E codes were assigned as additional codes to show the cause. In ICD-10-CM, the same code is used for adverse effects and poisonings to identify the substance. The fifth and sixth digits identify the circumstances, and the seventh digit identifies the encounter as initial, subsequent, or for treatment of sequelae.
- ICD-10-CM codes can be used to identify underdosing, taking less of a medication than is prescribed or less than the manufacturer's instructions, with a negative effect on health. A code for noncompliance or failure in dosage during surgical or medical care should also be assigned.
- The dummy placeholder or letter *x* is used in some codes in this chapter along with a seventh character.

ANATOMY AND PHYSIOLOGY

All areas of the body may be involved in an injury. These are outlined in their respective body system chapters.

DISEASE CONDITIONS

Injury, Poisoning, and Certain Other Consequences of External Causes (S00-T88), Chapter 19 in the ICD-10-CM code book, is divided into the following categories:

CATEGORY	SECTION TITLES
T20-T32	Burns and corrosions
T33-T34	Frostbite
T36-T50	Poisoning by, adverse effect of, and underdosing of drugs, medicaments, and biological substances
T51-T65	Toxic effects of substances chiefly nonmedicinal as to source
T66-T78	Other and unspecified effects of external causes

Burns and Corrosions (T20-T32) and Frostbite (T33-T34)

It may be necessary to transport burn victims to a hospital that has a specialized unit for care of the burn patient. Plastic surgeons, anesthesiologists, nurses, dietitians, and physical and occupational therapists assist the burn patient through the acute and recovery phases of their injury. As a result, many facilities only stabilize the burn patient in the emergency room and then transport to a burn unit, or only less critical burn patients are admitted for care.

According to the ICD-10-CM guidelines, the burn codes are assigned for thermal burns, except for sunburns, that come from a heat source such as a fire or hot appliance. **Corrosion** is a burn that is due to a chemical. The guidelines are the same for both types of burns. As with other injuries, it is necessary to assign separate codes for each burn site. Codes are

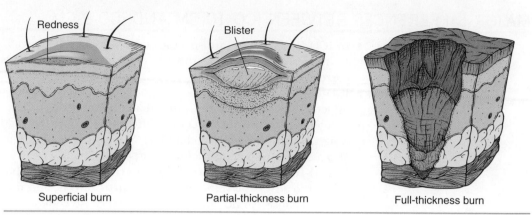

FIGURE 24-2. Depths of burns.

available for multiple sites, but these should be used only if the documentation is insufficient to allow assignment of more specific burn codes.

Burn severity is classified by degrees (Figure 24-2):

- First-degree burn: **erythema** or redness of the skin
- Second-degree burn: formation of blisters with epidermal loss
- Third-degree burn: full-thickness skin loss
- Fourth-degree burn: deep **necrosis** of underlying tissues or deep third-degree burn

The guidelines instruct the coder to sequence the code that reflects the highest degree of burn first.

EXAMPLE | Patient was seen in the ER for second-degree burns of the left calf and first-degree burns of the right foot due to uncontrolled grass fire in forest, T24.232A, T25.121A, X01.0xxA, Y92.821.

Often, a burn will be described as having different degrees at the same site. It is only necessary to assign the code that identifies the highest degree of burn.

EXAMPLE | Examination of the patient shows erythema and blisters to the right wrist due to burn from an iron. The accident occurred at the patient's house, T23.271A, X15.8xxA, Y92.019, Y93.e4.

EXAMPLE | Patient was seen in the ER with erythema and blisters on left hand due to accidental chemical burn from hydrochloric acid. Patient works in an industrial factory, T54.2x1A, T23.602A, Y92.63, Y99.0.

Although the physician did not state first- or second-degree burn, by the description, this burn is a first- (erythema) and second-degree (blister) burn, so it would be coded to the most severe burn, which is second-degree.

For a variety of reasons, a burn may not heal quickly, or it may become infected. A nonhealing burn is coded as an acute burn. It is possible to have burns that occurred at the same time, and some may have healed completely while others have not yet healed. If the burn contains necrotic tissue, it is coded as an acute burn. It is possible to have late effects (e.g., scar, contracture) of a burn along with a nonhealing burn. Sometimes, late effects remain after the burn has healed, and these still require treatment.

EXAMPLE | Patient has third-degree burn on chest wall due to house fire, T21.31xA, X00.0xxA, Y92.019.

EXAMPLE | Active treatment for patient who has a nonhealing third-degree burn of abdominal wall with keloid scar forming on right shoulder burn. Burns due to accidental injury in house fire, T21.32xA, L91.0, T22.051S, X00.0xxA, X00.0xxS, Y92.019.

EXAMPLE | Patient is being treated for an infected burn right palm from a hot light bulb, T23.051A, T79.8xxA, L08.9, X15.8xxA.

T31 and T32 categories are provided to identify the extent of body surface that is involved by burns and to indicate the percentage of body surface that has third-degree burns. According to the classic "rule of nines," in estimating involved body surface, head and neck are assigned 9%, each arm 9%, each leg 18%, anterior trunk 18%, posterior trunk 18%, and genitalia 1%. These percentage assignments may change as necessary to accommodate infants and children who have proportionately larger heads than adults and patients who have large buttocks, thighs, or abdomen that involve burns (Figure 24-3). The percentages of body surface involvement must be documented by a healthcare professional for code assignment. Percentages should not be calculated by the coder.

Category (T30) can be used when the site of the burn is not specified. In some instances, the burns may be so extensive that detailed documentation is not provided. A specialized burn assessment form to document burn location, type, and body percentage is often used in burn centers.

EXAMPLE | Patient has second- (3%) and third-degree (5%) burns of the trunk and first-degree burns (2%) of the right arm due to fire from a street car accident, T21.30xA, T22.10xA, T31.10, V82.8xxA, Y92.818.

Frostbite

Frostbite occurs when skin and the underlying tissues freeze due to extreme cold. The areas that are most likely to be affected are the cheeks, nose, ears, fingers, and toes. The blood vessels close to the skin start to constrict to sustain the core body temperature. The skin and underlying tissues are affected due to the lack of blood supply to these areas. There are four degrees of frostbite.

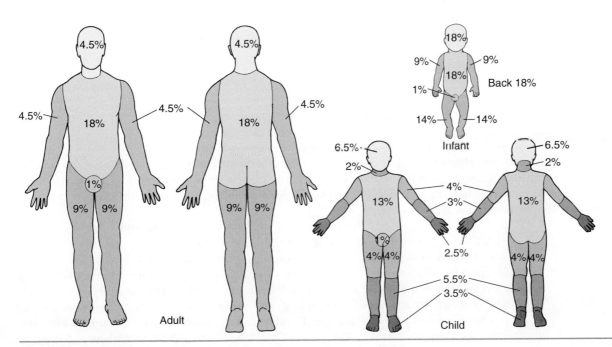

FIGURE 24-3. Rule of nines.

- First degree—only affects the skin surface. Usually no permanent damage but may be affected by heat and cold sensitivity.
- Second degree—blisters will form within 1 to 2 days. Blisters will become hard and are black. These areas will be insensitive to heat and cold.
- Third and fourth degree—the frostbite goes deep into the muscles, tendons, blood vessels, and nerves. Nerve damage will result in loss of feeling. Affected areas may develop gangrene, and amputation may be necessary.

EXAMPLE

Patient was seen in the ER for superficial frostbite, both ears. Patient was exposed to cold weather, T33.011A, T33.012A, X31.xxxA.

EXERCISE 24-1

Assign codes to the following conditions. (If percentage of the body burned is not documented do not assign a code from category T31 or T32).

1. Nonhealing second-degree burn left thigh due to hot coffee spill, subsequent encounter   _____

2. Second- and third-degree burns trunk, and second- and third-degree burns both legs due to fire at night club; in all, 35% of the body was burned, 25% third degree   _____

3. First-degree burn right wrist and second-degree burns right fingers and right hand due to firework explosion while playing in backyard   _____

4. Infected second-degree burn buttock, subsequent encounter   _____

5. Alkaline burn left cornea due to caustic soda while working in a paper manufacturing factory   _____

6. Hypertrophic scar of burn to right cheek   _____

7. Friction burn left elbow due to accidental fall on carpeted stairs at patient's home   _____

8. Patient in house fire with multiple burns over 60% of body, 30% third degree; patient was stabilized and prepared for transport to burn unit; fire was due to accidental causes   _____

9. Frostbite toes and fingers due to spending night outdoors in blizzard   _____

Poisoning by, Adverse Effect of, and Underdosing of Drugs, Medicaments, and Biological Substances (T36-T50)

An **adverse effect** can occur due to ingestion or exposure to drugs or other medicinal and biologic substances. It is a reaction to a drug that has been taken according to the prescription or instructions on the label of over-the-counter drugs. To code an adverse effect, at least two codes are required.

The Table of Drugs and Chemicals (Figure 24-4) is used to identify one code from categories T36-T50 to identify the drug and then additional code(s) to identify the manifestations of the adverse effect. The drug responsible for the adverse effect must first be identified and then located in the Table under the adverse effect column. If a specific drug cannot be located, the generic name should be determined or the category of the drug identified (e.g., antihypertensive, antianginal, antineoplastic). Once the drug or drug category has been located in the index, the T code from the adverse effect column is assigned after verification in the Tabular. Refer to the guidelines for assistance with sequencing of the manifestation(s) and assignment of the appropriate T code(s).

Substance	External Cause (T-Code)					
	Poisoning, Accidental (Unintentional)	Poisoning, Intentional Self-Harm	Poisoning, Assault	Poisoning, Undetermined	Adverse Effect	Underdosing
#						
1-propanol	T51.3X1	T51.3X2	T51.3X3	T51.3X4	—	—
2-propanol	T51.2X1	T51.2X2	T51.2X3	T51.2X4	—	—
2,4-D (dichlorophen-oxyacetic acid)	T60.3X1	T60.3X2	T60.3X3	T60.3X4	—	—
2,4-toluene diisocyanate	T65.0X1	T65.0X2	T65.0X3	T65.0X4	—	—
2,4,5-T (trichloro-phenoxyacetic acid)	T60.1X1	T60.1X2	T60.1X3	T60.1X4	—	—
14-hydroxydihydro-morphinone	T40.2X1	T40.2X2	T40.2X3	T40.2X4	T40.2X5	T40.2X6
A						
ABOB	T37.5X1	T37.5X2	T37.5X3	T37.5X4	T37.5X5	T37.5X6
Abrine	T62.2X1	T62.2X2	T62.2X3	T62.2X4	—	—
Abrus (seed)	T62.2X1	T62.2X2	T62.2X3	T62.2X4	—	—
Absinthe	T51.0X1	T51.0X2	T51.0X3	T51.0X4	—	—
beverage	T51.0X1	T51.0X2	T51.0X3	T51.0X4	—	—
Acaricide	T60.8X1	T60.8X2	T60.8X3	T60.8X4	—	—
Acebutolol	T44.7X1	T44.7X2	T44.7X3	T44.7X4	T44.7X5	T44.7X6
Acecarbromal	T42.6X1	T42.6X2	T42.6X3	T42.6X4	T42.6X5	T42.6X6
Aceclidine	T44.1X1	T44.1X2	T44.1X3	T44.1X4	T44.1X5	T44.1X6
Acedapsone	T37.0X1	T37.0X2	T37.0X3	T37.0X4	T37.0X5	T37.0X6
Acefylline piperazine	T48.6X1	T48.6X2	T48.6X3	T48.6X4	T48.6X5	T48.6X6
Acemorphan	T40.2X1	T40.2X2	T40.2X3	T40.2X4	T40.2X5	T40.2X6
Acenocoumarin	T45.511	T45.512	T45.513	T45.514	T45.515	T45.516
Acenocoumarol	T45.511	T45.512	T45.513	T45.514	T45.515	T45.516
Acepifylline	T48.6X1	T48.6X2	T48.6X3	T48.6X4	T48.6X5	T48.6X6
Acepromazine	T43.3X1	T43.3X2	T43.3X3	T43.3X4	T43.3X5	T43.3X6
Acesulfamethoxypyridazine	T37.0X1	T37.0X2	T37.0X3	T37.0X4	T37.0X5	T37.0X6
Acetal	T52.8X1	T52.8X2	T52.8X3	T52.8X4	—	—
Acetaldehyde (vapor)	T52.8X1	T52.8X2	T52.8X3	T52.8X4	—	—
liquid	T65.891	T65.892	T65.893	T65.894	—	—
P-Acetamidophenol	T39.1X1	T39.1X2	T39.1X3	T39.1X4	T39.1X5	T39.1X6
Acetaminophen	T39.1X1	T39.1X2	T39.1X3	T39.1X4	T39.1X5	T39.1X6
Acetaminosalol	T39.1X1	T39.1X2	T39.1X3	T39.1X4	T39.1X5	T39.1X6
Acetanilide	T39.1X1	T39.1X2	T39.1X3	T39.1X4	T39.1X5	T39.1X6
Acetarsol	T37.3X1	T37.3X2	T37.3X3	T37.3X4	T37.3X5	T37.3X6
Acetazolamide	T50.2X1	T50.2X2	T50.2X3	T50.2X4	T50.2X5	T50.2X6
Acetiamine	T45.2X1	T45.2X2	T45.2X3	T45.2X4	T45.2X5	T45.2X6
Acetic						
acid	T54.2X1	T54.2X2	T54.2X3	T54.2X4	—	—
with sodium acetate (ointment)	T49.3X1	T49.3X2	T49.3X3	T49.3X4	T49.3X5	T49.3X6
ester (solvent) (vapor)	T52.8X1	T52.8X2	T52.8X3	T52.8X4	—	—

FIGURE 24-4. Excerpt from the Table of Drugs and Chemicals.

Because drugs have generic and brand names, and these are used interchangeably, it may be difficult to locate the drug in the index. A drug reference book or an Internet search can be used to determine the generic name or category of the drug.

EXAMPLE

Hematuria due to Coumadin, which is taken for atrial fibrillation, R31.9, T45.515A, I48.91. Hematuria in this case is the adverse effect of medication that was properly prescribed and properly taken.

EXAMPLE

Patient presented with hypokalemia due to long-term use of diuretics, E87.6, T50.2x5A. Hypokalemia is the adverse effect of the diuretic.

EXAMPLE

Dizziness caused by Claritin, which was taken per instructions on the label, R42, T45.0x5A. Claritin is not listed in the Table of Drugs and Chemicals, but an Internet search reveals that loratadine is the generic name, and this is not listed either. Claritin is classified as an antihistamine that can be located in the Table.

EXERCISE 24-2

Using a drug reference book or the Internet, specify drug category or generic name for the following drugs.

1. Lunesta   _____
2. Cardizem   _____
3. Bactrim   _____
4. Zoloft   _____
5. Ditropan   _____

It is possible that an adverse effect to some drugs may be based on an abnormal laboratory result. Sometimes a physician will document "toxicity" based on these laboratory results. For a drug toxicity with no documented adverse reaction assign code R89.2. The appropriate 7th character will need to be added to the code to identify whether this is an initial encounter, subsequent encounter, or a sequela of an adverse effect. If the patient has any symptoms, then the symptom codes are assigned along with the appropriate T code for adverse effect.

EXAMPLE

Dilantin toxicity per laboratory report. Patient is asymptomatic. The Dilantin dosage will be adjusted and Dilantin levels monitored. Patient takes Dilantin for seizure disorder, R89.2, T42.0x5A, G40.909.

Underdosing is taking less of a medication than is prescribed by a provider or a manufacturer's instructions. Occasionally a patient will be admitted to the hospital for a relapse or exacerbation of the medical condition for which that drug was prescribed. According to the guidelines, a code for the medical condition should be assigned first, then a code from categories T36-T50 to indicate underdosing. Additional codes to further explain the reason for underdosing such as noncompliance because of financial hardship should also be assigned.

EXERCISE 24-3

Assign codes to the following conditions.

1. Hives due to Bactrim taken to treat UTI (urinary tract infection) _____

2. Diarrhea due to erythromycin used to treat acute bronchitis _____

3. Headache due to Nitrostat taken for angina _____

4. Constipation due to narcotics used after surgery _____

5. Decreased sex drive due to treatment with Zoloft for depression _____

6. Lab results show Digoxin toxicity. Digoxin taken for congestive heart failure; drug was taken as prescribed _____

7. Dizziness and irregular heartbeat due to Inderal, which was taken for hypertension _____

8. Tachycardia due to albuterol, which was administered for asthma _____

9. CHF exacerbation due to noncompliance with lasix. Not taking required dosage because patient has trouble getting to bathroom due to osteoarthritis _____

Poisonings

It is sometimes confusing to determine the difference between an adverse effect and a poisoning. Poisoning from medication(s) occurs when:

■ The wrong medication is taken—patient took a medication that is not currently prescribed for them

■ The wrong dose is taken—patient took 2 tablets instead of 1 (double the dosage)

■ Overdose—patient took large amount of medication or other drug or chemical

■ Nonprescribed drug (including illegal drugs and alcohol) interacts with a prescription medication—patient took an over-the-counter medication that causes some reaction with prescribed medication

The poisoning T code is always sequenced first and is found in the Table of Drugs and Chemicals under the heading for "poisoning." It is possible to assign more than one poisoning code, to describe a poisoning if more than one substance or drug is responsible. A poisoning requires at least two codes.

The selection of the appropriate T code for poisonings can be confusing. Unlike adverse effects where the only option for T code assignment from the "adverse effect" column, poisoning T codes are assigned according to circumstances surrounding this poisoning. The circumstances (intent) include the following:

■ Accidental

■ Intentional Self-Harm

■ Assault

■ Undetermined

According to the guidelines:

■ If the intent (accident, self-harm, assault) of the cause of an injury or poisoning is unknown or unspecified, code the intent as accidental.

■ Undetermined intent is only for use if the documentation specifies that the intent cannot be determined.

If the manifestation(s) of the poisoning is documented, it should be coded as a secondary diagnosis. Manifestations could include chest pain, vomiting, lethargy, coma, and so forth.

Chronic medical conditions related to alcohol and/or drug abuse or dependence would not be considered a poisoning. In these cases, the chronic medical condition should be coded along with a code to identify the type of abuse or dependence.

EXAMPLE | Alcoholic cardiomyopathy in patient with alcohol dependence, I42.6, F10.20.

EXAMPLE | Patient admitted for a suicide attempt with multiple medications, including Naproxen, Keppra, and acetaminophen mixed with beer. Patient was somnolent on arrival in the ER, T39.312A, T42.6x2A, T39.1x2A, T51.0x2A, R40.0.

EXAMPLE | Patient became weak, had labored breathing, and had altered mental status caused by an accidental overdose of codeine, T40.2x1A, R53.1, R06.4, R41.82.
  The manifestations of the overdose are the weakness, breathing problems, and alteration in mental status.

EXERCISE 24-4

Assign codes to the following conditions.

1. Patient took ampicillin that belonged to his wife; patient developed hives caused by the ampicillin _____

2. Patient became stuporous and lethargic after taking Valium according to prescription, then drinking a couple of beers; accidental intent _____

3. The patient accidentally received the higher dosage of potassium while in hospital; no effects were noted _____

4. Cocaine-induced chest pain; patient is a known cocaine abuser with a daily habit; accidental intent _____

5. Suicide attempt with acetaminophen; patient has nausea and vomiting with abdominal pain _____

6. Toddler accidentally drank bottle of Visine; the toddler was having labored breathing and was very irritable _____

7. Patient was taking extra doses of Lasix to reduce swelling of lower extremities; patient is hypokalemic and takes Lasix for congestive heart failure _____

8. Patient became dizzy and very drowsy after taking one of spouse's Vicodin tablets and drinking a couple of alcoholic beverages and smoking marijuana _____

Toxic Effects of Substances Chiefly Nonmedicinal as to Source (T51-T65)

Numerous toxic substances can cause ill effects. Categories T51 to T65 identify these types of reactions. Reactions range from mild events such as headache to life-threatening conditions. At the beginning of this section, instructions are provided on the use of additional codes for all associated manifestations of toxic effect.

EXAMPLE | Patient admitted with alcohol poisoning due to intake of vodka, T51.0x1A.

EXERCISE 24-5

Assign codes to the following conditions.

1. Nausea and vomiting due to ingestion of holly berries _____

2. Accidental lead poisoning from paint with anemia and muscle weakness _____

> 3. Unconscious due to carbon monoxide poisoning caused by _____
>   motor vehicle fumes, suicide attempt
>
> 4. Tremors, low-grade fever, weight loss, and extreme fatigue _____
>   due to mercury toxicity caused by exposure while working
>   with dental fillings

Other and Unspecified Effects of External Causes (T66-T78)

Categories T66 to T78 are used to identify the effects that external causes such as radiation, temperature, heat, light, and air pressure may have on the human body.

Adult/Child Abuse

Domestic violence, elder abuse, and child abuse occur more often than one might think. Healthcare providers are required to report to the proper authorities any suspicions of abuse and/or neglect. Four major types of abuse have been identified:
1. Physical abuse
2. Sexual abuse
3. Emotional or psychological abuse
4. Neglect or abandonment

There are specific ICD-10-CM T codes that identify "suspected" abuse or neglect. It is not necessary to assign external cause codes or perpetrator codes with these codes. If the suspected abuse or neglect has been ruled out during an encounter, Z04.71 should be assigned for adults and Z04.72 for children. A code from category T76 should not be assigned. Shaken infant syndrome is the exception to this rule and defaults to code T74.4.

ICD-10-CM classifies confirmed cases of abuse or neglect to code category T74. The fourth character of the T74 and T76 codes indicates the type of abuse. The fifth character identifies if the patient is a child or adult.

The code book gives instructions on the use of additional code(s), if applicable, to identify any associated injuries (Figure 24-5) and the appropriate External cause code to identify the perpetrator.

EXAMPLE

> The child was admitted for moderate malnutrition because of neglect by the mother, T74.02xA, E44.0, Y07.12.

Systemic Inflammatory Response Syndrome (SIRS)

Systemic inflammatory response syndrome (SIRS) is a serious medical condition that can occur in response to an infection or to noninfectious causes, such as severe trauma, burns, and complications of surgery. It may also occur in diseases such as pancreatitis and AIDS.

SIRS may be diagnosed when two or more of the following criteria are present:
- Heart rate >90 beats per minute
- Body temperature <36°C or >38°C
- Tachypnea (high respiratory rate) >20 breaths per minute or, on blood gas, a $PaCo_2$ <4.3 kPa (32 mm Hg)
- White blood cell count <4000 cells/mm^3 or >12,000 cells/mm^3 (<4 × 10^9 or >12 × 10^9 cells/L), or the presence of greater than 10% immature neutrophils.

Because of instructional notes in the code book to "code first underlying condition," the SIRS codes will generally not be the principal diagnosis. In patients with trauma, the most severe injury would be the principal diagnosis and the SIRS code would be assigned as a secondary code. It is possible for organ dysfunction to occur as a result of trauma, and this would be coded to SIRS due to noninfectious process with acute organ dysfunction.

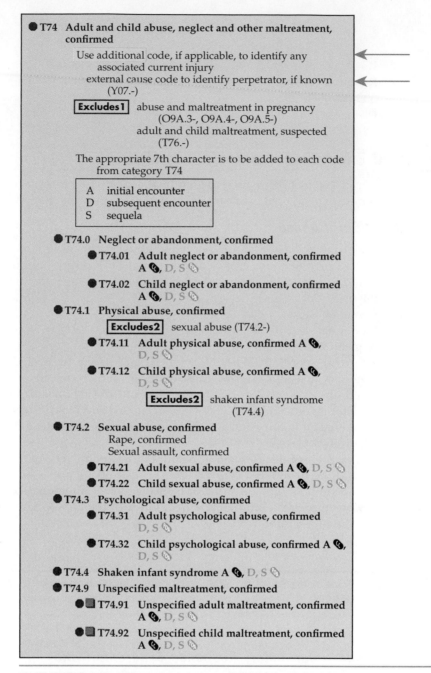

FIGURE 24-5. Instructions to use additional code(s) to identify any current injury and external cause code for perpetrator.

EXAMPLE Patient has SIRS due to accidental burns in an accident in which a street car caught on fire. Patient has second- (3%) and third-degree (5%) burns of the trunk and first-degree burns of the right arm, T21.30xA, T22.10xA, T31.0, R65.10, V82.8xxA, Y92.818.

Rhabomyolysis

Rhabomyolysis is the breakdown of muscle fibers that results in the release of muscle fiber contents into the circulation. Some of these contents are toxic to the kidney, frequently resulting in kidney damage. Some inherited disorders such as carnitine palmityltransferase, phosphofructokinase deficiency, and phosphoglycerate kinase deficiency can lead to muscle injury with exercise and rhabdomyolysis. Some of the most common causes include the following:

■ Muscle exertion (physical, related to convulsions or to heat injury)
■ Trauma-crush syndromes and pseudo-crush syndrome
■ Muscle ischemia related to arterial occlusion or insufficiency
■ Burns
■ Repetitive muscle injury (bongo drumming, torture)
■ Status epilepticus
■ Drug overdose
■ Extended periods of muscle pressure

EXAMPLE

Traumatic rhabdomyolysis due to intractable status epilepticus
        Patient was diagnosed with epilepsy 2 years ago, G40.911, T79.6xxA.

EXERCISE 24-6

Assign codes to the following conditions.

1. Heatstroke due to high temperature while at beach   _____

2. Anaphylactic shock due to peanut butter   _____

3. Seasickness while on cruise   _____

4. Shaken baby syndrome with subdural hematoma and retinal   _____
   hemorrhages. The baby was shaken by the babysitter

5. Diarrhea, drowsiness, and seizure caused by arsenic   _____
   poisoning. Wife was trying to harm the patient

Late Effects of Injuries, Poisonings, Toxic Effects, and Other External Causes

Once the acute nature of an injury, adverse effect, or poisoning has resolved, some residual effects or sequela that have remained may require medical treatment. In Chapter 5, the coding and sequencing of late effects were discussed. Remember, a late effect may occur at any time after the acute injury has resolved. No specific time frames are required.

To assign a code for a late effect or sequela of a traumatic injury, adverse effect, or poisoning, the code that identifies the type of injury, adverse effect, or poisoning is assigned with a 7th character of "S" which identifies "sequela." Code(s) are also assigned to identify the late effect or sequela. Usually there will be at least two codes when coding a late effect with the sequela code(s) sequenced first. There are also external cause codes for late effects, which can be found under the main term sequelae in the Alphabetic Index for External Causes (Figure 24-6). A 7th character of "K" may be used to identify encounters for fractures with nonunion.

EXAMPLE

The patient was diagnosed five years ago with drug-induced Parkinson's due to perphenazine, which was taken for schizophrenia, G21.11, T43.3x5S, F20.9.

EXAMPLE

Scar on left wrist due to previous burn by fire, L90.5, T23.072S.

EXAMPLE

Patient is being treated for avascular necrosis following previous left scaphoid fracture due to old sports injury with fall, M87.242, S62.002S.

Sequelae (of)
  accident NEC —*see* W00-X58 with 7th
    character S
  assault (homicidal) (any means) —*see*
    X92-Y08 with 7th character S
  homicide, attempt (any means) —*see*
    X92-Y08 with 7th character S
  injury undetermined whether
    accidentally or purposely
    inflicted —*see* Y21-Y33 with 7th
    character S
  intentional self-harm (classifiable to
    X71-X83) —*see* X71-X83 with 7th
    character S
  legal intervention (*see* with 7th
    character S Y35)
  motor vehicle accident —*see* V00-V99
    with 7th character S
  suicide, attempt (any means) —*see*
    X71-X83 with 7th character S
  transport accident —*see* V00-V99 with
    7th character S
  war operations —*see* War operations

FIGURE 24-6. Alphabetic Index entry for Sequelae.

EXERCISE 24-7

Assign codes to the following conditions.

1. Nonunion of left lateral humeral condylar fracture; patient fell _____
   2 months ago (accidental injury)

2. Traumatic arthritis due to severe sprain of right ankle 3 years _____
   ago (accidental injury)

3. Phantom limb pain due to traumatic AKA (above knee _____
   amputation); patient was in a motorcycle accident 6 months
   ago

4. Spastic quadriplegia due to complete C3 spinal cord injury _____
   from diving accident 5 years ago

5. Hypoxic brain injury due to suicide attempt by strangulation _____
   1 year ago

FACTORS INFLUENCING HEALTH STATUS AND CONTACT WITH HEALTH SERVICES (Z CODES)

As was discussed in Chapter 8, it may be difficult to locate Z codes in the index. Coders often say, "I did not know there was a Z code for that." It is important for the coder to be familiar with different types and uses of Z codes. Refer to Chapter 8 for a listing of common main terms used to locate Z codes. See Chapter 23 for Z codes used for injuries.

Z03.6	Encounter for observation for suspected toxic effect from ingested substance ruled out
Z03.810	Encounter for observation for suspected exposure to anthrax ruled out

Z03.818	Encounter for observation for suspected exposure to other biological agents ruled out
Z04.71	Encounter for examination and observation following alleged adult physical abuse
Z04.72	Encounter for examination and observation following alleged child physical abuse
Z13.88	Encounter for screening for disorder due to exposure to contaminants
Z18.01	Retained depleted uranium fragments
Z18.09	Other retained radioactive fragments
Z57.1	Occupational exposure to radiation
Z57.39	Occupational exposure to other air contaminants
Z57.4	Occupational exposure to toxic agents in agriculture
Z57.5	Occupational exposure to toxic agents in other industries
Z57.6	Occupational exposure to extreme temperature
Z62.810	Personal history of physical and sexual abuse in childhood
Z62.811	Personal history of psychological abuse in childhood
Z62.812	Personal history of neglect in childhood
Z62.819	Personal history of unspecified abuse in childhood
Z77.010	Contact with and (suspected) exposure to arsenic
Z77.011	Contact with and (suspected) exposure to lead
Z77.012	Contact with and (suspected) exposure to uranium
Z77.018	Contact with and (suspected) exposure to other hazardous metals
Z77.020	Contact with and (suspected) exposure to aromatic amines
Z77.021	Contact with and (suspected) exposure to benzene
Z77.028	Contact with and (suspected) exposure to other hazardous aromatic compounds
Z77.090	Contact with and (suspected) exposure to asbestos
Z77.098	Contact with and (suspected) exposure to other hazardous, chiefly nonmedicinal, chemicals
Z77.110	Contact with and (suspected) exposure to air pollution
Z77.111	Contact with and (suspected) exposure to water pollution
Z77.112	Contact with and (suspected) exposure to soil pollution
Z77.118	Contact with and (suspected) exposure to other environmental pollution
Z77.120	Contact with and (suspected) exposure to mold (toxic)
Z77.121	Contact with and (suspected) exposure to harmful algae and algae toxins
Z77.123	Contact with and (suspected) exposure to radon and other naturally occurring radiation
Z77.128	Contact with and (suspected) exposure to other hazards in the physical environment
Z77.29	Contact with and (suspected) exposure to other hazardous substances
Z77.9	Other contact with and (suspected) exposures hazardous to health
Z87.892	Personal history of anaphylaxis
Z88.0	Allergy status to penicillin
Z88.1	Allergy status to other antibiotic agents status
Z88.2	Allergy status to sulfonamides status
Z88.3	Allergy status to other anti-infective agents status
Z88.4	Allergy status to anesthetic agent status
Z88.5	Allergy status to narcotic agent status
Z88.6	Allergy status to analgesic agent status
Z88.7	Allergy status to serum and vaccine status
Z88.8	Allergy status to other drugs, medicaments, and biological substances status
Z88.9	Allergy status to unspecified drugs, medicaments and biological substances status
Z91.010	Allergy to peanuts
Z91.011	Allergy to milk products

Z91.012	Allergy to eggs
Z91.013	Allergy to seafood
Z91.018	Allergy to other foods
Z91.02	Food additives allergy status
Z91.030	Bee allergy status
Z91.038	Other insect allergy status
Z91.040	Latex allergy status
Z91.041	Radiographic dye allergy status
Z91.048	Other nonmedicinal substances allergy status
Z91.09	Other allergy status, other than to drugs and biological substances
Z91.120	Patient's intentional underdosing of medication regimen due to financial hardship
Z91.128	Patient's intentional underdosing of medication regimen for other reason
Z91.130	Patient's unintentional underdosing of medication regimen due to age-related debility
Z91.138	Patient's unintentional underdosing of medication regimen for other reason
Z91.14	Patient's other noncompliance with medication regimen
Z91.19	Patient's noncompliance with other medical treatment and regimen
Z91.410	Personal history of adult physical and sexual abuse
Z91.411	Personal history of adult psychological abuse
Z91.412	Personal history of adult neglect
Z91.419	Personal history of unspecified adult abuse
Z91.5	Personal history of self-harm

EXERCISE 24-8

Assign codes to the following conditions.

1. History of allergy to latex _____
2. History of allergy to Bactrim _____
3. Patient has a history of anaphylactic shock due to bee sting _____
4. History of rape. Patient is an adult _____
5. History of hives due to contrast media or radiologic dye _____
6. Observation for suspected physical abuse (adult), which was ruled out _____

EXAMPLE Patient was exposed to asbestos while working in a shipyard years ago, Z77.090.

EXAMPLE Patient wears a bracelet because of allergy to penicillin, Z88.0.

COMMON TREATMENTS

Treatment will depend on the type and severity of the injury. Pain medications, anti-inflammatories, corticosteroids, and antibiotics may be necessary to alleviate pain and inflammation and to prevent or fight infection.

PROCEDURES

Debridement

Debridement of burns is probably the most common procedure that will be assigned in this chapter. The root operation for debridement is excision (cutting out/off without replacement some of a body part). Debridements can be performed in many settings in the hospital including at the bedside, so documentation may be difficult to locate. Debridements do not have to be performed in the operating room. Debridements may also be performed by physical therapists, wound care nurses, and other healthcare professionals in addition to physicians.

According to the ICD-10-PCS guidelines, when an excision is performed on overlapping layers, the body part specifying the deepest layer is coded. If a patient had a debridement of skin, subcutaneous tissue, muscle, and bone, the bone is the deepest layer and debridement of the bone is the only procedure code assigned. If a nonexcisional debridement is performed the root operation is extraction.

Examples of nonexcisional debridement include brushing, irrigation, scrubbing, washing of tissue, or utilization of a Versajet device. Documentation of sharp debridement does not always mean that an excisional debridement was performed. Definite cutting away of tissue and not just removal of loose tissue fragments with a sharp instrument must be documented in order to code excisional debridement.

EXAMPLE Excisional debridement of infected burn right palm performed by physician. Patient was burned by hot light bulb, T23.051A, T79.8xxA, L08.9, X15.8xxA, 0HBFXZZ.

EXAMPLE Excisional debridement subcutaneous tissue of fourth-degree burn lower back by physician, T21.34xA, 0JB70ZZ.

Hyperbaric Oxygen Therapy

Hyperbaric oxygen therapy (HBOT) is a treatment in which the patient's entire body is placed in a transparent, airtight chamber at increased atmospheric pressure. The patient breathes in 100% pure oxygen. This increased oxygen flow in the body helps to improve healing within the tissues and helps to get rid of toxic gases in the case of a poisoning. The ICD-10-PCS codes for HBOT can be found in the extracorporeal assistance and performance section.

HBOT is helpful in treating medical conditions such as the following:

- Air or gas embolism (in divers or following bypass surgery)
- Decompression sickness in divers (bends)
- Burns and other wounds
- Carbon monoxide poisoning
- Smoke inhalation
- Near drowning, near electrocution, or near hanging
- Diabetic ulcers/skin ulcers

EXAMPLE Patient is being treated with HBOT for decompression sickness while surfacing while scuba diving in the ocean, T70.3xxA, W94.21xA, Y92.832, Y93.15, 6A150ZZ.

EXERCISE 24-9

Assign codes for all diagnoses and procedures.

1. Z-plasty to release scar contracture left forearm _____

2. Debridement of skin in patient with second-degree burn right knee _____

3. Excisional debridement of subcutaneous tissue in patient with second- and third-degree burns back performed at the patient's bedside _____

4. Debridement to the soft tissue of deep burns left thigh   _____

5. Full-thickness skin graft to deep third-degree burn area of the   _____
   right hand. Graft from patient

DOCUMENTATION/REIMBURSEMENT/MS-DRGs

Often, coding challenges are due to lack of documentation. Sometimes radiology and other test results are not available at the time of discharge or when the physician is dictating the discharge summary or is reporting the final diagnoses.

Documentation of how, when, and where an injury occurred, along with good descriptions of the injury, is often lacking. It may not be important to the physician that the accident occurred on the school playground instead of the backyard of the patient's home. Surgical procedures such as skin grafting, excisional debridement, or mechanical ventilation can make a difference in reimbursement.

Burns have their own major diagnostic category, or MDC—22. The following Medicare Severity diagnosis-related groups (MS-DRGs) fall into the burn MDC:

- 927   Extensive burns or full-thickness burns with mechanical ventilation 96 hours with skin graft
- 928   Full-thickness burn with skin graft or inhalation injury with CC/MCC
- 929   Full-thickness burn with skin graft or inhalation injury without CC/MCC
- 933   Extensive burns or full-thickness burns with mechanical ventilation 96 hours without skin graft
- 934   Full-thickness burn without skin graft of inhalation injury
- 935   Nonextensive burns

By the titles of these MS-DRGs, it is evident that the type of burn, mechanical ventilation, skin graft procedure, presence of an inhalation injury, and/or CC/MCC determines the MS-DRG assignment.

Frequently missed complications/comorbidities from this chapter are difficult to pinpoint. The CC/MCC listing contains numerous injury codes. It is important to code all injuries with the most serious injury as the principal diagnosis. Codes for complications related to trauma are also important.

Correct Procedure Code

EXAMPLE   A patient was admitted with third-degree burns to the abdomen and second-degree burns to the face with burn injury to the lungs. The patient was on a mechanical ventilator for 5 days. Documentation of mechanical ventilation may be difficult to find within the health record. The calculation of ventilation hours can also affect the MS-DRG assignment.

DIAGNOSES	CODES	MS-DRG	RW
Burns abdomen, face, and lungs Ventilation 96+ hours	T27.1xxA, T21.32xA, T20.20xA 5A1955Z	207	5.2933
Burns abdomen, face, and lungs Ventilation less than 96 hours (30 hours)	T27.1xxA, T21.32xA, T20.20xA 5A1945Z	208	2.2704
Burns abdomen and face No ventilation	T21.32xA, T20.20xA	934	1.3998

The MS-DRG assignment is affected by the burn injury to the lung and the use of mechanical ventilation.

Adverse Effect versus Poisoning

If an adverse effect is incorrectly coded as a poisoning, or if a poisoning is incorrectly coded as an adverse effect, reimbursement can be affected.

EXAMPLE

The patient's physician recently adjusted the dosage of the patient's digitalis, which the patient takes for congestive heart failure. The patient took the medication as directed by the physician but became severely nauseated. This is an adverse effect associated with digitalis because the patient took the medication as prescribed by the physician. The physician documents digitalis toxicity.

DIAGNOSES	CODES	MS-DRG	RW
Coded as Adverse Effect			
Nausea due to digitalis toxicity with congestive heart failure	R11.0, T46.0x5A, I50.9	392	0.7241
Coded as Poisoning			
Nausea due to digitalis toxicity with congestive heart failure	T46.0x1A, R11.0, I50.9	918	0.6228

The term "toxicity" does not necessarily indicate a poisoning. This case should be coded as an adverse effect. If this case had been coded as a poisoning, the facility would have received a lower reimbursement than was supported by the documentation in the health record.

CHAPTER REVIEW EXERCISE

Assign codes for all diagnoses and procedures. Explain why it is an adverse effect or a poisoning.

1. Alcoholic drank rubbing alcohol, undetermined circumstances _____

_____

2. Anaphylactic shock due to shellfish _____

_____

3. Gastrointestinal bleeding due to excessive use of aspirin for chronic low back pain (accidental)

_____

4. Orthostatic hypotension due to Nitro-Bid taken for stable angina _____

_____

5. Depression due to Keppra, which was taken for a seizure disorder _____

_____

6. Accidental ingestion of Drano with burns of the mouth and esophagus _____

_____

7. Drug-induced dementia due to Lithium. Lithium is taken for bipolar disorder_____

_____

8. Coma due to accidental alcohol poisoning with blood alcohol of 400 mg/100 mL _____

_____

9. Abnormal level of mercury in blood indicating poisoning. No symptoms_____

_____

10. Accidental injury with chemical burns to eyelids from Roundup chemical used on the job doing farm work _____

_____

11. Weakness and tremor due to Lithium toxicity. Patient has bipolar affective disease and is currently depressed. Lithium taken as prescribed_____

_____

12. Drug-induced hepatitis due to isoniazid, which is being taken because of exposure to tuberculosis _____

_____

13. Bite by poisonous rattlesnake _____

_____

14. Steroid-induced hyperglycemia due to prednisone _____

_____

15. Paralytic ileus due to interaction of anticholinergics and codeine _____

_____

16. Patient admitted with uncontrolled diabetes due to unintentional underdosing of metformin. Patient has dementia, which interferes with taking medications as prescribed _____

_____

Assign codes for all diagnoses and procedures.

17. Chemical burn on right knee due to leaking ice pack that was used for knee injury. The skin is reddened with no blister formation _____

18. History of exposure to lead. No apparent symptoms _____

19. Malunion of left radial shaft fracture. Previous accidental injury _____

20. Firefighter suffers smoke inhalation after fighting warehouse fire _____

21. Hypothermia due to cold weather. Patient is homeless and lives in alley _____

22. Second-degree burns to left foot due to accidental scald injury with hot water from bathroom sink at home _____

23. Toddler with third- and fourth-degree burns buttocks, lower legs, and feet. Patient was put into boiling water by the mother's boyfriend. Twenty percent of his body was affected _____

24. Extensive burns 50% of body with 18% third degree. Patient was in a motor vehicle accident (MVA) that occurred on Interstate highway _____

25. SIRS due to crush injury to chest. Patient driver of MV that hit deer on roadway_____

26. Second-degree burns right hand and third-degree burns left hand due to grease fire while working as employee at restaurant. Excisional debridement of the subcutaneous tissue of left hand done in the Operating Room_____

Write the correct answer(s) in the space(s) provided.

27. Name two things that can make a difference in the assignment of a burn MS-DRG.

_____

_____

28. Describe the code assignment for underdosing of a medication.

_____

29. What degree of burn results in full-thickness skin loss?

_____

30. Define adverse effect of a drug.

_____

CHAPTER GLOSSARY

Adverse effect: pathologic manifestation due to ingestion or exposure to drugs or other chemical substances.

Corrosion: burn due to a chemical.

Erythema: redness of the skin.

Frostbite: occurs when skin and underlying tissues freeze due to extreme cold.

Hyperbaric oxygen therapy (HBOT): treatment in which the patient's entire body is placed in a transparent, airtight chamber at increased atmospheric pressure.

Necrosis: death of cells.

Residual condition or effect: when the acute phase of an illness or injury has passed, but a residual condition or health problem remains.

Rhabdomyolysis: breakdown of muscle fibers that results in the release of muscle fiber contents into the circulation.

Systemic inflammatory response syndrome: a serious medical condition that can occur in response to infectious or noninfectious causes, such as severe trauma, burns, or complications of surgery.

Underdosing: taking less of a medication than is prescribed by a provider or a manufacturer's instructions.

Complications of Surgical and Medical Care

LEARNING OBJECTIVES

1. Apply and assign the correct ICD-10-CM/PCS codes in accordance with Official Guidelines for Coding and Reporting

2. Identify major differences between ICD-10-CM/PCS and ICD-9-CM related to complications of surgical and medical care

3. Identify complications of surgical and medical care

4. Assign the correct Z codes, codes, and procedure codes related to complications of surgical and medical care

5. Explain the importance of documentation in relation to MS-DRGs for reimbursement

ABBREVIATIONS/ ACRONYMS

CKD chronic kidney disease

DVT deep vein thrombosis

ECT electroconvulsive therapy

ESRD end-stage renal disease

HAP hospital acquired pneumonia

ICD-9-CM *International Classification of Diseases, 9th Revision, Clinical Modification*

ICD-10-CM *International Classification of Diseases, 10th Revision, Clinical Modification*

ICD-10-PCS *International Classification of Diseases, 10th Revision, Procedure Coding System*

IUD intrauterine device

MS-DRG Medicare Severity diagnosis-related group

PE pulmonary embolism

THR total hip replacement

TPN total parenteral nutrition

TURP transurethral resection of the prostate

UTI urinary tract infection

VAP ventilator assisted pneumonia

VSD ventricular septal defect

ICD-10-CM

Official Guidelines for Coding and Reporting

Please refer to the companion Evolve website for the most current guidelines.

Section II. Selection of a Principal Diagnosis

G. Complications of surgery and other medical care

When the admission is for treatment of a complication resulting from surgery or other medical care, the complication code is sequenced as the principal diagnosis. If the complication is classified to the T80-T88 series and the code lacks the necessary specificity in describing the complication, an additional code for the specific complication should be assigned.

Section I. Conventions, general coding guidelines and chapter specific guidelines

C. Chapter Specific Guidelines

  1. **Chapter 1: Certain Infectious and Parasitic Diseases (A00-B99)**

    d. **Sepsis, Severe Sepsis, and Septic Shock**

      5) **Sepsis due to a postprocedural infection**

        (a) **Documentation of causal relationship**

          As with all postprocedural complications, code assignment is based on the provider's documentation of the relationship between the infection and the procedure.

        (b) **Sepsis due to a postprocedural infection**

          For such cases, the postprocedural infection code, such as, T80.2, Infections following infusion, transfusion, and therapeutic injection, T81.4, Infection following a procedure, T88.0, Infection following immunization, or O86.0, Infection of obstetric surgical wound, should be coded first, followed by the code for the specific infection. If the patient has severe sepsis the appropriate code from subcategory R65.2 should also be assigned with the additional code(s) for any acute organ dysfunction.

        (c) **Postprocedural infection and postprocedural septic shock**

          In cases where a postprocedural infection has occurred and has resulted in severe sepsis and postprocedural septic shock, the code for the precipitating complication such as code T81.4, Infection following a procedure, or O86.0, Infection of obstetrical surgical wound should be coded first followed by code R65.21, Severe sepsis with septic shock and a code for the systemic infection.

EXAMPLE

The patient was readmitted after undergoing surgery last week; the patient is being treated for postoperative sepsis, T81.4xxA, A41.9, Y83.9.

---

  2. **Chapter 2: Neoplasms (C00-D49)**

    c. **Coding and sequencing of complications**

      4) **Treatment of a complication resulting from a surgical procedure**

        When the admission/encounter is for treatment of a complication resulting from a surgical procedure, designate the complication as the principal or first-listed diagnosis if treatment is directed at resolving the complication.

l. Sequencing of neoplasm codes

5) Complication from surgical procedure for treatment of a neoplasm

When an encounter is for treatment of a complication resulting from a surgical procedure performed for the treatment of the neoplasm, designate the complication as the principal/first-listed diagnosis. See guideline regarding the coding of a current malignancy versus personal history to determine if the code for the neoplasm should also be assigned.

r. Malignant neoplasm associated with transplanted organ

A malignant neoplasm of a transplanted organ should be coded as a transplant complication. Assign first the appropriate code from category T86.-, Complications of transplanted organs and tissue, followed by code C80.2, Malignant neoplasm associated with transplanted organ. Use an additional code for the specific malignancy.

EXAMPLE Hernia of colostomy with repair of parastomal hernia. The colostomy was performed 1 year ago during colon cancer resection. The patient is no longer receiving treatment, and the cancer was completely resected, K43.5, Z85.038, Y83.3, OWQFXZ2.

EXAMPLE Patient is admitted with abdominal pain. The patient had previously received a kidney transplant. After study it is determined that the patient had renal carcinoma of the right kidney, T86.19, C80.2, C64.1.

---

4. Chapter 4: Endocrine, Nutritional, and Metabolic Diseases (E00-*E89*)

a. Diabetes mellitus

5) Complications due to insulin pump malfunction

(a) Underdose of insulin due *to* insulin pump failure

An underdose of insulin due to an insulin pump failure should be assigned to a code from subcategory T85.6, Mechanical complication of other specified internal and external prosthetic devices, implants and grafts, that specifies the type of pump malfunction, as the principal or first listed code, followed by code T38.3x6-, Underdosing of insulin and oral hypoglycemic [antidiabetic] drugs. Additional codes for the type of diabetes mellitus and any associated complications due to the underdosing should also be assigned.

(b) Overdose of insulin due to insulin pump failure

The principal or first-listed code for an encounter due to an insulin pump malfunction resulting in an overdose of insulin, should also be T85.6-, Mechanical complication of other specified internal and external prosthetic devices, implants and grafts, followed by code T38.3x1-, Poisoning by insulin and oral hypoglycemic [antidiabetic] drugs, accidental (unintentional).

6) Secondary *Diabetes Mellitus*

(b) Assigning and Sequencing secondary diabetes codes and its causes

(i) Secondary diabetes mellitus due to pancreatectomy

For postpancreatectomy diabetes mellitus (lack of insulin due to the surgical removal of all or part of the pancreas), assign code E89.1, Postprocedural hypoinsulinemia. Assign a code from category E13 and a code from subcategory Z90.41-, Acquired absence of pancreas, as additional codes.

EXAMPLE Patient presents with a kink in the tubing of the insulin pump. This has resulted in diabetic ketoacidosis, T85.694A, E10.10, Y84.8, Z79.4.

6. Chapter 6: Diseases of Nervous System and Sense Organs (G00-G99)
   b. Pain—Category G89
   2) Pain due to devices, implants and grafts
   See Section I.C.19. Pain due to medical devices
   3) Postoperative Pain
   The provider's documentation should be used to guide the coding of postoperative pain, as well as *Section III. Reporting Additional Diagnoses* and *Section IV. Diagnostic Coding and Reporting in the Outpatient Setting*.
   The default for post-thoracotomy and other postoperative pain not specified as acute or chronic is the code for the acute form.
   Routine or expected postoperative pain immediately after surgery should not be coded.
   (a) Postoperative pain not associated with specific postoperative complication
   Postoperative pain not associated with a specific postoperative complication is assigned to the appropriate postoperative pain code in category G89.
   (b) Postoperative pain associated with specific postoperative complication
   Postoperative pain associated with a specific postoperative complication (such as painful wire sutures) is assigned to the appropriate code(s) found in Chapter 19, Injury, poisoning, and certain other consequences of external causes. If appropriate, use additional code(s) from category G89 to identify acute or chronic pain (G89.18 or G89.28).

EXAMPLE Patient presents to doctor's office with the chief complaint of acute postoperative pain. Patient is 2 weeks status post a laparoscopic appendectomy, G89.18.

9. Chapter 9: Diseases of Circulatory System (I00-I99)
   c. Intraoperative and Postprocedural Cerebrovascular Accident
   Medical record documentation should clearly specify the cause- and-effect relationship between the medical intervention and the cerebrovascular accident in order to assign a code for intraoperative or postprocedural cerebrovascular accident. Proper code assignment depends on whether it was an infarction or hemorrhage and whether it occurred intraoperatively or postoperatively. If it was a cerebral hemorrhage, code assignment depends on the type of procedure performed.

EXAMPLE The patient had a postoperative cerebrovascular accident, which was embolic in nature. The patient initially had been admitted for treatment of coronary artery arteriosclerosis with CABG (left internal mammary artery and two greater saphenous vein grafts from the left were used). Cardiopulmonary bypass was used during the surgery, I25.10, I97.820, I63.40, 021109W, 02100A9, 5A1221Z, 06BQ0ZZ.

10. Chapter 10: Diseases of Respiratory System (J00-J99)
   d. Ventilator associated Pneumonia
   1) Documentation of Ventilator associated Pneumonia
   As with all procedural or postprocedural complications, code assignment is based on the provider's documentation of the relationship between the condition and the procedure.
   Code J95.851, Ventilator associated pneumonia, should be assigned only when the provider has documented ventilator associated pneumonia (VAP). An additional code to identify the organism (e.g., Pseudomonas aeruginosa, code B96.5) should also be assigned. Do not assign an additional code from categories J12-J18 to identify the type of pneumonia.

Code J95.851 should not be assigned for cases where the patient has pneumonia and is on a mechanical ventilator but the provider has not specifically stated that the pneumonia is ventilator-associated pneumonia. If the documentation is unclear as to whether the patient has a pneumonia that is a complication attributable to the mechanical ventilator, query the provider.

2) **Ventilator associated Pneumonia Develops after Admission**

A patient may be admitted with one type of pneumonia (e.g., code J13, Pneumonia due to Streptococcus pneumonia) and subsequently develop VAP. In this instance, the principal diagnosis would be the appropriate code from categories J12-J18 for the pneumonia diagnosed at the time of admission. Code J95.851, Ventilator associated pneumonia, would be assigned as an additional diagnosis when the provider has also documented the presence of ventilator associated pneumonia.

EXAMPLE | Patient was hospitalized last month and was on a ventilator for exacerbation of COPD. She presents to the hospital today with pneumonia, J18.9, J44.9.

EXAMPLE | Patient was recently admitted for an acute exacerbation of CHF for which she was placed on a ventilator. She presents to the hospital today with ventilator associated pneumonia. Sputum cultures were taken and this pneumonia was found to be due to MRSA, J95.851, I50.9, B95.62, Y92.239.

EXAMPLE | Patient was admitted to the hospital in acute respiratory failure due to pneumonia. She is placed in the ICU intubated and on a vent for 120 hours. She is transferred to the floor after 3 days where she develops a high fever. The physician documents ventilator associated pneumonia due to *Pseudomonas aeruginosa,* J96.00, J18.9, J95.851, B96.5, Y84.8, Y92.230, 0BH17EZ, 5A1955Z.

19. **Chapter 19: Injury, poisoning, and certain other consequences of external causes (S00-T88)**
    g. **Complications of care**
       1) *General guidelines for* **complications of care**
          (a) **Documentation of complications of care**
              As with all procedural or postprocedural complications, code assignment is based on the provider's documentation of the relationship between the condition and the procedure.
       2) **Pain due to medical devices**
          Pain associated with devices, implants or grafts left in a surgical site (for example painful hip prosthesis) is assigned to the appropriate code(s) found in Chapter 19, Injury, poisoning, and certain other consequences of external causes. Specific codes for pain due to medical devices are found in the T code section of the ICD-10-CM. Use additional code(s) from category G89 to identify acute or chronic pain due to presence of the device, implant or graft (G89.18 or G89.28).

EXAMPLE | Patient presents with acute pain secondary to a displaced nail in the right femur, T84.124A, G89.18, M79.604, Y83.1.

       3) **Transplant complications**
          (a) **Transplant complications other than kidney**
              Codes under category T86, Complications of transplanted organs and tissues, are for use for both complications and rejection of transplanted organs. A transplant complication code is only assigned if the complication affects the function of the transplanted organ. Two codes are required to fully describe a transplant complication: the appropriate code from category T86 and a secondary code that identifies the complication.

Pre-existing conditions or conditions that develop after the transplant are not coded as complications unless they affect the function of the transplanted organs.

See *I.C.21.c.3 for transplant organ removal status*

See *I.C.2.r for malignant neoplasm associated with transplanted organ.*

EXAMPLE | A patient with a previous intestinal transplant presents with diarrhea which has been diagnosed as acute graft versus host disease, T86.858, D89.810, R19.7, Y83.0.

(b) *Kidney transplant complications*

Patients who have undergone kidney transplant may still have some form of chronic kidney disease (CKD) because the kidney transplant may not fully restore kidney function. Code T86.1- should be assigned for documented complications of a kidney transplant, such as transplant failure or rejection or other transplant complication. Code T86.1- should not be assigned for post kidney transplant patients who have chronic kidney (CKD) unless a transplant complication such as transplant failure or rejection is documented. If the documentation is unclear as to whether the patient has a complication of the transplant, query the provider.

Conditions that affect the function of the transplanted kidney, other than CKD, should be assigned a code from subcategory T86.1, Complications of transplanted organ, Kidney, and a secondary code that identifies the complication.

For patients with CKD following a kidney transplant, but who do not have a complication such as failure or rejection, *see section I.C.14. Chronic kidney disease and kidney transplant status.*

EXAMPLE | Patient with history of kidney transplant presents to the ER with gastroenteritis. His review of systems documents CKD and hypertension, K52.9, N18.9, I12.9, Z94.0.

EXAMPLE | Patient with history of kidney transplant presents to hospital in acute renal failure due to rejection, T86.11, N17.9, Y83.0.

---

4) Complication codes that include the external cause

As with certain other T codes, some of the complications of care codes have the external cause included in the code. The code includes the nature of the complication as well as the type of procedure that caused the complication. No external cause code indicating the type of procedure is necessary for these codes.

5) Complications of care codes within the body system chapters

Intraoperative and postprocedural complication codes are found within the body system chapters with codes specific to the organs and structures of that body system. These codes should be sequenced first, followed by a code(s) for the specific complication, if applicable.

EXAMPLE | Patient recently had a below the knee amputation of his right leg. He now presents to the surgeon's office with an infection of the amputation stump, T87.43, Y83.5.

EXAMPLE | Patient presents to the ER with a nonfunctioning colostomy, K94.03, Y83.3.

Apply the General Coding Guidelines as found in Chapters 5, 6, and 7.

MAJOR DIFFERENCES BETWEEN ICD-10-CM AND ICD-9-CM

- The section on foreign bodies left behind during a procedure has been expanded to include the type of procedure.
- Many more complications of care are located in specific body system chapters.
- The coding for complications of kidney transplants has been expanded to include specific types of complications.
- Many ICD-10-CM complications of care include the external cause within the code.
- Pain due to a medical device is assigned codes found in the T-code section.

ANATOMY AND PHYSIOLOGY

Complications of surgical or medical care can affect any of the body systems. The anatomy and physiology of these body systems are outlined in their respective chapters. Find below some general guidelines that apply to complications.

CODING COMPLICATIONS

Several general guidelines should be kept in mind when coding complications.

- No time limit: can occur after medical care or surgery, either immediately or years later.
- Complications after surgery or medical care should be documented as such. Routine events such as fever in the immediate postoperative period are not considered postoperative complications.
- Coding of complications does not imply that poor care or improper care has been delivered.
- Codes for complications may be located in the chapter for specified body sites or under abortion and pregnancy.
- Codes for complications that affect multiple sites or body systems are usually located in codes T80-T88.
- "Iatrogenic" is a term that is used to signify that a condition is a result or complication of treatment.
- When in doubt as to whether the condition occurred as the result of a procedure or medical care, it is best practice to query the physician.
- Complications of surgical and medical care may require an External cause code in the range of Y83-Y84 for abnormal reactions or later complications, or Y62-Y69 if misadventure is stated.
- When the admission is for treatment of a complication resulting from surgery or other medical care, the complication code is sequenced as the principal diagnosis.
- If the complication is classified to T80-T88 and the code lacks necessary specificity to describe the complication, an additional code should be assigned for the specific complication.

Locating Complication Codes in the Alphabetic Index

When looking for a complication code in the index, the condition for which the patient is admitted should be referred to first (Figures 25-1 and 25-2).

| EXAMPLE | Patient was readmitted for treatment of postoperative intestinal obstruction following appendectomy, K91.3, Y83.6. |

Obstruction, obstructed, obstructive
(Continued)
intestine *(Continued)*
by gallstone K56.3
congenital (small) Q41.9
large Q42.9
specified part NEC Q42.8
neurogenic K56.0
Hirschsprung's disease or megacolon Q43.1
newborn P76.9
due to
fecaliths P76.8
inspissated milk P76.2
meconium (plug) P76.0
in mucoviscidosis E84.11
specified NEC P76.8
postoperative K91.3

FIGURE 25-1. Obstruction, intestine, postoperative.

Anemia *(Continued)*
paludal (*see also* Malaria) B54 *[D63.8]*
pernicious (congenital) (malignant) (progressive) D51.0
pleochromic D64.89
of sprue D52.8
posthemorrhagic (chronic) D50.0
acute D62
newborn P61.3
postoperative (postprocedural)
due to (acute) blood loss D62
chronic blood loss D50.0
specified NEC D64.9
postpartum O90.81

FIGURE 25-2. Postoperative blood loss anemia.

EXAMPLE
Anemia due to acute blood loss following a right total knee replacement using metal and plastic components for osteoarthritis, M17.9, D62, Y83.1, Y92.239, 0SRC0JZ.

When no entry is found under the main term for the condition, the term "complication" should be referenced (Figures 25-3 and 25-4).

EXAMPLE
Patient is admitted with tracheal stenosis of tracheostomy site, J95.03, Y83.3.
Note that this complication code is located in the respiratory chapter.

EXAMPLE
Patient admitted with cystitis due to indwelling urinary catheter, T83.51xA, N30.90, Y84.6.

Locating External Causes of Injury and Poisoning to Correspond With Complication Coding

To locate the corresponding external cause code for complications, begin by locating the Alphabetic Index to External Causes. This index follows the Alphabetic Index to Diseases. Locate the term *complication* to see the cross-references to other index entries (Figure 25-5).

For further detail on external cause codes, refer to Chapter 23 of this textbook.

Complication(s) *(Continued)*
  suture, permanent (wire) NEC *(Continued)*
    mechanical
      breakdown T85.612
      displacement T85.622
      malfunction T85.612
      malposition T85.622
      obstruction T85.692
      perforation T85.692
      protrusion T85.692
      specified NEC T85.692
    pain T85.84
    specified type NEC T85.89
    stenosis T85.85
    thrombosis T85.86
  tracheostomy J95.00
    granuloma J95.09
    hemorrhage J95.01
    infection J95.02
    malfunction J95.03
    mechanical J95.03
    obstruction J95.03
    specified type NEC J95.09
    tracheo-esophageal fistula
      J95.04

FIGURE 25-3. Tracheostomy complication.

Complication(s) *(Continued)*
  catheter (device) NEC *(Continued)*
    urethral, indwelling T83.89
      embolism T83.81
      fibrosis T83.82
      hemorrhage T83.83
      infection and inflammation T83.51
      mechanical
        breakdown T83.018
      pain T83.84

FIGURE 25-4. Urinary catheter complications, indwelling.

Complication (delayed) **of or following**
    (medical or surgical procedure) Y84.9
  with misadventure - *see* Misadventure
  amputation of limb(s) Y83.5
  anastomosis (arteriovenous) (blood
      vessel) (gastrojejunal) (tendon)
      (natural or artificial material) Y83.2
  aspiration (of fluid) Y84.4
    tissue Y84.8
  biopsy Y84.8

FIGURE 25-5. Cross-reference to other index entries under *complication* in the External cause index.

EXAMPLE During spinal surgery, the surgeon accidentally nicks the dura due to the amount of adhesions present in the spinal canal, G97.41, G96.12, Y83.8, Y92.234 (Figure 25-6).

CHAPTER-SPECIFIC COMPLICATIONS

In ICD-10-CM, many complications are found in specific chapters. Intraoperative and post procedural complications may be found within the body system chapters.

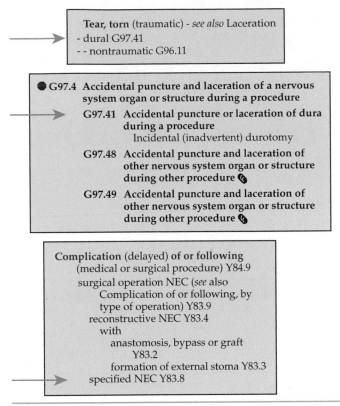

FIGURE 25-6. ICD-10-CM excerpts showing correct code assignment for accidental dural tear.

Complications of the Digestive System

Patients who have had some or part of their stomach removed or who have undergone gastric bypass surgery may be susceptible to a condition known as "**dumping syndrome.**"

This condition occurs when undigested contents of the stomach are transported to the small intestine too quickly. The symptoms of this condition may include abdominal cramping, nausea, and diarrhea, to name a few. Dumping syndrome may in turn result in weight loss or malnutrition. This syndrome may be treated with dietary changes, as well as with medications.

EXAMPLE   Patient presents with significant weight loss and abdominal pain following a gastric bypass performed for obesity. It is determined that she suffers from dumping syndrome, and dietary changes are suggested, K91.1, Z98.84, R63.4.

Complications of Gastrostomy, Colostomy, Enterostomy

Ostomies are surgically created openings into the body (Figure 25-7). Enterostomies and colostomies are created to discharge waste products from the body; gastrostomies are typically used for feeding or aspirating the contents of the stomach. Often, these surgically created openings result in complications. Complications associated with these openings are caused by a variety of problems such as infection, blockage of the opening, drainage or leakage around the opening, breakage of the device, and granulation of tissue.

If a patient presents to the hospital with a chief complaint of a percutaneous endoscopic gastrostomy (PEG) tube falling out, the principal diagnosis would be Z43.1, or attention to gastrostomy, because no complications resulted from the gastrostomy itself.

EXAMPLE   Patient is admitted for a clogged gastrostomy tube, Z43.1.

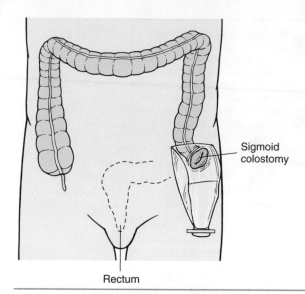

FIGURE 25-7. Colostomy. The opening in the colon is brought to the surface of the skin to divert feces into an external pouch worn by the patient.

EXAMPLE Patient is being treated for an enterocutaneous fistula in the colostomy, K94.09, Y83.3.

EXAMPLE Patient presents with cellulitis of the abdominal wall due to an infected colostomy site. The organism responsible for the cellulitis is *Staph aureus,* K94.02, L03.311, B95.61, Y83.3.

Complications of the Genitourinary System

Occasionally, hematuria occurs as the result of a traumatic injury due to forceful removal of a urinary catheter. This is coded as injury of the urethra, with hematuria assigned as an additional code. In some cases, it may be appropriate to assign an External cause code to indicate the cause and intent of the injury.

EXAMPLE Hematuria due to patient pulling out indwelling urinary catheter, S37.30xA, R31.9, X58.xxxA.

Hematuria is expected after many urinary procedures and should not be coded unless it is excessive and has been documented as such by the physician.

Complications of Dialysis

Several complications may result from dialysis treatment. Many of these conditions are included in other chapters of the ICD-10-CM book. **Dialysis disequilibrium syndrome**, which is characterized by weakness, dizziness, headache, and, in severe cases, mental status changes, is a complication of dialysis. Electrolyte imbalances such as hyperkalemia, hyponatremia, hypocalcemia, hypermagnesemia, and acidosis may also occur. Hypotension and fluid overload can complicate the care of the patient on dialysis. Occasionally, some of these conditions occur because the patient has been noncompliant with dialysis treatment and/or medications and diet. Complications associated with dialysis catheters may be due to infection or mechanical malfunction. If an infection is present, an additional code may be needed to identify specified infections and causative organisms.

EXAMPLE | Patient with ESRD was admitted to the hospital with noncardiogenic fluid overload due to noncompliance with dialysis treatment. Patient has a history of CHF and is on Lasix, E87.79, I50.9, N18.6, Z91.15, Z99.2.

EXAMPLE | Patient has dialysis disequilibrium syndrome due to hemodialysis for end-stage renal failure, E87.8, N18.6, Z99.2, Y84.1.

EXAMPLE | Leakage of peritoneal dialysis catheter. Patient is on dialysis for end-stage renal disease. Peritoneal catheter was removed, T85.631A, N18.6, Z99.2, Y84.1, 0WPGX0Z.

Complications of the Musculoskeletal System

Common complications of joint replacement include infection, blood clot, nerve injury, loosening, dislocation, wear and tear, and breakage of the prosthesis. It may be necessary to remove the prosthesis and insert a new prosthesis. Any time the joint is replaced or revised after the initial replacement this would be considered a revision.

EXAMPLE | Patient presents with dislocation of a right hip replacement. An open revision must be performed, T84.020A, Y83.1, 0SW90JZ (Figure 25-8).

Malunion/Nonunion of Fractures

Malunion of a fracture occurs when the fracture fragments have united but are not properly aligned. Incorrectly positioned bones may demonstrate angulation, rotation, and shortening. The degree and severity of the malunion will determine the selection of treatment, which may include surgery (Figure 25-9).

Nonunion of a fracture occurs when bony healing is not achieved at the fracture site. A fracture site that fails to heal within approximately 6 to 9 months of the injury represents a nonunion (Figure 25-10).

joint prosthesis, internal T84.9
  breakage (fracture) T84.01-
  dislocation T84.02-
  fracture T84.01-
  instability T84.02-
  subluxation T84.02-
  infection or inflammation
      T84.50
    hip T84.5-
    knee T84.5-
    specified joint NEC T84.59
  malposition - *see* Complications,
      joint prosthesis, mechanical,
      displacement
  mechanical
    breakage, broken T84.01-
    dislocation T84.02-
    fracture T84.01-
    instability T84.02-
    subluxation T84.02-

FIGURE 25-8. Complication of hip replacement.

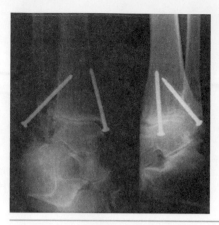

FIGURE 25-9. Surgical correction of malunion ankle fracture.

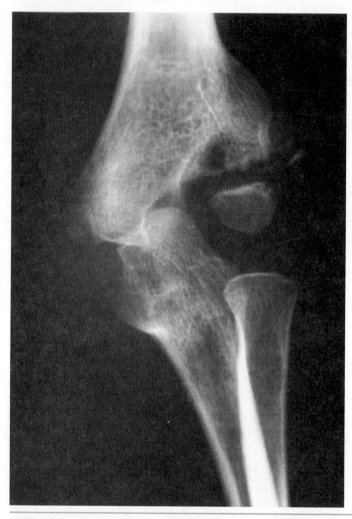

FIGURE 25-10. Nonunion of the lateral humeral condyle.

Malunion or nonunion may occur as the result of insufficient or improper reduction and immobilization, infection, metabolic bone disease, poor nutrition, and/or inadequate blood supply. Improper healing may be noted in cases of traumatic fracture and pathologic fracture and is considered a "late effect" of a fracture.

EXAMPLE	Patient's x-rays showed nonunion of left tibial shaft fracture which is a late effect of a fall, S82.202K, W19xxxS.

EXAMPLE	Patient presents with pain and swelling in the ankle status post casting 3 weeks ago. Patient suffered a closed fracture of the left ankle from falling down the stairs. It is determined that the patient has a malunion of the fracture, and the patient is scheduled next week for surgery to correct the malunion, S82.892P, W10.9xxD.

Complications of the Nervous System and Sense Organs

One of the most common complications discussed in this chapter is a spinal headache. A spinal headache, which is also known as a postdural puncture headache, may occur following a spinal tap (lumbar puncture) or spinal anesthesia. These headaches are caused by spinal fluid that is leaking from the puncture site of the procedure. The patient may experience nausea, vomiting, dizziness, ringing in the ears, and/or sensitivity to light. Treatment for the headache consists of lying flat and drinking fluids, particularly those that include caffeine. If these conservative treatments do not help, an epidural blood patch to seal the puncture hole may be required.

EXAMPLE	Patient develops a severe headache 1 day post lumbar puncture performed because of high fever and stiff neck to rule out meningitis, attending documents post-procedural headache, G97.1, R50.9, M43.6, Y83.4, 009U3ZX.

Complications of the Respiratory System

A **pulmonary embolism** (PE) is a blockage in an artery of the lung that can be life threatening. This blockage commonly is caused by a blood clot that started in the leg and then traveled to the lung. A pulmonary embolism may occur as a result of a surgical procedure. If a patient has recently had surgery and presents with sudden shortness of breath, chest pain, or cough, a pulmonary embolism may be suspected. To determine whether a patient has a PE, scans or angiograms may be performed. Treatment consists of anticoagulant drugs such as heparin. When a condition is the result of treatment, it is referred to as iatrogenic.

EXAMPLE	Patient presents with shortness of breath and chest pain. Two weeks before presentation, the patient had a right total hip replacement. A pulmonary angiogram is performed, as is a Doppler ultrasound of the legs. The attending documents that the patient is positive for both a pulmonary embolism in the pulmonary artery and a right lower leg deep vein thrombosis secondary to recent surgery, T81.718A, T81.72xA, I26.99, I82.401, I97.89, Z96.649, Y83.1.

A pneumothorax is another condition that can result from medical treatment. A **pneumothorax** is air in the space around the lung. Procedures such as central venous lines, chest tubes, and mechanical ventilation may inadvertently cause a traumatic pneumothorax. A patient may have symptoms of chest pain or shortness of breath. A chest x-ray or CT scan can be used to diagnose this condition.

EXAMPLE	Patient with a chronic cough undergoes a left transbronchial right lung biopsy. A chest x-ray is performed following this procedure, and a pneumothorax is noted. Attending physician decides that since the pneumothorax is small, the condition will be monitored by chest x-ray, R05, J95.811, Y83.8, Y92.234, 0BBK8ZX.

Patients with tracheostomies often develop complications related to the tracheostomy site. A patient can have infection or bleeding or mechanical complications at the site.

EXAMPLE | Patient presents with cellulitis of the neck secondary to an infected tracheostomy site, J95.02, L03.221, Y83.3.

Ventilator associated pneumonia is a type of hospital acquired pneumonia (HAP) that may occur in people who have been on a ventilator.

As with any postprocedural complication, code assignment must be based on provider documentation of the relationship between the procedure and condition. In the case of ventilator associated pneumonia, the provider must document the association of the use of a ventilator with the pneumonia. If the documentation is unclear about the association, the provider may be queried. An additional code may be used to identify the organism (B95-, B96-, B97-).

It is possible for a patient to be admitted with pneumonia and later develop ventilator associated pneumonia. In this case, the code for pneumonia would be assigned as the principal diagnosis with the complication code for the VAP assigned as a secondary diagnosis.

Ventilation pneumonitis is not the same as ventilator associated pneumonia. Ventilation pneumonitis is the result of inhalation of organisms growing in air conditioning systems.

EXAMPLE | Patient is admitted to the hospital with pneumonia. After reviewing the records from an outside hospital, the physician documents that it appears this pneumonia is due to the use of a ventilator on the previous admission, J95.851, Y84.8, Y92.239.

EXERCISE 25-1

Assign codes to the following conditions.

1. Patient is seen in the office after placement of a gastrostomy tube that is now malfunctioning _____

2. Two weeks prior to this admission patient had a resection of the intestine. The patient is now being seen for excessive vomiting following this surgery _____

3. Patient presents following a hysterectomy with pelvic pain and is now diagnosed with residual ovary syndrome _____

4. One month prior to this visit the patient had a left total knee replacement. The patient presents with pain and swelling of the knee and is diagnosed with an infection of the knee prosthesis _____

5. Patient is noted to have cerebral spinal fluid (CSF) leaking from the nose following a lumbar puncture _____

6. Patient with peritoneal dialysis catheter presents with inflammation of the skin around the catheter; patient had ESRD, initial encounter _____

7. Patient with pelvic inflammatory disease attributed to an intrauterine device (IUD), subsequent encounter _____

8. Patient is admitted for removal of her intramedullary rod because of acute leg pain, subsequent encounter _____

9. Cellulitis of the skin of the right knee due to right knee replacement, initial encounter _____

10. Patient with a transplanted lung presents with pneumonia _____

11. Patient is rejecting transplanted kidney _____

12. Patient has graft-versus-host disease; status post bone marrow transplant _____

13. Patient with an intestine transplant presents with dehydration _____

14. Patient with a ventricular shunt presents with severe headache due to stenosis of the shunt; patient has hydrocephalus _____

15. Patient with an abscess of a gastrostomy tube site due to *Staph aureus* _____

16. Patient with left pleural effusion develops iatrogenic pneumothorax following insertion of a chest tube _____

COMPLICATIONS OF SURGICAL AND MEDICAL CARE NOT ELSEWHERE CLASSIFIED (T80-T88)

Complications of Surgical and Medical Care, codes T80-T88 are found in ICD-10-CM, in Chapter 19 (Figure 25-11).

It is important to note that the instructional notes for this section remind the user to use an additional code to identify the specified condition that results from the complication, as well as an additional code from Y62-Y82 to identify the devices involved and the details of the circumstances. It is also important to note the many excludes2 notes in this section.

Complications of surgical and medical care, not elsewhere classified (T80-T88)
Use additional code for adverse effect, if applicable, to identify drug (T36-T50 with fifth or sixth character 5)
Use additional code(s) to identify the specified condition resulting from the complication
Use additional code to identify devices involved and details of circumstances (Y62-Y82)
Excludes2: any encounters with medical care for postprocedural conditions in which no complications are present, such as:
    artificial opening status (Z93.-)
    closure of external stoma (Z43.-)
    fitting and adjustment of external prosthetic device (Z44.-)
    burns and corrosions from local applications and irradiation (T20-T32)
    complications of surgical procedures during pregnancy, childbirth and the puerperium (O00-O9A)
    mechanical complication of respirator [ventilator] (J95.850)
    poisoning and toxic effects of drugs and chemicals (T36-T65 with fifth or sixth character 1-4 or 6)
    postprocedural fever (R50.82)
    specified complications classified elsewhere, such as:
    cerebrospinal fluid leak from spinal puncture (G97.0)
    colostomy malfunction (K94.0-)
    disorders of fluid and electrolyte imbalance (E86-E87)
    functional disturbances following cardiac surgery (I97.0-I97.1)
    intraoperative and postprocedural complications of specified body systems (D78.-, E36.-, E89.-, G97.3-, G97.4, H59.3-, H59.-, H95.2-, H95.3, I97.4-, I97.5, J95.6-, J95.7, K91.6-, L76.-, M96.-, N99.-)
    ostomy complicatons (J95.0-, K94-, N99.5-)
    postgastric surgery syndromes (K91.1)
    postlaminectomy syndrome NEC (M96.1)
    postmastectomy lymphedema syndrome (I97.2)
    postsurgical blind-loop syndrome (K91.2)
    ventilator associated pneumonia (J95.851)

FIGURE 25-11. Instruction notes for Complications of Surgical and Medical Care.

Complications Following Infusion, Transfusion, and Therapeutic Injection

There are many and varied risks that can be associated with infusions, transfusions, and injections. Some reactions may be minor and consist of fevers or urticarial reactions. Others can be more serious such as thrombosis, infections, and even shock.

There are codes in ICD-10-CM that cover the **extravasation** (i.e., the leakage of infused substances into the vasculature or into the subcutaneous tissue). If this occurs, there can be significant complications or tissue breakdown. Medicinal drugs that may cause only slight damage if extravasated are called irritants, and medicinal drugs that may cause severe damage, up to tissue necrosis, if extravasated are called vesicants. Common chemotherapeutic irritant drugs are bleomycin, carboplatin, cisplatin, and doxorubicin. Common chemotherapeutic vesicant drugs are doxorubicin, paclitaxel, and vinicristine.

EXAMPLE | Patient received her first infusion of chemotherapy yesterday. She returns to the office today with blistering on the right forearm. It appears that the chemotherapeutic agent has infiltrated, T80.810A, T22.611A, Y84.8.

EXAMPLE | After transfusion, patient presents with thrombophlebitis of right arm, T80.1xxA, I80.8, Y84.8.

EXAMPLE | Sepsis due to central line, T80.211A, A41.9, Y84.8.

Complications of Procedures, Not Elsewhere Classified

This category describes complications that may occur as the result of procedures but are not described by other specific codes. A second code to identify the exact type of complication may be required with this category.

EXAMPLE | Patient is admitted for treatment of a postoperative wound infection. The patient has developed cellulitis of the abdominal wound, T81.4xxA, L03.311, Y83.8.

EXAMPLE | Dehiscence of an external abdominal wound following cholecystectomy, T81.31xA, Y83.6.

EXAMPLE | Patient presents to the ER with terrible abdominal pain and fever. After performing abdominal x-rays it was discovered that she had a foreign object in her abdomen. She had a cesarean section 6 months prior to this presentation. It appears that the intestine has been perforated by this foreign object, T81.530A, K63.1, Y83.8.

EXAMPLE | Patient has acute osteomyelitis of femur secondary to infected right hip replacement, T84.51xA, M86.151, Z96.641, Y83.1.

Complications of Internal Prosthetic Devices, Implants, and Grafts

Categories T82-T85 are concerned with mechanical complications of prosthetic devices, implants, and grafts, as well as infection and inflammatory reactions due to other internal prosthetic devices, implants, and grafts. Mechanical complications may include items such as breakdown, displacement, leakage, and obstruction of the device implant or graft. For example:

- T82 Complications of cardiac and vascular prosthetic devices, implants, and grafts
- T82.1- through T82.5- Mechanical complications of cardiac and vascular prosthetic devices, implants, and grafts
  - Breakdown
  - Displacement

- Leakage
- Obstruction

■ T82.6- through T82.7- Infection and inflammatory reaction to cardiac and vascular devices, implants, and grafts

■ T82.8- Other specified complications of cardiac and vascular devices, implants, and grafts
  - Embolism
  - Fibrosis
  - Hemorrhage
  - Pain
  - Stenosis
  - Thrombosis
  - Other

■ T82.9- Unspecified complications of cardiac and vascular prosthetic devices, implants, and grafts

Mechanical Complications

Mechanical complications involve equipment malfunctions. If a device is causing a problem or complication such as breakdown, displacement, leakage, obstruction, perforation, or protrusion, the code assigned would be from the section on mechanical complications.

EXAMPLE

Patient has ascending cholangitis related to clogged biliary stent, T85.590A, K83.0, Y83.8 (Figure 25-12).

EXAMPLE

Patient has a leaking breast implant, T85.43xA, Y83.1.

Infections and Inflammatory Reactions Due to Prosthetic Device, Implants, and Grafts

The presence of a device, implant, or graft carries a risk of infection. It is important to note that the codes in this section may give instruction to use an additional code to identify specified infections.

Complication(s) *(Continued)*
  bile duct implant (prosthetic) T85.89
    embolism T85.81
    fibrosis T85.82
    hemorrhage T85.83
    infection and inflammation T85.79
    mechanical
      breakdown T85.510
      displacement T85.520
      malfunction T85.510
      malposition T85.520
      obstruction T85.590
      perforation T85.590
      protrusion T85.590
      specified NEC T85.590
    pain T85.84
    specified type NEC T85.89
    stenosis T85.85
    thrombosis T85.86

FIGURE 25-12. Complications of devices.

EXAMPLE | Patient has sepsis due to a dialysis catheter, T82.7xxA, A41.9, Y84.1.

Other Specified Complications

Devices can also cause embolisms, thrombosis, stenosis, and fibrosis, as well as hemorrhage and pain. When these conditions are documented they will be found in "Other specified complications."

EXAMPLE | Patient is admitted to remove prosthetic right hip because of severe hip pain, T84.84xA, Y83.1, 0SP90JZ.

EXAMPLE | Patient with a right arm dialysis graft in place is admitted because of an embolism in the graft, Patient has ESRD. An upper vein thrombectomy was performed, T82.818A, I82.601, N18.6, Y84.1, 05CY0ZZ.

EXAMPLE | Patient with CAD is admitted because of coronary artery stent restenosis and to percutaneously insert new drug-eluting stent, T82.857A, I25.10, Y83.8, 027034Z.

Complications of Transplanted Organs and Tissue

Complications of a transplanted organ include rejection or any posttransplant illnesses that affect the function of a transplanted organ. If illness affects the transplanted organ, two codes are required. The exceptions per guidelines are those patients with a kidney transplant and chronic kidney disease (CKD). In those cases, T86.1- should be used only for complications such as rejection, failure, or a medical condition such as infection affecting the transplanted organ. If documentation is unclear as to whether the CKD is a complication the provider should be queried.

EXAMPLE | Acute pyelonephritis of transplanted kidney, T86.13, N39.0, Y83.0.

Posttransplant surgical complications that do not affect the function of the transplanted organ are coded to the specific surgical complications.

EXAMPLE | Patient presents for heart transplant (donor is a victim of a car accident) due to primary cardiomyopathy and postoperatively develops renal failure, I42.9, N99.0, N19, Y83.0, Y92.239, 02YA0Z0.
   In this case, the complication is affecting the urinary system, not the heart, which is the transplanted organ.

Preexisting conditions or medical conditions that develop after transplant are not coded as complications unless they affect the transplanted organ. Code Z94.- is used as an additional code to identify transplant status when no complications are associated with the transplanted organ. Codes Z94.- and T86 are **NEVER** used together.

EXAMPLE | Patient is admitted for treatment of primary liver cancer. Patient had a liver transplant 2 years ago, T86.49, C80.2, C22.8, Y83.0.

Complications Peculiar to Reattachment and Amputation

Some common complications of amputations include infections, neuromas, necrosis, and contractures.

- **Neuroma** is a growth made up of a bundle of nerve fibers.
- **Contracture** is a tightening of muscle and skin that prevents normal movement.
- **Necrosis** is the decay of tissue.

EXAMPLE | Patient is seen in the physician's office following a below-the-knee amputation of the left leg. The patient is complaining of a burning pain in the leg. The physician documents a neuroma of the stump, T87.34, Y83.5.

Other Complications of Surgical and Medical Care, Not Elsewhere Classified

This category contains some anesthesia complications as well as some codes that don't fall into other more specified categories.

EXAMPLE | Hospitalist is called to the ER because of a difficult intubation, T88.4xxA.

EXAMPLE | Patient is in the OR for a colonoscopy. Versed and Demerol are administered via IV, and the patient immediately goes into shock, T88.6xxA, T41.1x5A.

EXERCISE 25-2

Assign diagnostic codes to the following conditions.

1. During a surgical procedure, patient goes into cardiac arrest   _____

2. After a surgical procedure, patient develops aspiration pneumonia   _____

3. Patient has a hemicolectomy and is readmitted to the hospital for intractable postoperative vomiting   _____

4. After spine surgery, patient becomes oliguric   _____

5. Patient is admitted for a *Staphylococcus aureus* infection of a right amputation stump of the lower extremity   _____

6. Patient is admitted for removal of a sponge left in during a hysterectomy, initial encounter   _____

7. Patient develops a hematoma of the operative wound, initial encounter, following an appendectomy   _____

8. Patient develops anaphylactic shock after a blood transfusion, initial encounter   _____

9. Patient develops seizures after electroconvulsive therapy (ECT)   _____

DOCUMENTATION/REIMBURSEMENT/MS-DRGs

Often, coding difficulties are due to lack of documentation. Sometimes pathology and other test results are not available at the time of discharge or when the physician is dictating the discharge summary or reporting the final diagnoses. Significant MS-DRG differences may result should the wrong principal diagnosis be selected.

UTI as a Principal Diagnosis versus UTI as a Postoperative Complication

EXAMPLE | A patient presents with UTI and the physician states status post prostatectomy 2 days prior to this admit.

DIAGNOSES	CODES	MS-DRG	RW
UTI	N39.0	690	0.7870
UTI as a postop infection	T81.4xxA	699	0.9998
	N39.0		
	Y83.9		

When patients have central lines, dialysis catheters, ports, or indwelling urinary catheters, to name a few, and they present with bacteremia/sepsis, it is important for the coder to verify whether the bacteremia/sepsis is due to the presence of these devices.

It is also important to realize that physicians do not often use the term "complication." If it is stated as UTI following appendectomy, it may be necessary to query the physician as to whether this is a postop complication, complication of a catheter, or not related to the surgery.

Pneumonia as a Principal Diagnosis versus Pneumonia as a Transplant Complication

EXAMPLE | Patient with a transplanted lung presents with pneumonia.

DIAGNOSES	CODES	MS-DRG	RW
Pneumonia h/o Kidney transplant	J18.9	194	1.0026
	Z94.0		
Pneumonia in transplanted lung	T86.812	205	1.3324
	J18.9		

In this case, if the transplant guideline was not applied, "a transplant code is only assigned if the complication affects the function of the transplant organ," a significant difference in payment would occur.

CHAPTER REVIEW EXERCISE

Where applicable, assign codes for diagnoses, procedures, and Z codes and external cause codes.

1. Postoperative septicemia, initial encounter _____

2. Internal wound dehiscence, initial encounter _____

3. Patient with abdominal adhesions due to surgical instrument left in body cavity, initial encounter _____

4. Perforation of coronary artery due to coronary artery stent insertion _____

5. During hemicolectomy, doctor inadvertently makes a rent in the intestine _____

6. Inflammation of the external stoma of the urinary tract _____

7. Rejection of a skin graft _____

8. Failure of an insulin pump. Patient has type 1 diabetes, initial encounter _____

9. Thrombophlebitis of the superficial vessels right lower extremity as the result of saphenous vein graft harvest, initial encounter _____

10. Patient had an outpatient cholecystectomy today. She is admitted _____
    this evening suffering with a postoperative embolic stroke.

11. Acute renal failure after surgery _____

12. Shock due to surgery, initial encounter _____

13. Severe hypertension after surgery _____

14. Hematoma of surgical site _____

15. After a transfusion of PRBC via the peripheral left arm vein, done _____
    percutaneously, patient develops high fever

16. Cytomegalovirus infection in transplanted kidney _____

17. Patient had a traumatic amputation of the right upper extremity 1 _____
    year ago after a farm accident. He presents with a neuroma of the
    amputation stump

CHAPTER GLOSSARY

Contracture: a tightening of muscle and skin that prevents normal movement.

Dialysis disequilibrium syndrome: characterized by weakness, dizziness, headache, and, in severe cases, mental status changes.

Dumping syndrome: occurs when undigested contents of the stomach are transported to the small intestine too quickly.

Extravasation: leakage of infused substance into vasculature or subcutaneous tissue.

Iatrogenic: caused by medical treatment.

Malunion: of a fracture occurs when the fracture fragments have united but are not properly aligned. Incorrectly positioned bones may demonstrate angulation, rotation, and shortening.

Mechanical complication: when a device or equipment malfunctions.

Necrosis: the decay of tissue.

Neuroma: a growth made up of a bundle of nerve fibers.

Nonunion: of a fracture occurs when bony healing is not achieved at the fracture site. A fracture site that fails to heal within approximately 6 to 9 months of the injury represents a nonunion.

Ostomies: surgically created openings in the body.

Pneumothorax: air in space around the lung.

Pulmonary embolism: blood clot(s) in the pulmonary artery that causes blockage in the artery.

26

Reimbursement Methodologies

LEARNING OBJECTIVES

1. Describe the complexities of MS-DRGs and hospital reimbursement
2. Explain the difference between optimization and maximization
3. Identify key elements of a UB-04
4. Describe the elements and purpose of the charge description master (CDM)
5. Explain medical necessity
6. Calculate case-mix index (CMI)
7. Explain the role of Quality Improvement Organizations (QIOs)
8. Explain the purpose of PEPPER
9. Explain the purpose of Recovery Audit Contract (RAC)
10. Describe the purpose of a clinical documentation improvement program

ABBREVIATIONS/ ACRONYMS

AHIMA American Health Information Management Association

ALOS average length of stay

CC complication/comorbidity

CDIP Clinical Documentation Improvement Program

CDM charge description master

CHF congestive heart failure

CMI case-mix index

CMS Centers for Medicare and Medicaid Services

**ABBREVIATIONS/
ACRONYMS**—*cont'd*

COPD chronic obstructive pulmonary disease

CPT *Current Procedural Terminology*

DHHS U.S. Department of Health and Human Services

DRA Deficit Reduction Act

GMLOS geometric length of stay

HAC hospital acquired condition

HCPCS Healthcare Common Procedure Coding System

HH Home Health

HMO Health Maintenance Organization

HPR hospital payment rate

ICD-9-CM *International Classification of Diseases, 9th Revision, Clinical Modification*

ICD-10-CM *International Classification of Diseases, 10th Revision, Clinical Modification*

ICD-10-PCS *International Classification of Diseases, 10th Revision, Procedure Coding System*

IPPS Inpatient Prospective Payment System

LCDs local coverage determinations

LMRP local medical review policies

LOS length of stay

LTC long-term care

MAC Medicare Administrative Contractor

MDC major diagnostic category

MI myocardial infarction

MIC Medicaid Integrity Contractor

MS-DRG Medicare Severity diagnosis-related group

NCDs national coverage determinations

NPI National Provider Identifier

PEPPER Program for Evaluating Payment Patterns Electronic Report

POA present on admission

PPO Preferred Provider Organization

PPS Prospective Payment System

QIO Quality Improvement Organization

RAC Recovery Audit Contract

RPS retrospective payment system

RW relative weight

SNF skilled nursing facility

SOW scope of work

TEFRA Tax Equity and Fiscal Responsibility Act

UB-04 Uniform Bill-04

ZPIC Zone Program Integrity Contractor

INTRODUCTION TO REIMBURSEMENT

Reimbursement or payment for healthcare services has evolved over time into a complicated system with many rules and guidelines that must be followed if proper payment is to be received from third party payers. Rules and guidelines vary, depending on which healthcare setting or third party payer is involved. A **third party payer** makes payments on behalf of the patient for health services. Third party payers may include government programs, insurance companies, and managed care plans.

Private Plans

A variety of private plans (commercial payer) are provided by companies such as Blue Cross/Blue Shield, Aetna, Cigna, and Travelers. These plans are available in different formats, including the following:

- **Self-insured plans**—self-insurance fund set up by an employer to provide health claim benefits for employees.
- **Health Maintenance Organization (HMO)**—type of managed care in which hospitals, physicians, and other providers contract to provide health care for patients, usually at a discounted rate.
- **Preferred Provider Organization (PPO)**—type of managed care in which hospitals, physicians, and other providers have an arrangement with a third party payer to provide health care at discounted rates to third party payer clients.

Because Medicare is the predominant payer for healthcare services, this text focuses on Medicare's reimbursement system. Of note, many private and commercial payers have adopted the Medicare reimbursement system.

Government Plans

Medicare is a federal entitlement program administered by the Centers for Medicare and Medicaid Services (CMS) for patients over 65 years of age, certain disabled individuals, and those with end-stage renal disease.

Medicaid is a federal and state insurance plan, administered by the states and managed by the Social Security Administration of the federal government for patients whose income and resources are insufficient to pay for health care.

TRICARE, previously known as CHAMPUS (Civilian Health and Medical Program for the Uniformed Services), is a medical program for active duty military members, qualified family members, non–Medicare-eligible retirees and their family members.

Workers' Compensation is a requirement of the federal government for employers to cover employees who are injured or become sick on the job. It is managed by various plans chosen by the employer or by state governments.

Medicare

After many years of debate in Congress, in July 1965, the House and Senate passed the bill that established Medicare, an insurance program designed to provide all older adults with comprehensive health care coverage at an affordable cost. In 1972, Medicare eligibility was extended to people with disabilities and those with end-stage renal disease.

The Social Security Act was responsible for the establishment of the Medicare program. As a result of this, the government became more involved in the delivery of health care. The government wanted to ensure that Medicare participants received both quality health care and medically necessary services.

Medicare is a federal health insurance program that is divided into parts according to the type of coverage.

Part A: Hospital Insurance. To be eligible for Part A hospital insurance, one must have worked or must have had a spouse who worked a minimum of 40 quarters of Medicare-covered employment. Part A of Medicare pays for inpatient hospital, skilled nursing facility, and some home health care. Medicare pays all costs for each benefit period (60 days), except for the deductible (which changes each year).

Part B: Medical Insurance. To be eligible for Part B insurance, one must meet the same requirements as for Part A. A premium (that changes each year) is deducted from a person's Social Security check for Part B coverage. Part B Medicare covers Medicare-eligible physician services, outpatient hospital services, certain home health services, and durable medical equipment. A yearly deductible (that changes each year) and a 20% co-payment amount are applied to these services.

Part C: Medicare Advantage Plans. Medicare Advantage Plans are run by private companies and are similar to HMOs and PPOs. They provide more choices and sometimes additional benefits. They offer all the benefits provided by Part A and Part B, but some also may provide prescription drug coverage (Part D). Patients may be required to use certain hospitals and physicians in the service area.

Part D: Prescription Drug Coverage. This is an optional program for prescription drug coverage. Medicare prescription drug coverage is available to anyone who is covered by Medicare.

DIAGNOSIS-RELATED GROUPS/MEDICARE SEVERITY DIAGNOSIS-RELATED GROUPS

DRGs were developed at Yale University in the late 1960s to monitor quality of care and utilization of services. DRGs were not intended to be a means of determining hospital reimbursement. In 1982, the Tax Equity and Fiscal Responsibility Act (TEFRA) mandated limits on Medicare payments to hospitals. The government decided to use the DRG classification system, a prospective payment system (PPS), to pay for services rendered to Medicare inpatients. A **prospective payment system** is a method of reimbursement in which payment is made according to a predetermined, fixed amount rather than on the basis of billed charges.

The government implemented a prospective payment system in an effort to control the costs of inpatient hospital stays. The DRG system had some inequities in that a patient with multiple complication(s) or comorbid condition(s) is assigned that same DRG and receives the same payment as the patient who has just one complication or comorbid condition. Larger hospitals and tertiary care centers may present greater financial risks because they routinely care for patients who are severely ill. As a result, CMS implemented the Medicare Severity diagnosis-related groups (MS-DRGs), which became effective on October 1, 2007.

ICD-10-CM/PCS codes will be used to determine the Medicare Severity diagnosis-related group (MS-DRG). First, a patient is assigned to an MDC (Figure 26-1) on the basis of the principal diagnosis code; next, it is determined whether the case is a "medical" or a

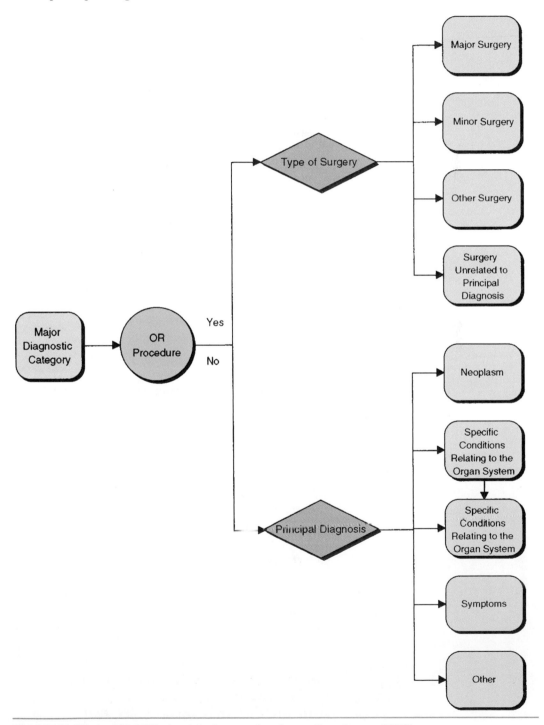

FIGURE 26-1. MS-DRG structure for a major diagnostic category (MDC).

"surgical" case. If no procedures are identified, a medical MS-DRG is assigned. Patients who undergo a valid operating room procedure or another non–operating room procedure that affects MS-DRG assignment are assigned a surgical MS-DRG. It is logical that a patient who has undergone a surgical procedure would use more resources because of costs associated with anesthesia, operating and recovery rooms, and additional nursing care.

The MS-DRG classification system is divided into 25 major diagnostic categories (MDCs), which are based on all possible principal diagnoses that often correspond with an organ system.

MDC 1	Diseases and Disorders of the Nervous System
MDC 2	Diseases and Disorders of the Eye
MDC 3	Diseases and Disorders of the Ear, Nose, Mouth, and Throat
MDC 4	Diseases and Disorders of the Respiratory System
MDC 5	Diseases and Disorders of the Circulatory System
MDC 6	Diseases and Disorders of the Digestive System
MDC 7	Diseases and Disorders of the Hepatobiliary System and Pancreas
MDC 8	Diseases and Disorders of the Musculoskeletal System and Connective Tissue
MDC 9	Diseases and Disorders of the Skin, Subcutaneous Tissue, and Breast
MDC 10	Endocrine, Nutritional, and Metabolic Diseases and Disorders
MDC 11	Diseases and Disorders of the Kidney and Urinary Tract
MDC 12	Diseases and Disorders of the Male Reproductive System
MDC 13	Diseases and Disorders of the Female Reproductive System
MDC 14	Pregnancy, Childbirth, and the Puerperium
MDC 15	Newborns and Other Neonates with Conditions Originating in the Perinatal Period
MDC 16	Diseases and Disorders of the Blood and Blood-Forming Organs and Immunologic Disorders
MDC 17	Myeloproliferative Diseases and Disorders, and Poorly Differentiated Neoplasms
MDC 18	Infectious and Parasitic Diseases (Systemic or unspecified sites).
MDC 19	Mental Diseases and Disorders
MDC 20	Alcohol/Drug Use and Alcohol/Drug-Induced Organic Mental Disorders
MDC 21	Injuries, Poisonings, and Toxic Effects of Drugs
MDC 22	Burns
MDC 23	Factors Influencing Health Status and Other Contacts with Health Services
MDC 24	Multiple Significant Trauma
MDC 25	Human Immunodeficiency Virus Infections

Pre MDC	MS-DRG	
	Heart transplant or implant of heart assist system with MCC	001
	Heart transplant or implant of heart assist system without MCC	002
	ECMO or trach with mechanical ventilation 96+ hr or PDX except face, mouth, and neck with major OR	003
	Trach with mechanical ventilation 96+ hr or PDX except face, mouth, and neck without major OR	004
	Liver transplant with MCC or intestinal transplant	005
	Liver transplant without MCC	006
	Lung transplant	007
	Simultaneous pancreas/kidney transplant	008
	Pancreas transplant	010
	Tracheostomy for face, mouth, and neck diagnoses with MCC	011
	Tracheostomy for face, mouth, and neck diagnoses with CC	012
	Tracheostomy for face, mouth, and neck diagnoses without CC/MCC	013
	Allogeneic bone marrow transplant	014
	Autologous bone marrow transplant with CC/MCC	016
	Autologous bone marrow transplant without CC/MCC	017

Other factors influencing MS-DRG assignment include:

- Patient's sex
- Patient's discharge disposition or status
- Secondary diagnoses and the presence or absence of complications or comorbidities (CC) or major complication or comorbidities (MCC)
- Birth weight for neonates
- Procedures used as proxy for CC/MCC

There are 751 MS-DRGs which group patients who have similar diagnoses, lengths of stay, and need for resources into a particular MS-DRG with a set payment rate. Specialized software called a **grouper** is used to assign the appropriate MS-DRG. Groupers are often included in the **encoder** or coding software that is used to assign diagnosis and procedure codes.

After completing a thorough review of the health record, the coder must determine the principal diagnosis on the basis of the UHDDS definition. The **principal diagnosis** is "the condition established after study to be chiefly responsible for occasioning the admission of the patient to the hospital for care." Then, codes for all secondary diagnoses and procedures can be assigned. Grouper software is used to determine the appropriate MS-DRG.

Changes may be made to ICD-10-CM/PCS codes each year. The government also makes changes to the MS-DRG system annually on October 1. These changes are published in the *Federal Register*, which is the official daily publication for rules, proposed rules, and notices of U.S. federal agencies and organizations, as well as for Executive Orders and other Presidential documents. MS-DRG changes are first published as a proposed rule, and a comment period is generally provided for the public prior to publishing of the final rule. The conversion of the MS-DRGs to ICD-10-CM/PCS was completed, and the *ICD-10 Definitions Manual* was posted in October of 2009. A team of researchers, physicians, clinical coding experts, MS-DRG analysts, and software programmers were involved in this conversion project.

MS-DRG OPTIMIZATION

Optimization is the process of striving to obtain optimal reimbursement or the highest possible payment to which the facility is legally entitled on the basis of coded data supported by documentation in the health record. It is often said that "If it is not documented, it was not done." If services were performed and not documented, payment for these services may be denied. On the other hand, **maximization** is the manipulation of codes to receive maximum reimbursement without supporting documentation in the health record or with disregard for coding conventions, guidelines, and UHDDS definitions. Maximization is unethical and is addressed in the American Health Information Management Association (AHIMA) Standards of Ethical Coding, which can be found in Chapter 1.

Not all MS-DRGs are affected by the presence of a secondary diagnosis. It can be determined by the MS-DRG title whether the MS-DRG is affected by the absence or presence of a CC or MCC. A **complication** is a condition that arises during a patient's hospitalization which may lead to increased resource use. A **comorbidity** is a preexisting condition (is present on admission) which may lead to increased resource use. The fact that a physician documents that a diagnosis is a complication during a patient's stay does not necessarily mean that diagnosis will fit the definition of a complication in the MS-DRG assignment. A physician may also document that the patient had no complications during hospital stay, and an assigned secondary diagnosis may qualify as a CC or MCC for that particular MS-DRG.

EXAMPLE

MS-DRG 193, Simple pneumonia and pleurisy with MCC, 1.4948
    MS-DRG 194, Simple pneumonia and pleurisy with CC, 1.0026
    MS-DRG 195, Simple pneumonia and pleurisy without MCC/CC, 0.7037

In the above example, one way to optimize MS-DRG 195 would be to review the record further for documentation of a secondary diagnosis that would qualify as CC or MCC.

Other ways to optimize in this case would be to review the record for the following:
- An organism that is responsible for the pneumonia
- Respiratory neoplasm
- Septicemia
- Mechanical ventilation
- Opportunistic lung infection in a patient with HIV
- Tracheostomy with mechanical ventilation over 96 hours

Remember, to optimize, supporting documentation must be included in the health record, and the definition for principal diagnosis must be met.

Some of the most commonly missed CCs or MCCs include the following:
- Atrial flutter
- Atelectasis
- Cachexia
- Cardiogenic shock
- Cardiomyopathy
- Cellulitis
- Chronic kidney disease, stages 4-5, including end-stage
- Chronic obstructive pulmonary disease (COPD)—exacerbation
- Diabetes mellitus with metabolic complications
- Hematemesis
- Hyponatremia
- Malnutrition
- Melena
- Pleural effusion
- Pneumothorax
- Respiratory failure
- Urinary tract infection

MS-DRG REIMBURSEMENT

Each MS-DRG payment is determined by two basic factors:
1. Relative weight of assigned MS-DRG
2. Individual hospital payment rate or base rate

Each MS-DRG is assigned a relative weight. The average relative weight factor is 1.0000. If a particular MS-DRG used twice as many resources as the average, it would be assigned a relative weight of 2.0000. If a particular MS-DRG used half as many resources as the average, it would be assigned a relative weight of 0.5000. Each year, MS-DRG relative weights are updated to reflect the following:
- Changes in treatment patterns
- Technology
- Any other factors that may change the use of hospital resources

Each hospital is assigned a base dollar amount as the hospital payment rate for a relative weight of 1.0000. Larger facilities that have more complicated cases and provide additional services may have higher hospital payment rates than smaller rural facilities. The individual hospital payment rate or base dollar amount is determined by the following:
- A regional or national adjusted standardized amount that considers the type of hospital
- Designation of large urban, urban, or rural hospital
- Wage index for the geographic area where the hospital is located

A hospital payment rate can change from time to time. It usually changes once a year, effective on October 1.

Relative weight (RW) is multiplied by the hospital's payment rate (HPR), to equal that hospital's MS-DRG reimbursement.

$$RW \times HPR = \text{MS-DRG payment}$$

EXAMPLE
> A patient who is admitted with pneumonia and is being treated for a urinary tract infection, which is a CC, is assigned to MS-DRG 194.
>
> Simple pneumonia and pleurisy with CC are assigned. If this hospital's payment rate is $6000.00, the MS-DRG payment would be calculated as follows. MS-DRG 194 has a relative weight of 1.0026.
>
> $$1.0026 \ (RW) \times \$6000.00 \ (HPR) = \$6015.60 \ (MS\text{-}DRG \ payment)$$

The MS-DRG payment is not based on actual charges for that patient during the hospital stay. If the patient had actual charges that totaled more than $10,000.00, the hospital would be paid only the MS-DRG payment. The hospital would not be able to bill the patient for any additional charges other than deductible and/or coinsurance amounts. If the patient had a hospital bill that totaled $5500.00, the hospital would still be paid the MS-DRG payment. The hospital would lose reimbursement in the first scenario but would gain reimbursement in the second case scenario.

The intent with a PPS system is that hospitals would know what they are going to be reimbursed for a particular type of patient before they render any services. The old payment method, or a retrospective payment system (RPS), was based on actual charges or a percentage of charges; this did not promote best practices and quality care because the hospital was paid on the basis of charges, and the higher the charges, the higher the payment. The amount of the payment is determined after the patient has been cared for and the charges assessed. If a patient experienced complications and the hospital bill went higher, the hospital was still paid. PPS provides incentive to decrease patient complications. Hospitals must provide quality care in an efficient manner to maintain a healthy bottom line.

Each hospital stay will fit into one and only one MS-DRG category. For example, if a patient was admitted because of osteoarthritis for a hip replacement and had a myocardial infarction (MI) 2 days after the procedure, the hip replacement MS-DRG is the one that will be assigned. No additional MS-DRG is assigned to pay for the costs associated with the MI. However, the MI is an MCC, and increased reimbursement would be received because of the assignment of an MS-DRG with MCC.

If more than one procedure is performed, the procedure in the highest surgical group will determine the MS-DRG assignment. For example, if the patient had a breast biopsy and a mastectomy during the same hospital stay, the mastectomy would determine the surgical MS-DRG.

PRESENT ON ADMISSION

The **Deficit Reduction Act** (DRA) mandates that as of October 1, 2007, all acute-care facilities reimbursed under Medicare Severity diagnosis-related groups (MS-DRGs) must identify and report diagnoses that are present at the time of a patient's admission. This policy change was implemented to save lives and dollars by no longer paying the extra costs of treating preventable errors, injuries, and infections that occur in hospitals. Medicare does not want to pay for conditions they consider preventable, such as pressure ulcers, injuries due to falls, infections caused by genitourinary catheters and central venous lines, or complications such as a sponge left in a patient during surgery.

The **present on admission** (POA) indicator (which follows) is to differentiate between conditions that develop during a particular hospital encounter and conditions that were present at the time of admission. Hospitals had 1-year grace period before their payment was affected by conditions that were not present at the time of admission. Most of these conditions will be identified by a particular ICD-9-CM diagnosis code, and the POA indicator on the UB-04. Coding staff will have to assign POA indicators to the ICD-9-CM codes that are assigned. This requirement places even more importance on accurate and complete documentation within the health record. In some instances it may be necessary to query the physician about whether a condition was present at the time of admission.

The Cooperating Parties have developed POA guidelines that are supplemental to the *ICD-9-CM Official Guidelines for Coding and Reporting* to assist with the application of the POA requirement. The indicators that are reported are the following:

- Y = Yes (present at the time of inpatient admission)
- N = No (not present at the time of inpatient admission)
- U = Unknown (documentation is insufficient to determine whether condition is present on admission)
- W = Clinically undetermined (provider is unable to clinically determine whether condition was present on admission)
- Unreported/Not used (Exempt from POA reporting). Electronic claims will have a "1."

The Centers for Medicare and Medicaid Services (CMS) has identified certain hospital-acquired conditions (HAC) and will no longer reimburse for the extra costs that are incurred as a result of these conditions. These conditions include the following:

- Catheter-associated urinary tract infection (UTI)
- Pressure ulcers (decubitus) stages 3 and 4
- Object left in the body during surgery
- Blood incompatibility (transfusion)
- Vascular catheter–associated infections (central line)
- Falls and trauma in the hospital
- Inadequate glycemic control
- Deep vein thrombosis and pulmonary embolism after orthopedic surgery
- Drug-induced delirium
- Surgical site infections following some orthopedic procedures and bariatric surgery for obesity
- Mediastinitis following coronary artery bypass graft (CABG)

As of October 1, 2008, these diagnoses do not count as an MCC/CC (major complication/comorbidity and complication/comorbidity) if they developed after the patient's admission to the hospital.

See the companion Evolve website for POA examples, which have been removed from the guidelines and will be published in *Coding Clinic* in the future. See the companion Evolve website for a listing of the categories and codes that are exempt from the diagnosis present on admission requirement.

Appendix I
Present on Admission Reporting Guidelines
(Effective with 2011 update)

Introduction

These guidelines are to be used as a supplement to the *ICD-10-CM Official Guidelines for Coding and Reporting* to facilitate the assignment of the Present on Admission (POA) indicator for each diagnosis and external cause of injury code reported on claim forms (UB-04 and 837 Institutional).

These guidelines are not intended to replace any guidelines in the main body of the *ICD-10-CM Official Guidelines for Coding and Reporting*. The POA guidelines are not intended to provide guidance on when a condition should be coded, but rather, how to apply the POA indicator to the final set of diagnosis codes that have been assigned in accordance with Sections I, II, and III of the official coding guidelines. Subsequent to the assignment of the ICD-10-CM codes, the POA indicator should then be assigned to those conditions that have been coded.

As stated in the Introduction to the ICD-10-CM Official Guidelines for Coding and Reporting, a joint effort between the healthcare provider and the coder is essential to achieve complete and accurate documentation, code assignment, and reporting of diagnoses and procedures. The importance of consistent, complete documentation in the medical record cannot be overemphasized. Medical record documentation from any provider involved in the care and treatment of the patient may be used to support the determination of whether a condition was present on admission or not. In the context of the official coding guidelines, the term "provider" means a physician or any qualified healthcare practitioner who is legally accountable for establishing the patient's diagnosis.

These guidelines are not a substitute for the provider's clinical judgment as to the determination of whether a condition was/was not present on admission. The provider should be queried regarding issues related to the linking of signs/symptoms, timing of test results, and the timing of findings.

General Reporting Requirements

All claims involving inpatient admissions to general acute care hospitals or other facilities that are subject to a law or regulation mandating collection of present on admission information.

Present on admission is defined as present at the time the order for inpatient admission occurs—conditions that develop during an outpatient encounter, including emergency department, observation, or outpatient surgery, are considered as present on admission.

POA indicator is assigned to principal and secondary diagnoses (as defined in Section II of the Official Guidelines for Coding and Reporting) and the external cause of injury codes.

Issues related to inconsistent, missing, conflicting or unclear documentation must still be resolved by the provider.

If a condition would not be coded and reported based on UHDDS definitions and current official coding guidelines, then the POA indicator would not be reported.

Reporting Options

Y—Yes

N—No

U—Unknown

W—Clinically undetermined

Unreported/Not used (or "1" for Medicare usage)—(Exempt from POA reporting)

Reporting Definitions

Y = present at the time of inpatient admission

N = not present at the time of inpatient admission

U = documentation is insufficient to determine if condition is present on admission

W = provider is unable to clinically determine whether condition was present on admission
or not

Timeframe for POA Identification and Documentation

There is no required timeframe as to when a provider (per the definition of "provider" used in these guidelines) must identify or document a condition to be present on admission. In some clinical situations, it may not be possible for a provider to make a definitive diagnosis (or a condition may not be recognized or reported by the patient) for a period of time after admission. In some cases it may be several days before the provider arrives at a definitive diagnosis. This does not mean that the condition was not present on admission. Determination of whether the condition was present on admission or not will be based on the applicable POA guideline as identified in this document, or on the provider's best clinical judgment.

If at the time of code assignment the documentation is unclear as to whether a condition was present on admission or not, it is appropriate to query the provider for clarification.

Assigning the POA Indicator

Condition is on the "Exempt from Reporting" list

Leave the "present on admission" field blank if the condition is on the list of ICD-10-CM codes for which this field is not applicable. This is the only circumstance in which the field may be left blank.

POA Explicitly Documented

Assign Y for any condition the provider explicitly documents as being present on admission.

Assign N for any condition the provider explicitly documents as not present at the time of admission.

Conditions diagnosed prior to inpatient admission

Assign "Y" for conditions that were diagnosed prior to admission (example: hypertension, diabetes mellitus, asthma)

Conditions diagnosed during the admission but clearly present before admission

Assign "Y" for conditions diagnosed during the admission that were clearly present but not diagnosed until after admission occurred.

Diagnoses subsequently confirmed after admission are considered present on admission if at the time of admission they are documented as suspected, possible, rule out, differential diagnosis, or constitute an underlying cause of a symptom that is present at the time of admission.

Condition develops during outpatient encounter prior to inpatient admission

Assign Y for any condition that develops during an outpatient encounter prior to a written order for inpatient admission.

Documentation does not indicate whether condition was present on admission

Assign "U" when the medical record documentation is unclear as to whether the condition was present on admission. "U" should not be routinely assigned and used only in very limited circumstances. Coders are encouraged to query the providers when the documentation is unclear.

Documentation states that it cannot be determined whether the condition was or was not present on admission

Assign "W" when the medical record documentation indicates that it cannot be clinically determined whether or not the condition was present on admission.

Chronic condition with acute exacerbation during the admission

If a single code identifies both the chronic condition and the acute exacerbation, see POA guidelines pertaining to combination codes.

If a single code only identifies the chronic condition and not the acute exacerbation (e.g., acute exacerbation of chronic leukemia), assign "Y."

Conditions documented as possible, probable, suspected, or rule out at the time of discharge

If the final diagnosis contains a possible, probable, suspected, or rule out diagnosis, and this diagnosis was based on signs, symptoms or clinical findings suspected at the time of inpatient admission, assign "Y."

If the final diagnosis contains a possible, probable, suspected, or rule out diagnosis, and this diagnosis was based on signs, symptoms or clinical findings that were not present on admission, assign "N".

Conditions documented as impending or threatened at the time of discharge

If the final diagnosis contains an impending or threatened diagnosis, and this diagnosis is based on symptoms or clinical findings that were present on admission, assign "Y".

If the final diagnosis contains an impending or threatened diagnosis, and this diagnosis is based on symptoms or clinical findings that were not present on admission, assign "N".

Acute and Chronic Conditions

Assign "Y" for acute conditions that are present at time of admission and N for acute conditions that are not present at time of admission.

Assign "Y" for chronic conditions, even though the condition may not be diagnosed until after admission.

If a single code identifies both an acute and chronic condition, see the POA guidelines for combination codes.

Combination Codes

Assign "N" if any part of the combination code was not present on admission (e.g., COPD with acute exacerbation and the exacerbation was not present on admission; gastric ulcer that does not start bleeding until after admission; asthma patient develops status asthmaticus after admission)

Assign "Y" if all parts of the combination code were present on admission (e.g., patient with acute prostatitis admitted with hematuria)

If the final diagnosis includes comparative or contrasting diagnoses, and both were present, or suspected, at the time of admission, assign "Y".

For infection codes that include the causal organism, assign "Y" if the infection (or signs of the infection) was present on admission, even though the culture results may not be known until after admission (e.g., patient is admitted with pneumonia and the provider documents pseudomonas as the causal organism a few days later).

Same Diagnosis Code for Two or More Conditions

When the same ICD-10-CM diagnosis code applies to two or more conditions during the same encounter (e.g. two separate conditions classified to the same ICD-10-CM diagnosis code):

Assign "Y" if all conditions represented by the single ICD-10-CM code were present on admission (e.g. bilateral unspecified age-related cataracts).

Assign "N" if any of the conditions represented by the single ICD-10-CM code was not present on admission (e.g. traumatic secondary and recurrent hemorrhage and seroma is assigned to a single code T79.2, but only one of the conditions was present on admission).

Obstetrical conditions

Whether or not the patient delivers during the current hospitalization does not affect assignment of the POA indicator. The determining factor for POA assignment is whether the pregnancy complication or obstetrical condition described by the code was present at the time of admission or not.

If the pregnancy complication or obstetrical condition was present on admission (e.g., patient admitted in preterm labor), assign "Y".

If the pregnancy complication or obstetrical condition was not present on admission (e.g., 2nd degree laceration during delivery, postpartum hemorrhage that occurred during current hospitalization, fetal distress develops after admission), assign "N".

If the obstetrical code includes more than one diagnosis and any of the diagnoses identified by the code were not present on admission assign "N".

(e.g., Category O11, Pre-existing hypertension with pre-eclampsia)

Perinatal conditions

Newborns are not considered to be admitted until after birth. Therefore, any condition present at birth or that developed in utero is considered present at admission and should be assigned "Y". This includes conditions that occur during delivery (e.g., injury during delivery, meconium aspiration, exposure to streptococcus B in the vaginal canal).

Congenital conditions and anomalies

Assign "Y" for congenital conditions and anomalies except for **categories** Q00-Q99, **Congenital anomalies**, which are **on the** exempt **list**. Congenital conditions are always considered present on admission.

External cause of injury codes

Assign "Y" for any external cause code representing an external cause of morbidity that occurred prior to inpatient admission (e.g., patient fell out of bed at home, patient fell out of bed in emergency room prior to admission)

Assign "N" for any external cause code representing an external cause of morbidity that occurred during inpatient hospitalization (e.g., patient fell out of hospital bed during hospital stay, patient experienced an adverse reaction to a medication administered after inpatient admission)

POST–ACUTE CARE TRANSFER POLICY

The U.S. Congress, through the Balanced Budget Act of 1997, required CMS to begin applying a slightly different payment methodology when transferring from acute care to a post–acute care setting. This payment methodology was already in place for transfers from an acute facility to another short-term acute care facility. Complicated formulas are used to determine the transfer-adjusted payment.

It was found that shortly after admission, many patients were transferred to other post–acute care settings, so CMS figured it was overpaying the hospitals for these patients. CMS created special rules for certain MS-DRGs when patients were discharged immediately after their hospitalization to a rehabilitation hospital, a skilled nursing facility (SNF), a long-term care (LTC) hospital, or home health care. These MS-DRGs are called "transfer MS-DRGs." This started in 1999 with 10 transfer MS-DRGs. It has expanded to 275 transfer MS-DRGs. Although a patient may be grouped in a transfer MS-DRG, a payment reduction occurs only if all of the following conditions are met:

- The patient is in a transfer MS-DRG.
- The patient was a "short-stay" or early discharge (LOS+1 < GMLOS).
- The patient was transferred to a SNF, home health care, a rehab hospital, or a long-term care hospital.

CASE-MIX INDEX

MS-DRGs provide a means of defining and measuring a hospital's **case-mix index** (CMI), in other words, how sick its patients are. Following are interrelated parts of case-mix:

- Severity of illness
- Prognosis

- Treatment difficulty
- Need for intervention
- Resource intensity

To calculate case-mix, add the relative weight of the MS-DRG assigned to each patient discharged during a specific time period. Then divide the total relative weight by the number of patients in that time period. The resultant value represents the case-mix index. Some facilities may calculate their Medicare case-mix, along with overall case-mix, which includes all patients. This value may be calculated each month, quarterly, and/or at the end of each fiscal year. If great variations in the case-mix are seen from month to month, hospital administration may want an explanation. For example, if the hospital was undergoing renovations in the surgery department and the number of surgeries for the month was significantly lower than usual, this change may cause a facility's case-mix to drop.

EXAMPLE

During the month of June, the following Medicare patients were discharged from Hospital A:

2 patients	MS-DRG 194	RW 1.0026
2 patients	MS-DRG 292	RW 1.0214
1 patient	MS-DRG 192	RW 0.7081
3 patients	MS-DRG 302	RW 1.0029
2 patients	MS-DRG 065	RW 1.1485

A total of 10 patients are included. To perform a manual calculation, add the following:

1.0026	
1.0026	
1.0214	
1.0214	
0.7081	
1.0029	
1.0029	
1.0029	
1.1485	
1.1485	
TOTAL	10.0618 is the total of the relative weights of the 10 patients listed above.

The next step is to divide the total relative weight by the number of patients. 10.0618 divided by 10 = 1.0062. This is the CMI for this group of patients.

Usually, these figures are calculated with the use of software programs and can be calculated using certain parameters such as specific third party payer, by date, by physician, or by clinical service. If significant coding errors and/or errors in MS-DRG assignment occur, the CMI may not be accurate.

UB-04

Uniform Bill-04, or UB-04, or CMS-1450 is the claim form (Figure 26-2) that is used to submit bills to Medicare and other third party payers. The first uniform bill was introduced in 1982 and was called the UB-82. Prior to that time, each and every insurance or third party payer had its own forms. The uniform bill made it much easier for patients and hospital billing offices to submit claims to all insurance companies in a timely manner. Some different completion requirements may apply for an individual payer.

The UB-04 consists of fields for 12 diagnosis codes (9 diagnosis codes and 3 E codes) and 6 procedure codes. Codes affecting reimbursement need to be sequenced in the top

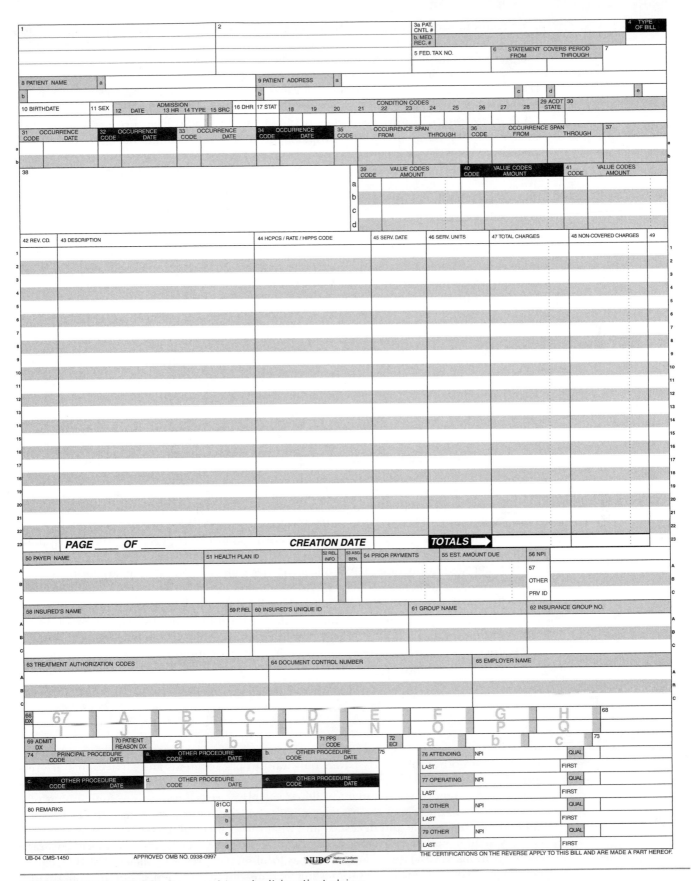

FIGURE 26-2. UB-04—form used to submit inpatient claims.

nine codes in order for codes to be submitted on the UB-04. The same applies to the top six procedure codes. A code for the admitting diagnosis is also required. The admitting diagnosis does not have to be the same as the principal diagnosis.

When errors in coding occur, the hospital may resubmit the billing data with revised codes on the claim or UB-04. For Medicare patients, the hospital has 60 days from the date of the MS-DRG payment to request a review of the original MS-DRG assignment. After 60 days, no resubmissions for higher payment can be made. If an error was found that meant a lower payment for the hospital, the adjustment should be made as soon as possible.

For the most part, hospital billing or claim forms are submitted electronically. There are specific formats that are required by HIPAA (Health Insurance Portability and Accountability Act). Most healthcare organizations use the HIPAA-approved ANSI (American National Standards Institute) ASC (Accredited Standards Committee) X12 standards as the format for various electronic documents. Because of ICD-10 and other industry changes, the current 4010 X12 standards need to be upgraded. All providers, payers, and clearinghouses will need to comply with the version 5010 X12 standards for electronic claims processing by January 1, 2012. Enforcement of these standards were initiated March 30, 2012.

CHARGE DESCRIPTION MASTER

The **chargemaster** or **charge description master** (CDM) is a listing of the services, procedures, drugs, and supplies that can be applied to a patient's bill. A chargemaster often contains many data items to properly identify a particular charge. Some of those data items include:

- **Department number**—Ancillary departments such as radiology, laboratory, and emergency room will have a specific hospital departmental number.
- **Charge description number**—This is a number that designates a particular service or procedure; it is used to generate a charge on a patient bill.
- Description of service, procedure, drug, or supply—This is a brief description of the procedure or service. If there is a corresponding HCPCS code, the description should match the code description.
- HCPCS code (includes CPT codes)—Codes will be assigned to all applicable CDM items. Not all items will have an HCPCS code.
- **Revenue code**—This four-digit code is utilized on the UB-04 to indicate a particular type of service. Revenue code 0351 would be used when billing a CT scan of the head, and code 0352 would be used for a CT scan of the body.
- Price or charge of the service, procedure, drug, or supply—The charge for the item is also shown.

MEDICAL NECESSITY

Medicare and other third-party payers only want to pay for items and services that are reasonable and necessary. Medicare may only pay for services that are "reasonable and necessary for the diagnosis or treatment of illness or injury or to improve the functioning of a malformed body member." There are policies that outline the criteria for what is determined to be reasonable and necessary and what meets **medical necessity** guidelines. These policies include **national coverage determinations** (**NCDs**; Figure 26-3) and **local coverage determinations (LCDs)**, previously known as local medical review policies (LMRPs). These may include certain time frames for testing, certain age requirements, and that a particular diagnosis or condition must be present for a procedure or treatment to be considered medically necessary.

220.4 - Mammograms
(Rev. 1, 10-03-03)
CIM 50-21

A diagnostic mammography is a radiologic procedure furnished to a man or woman with signs and symptoms of breast disease, or a personal history of breast cancer, or a personal history of biopsy – proven benign breast disease, and includes a physician's interpretation of the results of the procedure. A diagnostic mammography is a covered service if it is ordered by a doctor of medicine or osteopathy as defined in §1861 (r) (1) of the Act. A screening mammography is a radiologic procedure furnished to a woman without signs or symptoms of breast disease, for the purpose of early detection of breast cancer, and includes a physician's interpretation of the results of the procedure. A screening mammography has limitations as it must be, at a minimum a two-view exposure (cranio-caudal and a medial lateral oblique view) of each breast. Payment may not be made for a screening mammography performed on a woman under age 35. Payment may be made for only one screening mammography performed on a woman over age 34, but under age 40. For an asymptomatic woman over age 39, payment may be made for a screening mammography performed after at least 11 months have passed following the month in which the last screening mammography was performed.

A radiological mammogram is a covered diagnostic test under the following conditions:

• A patient has distinct signs and symptoms for which a mammogram is indicated;

• A patient has a history of breast cancer; or

• A patient is asymptomatic but, on the basis of the patient's history and other factors the physician considers significant, the physician's judgment is that a mammogram is appropriate.

Use of mammograms in routine screening of: (1) asymptomatic women aged 50 and over, and (2) asymptomatic women aged 40 or over whose mothers or sisters have had the disease, is considered medically appropriate, but would not be covered for Medicare purposes.

Cross-reference:

The Medicare Benefit Policy Manual, Chapter 15, "Covered Medical and Other Health Services," §80.

The Medicare Benefit Policy Manual, Chapter 1, "Inpatient Hospital Services," §50

FIGURE 26-3. An example of National Coverage Determinations.

QUALITY IMPROVEMENT ORGANIZATION

Quality improvement organizations (QIOs) work for consumers, healthcare providers, and hospitals to make sure that patients are getting the "right care at the right time in the appropriate setting." A total of 53 QIOs have been created, one for each state and territory and the District of Columbia. This network acts under the direction of CMS and is contracted to monitor the quality of health care, and to make sure that Medicare pays only for services that are reasonable and necessary. QIO functions under 3-year contract cycles called *scopes of work* (SOWs).

PEPPER

The Program for Evaluating Payment Patterns Electronic Report (PEPPER) is an electronic report that is sent to a hospital that contains hospital-specific information for 13 target areas. These target areas are specific MS-DRGs that have been identified as being at risk for payment errors. PEPPER was developed to assist QIOs with their Hospital Payment Monitoring Programs (HPMPs) to identify and prevent payment errors due to billing, MS-DRG assignment, coding, and/or admission necessity issues. CMS announced at the beginning of 2009 that it will continue to require the QIOs to provide hospitals with these reports.

RECOVERY AUDIT CONTRACT

The Recovery Audit Contract (RAC) Initiative was implemented as a result of section 306 of the Medicare Prescription Drug, Improvement, and Modernization Act of 2003 (MMA). Congress directed the Department of Health and Human Services (DHHS) to conduct a 3-year demonstration project using Recovery Audit Contractors (RACs) to detect and correct improper Medicare payments—both overpayments and underpayments. Under the demonstration project, RACs reviewed claims for hospital inpatient and outpatient, skilled nursing facility, physician, ambulance, laboratory, and durable medical equipment in California, Florida, New York, Massachusetts, South Carolina, and Arizona. At the conclusion of the project in March of 2008, over $900 million in overpayments were returned to the Medicare Trust Fund, and almost $38 million in underpayments were paid to healthcare providers/facilities. RACs are paid on a contingency fee basis, receiving a percentage of the improper payments collected from providers/facilities.

CMS is using lessons learned from the RAC demonstration project to improve its permanent program. A permanent RAC program is now in place for all 50 states.

Currently, four recovery audit contractors (RACs) are available:

- Region A: Diversified Collection Services, Inc., of Livermore, California
- Region B: CGI Technologies and Solutions, Inc., of Fairfax, Virginia
- Region C: Connolly Consulting Associates, Inc., of Wilton, Connecticut
- Region D: HealthDataInsights, Inc., of Las Vegas, Nevada

Other groups that are contracting with state and federal agencies to identify improper billing and overpayments include:

- Medicare Administrative Contractors (MACs) are the companies that process Part A and Part B Medicare claims. They are responsible for overseeing the accuracy of claims completion and the determination of correct payments for services. Because they review both Part A and Part B claims, they are able to review for discrepancies between the two sets of claims.
- Zone Program Integrity Contractors (ZPICs), who serve the same jurisdictions as the MCAs and are authorized to conduct investigations, provide support to law enforcement, and audit the Medicare advantage plans. They may also focus on Medicare billing targets.
- Medicaid Integrity Contractors (MICs) are in charge of reviewing and auditing Medicaid claims for inappropriate payments or fraud. They use a data-driven approach to identify some of the following target areas:
  - Services after the death of a beneficiary
  - Duplicate claims
  - Unbundling of services
  - Outpatient claims with service dates that overlap an inpatient stay

MICs also conduct medical record reviews to ensure that payment was made for medically necessary services, that services are covered, that payment was made correctly, and that the services were billed properly with the correct diagnosis and procedure codes.

DATA QUALITY

In Chapter 1, it was mentioned that coded data have many purposes.[1] In November 2007, AHIMA published a position statement on the "Consistency of Healthcare Diagnostic and Procedural Coding." It states that accurate and complete coded data are critical for:

- Healthcare delivery
- Research
- Public reporting
- Reimbursement
- Policy making

All users must consistently apply the same official coding rules, conventions, guidelines, and definitions. AHIMA promotes the idea that coding professionals are educated and certified to assign and validate codes and to assist with policy development related to coding accuracy.

As reimbursement and coding systems evolve, it is important to remember that the codes that are assigned today will have a role in the reimbursement system(s) of tomorrow, so it is imperative that each health record be coded accurately and completely.

CLINICAL DOCUMENTATION IMPROVEMENT PROGRAM

Incomplete, inaccurate, and illegible documentation has been a problem in health care for years. With the evolution of reimbursement systems that are based on documentation and coded data, it is imperative that hospitals make improvements in their clinical documentation. A clinical documentation improvement program (CDIP) will depend on the facility's needs and must work within the culture and framework of the organization. The success of any improvement type of program is dependent on the participation of the "right" team players. It is extremely important to get physician support and buy-in because physicians are responsible for much of the documentation within the health record.

One of the goals of a CDIP is to improve the facility's case-mix index (CMI). Case-mix data can be used for comparison with other facilities and for monitoring trends within the facility. Better documentation, along with accurate and complete coding of the health record, should lead to better reimbursement and increased CMI.

The manner in which documentation is collected should be analyzed, so improvements can be made to capture complete and accurate clinical documentation. As hospitals convert from paper to electronic records, the time is ideal for assessing all forms of documentation.

Many facilities are employing Clinical Documentation Specialists who concurrently review patient records and query the attending physician about documentation that may be missing or incomplete within the patient's record. Most documentation issues can be resolved before the patient is discharged, and the record will have more complete and accurate documentation for assigning codes. This should reduce the number of physician queries asked by the coder. Because greater specificity is required for ICD-10-CM and ICD-10-PCS, good documentation will be even more important.

Choose the best answer to the followings questions.

1. A preexisting condition that is present on admission and may lead to increased resource use
   A. Complication
   B. Comorbidity
   C. Morbidity
   D. Other diagnosis

2. The condition that, after study, is established as chiefly responsible for occasioning the admission of the patient to the hospital is called the
   A. Primary diagnosis
   B. Provisional diagnosis
   C. Principal diagnosis
   D. Major diagnosis

3. DRG stands for
   A. Drug-related gastritis
   B. Diagnostic related groups
   C. Diagnosis-related group
   D. Diagnostic regulation by government

4. The billing form that is currently in use in hospitals is
   A. UB-87
   B. UB-04
   C. UB-82
   D. UB-92

5. Calculate the case-mix for the following patients using the weights from the MS-DRG Table on the Evolve website:

2 patients	MS-DRG 690
3 patients	MS-DRG 292
1 patient	MS-DRG 069
2 patients	MS-DRG 378

Complete the following questions.

6. Identify four MS-DRGs that appear on the post-transfer policy listing.

   _____

   _____

   _____

   _____

7. List four commonly missed CCs or MCCs.

   _____

   _____

   _____

   _____

8. What organization is the QIO in your state?

   _____

9. Explain the purpose of a recovery audit contractor.

   _____

   _____

10. What date has been set to the full implementation of a permanent RAC program?

   _____

CHAPTER GLOSSARY

Case-mix index: a measurement used by hospitals to define how sick their patients are.

Chargemaster or **charge description master (CDM):** a listing of the services, procedures, drugs, and supplies that can be applied to a patient's bill.

Charge description number: a number that designates a particular service or procedure, used to generate a charge on a patient bill.

Comorbidity: a preexisting condition (it is present on admission) which may lead to increased resource use.

Complication: a condition that arises during a patient's hospitalization which may lead to increased resource use.

Department number: ancillary departments such as radiology, laboratory, and emergency room will have a specific hospital departmental number.

Deficit Reduction Act (DRA): requires all acute care facilities reimbursed under MS-DRGs to identify and report diagnoses that are present at the time of a patient's admission.

Encoder: coding software that is used to assign diagnosis and procedure codes.

Grouper: specialized software used to assign the appropriate MS-DRG.

Health Maintenance Organization (HMO): type of managed care in which hospitals, physicians, and other providers contract to provide health care for patients, usually at a discounted rate.

Local coverage determinations (LCDs): local policy that may include certain time frames for testing, certain age requirements, and that a particular diagnosis or condition must be present for a procedure or treatment to be considered medically necessary.

Maximization: the manipulation of codes to result in maximum reimbursement without supporting documentation in the health record or with disregard for coding conventions, guidelines, and UHDDS definitions.

Medical necessity: criteria or guidelines for what is determined to be reasonable and necessary for a particular medical service.

National coverage determinations (NCDs): national policy that may include certain time frames for testing, certain age requirements, and that a particular diagnosis or condition must be present for a treatment or procedure to be considered medically necessary.

Optimization: the process of striving to obtain optimal reimbursement or the highest possible payment to which a facility is legally entitled on the basis of documentation in the health record.

Preferred Provider Organization (PPO): type of managed care in which hospitals, physicians, and other providers have an arrangement with a third party payer to provide health care at discounted rates to third party payer clients.

Present on admission (POA): an indicator to differentiate between conditions that develop during a particular hospital encounter and conditions that were present at the time of admission.

Principal diagnosis: the condition established after study to be chiefly responsible for occasioning the admission of the patient to the hospital for care.

Prospective payment system: method of reimbursement in which payment is made on the basis of a predetermined, fixed amount rather than for billed charges.

Reimbursement: payment for healthcare services.

Revenue code: a four-digit code that is utilized on the UB-04 to indicate a particular type of service.

Self-insured plans: self-insurance fund is set up by an employer to provide health claim benefits for employees.

Third party payer: makes payments for health services on behalf of the patients; may be a government program, insurance company, or managed care plan.

REFERENCE   1. American Health Information Management Association (AHIMA). Statement on consistency of health care diagnostic and procedural coding (AHIMA Position Statement, December 2007).

27

Outpatient Coding

CHAPTER OUTLINE
Outpatient Terminology
ICD-10-CM Official Guidelines for Coding and Reporting
Major Differences Between ICD-10-CM and ICD-9-CM
Procedure Coding in the Outpatient Setting
APCs as Reimbursement
Chapter Review Exercise
Chapter Glossary
Reference

LEARNING OBJECTIVES

1. Explain terminology as related to the outpatient setting
2. Identify major differences between ICD-10-CM and ICD-9-CM related to outpatient conditions
3. Describe the difference between inpatient coding guidelines and outpatient coding guidelines
4. Describe what CPT coding is, when it is used, and the official guideline source
5. Apply Diagnostic Coding and Reporting Guidelines for Outpatient Services
6. Assign ICD-10-CM codes for outpatient services
7. Explain the purpose and use of APCs

ABBREVIATIONS/ ACRONYMS

AICD automatic implantable cardioverter-defibrillator

AMA American Medical Association

APC Ambulatory Payment Classification

COPD chronic obstructive pulmonary disease

CPT Current Procedural Terminology

CVA cerebrovascular accident

DEXA dual-energy x-ray absorptiometry

ER emergency room

HCPCS Healthcare Common Procedure Coding System

ICD-9-CM *International Classification of Diseases, 9th Revision, Clinical Modification*

ICD-10-CM *International Classification of Diseases, 10th Revision, Clinical Modification*

ICD-10-PCS *International Classification of Diseases, 10th Revision, Procedure Coding System*

MRI magnetic resonance imaging

MS-DRG Medicare Severity diagnosis-related group

OPPS Outpatient Prospective Payment System

PCP primary care provider

UTI urinary tract infection

OUTPATIENT TERMINOLOGY

Terminology in the outpatient setting is often confusing. Outpatient services may be provided in a variety of settings:

- Doctor's office
- Clinic, free standing or facility based
- Ambulatory surgery, which may also be called outpatient surgery, "in and out" surgery, same day surgery, or same day care

- Emergency room (ER)
- **Observation unit** (a unit to which unstable patients are admitted for a stay of less than 48 hours)
- **Ancillary service** visits/clinic visits (i.e., radiology, laboratory, chemotherapy, radiation therapy)

These outpatient services are called visits or **encounters**. Encounters may require hospital services and/or **professional services** (services rendered by a physician or a non-physician practitioner). For example, a patient receiving a chest x-ray in a hospital setting will have a hospital bill for the chest x-ray and a professional service bill from the radiologist for the reading of the x-ray.

The term "principal diagnosis" as used in the inpatient setting does not apply in the outpatient setting. The outpatient term that is synonymous with "principal diagnosis" is "first-listed diagnosis" or "primary diagnosis."

ICD-10-CM Official Guidelines for Coding and Reporting	Please refer to the companion Evolve website for the most current guidelines. **Section IV. Diagnostic Coding and Reporting Guidelines for Outpatient Services** These coding guidelines for outpatient diagnoses have been approved for use by hospitals/providers in coding and reporting hospital-based outpatient services and provider-based office visits. Information about the use of certain abbreviations, punctuation, symbols, and other conventions used in the ICD-10-CM Tabular List (code numbers and titles), can be found in Section IA of these guidelines, under "Conventions Used in the Tabular List." Information about the correct sequence to use in finding a code is also described in Section I. The terms encounter and visit are often used interchangeably in describing outpatient service contacts and, therefore, appear together in these guidelines without distinguishing one from the other. Though the conventions and general guidelines apply to all settings, coding guidelines for outpatient and provider reporting of diagnoses will vary in a number of instances from those for inpatient diagnoses, recognizing that: The Uniform Hospital Discharge Data Set (UHDDS) definition of principal diagnosis applies only to inpatients in acute, short-term, long-term care and psychiatric hospitals. Coding guidelines for inconclusive diagnoses (probable, suspected, rule out, etc.) were developed for inpatient reporting and do not apply to outpatients. **A. Selection of first-listed condition** In the outpatient setting, the term first-listed diagnosis is used in lieu of principal diagnosis. In determining the first-listed diagnosis the coding conventions of ICD-10-CM, as well as the general and disease specific guidelines take precedence over the outpatient guidelines.

In the outpatient setting, the first-listed diagnosis is the reason for the encounter. The first-listed diagnosis may often be a symptom.

EXAMPLE	Patient presents to physician's office with complaints of headache and slurred speech. Physician suspects that this patient is experiencing a transient ischemic attack (TIA) or a cerebrovascular accident (CVA). The patient is sent directly to the hospital. The first-listed diagnosis for the physician office visit is R51, headache, with a secondary diagnosis of R47.81, slurred speech.

      Diagnoses often are not established at the time of the initial encounter/visit. It may take two or more visits before the diagnosis is confirmed.

      The most critical rule involves beginning the search for the correct code assignment through the Alphabetic Index. Never begin searching initially in the Tabular List as this will lead to coding errors.

It is common in the outpatient setting for a patient to present to a physician's office with symptoms, for administrative reasons, for follow-up on conditions that no longer exist, or with abnormal findings. A code from the Chapter 21, Factors Influencing Health Status and Contact with Health Services (Z codes) may often be the most appropriate code. Refer to Chapter 8 for greater detail on assigning Z codes.

EXAMPLE

A child presents to his physician's office for a required camp physical, Z02.89
　　To locate this code in the Alphabetic Index, look under the main term "Examination, medical, admission to summer camp."

EXAMPLE

A healthcare worker is stuck by a needle used on a patient with acquired immunodeficiency syndrome (AIDS), Z20.6
　　To locate this code in the Alphabetic Index, look under the main term "Exposure to."

EXAMPLE

A patient is visiting her oncologist's office for her yearly visit 5 years status post left mastectomy for breast cancer. Z08, Z90.12, Z85.3
　　This code is located in the Alphabetic Index under "Exam for follow-up surgery malignant neoplasm" and "History, malignant neoplasms, breast."

EXAMPLE

A patient presents to her physician's office with a strong family history of breast cancer. She is interested in prophylactic removal of both breasts. Z80.3
　　This code is located in the Alphabetic Index under "History, family, malignant neoplasm."

1. Outpatient Surgery
When a patient presents for outpatient surgery, code the reason for the surgery as the first-listed diagnosis (reason for the encounter), even if the surgery is not performed due to a contraindication.

EXAMPLE

A patient reports to the outpatient surgery department for an arthroscopic meniscectomy for a bucket handle tear of the lateral meniscus of the right knee. The patient injured her meniscus when she tripped over the cat. The patient is administered anesthesia and is found to be in atrial fibrillation. The surgeon decides that it is best not to proceed with the procedure but wishes to consult with a cardiologist and reschedule. The primary diagnosis is the torn meniscus; atrial fibrillation is coded secondarily along with canceled surgery and the E code for the accident, S83.251A, I48.91, Z53.09, W01.0xxA.

2. Observation Stay
When a patient is admitted for observation for a medical condition, assign a code for the medical condition as the first-listed diagnosis.
　　When a patient presents for outpatient surgery and develops complications requiring admission to observation, code the reason for the surgery as the first reported diagnosis (reason for encounter), followed by codes for the complications as secondary diagnoses.

EXAMPLE

A patient is admitted to outpatient surgery with cholelithiasis and is scheduled for a laparoscopic cholecystectomy. The surgery proceeds uneventfully. In the recovery room, the patient is found to have hypotension. The surgeon decides to admit the patient for observation, K80.20, I95.9.

B. Codes from A00.0 through T88.9, Z00-Z99

The appropriate code(s) from A00.0 through T88.9, Z00-Z99 must be used to identify diagnoses, symptoms, conditions, problems, complaints, or other reason(s) for the encounter/visit.

EXAMPLE

When presenting to a doctor's office, a patient often presents with symptoms such as cough or leg pain. At the end of the visit, the physician may not know the cause of the leg pain and therefore may make the assessment that leg pain is probably the result of muscle strain. Therefore, in this case, the code would be M79.606 for leg pain.

C. Accurate reporting of ICD-10-CM diagnosis codes

For accurate reporting of ICD-10-CM diagnosis codes, the documentation should describe the patient's condition, using terminology which includes specific diagnoses as well as symptoms, problems, or reasons for the encounter. There are ICD-10-CM codes to describe all of these.

EXAMPLE

A patient is scheduled for cataract surgery and has congestive heart failure. The surgeon asks the patient's cardiologist for a preoperative consult, Z01.810, I50.9, H26.9.

D. Codes that describe symptoms and signs

Codes that describe symptoms and signs, as opposed to diagnoses, are acceptable for reporting purposes when a diagnosis has not been established (confirmed) by the provider. Chapter 18 of ICD-10-CM, Symptoms, Signs, and Abnormal Clinical and Laboratory Findings Not Elsewhere Classified (codes R00-R99) contain many, but not all codes for symptoms.

EXAMPLE

When a patient is seen in a physician's office for a problem-oriented visit, it is often a symptom that will be reported as the first-listed diagnosis. A patient may come to the office with abdominal pain, and the physician suspects it is due to diverticulitis. The patient is sent for testing. The first-listed diagnosis for this encounter is R10.9.

On the return visit, test results reveal that the patient does indeed have diverticulitis; therefore, the follow-up visit code would be K57.92.

E. Encounters for circumstances other than a disease or injury

ICD-10-CM provides codes to deal with encounters for circumstances other than a disease or injury. The Factors Influencing Health Status and Contact with Health Services codes (Z00-Z99) are provided to deal with occasions when circumstances other than a disease or injury are recorded as diagnosis or problems.

See Section I.C.21. Factors influencing health status and contact with health services.

EXAMPLE

A patient is planning on donating an organ and is seen by their family physician. The patient must be examined so it can be determined whether they qualify as a donor, Z00.5.

EXAMPLE

A patient who is on Coumadin therapy for history of DVT is required to visit a Coumadin clinic weekly until the levels of medication are adjusted, Z51.81, Z79.01, Z86.718.

F. Level of Detail in Coding
1. ICD-10-CM codes with 3, 4, 5, 6 or 7 characters
ICD-10-CM is composed of codes with either 3, 4, 5, 6 or 7 characters. Codes with three characters are included in ICD-10-CM as the heading of a category of codes that may be further subdivided by the use of fourth, fifth, sixth or seventh characters to provide greater specificity.
2. Use of full number of digits required for a code
A three-**character** code is to be used only if it is not further subdivided. A code is invalid if it has not been coded to the full number of characters required for that code, including the 7th character, if applicable.
G. ICD-10-CM code for the diagnosis, condition, problem, or other reason for encounter/visit
List first the ICD-10-CM code for the diagnosis, condition, problem, or other reason for encounter/visit shown in the medical record to be chiefly responsible for the services provided. List additional codes that describe any coexisting conditions. In some cases the first-listed diagnosis may be a symptom when a diagnosis has not been established (confirmed) by the physician.

It is important when coding outpatient services that codes for all coexisting conditions are also assigned.

EXAMPLE
A patient presents to his primary care provider (PCP) with a cough and a fever and a long history of chronic obstructive pulmonary disease (COPD). After reviewing the chest x-ray, the physician determines that the patient has pneumonia, J18.9, J44.9.

H. Uncertain diagnosis
Do not code diagnoses documented as "probable", "suspected," "questionable," "rule out," or "working diagnosis" or other similar terms indicating uncertainty. Rather, code the condition(s) to the highest degree of certainty for that encounter/visit, such as symptoms, signs, abnormal test results, or other reason for the visit.
Please note: This differs from the coding practices used by short-term, acute care, long-term care and psychiatric hospitals.

Coding Clinic for ICD-9-CM (2005:3Q:p21-2)[1] has also identified the term "compatible" to fall into the same category as possible and probable and a diagnosis described as "compatible with" is not coded in the outpatient setting. The condition should only be coded to the highest degree of certainty for that encounter.

EXAMPLE
A patient presents to her doctor with complaints of weight gain, decreased libido, and cold intolerance. The physician sends her to the laboratory for blood work with a diagnosis of probable hypothyroidism. She is to return in 2 weeks for results of the blood work, which comes back positive for hypothyroidism.
First visit: R63.5, R68.82, R68.89
Second visit: E03.9

I. Chronic diseases
Chronic diseases treated on an ongoing basis may be coded and reported as many times as the patient receives treatment and care for the condition(s)

EXAMPLE
A patient is scheduled for a return visit every 6 months for hypercholesterolemia, E78.0.

J. Code all documented conditions that coexist

Code all documented conditions that coexist at the time of the encounter/visit, and require or affect patient care treatment or management. Do not code conditions that were previously treated and no longer exist. However, history codes (categories Z80-Z87) may be used as secondary codes if the historical condition or family history has an impact on current care or influences treatment.

EXAMPLE

A patient presents to a physician's office with a complaint of low back pain and is on medications for hypertension and hypercholesterolemia. During the visit the patient's blood pressure is checked and blood was drawn to check cholesterol level, M54.5, I10, E78.0.

This case follows the rule of coding coexisting conditions that affect the management of the patient. The physician must take into account the patient's other history and medications before prescribing medication for the back pain.

K. Patients receiving diagnostic services only

For patients receiving diagnostic services only during an encounter/visit, sequence first the diagnosis, condition, problem, or other reason for encounter/visit shown in the medical record to be chiefly responsible for the outpatient services provided during the encounter/visit. Codes for other diagnoses (e.g., chronic conditions) may be sequenced as additional diagnoses.

For encounters for routine laboratory/radiology testing in the absence of any signs, symptoms, or associated diagnosis, assign Z01.89, Encounter for other specified special examinations. If routine testing is performed during the same encounter as a test to evaluate a sign, symptom, or diagnosis, it is appropriate to assign both the V code and the code describing the reason for the non-routine test.

EXAMPLE

A patient who presents to radiology for a chest x-ray may have a working diagnosis such as cough r/o pneumonia. The ordering physician documents that the patient also has a history of asthma for which he takes albuterol, prn. On reading the x-ray the radiologist documents COPD with no evidence of pneumonia, R05, J44.9.

For outpatient encounters for diagnostic tests that have been interpreted by a physician, and the final report is available at the time of coding, code any confirmed or definitive diagnosis(es) documented in the interpretation. Do not code related signs and symptoms as additional diagnoses.

Please note: This differs from the coding practice in the hospital inpatient setting regarding abnormal findings on test results.

EXAMPLE

As in the previous example, a patient presents to radiology for a cough/rule out pneumonia and history of asthma, and after the chest x-ray is performed, the radiologist interprets the x-ray as pneumonia and COPD, J18.9, J44.9.

The code for the symptom would not be assigned.

L. Patients receiving therapeutic services only

For patients receiving therapeutic services only during an encounter/visit, sequence first the diagnosis, condition, problem, or other reason for encounter/visit shown in the medical record to be chiefly responsible for the outpatient services provided during the encounter/visit. Codes for other diagnoses (e.g., chronic conditions) may be sequenced as additional diagnoses.

EXAMPLE Patient presents to the physician's office monthly for a vitamin B_{12} shot for pernicious anemia, D51.0.

The only exception to this rule is that when the primary reason for the admission/encounter is chemotherapy or radiation therapy, the appropriate Z code for the service is listed first, and the diagnosis or problem for which the service is being performed listed second.

EXAMPLE A patient presents to a physician's office for chemotherapy for pancreatic cancer, Z51.11, C25.9.

M. Patients receiving preoperative evaluations only

For patients receiving preoperative evaluations only, sequence first a code from subcategory Z01.81, Encounter for pre-procedural examinations, to describe the pre-op consultations. Assign a code for the condition to describe the reason for the surgery as an additional diagnosis. Code also any findings related to the pre-op evaluation.

EXAMPLE Patient who is planning surgery for an abdominal aortic aneurysm (AAA). The surgeon requests that the patient see her primary care provider for a preoperative evaluation. This patient is well known to her primary care provider and has additional chronic diagnoses of hypertension, hypercholesterolemia, and history of breast cancer, Z01.818, I10, E78.0, Z85.3, I71.4.

N. Ambulatory surgery

For ambulatory surgery, code the diagnosis for which the surgery was performed. If the postoperative diagnosis is known to be different from the preoperative diagnosis at the time the diagnosis is confirmed, select the postoperative diagnosis for coding, since it is the most definitive.

EXAMPLE A patient undergoes surgery to remove a left breast mass. The mass is sent to the pathology department, where a diagnosis of breast cancer is confirmed, C50.912.

O. Routine outpatient prenatal visits

   b. Selection of OB Principal or First-listed Diagnosis

      1) Routine outpatient prenatal visits

         For routine outpatient prenatal visits when no complications are present, a code from category Z34, Encounter for supervision of normal pregnancy, should be used as the first-listed diagnosis. These codes should not be used in conjunction with chapter 15 codes.

EXAMPLE

Patient was seen at 22 weeks for prenatal visit. There are no problems noted. Patient has a 3-year-old daughter, Z34.82.

P. Encounters for general medical examinations with abnormal findings

The subcategories for encounters for general medical examinations, Z00.0-, provide codes for with and without abnormal findings. Should a general medical examination result in an abnormal finding, the code for general medical examination with abnormal finding should be assigned as the first-listed diagnosis. A secondary code for the abnormal finding should also be coded.

Q. Encounters for routine health screenings

See Section I.C.21. Factors influencing health status and contact with health services, Screening

EXAMPLE

Patient presents to physician's office for routine yearly general exam, Z00.00.

EXAMPLE

Patient presents to physician's office for routine yearly exam. He complains of lightheadedness and rapid heart rate on occasion. The physician diagnoses the patient with atrial fibrillation and sends him for an echocardiogram, Z00.01, I48.91.

Apply the General Coding Guidelines as found in Chapter 5.

MAJOR DIFFERENCES BETWEEN ICD-10-CM AND ICD-9-CM

The guidelines for coding outpatient conditions in ICD-9-CM and ICD-10-CM are nearly identical. The only differences appear in ICD-10-CM where guidelines have been added for encounters for general medical exams with abnormal findings. There is now a code in ICD-10-CM for general medical exams with and without abnormal findings. There is also a cross reference in the guidelines directing the user to go to the Section on Factors influencing health status and contact with health services, Screening, to code encounters for routine health screenings.

PROCEDURE CODING IN THE OUTPATIENT SETTING

In ICD-10, procedures are coded from ICD-10-PCS for inpatient coding. In the outpatient setting, procedure codes are assigned from the **Current Procedural Terminology (CPT)** published by the American Medical Association (AMA). According to the Health Insurance Portability and Accountability Act (HIPAA), "The use of ICD-9-CM procedure codes is restricted to the reporting of inpatient procedures by the hospital." Hospitals may still elect to code outpatient visits with ICD-10-CM procedure codes for non–claim-related purposes. CPT is a coding system for reporting medical services and procedures performed by health-care providers. Physicians report office visits using CPT codes (Figure 27-1) to describe the service provided, along with diagnostic codes from ICD-10-CM to describe why the service was performed.

CPT is Level I of the Healthcare Common Procedure Coding System (HCPCS). CPT is published yearly by the AMA. Revisions are effective for dates of service after January 1 of each year. CPT codes are five-digit numeric codes.

Mastectomy Procedures

19300 Mastectomy for gynecomastia

19301 Mastectomy, partial (eg, lumpectomy, tylectomy, quadrantectomy, segmentectomy);

19302 with axillary lymphadenectomy

(For placement of radiotherapy afterloading balloon/brachytherapy catheters, see 19296-19298)

19303 Mastectomy, simple, complete

FIGURE 27-1. Example of CPT codes (Level I HCPCS).

Chemotherapy Drugs *J9000-J9999*

J9000 **Doxorubicin HCl, 10 mg**
Use this code for Adriamycin PFS, Adriamycin RDF, Rubex.
MED: 100-2, 15, 50

J9001 **Doxorubicin HCl, all lipid formulations, 10 mg**
Use this code for Doxil.
MED: 100-2, 15, 50

J9010 **Alemtuzumab, 10 mg**
Use this code for Campath.

J9015 **Aldesleukin, per single use vial**
Use this code for Proleukin, IL-2, Interleukin.
MED: 100-2, 15, 50

FIGURE 27-2. Example of HCPCS Level II codes.

Level II of HCPCS consists of alphanumeric codes (Figure 27-2). These codes, which are used to identify drugs, medical supplies, and durable medical equipment, are maintained by the HCPCS National Panel, which is composed of Blue Cross/Blue Shield, the Health Insurance Association of America, and Centers for Medicare and Medicaid Services (CMS).

EXAMPLE Patient with acute appendicitis had laparoscopic appendectomy, K35.80, 44970 (CPT code).

EXAMPLE Patient with right carpal tunnel syndrome had an endoscopic carpal tunnel release, G56.01, 29848-RT (CPT code).

APCs AS REIMBURSEMENT

Ambulatory Payment Classifications (APCs) became effective on August 1, 2000. APCs constitute a reimbursement system that is similar to Medicare Severity diagnosis-related groups (MS-DRGs), which are used in the inpatient setting. APCs categorize outpatient procedures into similar groups for payment purposes (Figure 27-3). This is Medicare's Outpatient Prospective Payment System (OPPS). Assignment to an APC is based primarily on CPT codes. One of the big differences between MS-DRGs and APCs is that more than one APC may be assigned per claim.

Addendum A.-OPPS APCs for CY 2010					National Unadjusted Copayment	Minimum Unadjusted Copayment
APC	Group Title	SI	Relative Weight	Payment Rate		
0001	Level I Photochemotherapy	S	0.5302	$35.65		$7.13
0002	Fine Needle Biopsy/Aspiration	T	1.5111	$101.61		$20.33
0003	Bone Marrow Biopsy/Aspiration	T	3.0998	$208.43		$41.69
0004	Level I Needle Biopsy/Aspiration Except Bone Marrow	T	4.5991	$309.25		$61.85
0005	Level II Needle Biopsy/Aspiration Except Bone Marrow	T	7.8145	$525.45		$105.09
0006	Level I Incision & Drainage	T	1.4557	$97.88		$19.58
0007	Level II Incision & Drainage	T	12.6217	$848.70		$169.74
0008	Level III Incision and Drainage	T	19.4063	$1,304.90		$260.98
0012	Level I Debridement & Destruction	T	0.4436	$29.83		$5.97
0013	Level II Debridement & Destruction	T	0.8789	$59.10		$11.82
0015	Level III Debridement & Destruction	T	1.5412	$103.63		$20.73
0016	Level IV Debridement & Destruction	T	2.7982	$188.15		$37.63
0017	Level VI Debridement & Destruction	T	21.2653	$1,429.90		$285.98
0019	Level I Excision/Biopsy	T	4.3625	$293.34	$64.35	$58.67
0020	Level II Excision/Biopsy	T	8.2028	$551.56		$110.32
0021	Level III Excision/Biopsy	T	17.4975	$1,176.55		$235.31
0022	Level IV Excision/Biopsy	T	23.3880	$1,572.63	$354.45	$314.53

FIGURE 27-3. Example of APCs.

CHAPTER REVIEW EXERCISE

Answer questions or assign ICD-10-CM codes for all diagnoses and CPT codes for procedures.

1. Outpatient visits are only visits to physicians' offices.
   A. True
   B. False

2. The same coding guidelines apply to inpatient and outpatient settings.
   A. True
   B. False

3. What is another name for "in and out" surgery?

   _____

4. What is the term in the outpatient setting for principal diagnosis?

   _____

5. Is an encounter the same as a visit?

   _____

6. A coder should always begin the search for the correct code in the Tabular List.
   A. True
   B. False

7. Patient presents to office with burning on urination. Physician performs a urinalysis, which is sent out to the laboratory. Physician prescribes antibiotics for presumed urinary tract infection (UTI).   _____

8. Patient presents to ER stating that she has been raped. A rape kit is used to determine whether the rape actually occurred. Results were negative.   _____

9. Patient presents to the gynecologist's office for a routine Pap and pelvic examination.   _____

10. Postmenopausal patient is sent for dual-energy x-ray absorptiometry (DEXA) scan to evaluate status of bone loss.   _____

11. Diabetic patient is sent to nutritionist for dietary counseling.   _____

12. Child presents to physician's office for routine vaccination. The physician decides not to administer because the child has a cold.   _____

13. Patient and husband present to clinical social worker for marriage counseling.   _____

14. Patient had a malignant neoplasm of the lung removed. She presents to the surgeon for routine aftercare.   _____

15. Patient presents to physician's office for reprogramming of an automatic implantable cardioverter-defibrillator (AICD).   _____

16. Patient presents to physician's office complaining of dizziness.   _____

17. Patient presents to physician's office complaining of testicular pain. Physician prescribes antibiotics and says the symptoms are compatible with epididymitis.   _____

18. Patient presents to physician's office as a possible bone marrow donor for her sister.   _____

19. Patient presents to physician's office with severe headache. Physician sends patient for magnetic resonance imaging (MRI) and notes to rule out cerebrovascular accident (CVA) in a patient with a history of hypertension and coronary artery disease. _____

20. Patient is seen in doctor's office for abdominal pain. After examination, the physician states that this is probably due to diverticulitis in that the patient has known diverticulum. He also notes that this patient has a history of alcohol abuse and is currently drinking on a daily basis. _____

21. Patient presents to doctor's office with fever, cough, and muscle aches and pains. Physician is uncertain as to whether these symptoms are an exacerbation of her COPD, or whether she has viral pneumonia. Laboratory work is ordered. _____

CHAPTER GLOSSARY

Ambulatory Payment Classifications (APCs): used for outpatient prospective payment.

Ancillary services: services provided by a hospital that are additional to a professional service, such as laboratory work and radiology and pathology services.

Current Procedural Terminology (CPT): a coding system for reporting medical services and procedures.

Encounter: face-to-face visit with a healthcare provider.

Level II of HCPCS: codes used to identify drugs, medical supplies, and durable medical equipment.

Observation unit: area outside the emergency department where unstable patients are admitted for a stay of less than 48 hours. The patient is observed for admission to the hospital or discharge to home.

Professional service: service rendered by a physician or a nonphysician practitioner.

REFERENCE

1. American Hospital Association. *Coding Clinic for ICD-9-CM* 2005:3Q:p21-22. Consistent with and compatible with.

Glossary

Ablation Correction of abnormal heart rhythm by burning of abnormal heart tissue through radiofrequency or other methods such as laser, microwave, or freezing.

Abortion Artificially terminating a pregnancy.

Abscess A localized collection of pus that causes swelling.

Abstracting Extracting data from the health record.

Acromegaly Condition that results when hypersecretion of human growth hormone (hGH) occurs after puberty, along with overgrowth of the face, hands, feet, and soft tissues.

Activities of daily living assessment Measurement of functional level for activities of daily living.

Activities of daily living treatment Exercise or activities to facilitate functional competence for activities of daily living.

Acute A short and relatively severe course.

Acute renal failure Sudden and severe impairment of renal function characterized by oliguria, increased serum urea, and acidosis.

Addison's disease Adrenocortical insufficiency that may be caused by neoplasms, surgical removal of the adrenal gland, autoimmune processes, tuberculosis, hemorrhage, and/or infection.

Adenocarcinomas Malignancies of epithelial glandular tissue such as those found in the breast, prostate, and colon.

Adhesion Scar tissue that forms an abnormal connection between body parts.

Adjunct codes Add-on codes to a primary procedure to provide additional information about the primary procedure that was performed.

Admission diagnosis Diagnosis that brings the patient to the hospital. This will often be a symptom.

Admitting diagnosis The condition that requires the patient to be hospitalized.

Adverse effect Pathologic manifestation due to ingestion or exposure to drugs or other chemical substances.

Affective disorders A category of mental health problems that includes major depressive disorders and bipolar disorders.

AIDS Acquired immunodeficiency syndrome, an incurable disease of the immune system caused by a virus.

Air embolism When air or gas bubbles get into the bloodstream and obstruct the circulation.

Alimentary canal Comprises the mouth, pharynx, esophagus, stomach, small intestine, and large intestine.

Allograft Graft of tissue between individuals of the same species.

Alopecia Hair loss.

Alphabetic Index The index found in the ICD-10-CM book for both disease conditions and procedures.

Alteration Modifying the natural anatomic structure of a body part without affecting the function of the body part (e.g., breast augmentation).

Alzheimer's disease Disorder of the brain that causes a progressive decline in mental and physical function.

Ambulatory Payment Classifications (APCs) Used for outpatient prospective payment.

Amnioinfusion The insertion of normal saline or lactated Ringer's solution into the amniotic sac.

Ancillary services Services provided by a hospital that are additional to a professional service, such as laboratory work and radiology and pathology services.

Anemia Occurs when hemoglobin drops, which interrupts the transport of oxygen throughout the body.

Aneurysm Bulging or ballooning out of a vessel.

Angiodysplasia Type of AVM characterized by dilated or fragile blood vessels.

Angioplasty A procedure performed to treat coronary artery disease. An inflated balloon compresses plaque against artery walls.

Anomaly A deviation from normal standards (e.g., as in congenital defects).

Anorexia Loss of appetite.

Antepartum Time from conception until delivery or childbirth with regard to the mother.

Anterior Front of the body or an organ.

Anthrax Bacterial infection usually found in wild or domestic animals.

Anticoagulant medications Medications that are used to prevent venous thrombi.

Antiplatelet medications Medications that are used to prevent clumping of platelets or formation of an arterial thrombus.

Apgar Test used to measure the condition of a newborn at birth.

Aphasia Impairment of speech expression and/or word understanding.

Apheresis Procedure that separates different components of blood and removes a certain part of the blood, such as occurs in leukapheresis, plateletpheresis, and plasmapheresis.

Aplastic anemia Reduction in red blood cells due to impairment or failure of bone marrow function.

Appendectomy Removal of the appendix.

Appendicitis Inflammation of the appendix.

Arteriovenous malformation Defect that arises during fetal development.

Arthropathy Disease that affects the joints.

Arthroscopic Minimally invasive surgery that involves the use of highly specialized instruments to perform surgery through very small incisions on joints.

Arthroscopic approach An arthroscope is used to examine and perform closed procedures within a joint.

Asbestosis Lung disease due to inhalation of asbestos.

Aspiration pneumonia Inflammation of the lungs and bronchial tubes due to aspiration of foreign material into the lung.

Assistance Taking over a portion of a physiological function by extracorporeal means.

Asthma Chronic disease that affects the airways that carry air into and out of the lungs.

Asthmatic bronchitis Underlying asthmatic problem in patients in whom asthma has become so persistent that clinically significant chronic airflow obstruction is present despite antiasthmatic therapy.

Asymptomatic Without any symptoms.

Atherosclerosis Type of arteriosclerosis wherein fatty substances such as plaque block or clog the arteries.

Atmospheric control Extracorporeal control of atmospheric pressure and composition.

Atrophy When a gland becomes smaller.

Attention deficit disorder A common childhood disorder characterized by inattention and impulsivity.

Attention deficit hyperactivity disorder A common childhood disorder characterized by inattention, hyperactivity, and impulsivity.

Autograft Graft of tissue from another site on the same individual.

Autoimmune disorder Disorder that occurs when the immune system attacks itself inappropriately.

Autologous Originating from the recipient, rather than from a donor; tissue transferred from the same individual's body (e.g., a skin graft taken from one part of the body and transferred to another part of the body on the same individual).

Autologous transfusion Transfusion of a patient's own blood. Blood may have been donated before an elective procedure.

Autonomic nervous system Consists of both sensory and motor functions that involve the central nervous system and internal organs.

Bacteremia Bacteria in blood, which is a laboratory finding.

Bariatrics Branch of medicine that is concerned with the management (prevention or control) of obesity and allied diseases.

Baritosis Lung disease due to inhalation of barium.

Barrett's esophagus Precancerous condition that usually occurs in people with chronic GERD.

Basal cell carcinoma (BCC) Most common type of skin cancer.

Benign Neoplasm or tumor; means that it is not malignant.

Benign prostatic hyperplasia Condition resulting in enlargement of the prostate gland; usually occurs in men older than 50 years of age.

Benign prostatic hypertrophy Condition resulting in enlargement of the prostate gland; usually occurs in men older than 50 years of age.

Bilateral procedure Operative procedure performed on paired anatomic organs or tissues during the same operative session.

Biological response modifiers (BRM) Immunotherapy that can destroy cancer cells, stimulate the immune system to destroy cancer cells, or change cancer cells to normal cells.

Biopsy Removal of a representative sample for pathologic examination and diagnosis.

Bipolar disorder Brain disorder that causes unusual shifts in a person's mood, energy, and ability to function. Different from the normal ups and downs that everyone goes through, the symptoms of bipolar disorder are severe.

Black lung Lung disease due to inhalation of coal dust.

Blalock-Taussig procedure Procedure used to treat patients with tetralogy of Fallot who have insufficient pulmonary arterial flow.

Blood Viscous fluid that circulates through the vessels of the circulatory system as a result of the pumping action of the heart.

Blood pressure The force that blood puts on the arterial walls when the heart beats.

BNP (Brain natriuretic peptide) A hormone that is produced by the heart; a BNP test measures the amount of BNP that is found in the heart.

Body mass index Uses weight and height to estimate body fat.

Body system An anatomic region or a general physiological system on which a procedure is performed.

Bone marrow biopsy Diagnostic procedure that is used to identify types of anemia and cell deficiencies, and to detect leukemia.

Bowel resection Removal of a portion of the bowel.

Brachytherapy Placement of radioactive material directly into or near the cancer.

Bradycardia Slow heart rate, generally fewer than 60 beats per minute.

Bronchi The two air tubes that branch off the trachea and deliver air to both lungs.

Bronchitis Lower respiratory tract or bronchial tree infection characterized by cough, sputum production, and wheezing.

Bronchopulmonary dysplasia Chronic lung disease that develops in babies during the first 4 weeks after birth.

Bronchoscopy Diagnostic endoscopic procedure in which a tube with a tiny camera on the end is inserted through the nose or mouth into the lungs.

Bursitis Inflammation of a bursa, which is a tiny, fluid-filled sac that is found between muscles, tendons, and bones that reduces friction and facilitates movement.

Bypass Altering the route of passage of the contents of a tubular body part (CABG).

Calculus A stone. Calculi, which vary in size, can develop anywhere in the urinary tract.

Candidiasis Fungal infection also known as a *yeast infection*.

Capillaries Smallest blood vessel through which material passes to and from the bloodstream.

Carbuncle Cluster of boils.

Carcinoma in situ Malignant cells that remain within the original site with no spread or invasion into neighboring tissue.

Carcinomas Malignant tumors originating from epithelial tissue (e.g., in the skin, bronchi, and stomach).

Cardiac arrest Sudden loss of heart function.

Cardiomyopathy A disorder of the muscles of the heart chambers that impedes heart function.

Caregiver training Training in activities to support patient's optimal level of function.

Carryover line Used when an entry will not fit on a single line.

Case-mix index A measurement used by hospitals to define how sick their patients are.

Cataract Clouding of the lens of the eye causing obstructed vision.

Category A single three-digit code that describes a disease or a similarly related group of conditions.

Caudal Toward the tail.

Cellulitis Inflammation of the tissue with possible abscess.

Cephalhematoma A condition of blood between the skull and periosteum of a newborn.

Cerebral edema An accumulation of water on the brain either intracellular or extracellular.

Cervical dysplasia Abnormal growth of cells on the surface of the cervix.

Cervical intraepithelial neoplasia (CIN) Dysplasia that is seen on a biopsy of the cervix.

Cervix The neck of the uterus that serves as an outlet from the uterus.

Chancre An ulcer that forms during the first stage of syphilis.

Change To take out or off a device from a body part and put back an identical or similar device, in or on the same body part, without cutting or puncturing the skin or a mucous membrane (e.g., change gastrostomy tube).

Charge description number A number that designates a particular service or procedure, used to generate a charge on a patient bill.

Chargemaster or Charge description master A listing of the services, procedures, drugs, and supplies that can be applied to a patient's bill.

Chemoembolization Intra-arterial administration of chemotherapy with collagen particles to enhance the delivery of chemotherapy to the targeted area.

Chemotherapy Use of drugs or medications to treat disease.

Chief complaint The reason, in the patient's own words, for presenting to the hospital.

Choledocholithiasis Stone lodged in the bile duct.

Cholelithiasis An abnormal condition of stones in the gallbladder.

Cholesteatoma Growth in the middle ear that usually results from repeated ear infections.

Chronic Persistent over a long period.

Chronic bronchitis Condition defined by a mucus-producing cough most days of the month, 3 months out of a year for 2 successive years, with no other underlying disease to explain the cough.

Chronic obstructive pulmonary disease General term used to describe a lung disease in which the airways become obstructed, making it difficult for air to get into and out of the lungs.

Chronic sinusitis Occurs when the sinuses become inflamed and swollen.

Chylothorax Milky fluid consisting of lymph and fat (chyle) that accumulates in the pleural space.

Cirrhosis Liver disease wherein scar tissue replaces healthy tissue and blocks blood flow.

Classification Grouping together of items as for storage and retrieval.

Cleft lip/palate Opening in the lip or palate of an infant that occurs in utero.

Closed fracture Injury in which the bone is broken, but the skin remains intact.

Closed head injuries Injuries that result from a blow to the head.

Closed reduction The surgeon manipulates or reduces fractured bones into anatomic alignment without making an incision through the skin and subcutaneous tissue.

Clostridium difficile Microorganisms that are a leading cause of pseudomembranous colitis; also known as *C. diff.*

Coagulation defect Breakdown in the clotting process of the blood.

Coal workers' pneumoconiosis Lung disease due to inhalation of coal dust.

Cognitive deficit Disorder in thinking, learning, awareness, or judgment.

Cognitive impairment Decline in mental activities associated with thinking, learning, and memory.

Colles' fracture Common fracture in adults in which the lower end of the radius is fractured, and the wrist and the hand are displaced backward.

Colostomy A procedure that uses the colon to create an artificial opening.

Combination code A single code used to classify two diagnoses; or a diagnosis with an associated secondary process (manifestation); or a diagnosis with an associated complication.

Communicable Easily spread from one person to another.

Community-acquired pneumonia Broad term used to define pneumonias that are contracted outside of the hospital or nursing home setting.

Comorbidities Preexisting diagnoses or conditions that are present on admission.

Comorbidity A preexisting condition (it is present on admission) which may lead to increased resource use.

Complete abortion Abortion in which all the products of conception are expelled.

Complete remission There are no signs or symptoms of the cancer.

Compliance Adherence to accepted standards.

Complicated fracture Fracture that causes injury to surrounding tissues.

Complication A condition that arises during a patient's hospitalization which may lead to increased resource use.

Compound fracture When the broken bone exits and is visible through the skin, or a deep wound exposes the broken bone through the skin.

Compression Putting pressure on a body region.

Computer assisted surgery (CAS) Adjunctive procedure that allows increased visualization and more precise navigation while remaining minimally invasive.

Computerized tomography (CT scans) Computer reformatted digital display of multiplanar images developed from the capture of multiple exposures of external ionizing radiation.

Concussion Injury to the brain that results from a significant blow to the head.

Conduction disorder Abnormalities of cardiac impulses.

Condylomata Wart-type growth found usually in the genital or anal area.

Congenital anomaly An abnormal condition present at birth.

Connecting words Subterms that denote a relationship between a main term or a subterm and an associated condition or etiology.

Consultant Healthcare provider who is asked to see the patient to provide expert opinion outside the expertise of the requestor.

Contaminant A cultured organism that a physician does not believe is responsible for causing a particular infection.

Continuous ambulatory peritoneal dialysis Type of peritoneal dialysis that takes about 15 minutes and is performed 3 to 4 times per day and once at night.

Continuous cycling peritoneal dialysis Type of peritoneal dialysis that uses a cycling machine and is performed while the patient sleeps.

Control Stopping, or attempting to stop, postprocedural bleeding (e.g., control of post-tonsillectomy hemorrhage)

Contusion Any mechanical injury that results in hemorrhage beneath unbroken skin.

Conventions General rules for use in classification that must be followed for accurate coding.

Conversion disorder Condition in which a person has some type of sensory or motor (neurologic) symptom(s) that cannot be explained.

Core biopsy Procedure in which a large needle is used to extract a core sample.

Coronary artery bypass graft Surgery performed to bypass an occluded coronary artery.

Corrosion Burn due to a chemical.

Cranial Toward the head.

Creation Making a new structure that does not take the place of a body part (creation of vagina in males for sex reassignment).

Credential Degree, certificate, or award that recognizes a course of study taken in a specific field and that acknowledges the competency required.

Crohn's disease Inflammation of the GI tract, especially the small and large intestine.

Crush injury When a body part is subjected to a high degree of force or pressure, usually after it has been squeezed between two heavy or immobile objects.

Current Procedural Terminology (CPT) A coding system for reporting medical services and procedures.

Cushing's syndrome Condition that results in excessive circulating cortisol levels caused by chronic hypersecretion of the adrenal cortex.

Cystic fibrosis Genetic (inherited) condition that affects the cells that produce mucus, sweat, saliva, and digestive juices. Instead of being thin and slippery, these secretions are thick and sticky, plugging up tubes, ducts, and passageways, especially in the pancreas and lungs.

Cystitis Lower tract infection that affects the bladder.

Cystocele When the bladder descends and presses into the wall of the vagina.

Cystoscopy Approach used for many procedures of the urinary tract.

Cystourethrocele A urethrocele in conjunction with a cystocele.

Debridement Removal of devitalized tissue, necrosis, or slough.

Debulking Procedures performed when it is impossible to remove the tumor entirely.

Decompression Extracorporeal elimination of undissolved gas from body fluids.

Decubitus ulcer Skin ulcer also known as a bed sore.

Deep brain stimulator A device implanted to control tremors.

Deep vein thrombosis A blood clot that forms in a deep vein.

Deficit Reduction Act (DRA) Mandates all acute-care facilities reimbursed under MS-DRGs to identify and report diagnoses that are present at the time of a patient's admission.

Dehiscence Opening of a surgical wound.

Dehydration When the body does not have as much water or fluids as it should.

Delirium tremens Life-threatening condition that may involve severe mental or neurologic changes, such as delirium and/or hallucinations.

Delivery Assisting the passage of the products of conception from the genital canal.

Dementia Progressive deterioration of mental faculties characterized by impaired memory and one or more cognitive impairments such as language, reasoning and judgment, or calculation and problem-solving ability.

Dengue fever A virus transmitted by an infected mosquito.

Department number Ancillary departments (e.g., radiology, laboratory, ER) that have a specific hospital departmental number.

Depression Affective disorder that is characterized by sadness, lack of interest in everyday activities and events, and a sense of worthlessness.

Destruction Physical eradication of all or a portion of a body part by the direct use of energy, force, or a destructive agent (e.g., ablation of endometriosis).

Dermatitis Inflammation of the skin.

Dermis Layer of skin below the epidermis.

Detachment Cutting off all or a portion of the upper or lower extremities (e.g., above-knee amputation).

Detoxification Active management of withdrawal symptoms in a patient who is physically dependent on alcohol or drugs.

Device fitting Fitting of a device designed to facilitate or support achievement of a higher level of function.

Diabetes insipidus Deficiency in the release of vasopressin by the posterior pituitary gland.

Diabetes mellitus Chronic syndrome of impaired carbohydrate, protein, and fat metabolism caused by insufficient production of insulin by the pancreas or faulty utilization of insulin by the cells.

Diagnosis Identification of a disease through signs, symptoms, and tests.

Dialysis disequilibrium syndrome Characterized by weakness, dizziness, headache, and in severe cases mental status changes.

Diaphragm Dome-shaped muscles at the bottom of the lungs that assist in the process of breathing and in the exchange of oxygen/carbon dioxide.

Differential diagnosis When a symptom may represent a variety of diagnoses.

Dilation Expanding an orifice or the lumen of a tubular body part (e.g., PTCA).

Discharge summary A review of the patient's hospital course. This summary details the reason for admission or tests or procedures performed and how the patient responded.

Dislocation Displacement of the bones that form a joint; separation of the end of a bone from the joint it meets.

Dissection A tear in wall of a vessel.

Disseminated intravascular coagulation Disorder that results in depletion of clotting factors in the blood.

Distal Farther from the median plane; term is often used to describe a location in the limbs.

Diverticula Small pouches in the lining of the mucous membranes of an organ.

Division Cutting into a body part, without draining fluids and/or gases from it, in order to separate or transect the part (e.g., osteotomy).

Dorsal Back of the body or an organ.

Dorsopathies Conditions or diseases that affect the back or spine.

Drainage Taking or letting out fluids and/or gases from a body part (e.g., paracentesis).

Dressing Putting material on a body region for protection.

Dumping syndrome Occurs when undigested contents of the stomach are transported to the small intestine too quickly.

Dyscalculia Learning disability that affects a child's ability to do mathematical calculations.

Dysgraphia Learning disability that affects a child's ability to coordinate movements such as writing.

Dyslexia Learning disability that affects a child's ability to understand or use spoken or written language.

Dysmetabolic Syndrome X Characterized by abdominal obesity, insulin resistance, dyslipidemia and elevated blood pressure or hypertension.

Eating disorders A group of conditions characterized by abnormal eating habits that may affect an individual's physical and psychological well-being. The most common eating disorders are binge-eating disorder, bulimia nervosa, and anorexia nervosa.

Eclampsia Complication of pregnancy characterized by hypertension, edema, proteinuria, and convulsions or seizures.

Ectopic Type of pregnancy that occurs when the egg is implanted outside the cavity of the uterus.

Eczema Type of dermatitis characterized by itching.

Edentulism The complete loss of teeth.

Effaced Cervical thinning.

Elderly obstetric patient 35 years or older at date of delivery.

Elective abortion Elective termination of pregnancy.

Electroconvulsive therapy Psychiatric treatment in which electricity is used to induce seizures.

Electromagnetic therapy Extracorporeal treatment by electromagnetic rays.

Electromyelogram Test that measures electrical activity in muscles and nerves.

Electrophysiologist Physician trained in electrical disorders of the heart.

Embolus Clot that travels to another part of the body.

Emphysema Chronic lung disease of gradual onset that can be attributed to chronic infection and inflammation or irritation from cigarette smoke.

Empiric Initiation of treatment prior to making a definite diagnosis.

Empyema Pus that accumulates in the pleural space.

Encoder Coding software that is used to assign diagnosis and procedure codes.

Encounter Face-to-face visit with a healthcare provider.

Endocarditis Inflammation of the lining of the heart chambers and valves.

Endocrine system Body system composed of many glands that secrete hormones that regulate bodily functions; it works with the nervous system to maintain body activities and homeostasis and to respond to stress.

Endogenous Type of dermatitis caused by something taken internally, such as medication.

Endometriosis A chronic condition in which endometrial material, the tissue that lines the inside of the uterus, grows outside the uterus and attaches to other organs in the pelvic cavity.

Endometritis Inflammation of the uterus.

Endoscopic Examinations and procedures performed with an instrument that examines any cavity of the body with a rigid or a flexible scope.

Endoscopic biopsy Biopsy that is performed during endoscopic examination.

Epidermis Outermost layer of skin.

Epilepsy Disorder of the brain that is characterized by abnormal electrical discharges from the brain cells.

Eponym Term for a disease, structure, procedure, or syndrome that has been named for a person.

Erythema Redness of the skin.

Erythrocytes Another name for red blood cells that are made in the marrow of bones; their main responsibility is to carry oxygen around the body and remove carbon dioxide. These are the cells that give blood its red color.

Ethics Moral standard.

Etiology Cause or origin of a disease or condition.

Euvolemia State of normal body fluid volume.

Excision Cutting out or off, without replacement, a portion of a body part (e.g., partial nephrectomy).

Excisional Removal by surgical cutting.

Excisional biopsy Total removal of local small masses or growths.

Exhibitionism Recurrent intense sexual urges and fantasies of exposing the genitals to an unsuspecting stranger.

Exogenous Type of dermatitis caused by contact with a substance.

Exophthalmos Bulging of the eyes.

External Procedures performed directly on the skin or mucous membrane, and procedures performed indirectly by the application of external force through the skin or mucous membrane (e.g., tonsillectomy).

External skeletal fixation Form of fracture treatment that involves insertion of percutaneous pins proximal and distal to the fracture and application of a frame that connects the pins externally.

Extirpation Taking or cutting out solid matter from a body part (e.g., thrombectomy).

Extracorporeal shock wave lithotripsy Used to break up kidney stones into small particles that can then pass through the urinary tract into the urine.

Extraction Pulling or stripping out or off all or portion of a body part by force (e.g., bone marrow biopsy).

Extravasation Leakage of infused substance into vasculature or subcutaneous tissue.

Facet joints Small, stabilizing joints located between and behind adjacent vertebrae.

Fallopian tube Delivers the mature egg to the uterus for fertilization.

Fascia Tissue just below the skin that covers and separates the underlying layers of muscle.

Fat embolism When fat enters the circulatory system after long bone or pelvic fractures.

Federal Register The official daily publication for rules, proposed rules, and notices of U.S. federal agencies and organizations.

Fetishism Recurrent intense sexual urges and fantasies of using inanimate objects for sexual arousal or orgasm. Objects commonly used include female clothing such as shoes, earrings, or undergarments.

Fibromas Neoplasms of fibrous connective tissue.

Fibromyalgia One of the most common diseases affecting the muscles; it is characterized by widespread muscle pain associated with chronic fatigue.

Fine needle aspiration Procedure in which a very small needle is used; works best for masses that are superficial or easily accessible.

Fistula Abnormal passage or communication between two internal organs, or leading from an organ to the surface of the body. It can also be an abnormal passage between an artery and a vein.

Fluid overload Occurs when there is too much fluid in the body.

Fluoroscopy Single plane or bi-plane real time display of an image developed from the capture of external ionizing radiation on a fluorescent screen. The image may also be stored by either digital or analog means.

Foregut Bronchi and stomach (sites of carcinoid neoplasm).

Fracture Break in a bone.

Fragmentation Breaking solid matter in a body part into pieces (e.g., extracorporeal shock wave lithotripsy).

Free flap Involves the cutting of skin, fat, blood vessels, and muscle free from its location and moving it to the chest area.

Frostbite Occurs when skin and underlying tissues freeze due to extreme cold.

Fundoplication Surgery in which the fundus of the stomach is wrapped around the esophagus.

Furuncle A boil.

Fusion Joining together portions of an articular body part, rendering the articular body part immobile (e.g., spinal fusion).

Gangrene Dead tissue usually associated with loss of vascular supply.

Gastroenteritis Inflammation of the stomach, small intestine, and large intestine.

Generalized anxiety disorder Chronic exaggerated worry, tension, and irritability that may occur without cause or that are more intense than the situation warrants.

Genetic Inherited.

Genital prolapse When pelvic organs such as the uterus, bladder, and rectum shift from their normal anatomic positions and protrude into the vagina or press against the wall of the vagina.

Gigantism Condition that occurs when hypersecretion of hGH occurs before puberty, along with proportionate overgrowth of all bodily tissues, especially the long bones.

Glaucoma Disorder of the optic nerve that may result in vision loss.

Glioma A primary malignant brain neoplasm that starts in the glial cells of the central nervous system.

Glomerulonephritis Inflammation of the glomeruli of the kidneys.

Goiter Enlargement of the thyroid gland.

Gonorrhea Disease caused by a bacterium and transmitted by sexual contact.

Grading Pathologic examination of tumor cells. Degree of cell abnormality determines the grade of cancer.

Graft-versus-host disease (GVHD) Common complication that can occur after a stem cell or bone marrow transplant in which the newly transplanted material attacks the transplant recipient's body.

Granulation Newly formed tissue that covers an open sore or a wound.

Graves' disease The most common form of hyperthyroidism; it occurs through an autoimmune response that attacks the thyroid gland, resulting in overproduction of the thyroid hormone thyroxine.

Gravid Pregnant.

Grouper Specialized software used to assign the appropriate MS-DRG.

Gustilo open fracture classification Based on the mechanism of the injury and the amount of soft tissue and skeletal injury and is useful in assessing risk of infection and possible amputation.

HAART Highly active antiretroviral therapy, a group of drugs given to AIDS patients for prophylaxis.

Habitual aborter A woman who miscarries at least three consecutive times.

Hashimoto's disease Inflammation of the thyroid gland that often results in hypothyroidism.

Health Maintenance Organizations (HMOs) Type of managed care in which hospitals, physicians, and other providers contract to provide health care for patients, usually at a discounted rate.

Healthcare provider Person who provides care to a patient.

Hearing aid assessment Measurement of the appropriateness and/or effectiveness of a hearing device.

Hearing aid treatment Application of techniques to improve the communication abilities of individuals with cochlear implant.

Hearing assessment Measurement of hearing and related functions.

Hearing treatment Application of techniques to improve, augment, or compensate for hearing and related functional impairment.

Heart failure Impaired function of the heart's pumping ability.

Helminthiases Another word for diseases caused by parasitic worms.

Hematemesis Vomiting of blood.

Hematochezia Bright red blood in stool.

Hematopoiesis Development of blood cells that occurs in the bone marrow and lymphatic tissue of normal adults.

Hematuria The presence of blood in the urine.

Hemiplegia Paralysis of half of the body.

Hemodialysis Process that uses a machine called a hemodialyzer to remove wastes from the blood.

Hemolysis The breaking down of red blood cells.

Hemolytic anemias Result from abnormal or excessive destruction of red blood cells.

Hemophilia A Most common type of hemophilia; deficiency or abnormality in clotting factor VIII.

Hemophilia B Another name for Christmas disease, which results from a deficiency of factor IX.

Hemophilia C Mild form of hemophilia with decreased factor XI.

Hemothorax Blood that accumulates in the pleural space.

Hepatitis An inflammation of the liver.

Hernia Protrusion of an organ or tissue through an abnormal opening in the body.

Herniorrhaphy Repair of a hernia.

Herpes simplex A virus also known as a *cold sore* or *fever blister*.

Herpes zoster A disease caused by the same virus that causes chicken pox.

Heterograft Graft of skin from another species, such as a graft from a pig to a human.

Hindgut Colon and rectum (sites of carcinoid neoplasms).

Histologic type Type of tissue or cell in which the neoplasm occurs.

Histoplasmosis A fungal disease that primarily affects the lungs.

HIV Human immunodeficiency virus is the virus that affects the immune system and can progress to AIDS.

Hives Skin condition also known as urticaria, wherein the skin reacts with welts; characterized by itching.

Homeostasis The ability of an organism or cell to maintain internal equilibrium by adjusting its physiological processes.

Homograft Graft from one individual to another of the same species; also known as an allograft.

Hormones Substances secreted by glands that can regulate bodily functions, such as urinary output, cellular metabolic rate, and growth and development.

Hybrid A combination of formats producing similar results (e.g., paper and electronic records).

Hydrocephalus Cerebrospinal fluid collection in the skull.

Hyperhidrosis Excessive sweating.

Hydronephrosis Abnormal dilatation of the renal pelvis caused by pressure from urine that cannot flow past an obstruction in the urinary tract.

Hydroureter Accumulation of urine in the ureters.

Hyperbaric oxygen therapy (HBOT) Treatment in which the patient's entire body is placed in a transparent, airtight chamber at increased atmospheric pressure.

Hyperemesis gravidarum Excessive vomiting in pregnancy.

Hyperglycemia Condition that results when glucose or blood sugar becomes abnormally high. This is a relatively common event in patients with diabetes.

Hyperparathyroidism Condition that results when an overactive parathyroid gland secretes excessive parathyroid hormone, causing increased levels of circulating calcium associated with loss of calcium in the bone.

Hyperpituitarism Increased production of the pituitary hormones, particularly the human growth hormone (hGH).

Hyperplasia Enlargement of a gland.

Hypersomnia Excessive sleep.

Hyperthermia Extracorporeal raising of body temperature.

Hyperthyroidism Abnormality of the thyroid gland in which secretion of thyroid hormone is usually increased and is no longer under the regulatory control of hypothalamic-pituitary centers.

Hypertrophy Enlargement of a gland.

Hypervitaminosis Toxicity resulting from an excess of any vitamin, especially fat-soluble vitamins such as A, D, and K.

Hypervolemia Occurs when there is too much fluid in the body.

Hypoglycemia Condition that results when glucose, or blood sugar, becomes abnormally low.

Hypomania Milder form of mania, but this "feel good" mood can change to depression or mania.

Hypoparathyroidism Underactive parathyroid gland that results in decreased levels of circulating calcium.

Hypopituitarism Condition caused by low levels of pituitary hormones. Hormones secreted by the pituitary gland can affect the functions of other glands.

Hypoplasia Atrophy; condition that results when a gland becomes smaller.

Hypothermia Extracorporeal lowering of body temperature.

Hypothyroidism Condition caused by low levels of pituitary hormones. Hormones secreted by the pituitary gland can affect the functions of other glands.

Hypovolemia Occurs due to decreased plasma volume.

Hypoxia Insufficient oxygen in the blood.

Iatrogenic Caused by medical treatment.

ICD-10-CM *International Classification of Diseases, 10th Revision Clinical Modification.*

ICD-10-PCS *International Classification of Diseases, 10th Revision-Procedure Coding System.*

Idiopathic Causative factor is unknown.

Ileostomy End of small intestine brought out through the abdominal wall.

Ileus Absence of normal movement within the intestine.

Immobilization Limiting or preventing motion of a body region.

Immune system Includes the bone marrow, lymph nodes, thymus, and spleen; its purpose is to protect the body from all types of infections, toxins, neoplastic cell growth and foreign blood or tissues from another person.

Immunotherapy Administration of agents that stimulate the immune system's response against tumors.

Impaction Condition that occurs when stool in the rectum becomes so hard that it cannot be passed normally.

Incidental appendectomy Appendectomy performed at the time of another procedure with no known disease process in the appendix.

Incisional biopsy Procedure in which a representative sample of a tumor mass is removed to permit pathologic examination.

Incomplete abortion Abortion in which not all of the products of conception are expelled.

Inevitable abortion Abortion that occurs when symptoms are present and a miscarriage will happen.

Infection Invasion of the body with organisms that have the potential to cause disease.

Inferior Position of the body or an organ relative to the vertical axis of the body.

Influenza Contagious viral infection of the respiratory tract that causes coughing, difficulty breathing, headache, muscle aches, and weakness.

Insertion Putting in a nonbiological appliance that monitors, assists, performs, or prevents a physiological function but does not physically take the place of a body part (e.g., insertion of pacemaker lead).

Inspection Visually and/or manually exploring a body part (e.g., diagnostic arthroscopy).

Integral Essential part of a disease process.

Integumentary Another name for skin.

Intellectual disabilities Disorder in which a person's overall intellectual functioning is well below average, with an intelligence quotient (IQ) around 70 or less.

Intertrigo Dermatitis in areas where friction may occur.

Interventionalist Physician trained in disease treatment via the use of catheter-based technique.

Intractable Not manageable.

Introduction Putting in or on a therapeutic, diagnostic, nutritional, physiological, or prophylactic substance except blood or blood products.

Insomnia Difficulty falling asleep, wakefulness, and early morning awakening.

Intussusception Bowel becomes obstructed when a portion of the intestine telescopes into another portion.

Irrigation Putting in or on a cleansing substance.

Joints Means of joining two bones together.

Juvenile rheumatoid arthritis Type of arthritis which affects children usually between the ages of 2 and 5 years.

Kaposi's sarcoma (KS) Cancer that develops from the lining of lymph or blood vessels.

Klinefelter's syndrome A sex chromosome disorder that occurs in males and is caused by an extra X chromosome.

Kwashiorkor Severe type of malnutrition resulting in dyspigmentation of the skin and hair, edema, and growth retardation.

Kyphoplasty Procedure to treat and stabilize fractures of the spine.

Kyphosis Excessive posterior curvature of the thoracic spine that may not be detected until a hump in the upper back is noticeable.

Labia Surrounds the vaginal opening.

Labor Process by which the products of conception are expelled from the uterus.

Laceration An injury that results in a tear in the skin.

Lactation Process of milk production from mammary glands.

Laparoscopic approach Uses a laparoscope to examine and perform closed procedures within the abdomen.

Lateral Position of a structure that is to the side of the body.

Legal blindness Severe or profound impairment in both eyes.

Leiomyoma Tumor or growth within the walls of the uterus. Also called *uterine fibroid.*

Leukemia Cancer of the white blood cells that begins in the blood-forming cells of the bone marrow.

Leukocytes White blood cells increase in number to battle infection, inflammation, and other diseases.

Leukocytosis Increase in the number of white cells in the blood; it may be a sign of infection or may indicate stress on the body.

Level II HCPCS Codes used to identify drugs, medical supplies, and durable medical equipment.

Ligaments Dense, fibrous bands of connective tissue that provide stability for the joint.

Limited coverage Procedures that are identified by the Medicare Code Editor as procedures covered under limited circumstances.

Lipoma Growth of fat cells within a capsule that usually is found just below the skin.

Lobar pneumonia Synonym for pneumococcal pneumonia or pneumonia due to *Streptococcus pneumoniae* pneumonia.

Local coverage determinations Local policy that may include certain time frames for testing, that a patient be a certain age, and that a particular diagnosis or condition is present to be considered medical necessary.

Lordosis Exaggerated inward curvature of the spine that may be caused by increased abdominal girth due to obesity, pregnancy, or abdominal tumor.

Loss of consciousness When a patient is unable to respond to people or other stimuli.

Lung abscess Infection that forms in the lung parenchyma.

Lyme disease An inflammatory disease caused by bacteria carried by ticks.

Lymphadenitis Inflammation of a lymph node that usually is caused by a bacterial infection.

Lymphoma Cancer of the lymphatic system.

Lysis Destruction of adhesions.

Macular degeneration Vision loss in the central portion of the eye, leaving the patient with peripheral vision or low vision.

Main term Term that identifies disease conditions or injuries, it is identified in bold print and set flush with the left margin of each column in the Alphabetic Index.

Magnetic resonance imaging (MRI) Computer reformatted digital display of multiplanar images developed from the capture of radio-frequency signals emitted by nuclei in a body site excited within a magnetic field.

Major depressive disorder Characterized by one or more major depressive episodes with a history of mania, hypomania, or mixed episodes.

Malignancy Neoplasm that has the ability to invade adjacent structures and spread to distant sites.

Malignant A neoplasm that invades surrounding structures and metastasizes to distant places in the body.

Malignant ascites Excess fluid that contains malignant cells and accumulates in the abdomen or peritoneum.

Malignant hypertension Rapidly rising blood pressure, usually in excess of 140 mm Hg diastolic, with findings of visual impairment and symptoms or signs of progressive cardiac failure.

Malignant melanoma Malignant neoplasm of the melanocytes; the most common place of occurrence is the skin.

Malignant mesothelioma Rare aggressive cancer that develops in the protective lining or mesothelium that surrounds and protects the internal organs.

Malignant pleural effusion Fluid accumulates in the pleural space and contains malignant cells.

Mallory-Weiss Bleeding laceration of the esophagogastric junction.

Malnutrition Nutrition disorder caused by primary deprivation of protein energy resulting from poverty or self-imposed starvation or associated with deficiency diseases such as cancer.

Malunion Occurs when fracture fragments have united but are not properly aligned. Incorrectly positioned bones may demonstrate angulation, rotation, and shortening.

Mania The other side of depression, in which a person feels so good, it is like a "high"; may do risky things.

Manifestation Symptom or condition that is the result of a disease.

Manipulation Manual procedure that involves a directed thrust to move a joint past the physiological range of motion without exceeding the anatomical limit.

Map Locating the route of passage of electrical impulses and/or locating functional areas in a body part (e.g., cardiac mapping).

Marfan syndrome An inherited condition that affects connective tissue and is caused by gene mutation.

Masochism The act or sense of gaining pleasure from experiencing physical or psychological pain.

Mastication Chewing of food.

Mastitis Inflammation or infection of the breast.

Mastoiditis Infection of the mastoid bone of the skull.

Maximization The manipulation of codes to result in maximum reimbursement without supporting documentation in the health record or with disregard for coding conventions, guidelines, and UHDDS definitions.

McBurney's point Area of the abdomen that, when touched, causes pain that may be indicative of appendicitis.

Measurement Determining the level of a physiological or physical function at a point in time.

Mechanical complication When a device or equipment malfunctions.

Mechanical ventilation Use of a machine to induce alternating inflation and deflation of the lungs, to regulate the exchange rate of gases in the blood.

Meconium Material in the intestine of a fetus.

Medial Position of a structure closer to the median plane than is another structure in the body.

Medical necessity Criteria or guidelines for what is determined to be reasonable and necessary for a particular medical service.

Medicare Code Editor Software that detects errors in coding on Medicare claims.

Melanomas Malignant changes of melanin cells.

Melena Dark blood in stool.

Meningitis An infection in the fluid of a person's spinal cord and brain.

Mental retardation A disorder in which a person's overall intellectual functioning is well below average, and intelligence quotient (IQ) is around 70 or less.

Metabolic encephalopathy Temporary or permanent damage to the brain due to lack of glucose, oxygen, metabolic agents, or organ dysfunction.

Metastasis Spread of a cancer from one part of the body to another, as in the appearance of neoplasms in parts of the body separate from the site of the primary tumor.

Midgut Small intestine and appendix (sites of carcinoid neoplasms).

Miscarriage Spontaneous termination of pregnancy before the fetus has reached 20 weeks.

Missed abortion Pregnancy with fetal demise before 20 weeks; products of conception are not expelled.

Mixed incontinence Combination of stress and urge incontinence.

Mixed mania/mood Alteration from mania and depression, back and forth, very quickly.

Molar pregnancy Fertilized ovum is converted to a mole.

Monitoring Determining the level of a physiological or physical function repetitively over a period of time.

Mood disorder Condition that occurs when there has been a change in mood for a prolonged time.

Morbid obesity Applies to patients who are 50% to 100% or 100 pounds above their ideal body weight. A BMI of 40 or higher defines morbid obesity.

Morbidity Pertaining to disease.

Morphology The study of neoplasms.

Morphology codes (M codes) Codes that identify the type of cell that has become neoplastic and its biological activity or behavior.

Mortality Pertaining to death.

Motor and/or nerve function assessment Measurement of motor, nerve, and related functions.

Motor treatment Exercise or activities to increase or facilitate motor function.

MS-DRG grouper Software that assigns MS-DRG using diagnosis and procedure codes.

Mucositis An inflammation/ulceration of the digestive tract commonly occurring in the oral cavity.

Multigravida/Multiparity A woman with two or more pregnancies.

Muscular dystrophy Type of myopathy.

Myasthenia gravis Chronic autoimmune disorder that manifests as muscle weakness of varying degrees.

Mycobacterium avium intercellulare Mycobacteria found in soil and water.

Mycosis Fungal infection.

Myeloma Malignancy that originates in the bone marrow.

Myelopathy Compression of the spinal cord.

Myocardial infarction Heart attack.

Myopathy Disorder that affects muscles, usually resulting in weakness or atrophy.

Myxedema Skin and tissue disorder that usually is due to severe prolonged hypothyroidism.

Nadir The lowest level.

National coverage determinations (NCDs) National policy that may include certain time frames for testing, certain age requirements, and that a particular diagnosis or condition be present for a procedure to be considered medically necessary.

NEC Abbreviation for "not elsewhere classifiable" that means "other specified."

Necrosis Death of cells.

Necrotic Dead tissue that lacks a blood supply.

Necrotizing fasciitis (or "flesh-eating disease") A rare but serious condition in which an infection occurs in the tissues below the skin.

Neoplasm Abnormal growth.

Nephrolithiasis Kidney stone.

Nephrotic syndrome Condition marked by proteinuria (protein in the urine), low levels of protein in the blood, hypercholesterolemia, and swelling of the eyes, feet, and hands.

Neutropenia Abnormal decrease in granular leukocytes in the blood.

Nomenclature System of names that are used as the preferred terminology.

Noncovered OR procedure A procedure code categorized by the Medicare Code Editor as a noncovered operating room procedure for which Medicare does not provide reimbursement.

Nonessential modifier Term that is enclosed in parentheses; its presence or absence does not affect code assignment.

Non-Hodgkin's lymphoma A type of cancer of the lymphatic system.

Nonimaging nuclear medicine assay Introduction of radioactive materials into the body for the study of body fluids and blood elements, by the detection of radioactive emissions.

Nonimaging nuclear medicine probe Introduction of radioactive materials into the body for the study of distribution and fate of certain substances by the detection of radioactive emissions from an external source.

Nonimaging nuclear medicine uptake Introduction of radioactive materials into the body for measurements of organ functions, from detection of radioactive emissions.

Noninvasive ventilation Ventilation without an invasive artificial airway (endotracheal tube or tracheostomy).

Non-OR procedure affecting DRG assignment Procedure code recognized by the MS-DRG Grouper as a non–operating room procedure that may affect MS-DRG assignment.

Nonunion Of a fracture occurs when the bony healing is not achieved at the fracture site. A fracture site that fails to heal within approximately 6 to 9 months of the injury represents a nonunion.

NOS Abbreviation for "not otherwise specified" that means "unspecified."

Nosocomial Hospital-acquired infection.

Nosocomial pneumonia Pneumonia that is acquired while the patient is residing in a hospital-type setting.

NSTEMI Non–ST elevation myocardial infarction.

Nursing home–acquired pneumonia Pneumonia that is acquired in a nursing home or extended care facility.

Nutritional marasmus Severe form of malnutrition that is characterized by severe tissue wasting, loss of subcutaneous fat, and maybe dehydration.

Obesity Condition defined as an increase in body weight beyond the limitation of skeletal and physical requirements, caused by excessive accumulation of fat in the body.

Observation unit Area outside the emergency department where unstable patients are admitted for a stay of less than 48 hours. The patient is observed for admission to the hospital or is discharged to home.

Occult blood Blood found only by laboratory inspection.

Occlusion Completely closing an orifice or lumen of a tubular body part (e.g., tubal ligation).

Omit code An instructional note found in Volume 3 that denotes that no code is to be assigned; it generally is used for coding approaches and closures that are integral to an operative procedure.

Oophoritis Inflammation of the ovaries.

Open Cutting through the skin, mucous membrane, and any other body layers necessary to expose the site of the procedure (e.g., abdominal hysterectomy).

Open fracture When the broken bone exits and is visible through the skin, or a deep wound exposes the broken bone through the skin.

Open reduction When the surgeon makes an incision at the fracture site to reduce or manipulate the fracture into anatomic position.

Open with percutaneous endoscopic assistance Cutting through the skin, mucous membrane, and any other body layers necessary to expose the site of the procedure; and entry of instrumentation, by puncture or minor incision, through the skin, mucous membrane, and any other body layers necessary to aid in the performance of the procedure (laparoscopically assisted vaginal hysterectomy).

Oppositional defiant disorder Pattern of uncooperative, defiant, and hostile behavior toward authority figures that does not involve major antisocial violations, is not accounted for by the child's developmental stage, and results in significant functional impairment.

Optimization The process of striving to obtain optimal reimbursement or the highest possible payment to which a facility is legally entitled on the basis of documentation in the health record.

Organic brain syndrome General term used to describe the decrease in mental function caused by other physical disease(s).

Osteoarthritis Type of arthritis that develops as the result of wear and tear on the joints.

Osteomyelitis Infection of the bone that often starts in another part of the body and spreads to the bone via the blood.

Osteoporosis Metabolic bone disorder that results in decreased bone mass and density.

Ostomies Surgically created openings into the body.

Other procedures Methodologies that attempt to remediate or cure a disorder or disease.

Otitis media Middle ear infection.

Ovaries Produce female hormones and eggs.

Overflow incontinence The constant dribbling of urine.

Packing Putting material in a body region or orifice.

Palliative Procedure performed to correct a condition that is causing problems for the patient.

Pancreatitis Inflammation of the pancreas often caused by gallstones or chronic heavy alcohol use.

Pancytopenia Decrease in production of erythrocytes (red blood cells), leukocytes (white blood cells), and thrombocytes (platelets).

Panic disorder Terrifying experience that occurs suddenly without warning. Physical symptoms include pounding heart, chest pains, dizziness, nausea, shortness of breath, trembling, choking, fear of dying, sweating, feelings of unreality, numbness, hot flashes or chills, and a feeling of going out of control or "crazy."

Parasitic Organism that lives on or takes nourishment from another organism.

Parenteral When medications are administered other than through the digestive tract, such as by intravenous or intramuscular injection.

Parkinson's disease Progressive and chronic motor system disorder.

Partial remission There are still a few signs and symptoms of the cancer, and the cancer cells have significantly decreased.

Pathologic fracture Break in a bone that occurs because of underlying disorders that weaken the bone, including malignancy, benign bone tumor, metabolic disorder, infection, and osteoporosis.

Pedicle graft/flap Involves identifying a flap that remains attached to its original blood supply and tunneling it under the skin to a particular area, such as the breast.

Pelvic inflammatory disease When vaginal or cervical infections spread and involve the uterus, fallopian tubes, ovaries, and surrounding tissues.

Pemphigus Autoimmune disorder causing blistering of skin and mucous membranes.

Percutaneous Entry of instrumentation, by puncture or minor incision, through the skin, mucous membrane, and any other body layers necessary to reach the site of the procedure (e.g., needle biopsy liver).

Percutaneous endoscopic Entry of instrumentation, by puncture or minor incision, through the skin, mucous membrane, and any other body layers necessary to reach and visualize the site of the procedure (e.g., laparoscopic cholecystectomy).

Percutaneous endoscopic gastrostomy A tube put through the abdominal wall into the stomach with the use of a scope.

Percutaneous nephrolithotomy Procedure in which the surgeon uses a nephroscope to remove a stone. At times, an ultrasonic or electrohydraulic probe is used to break up the stone, and the fragments are then removed.

Percutaneous vertebroplasty Technique in which x-ray guidance is used to inject an acrylic cement through a needle into a collapsed or weakened vertebra; procedure is performed to treat pain caused by compression fractures of the vertebrae.

Performance Completely taking over a physiological function by extracorporeal means.

Pericarditis Inflammation of the covering of the heart.

Perinatal period Before birth through the first 28 days of life.

Peristalsis Rhythmic muscle contractions that move food down the digestive tract.

Peritoneal dialysis When the peritoneal membrane in the patient's own body is used with a dialysate solution to filter out the wastes and excess fluids.

Peritonitis Inflammation of the peritoneum usually caused by bacteria or fungus.

Personality disorder A pattern of behavior that can disrupt many aspects of a person's life.

Phacoemulsification Incision that is made on the side of the cornea where the lens material is softened, broken, and suctioned out.

Pheresis Extracorporeal separation of blood products.

Phlebitis Inflammation of a vein.

Phobia Irrational anxiety or fear that can interfere with one's everyday life or daily routine.

Phototherapy Extracorporeal treatment by light rays.

Physician Licensed medical doctor.

Plain radiography Planar display of an image developed from the capture of external ionizing radiation on photographic or photoconductive plate.

Planar nuclear medicine imaging Introduction of radioactive materials into the body for single plane display of images developed from the capture of radioactive emissions.

Platelets Another name for thrombocytes. Platelets circulate in the blood and assist in the clotting process.

Pleural effusion Fluid that accumulates in the pleural space because of trauma or disease.

Pneumoconioses Lung diseases due to chronic inhalation of inorganic (mineral) dust that are often due to occupational exposure.

Pneumonia Infection of the lungs that may be caused by a variety of organisms, including viruses, bacteria, and parasites.

Pneumothorax Air in space around the lung.

Poliomyelitis A viral disease that affects the nerves.

Polymyalgia rheumatica Syndrome classified as a rheumatic disease that is characterized by severe aching and stiffness in the neck, shoulder girdle, and pelvic girdle.

Positron emission tomography (PET) Introduction of radioactive materials into the body for three-dimensional display of images developed from the simultaneous capture, 180 degrees apart, of radioactive emissions.

Posterior Back of the body or an organ.

Postlaminectomy syndrome Terms used to describe patients who have undergone spine surgery and have some degree of recurrent spinal and/or leg pain due to the build up of scar tissue.

Postpartum After delivery or childbirth.

Postterm pregnancy Pregnancy longer than 40 weeks up to 42 weeks.

Posttraumatic stress disorder Anxiety disorder that is triggered by memories of a traumatic event.

Precipitate labor Rapid labor and delivery.

Preeclampsia Pregnancy complication characterized by hypertension, edema, and/or proteinuria.

Preferred Provider Organizations (PPO) Type of managed care in which hospitals, physicians, and other providers have an arrangement with a third-party payer to provide health care at discounted rates to third party payer clients.

Pregestational Condition present prior to pregnancy.

Prenatal Before birth.

Present on admission (POA) An indicator to differentiate between a condition that developed during a particular hospital encounter and a condition present at the time of admission.

Preventive or prophylactic surgery Procedure performed to remove tissue that has the potential to become cancerous.

Primary osteoarthritis Idiopathic degenerative condition that occurs in previously intact joints, with no apparent initiating factor.

Primary site Site at which the neoplasm begins or originates.

Primigravida First pregnancy.

Principal diagnosis Condition established after study to be chiefly responsible for occasioning admission of the patient to the hospital for care.

Principal procedure Procedure performed for definitive treatment, rather than for diagnostic or exploratory purposes, or one that was necessary to take care of a complication.

Procedure A diagnostic or therapeutic process performed on a patient.

Products of conception All physical components of a pregnancy including the fetus, amnion, umbilical cord, and placenta, regardless of gestational age.

Professional service Service rendered by a physician or a nonphysician practitioner.

Progress notes Daily recordings by health care providers of patient progress.

Prolonged pregnancy Beyond 42 weeks of pregnancy.

Prone Lying on the stomach, face down.

Prophylactic Medication or treatment used to prevent a disease from occurring.

Prospective payment system Method of reimbursement in which payment is made on the basis of a predetermined, fixed amount rather than for billed charges.

Prostate-specific antigen (PSA) Protein produced by the prostate gland.

Prostatitis Inflammation of the prostate that can be acute and/or chronic in nature and is due to a bacterium or inflammation that is not caused by a bacterial infection.

Proteinuria Protein in urine.

Proximal Closer to the median plane.

Pruritus Itching.

Psoriasis Inflammation of skin caused by a fault in the immune system.

Psychosis Impaired mental state in which the perception of reality has become distorted.

Puerperium Time from delivery through the first 6 weeks postpartum.

Pulmonary edema Condition in which fluid accumulates in the lungs.

Pulmonary embolism A blood clot(s) in the pulmonary artery that causes blockage in the artery.

Pulmonary hypertension High blood pressure in the arteries that supply blood to the lungs.

Purpura Ecchymoses or small hemorrhages in the skin, mucous membranes, or serosal surfaces due to blood disorders, vascular abnormalities, or trauma.

Pyelonephritis Upper tract infection that involves the kidneys.

Radiation Use of high-energy radiation to treat cancer.

Radiculopathy Compression of a nerve root.

Reattachment Putting back in or on all or a portion of a separated body part to its normal location or other suitable location.

Rectocele Descent of the rectum and pressing of the rectum against the vaginal wall.

Rectovesical fistula A communication between the bladder and the rectum.

Rehabilitation Structured program with the goal to stop and recover from the use of alcohol and/or drugs.

Reimbursement Payment for healthcare services.

Release Freeing a body part from an abnormal physical constraint (e.g., lysis of adhesions) or location to a more suitable location (e.g., reattachment of finger).

Removal Taking out or off a device from a body part (e.g., removal of a chest tube).

Renal colic Intense pain associated with the body's efforts to try to force the stone through the ureters.

Repair Restoring, to the extent possible, a body part to its normal anatomic structure and function (herniorrhaphy).

Replacement Putting in or on biological or synthetic material that physically takes the place and/or fuction of all or a portion of a body part (total knee replacement).

Reposition Moving to its normal location or other suitable location all or a portion of a body part (e.g., fracture reduction).

Resection Cutting out or off, without replacement, all of a body part (e.g., total lobectomy of lung).

Residual condition or effect When the acute phase of an illness or injury has passed, but a residual condition or health problem remains.

Respiratory failure General term that describes ineffective gas exchange across the lungs by the respiratory system.

Respiratory system System that supplies the body with oxygen (O_2).

Restoration Returning, or attempting to return, a physiological function to its original state by extracorporeal means.

Restorative or reconstruction Surgery performed to restore function and enhance aesthetic appearance after surgery.

Restriction Partially closing an orifice or lumen of a tubular body part (e.g., Nissen fundoplication).

Revenue code A four-digit code that is utilized on the UB-04 to indicate a particular type of service.

Revision Correcting, to the extent possible, a malfunctioning of displaced device (e.g., adjustment of knee prosthesis).

Rhabdomyolysis Breakdown of muscle fibers resulting in the release of muscle fiber contents into the circulation.

Rheumatoid arthritis Chronic, inflammatory systemic disease that affects the joints, often causing deformity.

Robotic assisted surgery Minimally invasive technique that utilizes robotic arms to manipulate the surgical equipment and tools.

Rosacea Skin condition affecting cheeks, nose, and chin. It can be characterized by redness, a bulbous nose, or an increased number of blood vessels in the face.

Sadism The act or sense of gaining pleasure from inflicting physical or psychological pain on another.

Salpingitis Inflammation of the fallopian tubes, which are the most common site of pelvic inflammation.

Sarcomas Malignant growths of connective tissue (e.g., muscle, cartilage, lymph tissue, bone).

Scabies Contagious dermatitis caused by mites.

Schizoaffective disorder Condition in which a person experiences a combination of schizophrenia symptoms while exhibiting mood disorder symptoms, such as mania or depression.

Schizophrenia Disorder of the brain characterized by difficulty differentiating between real and unreal experiences, as well as in logical thinking, normal emotional responses to others, and appropriate behavior in social situations.

Scleroderma Chronic, progressive disease characterized by hardening of the skin and scarring of internal organs.

Scoliosis Deviation of the vertical line of the spine.

Screening examination One that occurs in the absence of any signs or symptoms. It involves examination of an asymptomatic individual to detect a given disease, typically by means of an inexpensive diagnostic test.

Sebum Substance secreted from the sebaceous gland.

Secondary diabetes mellitus Form of the disease that develops as a result of another disease or condition.

Secondary osteoarthritis Degenerative disease of the joints that results from some predisposing condition such as trauma or disease.

Secondary thrombocytopenia Decrease in the number of platelets due to specific diseases or external causes, such as drugs, blood transfusions, and overhydration.

Section Consists of a group of three-digit categories that represent diseases or conditions that are similar.

See A mandatory cross-reference that advises the coder to go to another main term.

See also Cross-reference that instructs the coder about the possibility that there may be a better main term elsewhere in the Alphabetic Index.

Self-insured plans Self-insurance fund is set up by an employer to provide health claim benefits for employees.

Sepsis A medical condition in which the immune system goes into overdrive, releasing chemicals into the blood to combat infection that trigger widespread inflammation.

Septic shock A condition caused by infection and sepsis. It can cause multiple organ failure and death.

Septicemia The presence in the blood of pathologic microorganisms that cause systemic illness.

Sequelae Late effect or residual of an acute disease.

Shock wave therapy Extracorporeal treatment by shock waves.

Shunting Procedure to drain fluid from the brain to relieve pressure.

Sialolithiasis Stones in the salivary glands.

Sickle cell anemia One of the most common hemolytic anemias, in which the shape of the red blood cell changes from a disc to a crescent or "sickle," causing obstruction of small blood vessels and eventual damage throughout the body.

Siderosis Lung disease due to inhalation of iron oxide.

Sign Objective evidence of a disease or of a patient's condition as perceived by the patient's examining physician.

Significant procedure A procedure is considered significant if it is surgical in nature, carries a procedural risk, carries an anesthetic risk, and/or requires specialized training.

Simple fracture Injury in which the bone is broken, but the skin remains intact.

Sinusitis A condition in which the linings of one or more sinuses become infected, usually because of viruses or bacteria.

SIRS Systemic inflammatory response syndrome, which can be caused by infection or trauma.

Sleep apnea Disorder characterized by breathing interruption during sleep.

Solar keratosis Precancerous scaly growth.

Somatic nervous system Sends sensory (taste, hearing, smell) information to the central nervous system.

Somnolence Sleepiness.

Specificity Coding to the greatest detail of a code. Coding to the fourth or fifth digit as necessary.

Speech assessment Measurement of speech and related functions.

Speech treatment Application of techniques to improve, augment, or compensate for speech and related functional impairment.

Spinal cord injury Damage to the spinal cord that causes loss of sensation and motor control.

Spinal decompression Surgical procedure that frees space for the nerves in the spinal canal.

Spinal fusion The creation of a solid bone bridge between two or more adjacent vertebrae to enhance stability between levels of the spine.

Spinal stenosis Narrowing of the central spinal canal or the areas of the spine where the nerve roots exit (neuroforamina).

Splenomegaly Enlarged spleen.

Spondylolisthesis Condition in which one vertebra slips on another.

Spondylosis (or spinal osteoarthritis) Degenerative disorder that may cause loss of normal spinal structure and function.

Spontaneous abortion Loss of a fetus due to natural causes; also known as *miscarriage*.

Spontaneous pneumothorax Pneumothorax that is not caused by trauma.

Sprain Stretch and/or tear of a ligament.

Squamous cell carcinoma (SCC) Second most common type of skin cancer and also occurs in areas of the body that have been exposed to the sun.

Squamous intraepithelial lesion (SIL) Dysplasia of the cervix that is identified on a Pap smear.

Staging Means of categorizing a particular cancer that assists in determination of a patient's treatment plan and the need for further therapy.

Staging surgeries Procedures performed to help the clinician determine the extent of disease; these generally are more accurate than laboratory and imaging tests.

Stannosis Lung disease due to inhalation of tin particles.

Stasis dermatitis Skin condition due to poor circulation (venous insufficiency) that is characterized by swelling, skin discoloration, weeping, itching, and scaly skin.

Stasis ulcer Ulcer associated with varicose veins.

STEMI ST elevation myocardial infarction.

Stenosis Abnormal narrowing.

Steroid-induced diabetes Diabetes that is caused by the use of steroids.

Stevens Johnson Syndrome Skin necrosis caused by a reaction to medication or infection.

Stillbirth Born dead.

Stoma An artificial opening.

Strain Injury to a muscle or a tendon.

Stress incontinence Involuntary loss of small amounts of urine due to increased pressure resulting from coughing, sneezing, or laughing.

Stroke Cerebrovascular accident or brain infarction.

Subacute Somewhat acute; between chronic and acute.

Subcategory A fourth-digit code that provides additional information or specificity.

Subclassification A fifth-digit code that provides even greater specificity.

Subcutaneous Inner layer of the skin that contains fat and sweat glands.

Subluxation Partial or incomplete dislocation.

Subterm Gives more specific information about a main term. Subterms identify site, type, or etiology of a disease condition or injury, they are indented to the right of the main term.

Superior Position of the body or an organ relative to the vertical axis of the body.

Supine Lying on the back, face up.

Supplement Putting in or on biological or synthetic material that physically reinforces and/or augments the function of a portion of a body part (e.g., herniorrhaphy with mesh).

Suture Method for closing cutaneous wounds.

Symptom Subjective evidence of a disease or of a patient's condition as perceived by the patient.

Syphilis A sexually transmitted disease (STD) that is caused by bacteria.

Systemic inflammatory response syndrome A serious medical condition that can occur in response to infectious or noninfectious causes, such as severe trauma, burns, or complications of surgery.

Systemic lupus erythematosus Chronic, inflammatory autoimmune disease that can damage connective tissue anywhere in the body.

Systemic nuclear medicine therapy Introduction of unsealed radioactive materials into the body for treatment.

Tabular List Section of the ICD-10-CM book that contains the code listing, along with exclusion or inclusion notes.

Tachycardia Fast heart rate, generally greater than 100 beats per minute.

Tachypnea Fast breathing.

Tendons Connective tissue that attaches muscle to bone.

Terminology Words and phrases that apply to a particular field.

Tetany A continuous muscle spasm.

Thalassemia Hereditary disease that is similar to sickle cell anemia and occurs in varying degrees.

Therapeutic Treating disease.

Therapeutic abortion Abortion performed when the pregnancy is endangering the mother's health, or when the fetus has a condition that is incompatible with life.

Third party payer Makes payments for health services on behalf of the patient; may be a government program, insurance company, or managed care plan.

Thoracentesis Puncture of the chest wall to remove fluid (pleural effusion) from the space between the lining of the outside of the lungs (pleura) and the wall of the chest.

Thoracoscopic approach A thoracoscope is used to examine and perform closed procedures within the thorax.

Threatened abortion Abortion that occurs when symptoms are present that indicate the possibility of a miscarriage.

Thrombocytes Another name for platelets. Thrombocytes circulate in the blood and assist in the clotting process.

Thrombus A blood clot that forms and remains in a vein.

Thyrotoxic crisis/storm Complication of hyperthyroidism associated with a sudden intensification of symptoms combined with fever, rapid pulse, and delirium.

TIPS (transjugular intrahepatic portosystemic shunt) A procedure in which the portal vein is connected to one of the hepatic veins and a stent is inserted.

Tomographic nuclear medicine imaging Introduction of radioactive materials into the body for three-dimensional display of images developed from the capture of radioactive emissions.

Toxemia Another term for preeclampsia, which is pregnancy complicated by hypertension, edema, or proteinuria.

Toxic effect When a harmful substance is ingested or comes in contact with a person, this is classified as a toxic effect.

Toxic hepatitis When liver is damaged by chemicals or drugs.

Trachea (windpipe) Body part that is responsible for filtering the air that we breathe.

Tracheostomy Procedure in which an artificial opening is made in the front of the windpipe (trachea) through the skin of the neck.

Traction Exerting a pulling force on a body region in a distal direction.

Transfer Moving, without taking out, all or a portion of a body part to another location to take over the function of all or a portion of a body part (e.g., pedicle skin flap).

Transfusion Putting in blood or blood products.

Transient ischemic attack A stroke that lasts for only a few minutes.

Transplantation Putting in or on all or a portion of a living body part taken from another individual or animal to physically take the place and/or function of all or a portion of a similar body part (kidney transplant).

Transurethral resection of the prostate Endoscopic removal of prostate tissue.

Transvestism Assuming the appearance, manner, or roles traditionally associated with members of the opposite sex (cross-dressing).

Traumatic brain injury Injury to the brain that may result in interference with the brain's normal functions.

Treatment Manual treatment to eliminate or alleviate somatic dysfunction and related disorders.

Trisomy Extra chromosome.

Tube thoracostomy Insertion of chest tube(s) to drain blood, fluid, or air and allow full expansion of the lungs.

Tuberculosis (TB) An infection caused by *Mycobacterium tuberculosis*.

Tumor lysis syndrome (TLS) Development of electrolyte and metabolic disturbances that can occur after treatment of cancer, usually lymphoma and leukemia, and sometimes even without treatment.

Ulcer Open sore of the skin.

Ulcerative colitis An inflammatory bowel disease.

Ultrasonography Real time display of images of anatomy or flow information developed from the capture of reflected and attenuated high frequency sound waves.

Ultrasound therapy Extracorporeal treatment by ultrasound.

Ultraviolet light therapy Extracorporeal treatment by ultraviolet light.

Underdosing Taking less of a medication than is prescribed by a provider or a manufacturer's instructions.

Undifferentiated Tumor cells that are highly abnormal (e.g., immature, primitive).

Ureterolithiasis Ureter stone.

Urethritis Infection of the urethra.

Urethrocele When the urethra presses into the vagina.

Urethrovaginal fistula Abnormal passage between the urethra and the vagina.

Urge incontinence Sudden and involuntary loss of large amounts of urine.

Urinary tract infection General term used to describe infection in any area of the urinary tract.

Urolithiasis A stone in the urinary tract.

Urosepsis Infection of urinary site.

Urticaria Another name for hives.

Uterine prolapse Descent of the uterus and the cervix into the vaginal canal.

Uterus A muscular organ that serves as an incubator for the developing fetus.

Vagal nerve stimulator A device to control seizures.

Vagina A muscular tube that extends from the vaginal opening to the uterus.

Vaginal vault prolapse Condition that may occur following a hysterectomy, when the top of the vagina descends.

Valid OR procedure A procedure that may affect MSG-DRG assignment.

Varicose veins Enlarged, twisted veins that usually occur in the legs.

Ventral Front of the body or an organ.

Ventriculoperitoneal shunt Procedure used to treat patient with hydrocephalus in whom drainage of the ventricle occurs through an artificial channel between the ventricle and the peritoneum.

Vesicoureteral reflux Abnormality in the flow of urine from the bladder into the ureters and/or kidneys.

Vesicouterine fistula Communication between the bladder and the uterus.

Vesicovaginal fistula Communication between the bladder and the vagina.

Vestibular assessment Measurement of vestibular system and related functions.

Vestibular treatment Application of techniques to improve, augment, or compensate for vestibular and related functional impairment.

Via natural or artificial opening Entry of instrumentation through a natural or artificial external opening to reach the site of the procedure (e.g., endotracheal intubation).

Via natural or artificial opening endoscopic Entry of instrumentation through a natural or artificial external opening to reach and visualize the site of the procedure (e.g., colonoscopy).

Viral meningitis An infection of the fluid in the spinal cord and around the brain.

Vitamin deficiency Condition caused by many different factors, such as poor nutrient absorption, associated with digestive tract disorders, lifestyle issues (e.g., alcohol, smoking, medication, over exercising), chronic illness, age, and many other factors.

Volume depletion May be the result of either dehydration or hypovolemia.

Vulvar intraepithelial neoplasia (VIN) Certain changes that can occur in the skin that covers the vulva.

Volvulus An abnormal twisting of the intestine that may impair blood flow to the intestine.

Voyeurism Recurrent intense sexual urges and fantasies involving observing unsuspecting people who are naked, disrobing, or engaging in sexual activity.

Vulva The external covering to the vagina.

Well differentiated Tumor cells that closely resemble mature, specialized cells.

West Nile A viral disease that is spread to individuals by a mosquito bite.

Whipple procedure A procedure that generally involves removal of the gallbladder, common bile duct, part of the duodenum, and head of the pancreas.

Young obstetric patient Younger than 16 years at date of delivery.

Xenograft Graft to an individual from another species; also known as a *heterograft*.

Abbreviations/ Acronyms

A&P anatomy and physiology

AAPC American Academy of Professional Coders

ABG arterial blood gas

ACS acute coronary syndrome

ADD attention deficit disorder

ADHD attention deficit hyperactivity disorder

AF atrial fibrillation

AGA appropriate for gestational age

AHA American Hospital Association

AHFS American Hospital Formulary Service

AHIMA American Health Information Management Association

AHQA American Health Quality Association

AICD automatic implantable cardioverter-defibrillator

AIDS acquired immunodeficiency syndrome

AKA above-knee amputation

ALL acute lymphocytic leukemia

ALOS average length of stay

AMA American Medical Association

AMI acute myocardial infarction

AML acute myeloid leukemia

APC Ambulatory Payment Classification

ARF acute renal failure

ARI acute renal insufficiency

AROM artificial rupture of membranes

ASA aspirin

ASCUS atypical squamous cells of undetermined significance

ATV all-terrain vehicle

AV arteriovenous

AV atrioventricular

AVM arteriovenous malformation

AVR aortic valve replacement

BCC basal cell carcinoma

BCG Bacille Calmette Guerin vaccine

BIPAP bilevel positive airway pressure

BMI body mass index

BMR biological response modifier

BMT bone marrow transplant

BP blood pressure

BPD biliopancreatic diversion

BPD bronchopulmonary dysplasia

BPH benign prostatic hypertrophy

BUN blood urea nitrogen

C. diff Clostridium *difficile*

CAB coronary artery bypass

CABG coronary artery bypass graft

CAD coronary artery disease

CAP community-acquired pneumonia

CAPD continuous ambulatory peritoneal dialysis

CAS computer-assisted surgery

CAT computerized axial tomography

CBC complete blood count

CC chief complaint

CC complication/comorbidity

CCA Certified Coding Associate

CCPD continuous-cycling peritoneal dialysis

CCS Certified Coding Specialist

CCS-P Certified Coding Specialist—Physician-Based

CCU coronary care unit

CD4 cluster of differentiation 4

CDC Centers for Disease Control and Prevention

CDIP Clinical Documentation Improvement Program

CDM charge description master

CEA cultured epidermal autograft

CEUs continuing education units

CF cystic fibrosis

CHB complete heart block

CHD congenital heart disease

CHF congestive heart failure

CHI closed head injury

CIN cervical intraepithelial neoplasia

CKD chronic kidney disease

CLL chronic lymphocytic leukemia

CM clinical modification

CMI case-mix index

CMS Centers for Medicare and Medicaid Services

CNS central nervous system

COPD chronic obstructive pulmonary disease

CPAP continuous positive airway pressure

CPC Certified Professional Coder

CPC-H Certified Professional Coder—Hospital-Based

CPD cephalopelvic disproportion

CPK creatine phosphokinase

CPK-MB creatine phosphokinase, isoenzyme MB

CPT Current Procedural Terminology

CRF chronic renal failure

CRI chronic renal insufficiency

CRT cardiac resynchronization therapy

CRT-D cardiac resynchronization treatment defibrillator

CRT-P cardiac resynchronization treatment pacemaker

CSF cerebrospinal fluid

CT computerized tomography

CVA cerebrovascular accident

CVL central venous line

CXR chest x-ray

CVS chorionic villus sampling

D&C dilatation and curettage

DBS deep brain stimulation

DCIS ductal carcinoma in situ

DES drug-eluting stent

DEXA dual-energy x-ray absorptiometry (bone density)

DHHS U.S. Department of Health and Human Services

DI diabetes insipidus

DIC disseminated intravascular coagulation

DIEP deep inferior epigastric perforator

DJD degenerative joint disease

DOE dyspnea on exertion

DM diabetes mellitus

DMAC disseminated *Mycobacterium avium-intracellulare* complex

DOB date of birth

DRA Deficit Reduction Act

DRG diagnosis-related group

DS discharge summary

DSM-IV-TR *Diagnostic and Statistical Manual of Mental Disorders, Fourth Edition, Text Revision*

DTs delirium tremens

DVT deep vein thrombosis

E. coli *Escherichia coli*

ECMO extracorporeal membrane oxygenation

ECT electroconvulsive therapy

ED Emergency Department

EDC estimated date of confinement

EEG electroencephalogram

EGD esophogastroduodenoscopy

EKG/ECG electrocardiogram

EP electrophysiologic

ER Emergency Room

ERCP endoscopic retrograde cholangiopancreatography

ESRD end-stage renal disease

ESWL extracorporeal shock wave lithotripsy

FB foreign body

FNA fine needle aspiration

FSG focal segmental glomerulosclerosis

FTSG full-thickness skin graft

FUO fever of unknown origin

GAP gluteal artery perforator

GBS group B strep

GDM gestational diabetes mellitus

GEMS General Equivalence Mappings

GERD gastroesophageal reflux disease

GFR glomerular filtration rate

GI gastrointestinal

GMLOS geometric length of stay

GN glomerulonephritis

GPO Government Printing Office

GVHD graft-versus-host disease

H. flu *Haemophilus influenzae*

H&P history and physical

HAART highly active antiretroviral therapy

HAC hospital acquired condition

HAP hospital acquired pneumonia

HBOT hyperbaric oxygen therapy

HCC hepatocellular carcinoma

hCG human chorionic gonadotropin

HCPCS Healthcare Common Procedure Coding System

Hct hematocrit

HCVD hypertensive cardiovascular disease

HELLP hemolysis, elevated liver enzymes, and low platelet count

HFMD hand, foot, and mouth disease

Hgb hemoglobin

HGSIL high-grade squamous intraepithelial lesion

HH home health

HIPAA Health Insurance Portability and Accountability Act

HIV human immunodeficiency virus

HIVAN HIV-associated nephropathy

HMO health maintenance organization

HPI history of present illness

HPR hospital payment rate

HPV human papillomavirus

HSV herpes simplex virus

HTN hypertension

I&D incision and drainage

ICD internal cardiac defibrillator

ICD *International Classification of Diseases*

ICD-9-CM *International Classification of Diseases, 9th Revision, Clinical Modification*

ICD-10-CM *International Classification of Diseases, 10th Revision, Clinical Modification*

ICD-O *International Classification of Diseases for Oncology*

ICD-10-PCS *International Classification of Diseases, 10th Revision, Procedure Coding System*

ICU intensive care unit

ICV implantable cardioverter

IDDM insulin-dependent diabetes mellitus

Ig immunoglobulin

IOL induction of labor

IOL intraocular lens

IOP intraocular pressure

IPPS Inpatient Prospective Payment System

IPPV intermittent positive-pressure ventilation

IQ intelligence quotient

IS information systems

ITP idiopathic thrombocytopenic purpura

IUD intrauterine device

IUGR intrauterine growth retardation

IV intravenous

IVDU intravenous drug use

JRA juvenile rheumatoid arthritis

KS Kaposi's sarcoma

LAD left anterior descending

LAVH laparoscopically assisted vaginal hysterectomy

LCA left coronary artery

LCDs local code determinations

LD learning disability/difficulty

LDMF latissimus dorsi musculocutaneous flap

LGA large for gestational age

LGIB lower gastrointestinal bleed

LLL lower left lobe

LMRP local medical review policies

LOC loss of consciousness

LOS length of stay

LP lumbar puncture

LSIL low-grade intraepithelial lesion

LTC long-term care

LTCS low transverse cesarean section

LUTS lower urinary tract symptoms

MAC Medicare administrative contractor

MAC *Mycobacterium avium-intracellulare* complex

MAI *Mycobacterium avium-intracellulare*

MAO monoamine oxidase

MAR medication administration record

MCE Medicare Code Editor

MCI mild cognitive impairment

MDC major diagnostic category

MEN multiple endocrine neoplasia

MI myocardial infarction

MIC Medicaid integrity contractor

MOD multiple organ dysfunction

MR mental retardation

MRA magnetic resonance angiography

MRCP mental retardation, cerebral palsy

MRI magnetic resonance imaging

MRSA methicillin-resistant *Staphylococcus aureus*

MSAFP maternal serum alpha-fetoprotein

MS-DRG Medicare Severity diagnosis–related group

MSSA methicillin-sensitive *Staphylococcus aureus*

MUGA multiple-gated acquisition

MVA motor vehicle accident

MVP mitral valve prolapse

NCDs national coverage determinations

NCHS National Center for Health Statistics

NEC not elsewhere classifiable

NHL non-Hodgkins' lymphoma

NICU neonatal intensive care unit

NIDDM non–insulin-dependent diabetes mellitus

NKF National Kidney Foundation

NOS not otherwise specified

NPH normal pressure hydrocephalus

NPI national provider identifier

NPPV noninvasive positive-pressure ventilation

NPRM Notice of Proposed Rule Making

NQMI non–Q wave myocardial infarction

NRFHT non-reassuring fetal heart rate

NSAIDs nonsteroidal antiinflammatory drugs

NSCLC non–small cell lung cancer

NST nonstress test

NSTEMI non–ST-elevation myocardial infarction

O$_2$ oxygen

OA osteoarthritis

OB obstetrics

OBS organic brain syndrome

OI osteogenesis imperfecta

OIG Office of the Inspector General

OM otitis media

OP note operative note

OPPS Outpatient Prospective Payment System

OR Operating Room

ORIF open reduction with internal fixation

OSA obstructive sleep apnea

Paco₂ partial pressure of carbon dioxide in arterial blood

Pao₂ partial pressure of oxygen in arterial blood

PCI percutaneous coronary intervention

PCP *Pneumocystis carinii* pneumonia

PCP primary care provider

PCS Procedure Classification System

PDA patent ductus arteriosus

PDA posterior descending artery

PDT photodynamic therapy

PE pulmonary embolism

PEG percutaneous endoscopic gastrostomy

PEPPER Program for Evaluating Payment Patterns Electronic Report

PET positron emission tomography

PICC peripherally inserted central catheter

PID pelvic inflammatory disease

PIH pregnancy-induced hypertension

PKU phenylketonuria

PMR polymyalgia rheumatica

POA present on admission

POCs products of conception

PPH primary pulmonary hypertension

PPN peripheral parenteral nutrition

PPO Preferred Provider Organization

PPROM preterm premature rupture of membranes

PPS Prospective Payment System

PROM premature rupture of membranes

PSA prostate-specific antigen

PT prothrombin time

PTA prior to admission

PTCA percutaneous transluminal coronary angioplasty

PTL preterm labor

PTSD posttraumatic stress disorder

PTT partial thromboplastin time

PUD peptic ulcer disease

PV percutaneous vertebroplasty

PVD peripheral vascular disease

PWS Prader–Willi syndrome

QIO Quality Improvement Organization

RA rheumatoid arthritis

RA right atrium

RAC recovery audit contract

RAD reactive airway disease

RBBB right bundle branch block

RCA right coronary artery

RCC renal cell carcinoma

RDS respiratory distress syndrome

RFA radiofrequency ablation

RHD rheumatic heart disease

RHIA Registered Health Information Administrator

RHIT Registered Health Information Technician

RPGN rapidly progressive glomerulonephritis

RPR rapid plasma reagin

RPS retrospective payment system

RSV respiratory syncytial virus

RUL right upper lobe

RW relative weight

SARS severe acute respiratory syndrome

SCC squamous cell carcinoma

SCI spinal cord injury

SCID severe combined immunodeficiency

SCLC small cell lung cancer

SGA small for gestational age

SIADH syndrome of inappropriate antidiuretic hormone secretion

SIDS sudden infant death syndrome

SIEA superficial inferior epigastric artery

SIL squmous intraepithelial lesion

SIRS systemic inflammatory response syndrome

SJS Stevens-Johnson Syndrome

SLAP superior labrum anterior–posterior

SLE systemic lupus erythematosus

SNF skilled nursing facility

SNOMED Systematized Nomenclature of Medicine

SOAP Subjective/Objective Assessment Plan

SOB shortness of breath

SOM serous otitis media

SOW scope of work

SSS sick sinus syndrome

Staph aureus *Staphylococcus aureus*

STD sexually transmitted disease

STEC shiga toxin-producing *E. coli*

STEMI ST-elevation myocardial infarction

STSG split-thickness skin graft

SVD spontaneous vaginal delivery

SVT supraventricular tachycardia

SZ seizure

TB tuberculosis

TBI traumatic brain injury

TEFRA Tax Equity and Fiscal Responsibility Act

TEN toxic epidermal neurolysis

THR total hip replacement

TIA transient ischemic attack

TIPS transjugular intrahepatic portosystemic shunt

TJC The Joint Commission

TLS tumor lysis syndrome

TOF tetralogy of Fallot

TPA tissue plasminogen activator

TPN total parenteral nutrition

TPR temperature, pulse, and respiration

TRALI transfusion-related acute lung injury

TRAM transverse rectus abdominis musculocutaneous

TSH thyroid-stimulating hormone

TTN transitory tachypnea of the newborn

TULIP transurethral ultrasound-guided laser-induced prostatectomy

TUMT transurethral microwave thermotherapy

TUNA transurethral needle ablation of the prostate

TURP transurethral resection of the prostate

UB-04 Uniform Bill 04

UGIB upper gastrointestinal bleed

UHDDS Uniform Hospital Discharge Data Set

UPIN Unique Physician Identification Number

UR utilization review

USA unstable angina

UTI urinary tract infection

VAD vascular access device

VAP ventilator assisted pneumonia

VATS video-assisted thoracic surgery

VBAC vaginal birth after cesarean section

VBG vertical banded gastroplasty

VDRL Venereal Disease Research Laboratory

VLAP visual laser ablation of the prostate

VNS vagal nerve stimulation

VPS ventriculoperitoneal shunt

VRE vancomycin-resistant *Enterococcus*

VSD ventricular septal defect

VUR vesicoureteral reflux

WBC white blood cell

WHO World Health Organization

ZPIC zone program integrity contractor

Illustration Credits

Chapter 1
Figure 1-1: Courtesy American Health Information Management Association. 1-2: Courtesy American Academy of Professional Coders.

Chapter 2
Figures 2-1, 2-9, 2-11, 2-12: From Abdelhak M, Grostick S, Hanken MA, Jacobs EB (eds). Health Information: Management of a Strategic Resource, 2nd ed. St. Louis, Saunders, 2001.

Chapter 6
Figures 6-6: A & C from Rothrock J. Alexander's Care of the Patient in Surgery, 13th ed. St. Louis, Elsevier, 2007. B from Spiro SG, Albert RK, Jett JR. Clinical Respiratory Medicine, 3rd ed. St. Louis, Elsevier, 2008. D from Sanders MJ, McKenna KD. Mosby's Paramedic Textbook, 3rd ed. St. Louis, Mosby/JEMS, 2007. E from Salvo SG. Mosby's Pathology for Massage Therapists, 2nd ed. St. Louis, Elsevier, 2009. F from Phillips N. Berry & Kohn's Operating Room Technique, 11th ed. St. Louis, Elsevier, 2007. G from Lovaasen KR, Schwerdtfeger J. 2012 ICD-9-CM Coding Theory and Practice with ICD-10. St. Louis, Elsevier, 2012.

Chapter 9
Figures 9-2: From Kumar V, Cotran RS, Robbins SJ. Robbins Basic Pathology, 7th ed. Philadelphia, Saunders, 2003. 9-3: Courtesy Dr. John J. Kepers, Kansas City, Kansas. 9-4: From Behrman RE, Kleigman RM, Arvin AM. Slide set for Nelson Textbook of Pediatrics, 15th ed. Philadelphia, Saunders, 1996. 9-5: From Frazier MS, Drzymkowski JW. Essentials of Human Diseases and Conditions, 4th ed. St. Louis, Saunders, 2009. 9-6: From Eichenfeld L. Textbook of Neonatal Dermatology, 2nd ed. Philadelphia, Saunders, 2008.

Chapter 10
Figure 10-1: From Chabner D. The Language of Medicine, 8th ed. St. Louis, Saunders, 2007. 10-5: From Odom RB, James WD, Berger TG. Andrews' Diseases of the Skin, 9th ed. Philadelphia, Saunders, 2000. 10-6: From Doughty DB, Jackson DB. Gastrointestinal Disorders—Mosby's Clinical Nursing Series, 5th ed. St. Louis, Mosby, 1993. 10-7: From Cotran RS, Kumar V, Collins T. Robbins Pathologic Basis for Disease, 6th ed. Philadelphia, Saunders, 1999. 10-8: From Kumar V, Abbas AK, Fausto N. Robbins & Cotran Pathologic Basis of Disease, 7th ed. Philadelphia, Saunders, 2005. 10-9, 10-10, 10-11, 10-13: From Damjanov I. Pathology for the Health Professions, 3rd ed. St. Louis, Saunders, 2006. 10-12: From Huether SE, McCance KL. Understanding Pathophysiology, 3rd ed. St. Louis, Mosby, 2004. 10-14: From Gould BE. Pathophysiology for the Health Professions, 3rd ed. St. Louis, Saunders, 2006. 10-15: Burkitt HG, Quick RG. Essential Surgery, 3rd ed. London, Churchill Livingstone, 2002.

Chapter 11
Figures 11-5, 11-9: From Chabner D. The Language of Medicine, 8th ed. St. Louis, Saunders, 2007. 11-7: From Lookingbill DP, Marks JG. Principles of Dermatology, 3rd ed. Philadelphia, Saunders, 2000.

Chapter 12
Figures 12-2, 12-7: From Chabner D. The Language of Medicine, 8th ed. St. Louis, Saunders, 2007. 12-3: From Swartz M. Textbook of Physical Diagnosis, 4th ed. Philadelphia, Saunders, 2002. 12-4: Courtesy Paul W. Ladenson, MD, The Johns Hopkins University and Hospital, Baltimore, Maryland. 12-5, 12-17, 12-21: From Damjanov I. Pathology for the Health Professions, 3rd ed. St. Louis, Saunders, 2006. 12-6: From Seidel HM, Ball JW, Dains JE, Benedict GW. Mosby's Guide to Physical Examination, 4th ed. St. Louis, Mosby, 1998. 12-14A: From Thibodeau GA. Anatomy and Physiology. 4th ed. St. Louis, Times Mirror/Mosby College Publishing, 1987. 12-13: Courtesy Dr. Edmund Beard, Cleveland, Ohio. 12-14B: From Beuschlein F, Strasburger CJ, Siegerstetter V, et al. Acromegaly caused by secretion of growth hormone by a non-Hodgkins lymphoma. N Engl J Med 2000;342:1871-1876. Copyright 2000, Massachusetts Medical Society. All rights reserved. 12-14C: From Little JW, Falace D, Miller C, Rhodus NL. Dental Management of the Medically Compromised Patient, 7th ed. St. Louis, Mosby, 2008. 12-16: From Mahan LK, Escott-Stump S. Krause's Food & Nutrition Therapy. St. Louis, Elsevier, 2008. 12-18: From Zitelli BJ, Davis HW. Atlas of Pediatric Physical Diagnosis, 4th ed. St. Louis, Mosby, 2002. 12-18: From Kumar V, Abbas AK, Fausto N. Robbins & Cotran Pathologic Basis of Disease, 7th ed. Philadelphia, Saunders, 2005. 12-22: Courtesy MiniMed Technologies, Sylmar, California; from Mosby's Medical, Nursing, and Allied Health Dictionary, 6th ed. St. Louis, Mosby, 2002.

Chapter 14
Figures 14-1, 14-2, 14-3, 14-4, 14-5, 14-14: From Chabner D. The Language of Medicine, 8th ed. St. Louis, Saunders, 2007. 14-7: From Damjanov I. Pathology for the Health Professions, 3rd ed. St. Louis, Saunders, 2006. 14-8, 14-9, 14-10, 14-11, 14-12, 14-16: From Frazier MS, Drzymkowski JW. Essentials of Human Diseases and Conditions, 4th ed. St. Louis, Saunders, 2009. 14-15: Courtesy Ophthalmic Photography at the University of Michigan, WK Kellogg Eye Center, Ann Arbor, Michigan. 14-18: From Lewis SM, Heitkemper MM, Dirksen SR. Medical-Surgical Nursing: Assessment and Management of Clinical Problems, 5th ed. St. Louis, Mosby, 2000.

Chapter 15
Figure 15-1: From Patton KT, Thibodeau GA. Mosby's Handbook of Anatomy and Physiology. St. Louis, Mosby, 2000. 15-2: From Applegate EJ. The Anatomy and Physiology Learning System, 2nd ed. Philadelphia, Saunders, 2000. 15-3, 15-9, 15-11, 15-14, 15-18: From Frazier MS, Drzymkowski JW. Essentials of Human Diseases and Conditions, 4th ed. St. Louis, Saunders, 2009. 15-5: From Gould BE. Pathophysiology for the Health Professions, 3rd ed. St. Louis, Saunders, 2006. 15-6: © Bayer Schering Pharma AG www.thrombosisadvisor.com. 15-8, 15-15: From Damjanov I. Pathology for the Health Professions, 3rd ed. St. Louis, Saunders, 2006. 15-10: Modified from

Ignatavicius DD, Workman ML. Medical-Surgical Nursing: Critical Thinking for Collaborative Care, 4th ed. Philadelphia, Saunders, 2002. 15-16, 15-17, 15-19, 15-20: From Chabner D. The Language of Medicine, 8th ed. St. Louis, Saunders, 2007. 15-22: From Drake RL, Vogl W, Mitchell AWM. Gray's Anatomy for Students. Philadelphia, Churchill Livingstone, 2005. 15-23: From Lewis SM, Heitkemper MM, Dirksen SR. Medical-Surgical Nursing: Assessment and Management of Clinical Problems, 5th ed. St. Louis, Mosby, 2000.

Chapter 16

Figure 16-1: From Gould BE. Pathophysiology for the Health Professions, 3rd ed. St. Louis, Saunders, 2006. 16-4A, B: From Kumar V, Abbas AK, Fausto N. Robbins & Cotran Pathologic Basis of Disease, 7th ed. Philadelphia, Saunders, 2005. 16-4C: Courtesy Paul Emmerson and Seneca College of Applied Arts and Technology, Toronto, Ontario, Canada. 16-5: Courtesy Dr. W. Thurlback, Vancouver, BC, Canada. 16-7, 16-8, 16-9A, 16-10: From Chabner D. The Language of Medicine, 8th ed. St. Louis, Saunders, 2007. 16-9B: From Black JM, Hawks JH, Keene AM. Medical-Surgical Nursing: Clinical Management for Positive Outcomes, 6th ed. Philadelphia, Saunders, 2001.

Chapter 17

Figure 17-1: Redrawn from Miller M. Pathophysiology: Principles of Disease. Philadelphia, Saunders, 1983. 17-2: From Buck CJ. Saunders 2010 ICD-9-CM, Volumes 1, 2, and 3. St. Louis, Saunders, 2010. 17-3: From Damjanov I. Pathology for the Health-Related Professions, 2nd ed. Philadelphia, Saunders, 2000. 17-5: From Damjanov I. Pathology for the Health Professions, 3rd ed. St. Louis, Saunders, 2006. 17-6, 17-8A, 17-13, 17-14: From Chabner D. The Language of Medicine, 8th ed. St. Louis, Saunders, 2007. 17-8: From Cotran RS, Kumar V, Collins T. Robbins Pathologic Basis for Disease, 6th ed. Philadelphia, Saunders, 1999. 17-9B: From Kumar V, Abbas AK, Fausto N. Robbins & Cotran Pathologic Basis of Disease, 7th ed. Philadelphia, Saunders, 2005. 17-10: From Patton KT, Thibodeau GA. Anatomy and Physiology, 7th ed. St. Louis, Mosby, 2010. 17-11: From Dorland's Illustrated Medical Dictionary, 31st ed. Philadelphia, Saunders, 2007. 17-11, 17-12: From Frazier MS, Drzymkowski JW. Essentials of Human Diseases and Conditions, 4th ed. St. Louis, Saunders, 2009.

Chapter 18

Figure 18-1: From Chabner D. The Language of Medicine, 8th ed. St. Louis, Saunders, 2007. 18-2A: From Lookingbill D, Marks J. Principles of Dermatology, 2nd ed. Philadelphia, Saunders, 1993. 18-2B: From Lawrence CM, Cox NH. Physical Signs in Dermatology: Color Atlas and Text. London, Mosby Europe, 1993. 18-3: From Murphy GF, Herzberg AJ. Atlas of Dermatopathology. Philadelphia, Saunders, 1996. 18-4: From Dorland's Illustrated Medical Dictionary, 31st ed. Philadelphia, Saunders, 2007. 18-5: From Callen J, Greer K, Hood A, et al. Color Atlas of Dermatology. Philadelphia, Saunders, 1993. 18-8: From McCarthy JG, et al (eds). Plastic Surgery, vol 7, Philadelphia, WB Saunders, 1990.

Chapter 19

Figure 19-1, 19-12: From Dorland's Illustrated Medical Dictionary, 31st ed. Philadelphia, Saunders, 2007. 19-2, 19-8AB: From Frazier MS, Drzymkowski JW. Essentials of Human Diseases and Conditions, 4th ed. St. Louis, Saunders, 2009. 19-3: Thibodeau GA, Patton KT: The Human Body in Health and Disease, 4th ed. St. Louis, Mosby, 2005. 19-6: From Chabner D. The Language of Medicine, 8th ed. St. Louis, Saunders, 2007. 19-4, 19-5, 19-12, 19-13: From Damjanov I. Pathology for the Health Professions, 3rd ed. St. Louis, Saunders, 2006. 19-11: From Mettler FA, Jr. Essentials of Radiology, 2nd ed. Philadelphia, Saunders, 2004. 19-15: From Zitelli BJ, Davis HW. Atlas of Pediatric Physical Diagnosis, 4th ed. St. Louis, Mosby, 2002. 19-13: From Buck CJ. Step-by-Step

Medical Coding, 2010 edition. St. Louis, Saunders, 2010. 19-14: From Duthie EH Jr, Katz PR, Malone M. Practice of Geriatrics, 4th ed. Philadelphia, Saunders, 2007.

Chapter 20

Figures 20-1, 20-6, 20-14, 20-15, 20-18: From Gould BE. Pathophysiology for the Health Professions, 3rd ed. St. Louis, Saunders, 2006. 20-2, 20-3: From Frazier MS, Drzymkowski JW. Essentials of Human Diseases and Conditions, 4th ed. St. Louis, Saunders, 2009. 20-4, 20-11, 20-19, 20-22, 20-23: From Chabner D. The Language of Medicine, 8th ed. St. Louis, Saunders, 2007. 20-5, 20-7, 20-8, 20-10, 20-12, 20-15: From Damjanov I. Pathology for the Health Professions, 3rd ed. St. Louis, Saunders, 2006. 20-18: From Dorland's Illustrated Medical Dictionary, 31st ed. Philadelphia, Saunders, 2007.

Chapter 21

Figures 21-1, 21-2, 21-4A, 21-9: From Frazier MS, Drzymkowski JW. Essentials of Human Diseases and Conditions, 4th ed. St. Louis, Saunders, 2009. 21-3, 21-10: From Dorland's Illustrated Medical Dictionary, 31st ed. Philadelphia, Saunders, 2007. 21-4B: From Damjanov I, Linder J. Pathology: A Color Atlas. St. Louis, Mosby, 1999. 21-5, 21-11: From Chabner D. The Language of Medicine, 8th ed. St. Louis, Saunders, 2007.

Chapter 22

Figures 22-1, 22-3: From Frazier MS, Drzymkowski JW. Essentials of Human Diseases and Conditions, 4th ed. St. Louis, Saunders, 2009. 22-2: From Gould BE. Pathophysiology for the Health Professions, 3rd ed. St. Louis, Saunders, 2006. 22-4: From Dorland's Illustrated Medical Dictionary, 31st ed. Philadelphia, Saunders, 2007. 22-5: From Behrman RE, Kleigman RM, Arvin AM. Slide set for Nelson Textbook of Pediatrics, 15th ed. Philadelphia, Saunders, 1996. 22-6: From Baralos M, Baramki TA. Medical Cytogenics. Baltimore, Lippincott Williams and Wilkins, 1967. 22-7: From Damjanov I. Pathology for the Health Professions, 3rd ed. St. Louis, Saunders, 2006. 22-8: Modified from O'Toole M (ed). Miller-Keane Encyclopedia of Medicine, Nursing, and Allied Health, 6th ed. Philadelphia, Saunders, 1997.

Chapter 23

Figure 23-2: From Gould BE. Pathophysiology for the Health Professions, 3rd ed. St. Louis, Saunders, 2006. 23-3, 23-5, 23-6, 23-7: From Drake RL, Vogl W, Mitchell AWM. Gray's Anatomy for Students. Philadelphia, Churchill Livingstone, 2005. 23-4: From Chabner D. The Language of Medicine, 8th ed. St. Louis, Saunders, 2007. 23-11, 23-12: From Henry MC, Stapleton ER. EMT Prehospital Care, 3rd ed. Philadelphia, Saunders, 2004. 23-16: Buck CJ. Step-by-Step Medical Coding, 2008. Philadelphia, Saunders, 2008.

Chapter 24

Figures 24-2, 24-3: From Frazier MS, Drzymkowski JW. Essentials of Human Diseases and Conditions, 4th ed. St. Louis, Saunders, 2009.

Chapter 25

Figures 25-7: From Frazier MS, Drzymkowski JW. Essentials of Human Diseases and Conditions, 4th ed. St. Louis, Saunders, 2009. 25-9: From Canale ST. Campbell's Operative Orthopaedics, 11th ed. Philadelphia, Mosby, 2008. 25-10: From Green NE, Swiontkowski MF. Skeletal Trauma in Children, 3rd ed. Philadelphia, Saunders, 2003.

Chapter 26

Figures 26-1: From Diagnosis Related Groups Definitions Manual, version 14.0. Wallingford, Conn, 3M Health Information Systems, 1996. 26-2: Courtesy U.S. Department of Health and Human Services, Public Health Service, Centers for Medicare and Medicaid Services.

Index

Note: Entries followed by "f" indicate figures, "t" tables.